PATHOPHYSIOLOGY

AN INTRODUCTION
TO THE MECHANISMS
OF DISEASE

PATHOPHYSIOLOGY
AN INTRODUCTION TO THE MECHANISMS OF DISEASE

Bernice L. Muir, R.N., M.Sc.

Formerly Instructor of Anatomy and Physiology and Pathophysiology
Nursing Department, Cariboo College
Kamloops, British Columbia

A Wiley Medical Publication
JOHN WILEY & SONS
New York • Chichester • Brisbane • Toronto • Singapore

COVER PHOTOGRAPH: Scanning electron micrograph of an erythrocyte enmeshed in fibrin. From E. Bernstein and E. Kairinen, *Science,* Vol. 173, 27 August 1971. Copyright © 1971 by the American Association for the Advancement of Science. Reprinted by permission of author and publisher.

Cover and Interior Design: Wanda Lubelska
Production Editor: Charles Kyreakou

Library of Congress Cataloging in Publication Data:
Muir, Bernice L
   Pathophysiology: an introduction to the mechanisms of disease.

   (A Wiley medical publication)
   Bibliography: p.
   Includes index.
   1. Physiology, Pathological. I. Title.
[DNLM: 1. Pathology—Nursing texts. 2. Physiology—Nursing texts. QZ140 M953p]
RB113.M84   616.07   79-27791
ISBN 0-471-03202-6

Printed in the United States of America

10 9 8 7 6 5

For my former students at Cariboo College, especially Jackie, who taught me about the Baha'i Faith

Preface

Some schools of nursing have taken the pathophysiology out of their nursing courses and offer it as a separate support course so that nursing courses can put more emphasis on nursing measures. I taught such a separate pathophysiology course at Cariboo College for two years. During that time I could not find a suitable pathophysiology book to adopt as a course text but had to draw material from many different sources. Therefore, with the urging of several of my colleagues and some of my students, I decided to write this pathophysiology textbook.

Most of the books that are currently available follow the medical model, organ system by organ system, and are oriented to specific diseases. Many nursing programs no longer follow the medical model, however, but base their curricula on the adaptation model or needs model. The purpose of this book is to present broad principles in an integrated manner, which cannot be done using an organ system approach. The focus is on mechanisms by which pathogenic agents disrupt homeostasis and mechanisms by which the body maintains or restores homeostasis. The intent is not to cover every disease, although many specific diseases are given as examples. My philosophy is to include sufficient facts and details to enable students to *understand* the mechanisms and principles involved, rather than to merely provide a list of signs and symptoms for them to *memorize*.

It is expected that the students using this book have had a previous course in anatomy and physiology. I have included a review of normal physiology in some sections, however, particularly in areas where I feel students may have difficulty understanding the pathophysiological concepts if they do not have a firm grounding in normal physiology. I expect that the people using this book have different levels of background knowledge. Therefore I have started each chapter or section with relatively simple explanations and definitions and proceeded from there to cover the topic in increasing depth. Those with more advanced levels of prior knowledge may wish to skip the beginning sections in each chapter, but I suspect many students will appreciate the review, even if they have learned the material previously.

I have placed considerable emphasis on genetics in this book, because diseases with a genetic component are assuming greater importance as infectious diseases and nutritional deficiency come under control. Since many nursing programs do not include a genetics course, two chapters are devoted to basic principles of genetics. On the other hand, I have not ignored infectious diseases or nutritional aspects of disease. In the discussion of infectious diseases, however, the emphasis is on general principles of host-microbe interactions rather than specific microorganisms and specific diseases. I have not included a separate discussion of aging, because I consider aging to be a normal process, not a pathophysiological one. Where pertinent, however, age-related aspects of disease have been discussed and all age groups have been covered.

This book can be used as a textbook for a separate pathophysiology course such as I taught or as a reference text where pathophysiology is integrated into a nursing course. The pathophysiological concepts presented here can provide the bases for subsequent nursing actions, although the application to nursing is not included in this book. In Unit One, I have attempted to point out that physiological processes represent only one aspect of a person. It is beyond the scope of this book, however, to include the many psychological, social, and cultural factors that influence individual responses. I leave it to nursing faculty to help students integrate the material in this text with knowledge learned from other courses and apply it to the nursing process.

Bernice L. Muir

Acknowledgments

Having never written a book before, I started on the adventure of writing this one thinking I was climbing a small mountain; when I got part way up the slope, I discovered it was Mt. Everest. I could not have reached the peak without the support, encouragement, and assistance of my family and friends. I am deeply indebted to all of them. I would especially like to thank Beverley Green, Valerie Macdonald, Hazel Thomas, my sister Shirley, and my parents. The help and encouragement of former colleagues Dawn Patterson, Claudette Kelly, and Pam Steuart was also greatly appreciated.

Several people offered suggestions and criticisms as the book was being written; I appreciated the comments, even if I did not always follow the advice. In addition, I am indebted to the people who generously provided the photographs that appear in this book. Specific credit is cited where the illustrations appear.

My typist, Louise Hunter, deserves special thanks, not only for doing an excellent job of typing and retyping the manuscript but also for rendering services above and beyond the call of duty. I would also like to thank her husband, Bob, who helped check the manuscript for typographical errors and thought of the "please sign here" example for Chapter 3.

I should also like to thank the staff at Wiley. I am particularly grateful to Cathy Somer, Nursing Editor, for her kind and patient help and encouragement.

Contents

CONTENTS

UNIT ONE

BASIC CONCEPTS OF HEALTH AND DISEASE

1
Homeostasis and Adaptation

All living cells must exchange substances with their environment. Nutrients are taken into cells and wastes are eliminated. Respiratory gases are exchanged. For unicellular organisms these exchanges occur directly with the surrounding environment, but in complex multicellular organisms, such as human beings, relatively few cells are in direct contact with the external environment. The interior cells still require nutrients and still must eliminate wastes. They need oxygen and must be rid of carbon dioxide. Internal cells cannot carry out this exchange directly with the outer world. They must have some intermediate means of exchanging substances with the external environment in which the whole organism exists.

The spaces between the body cells contain *extracellular fluid* (i.e., fluid outside the cells), which bathes the cells and provides a medium for the exchange of nutrients and wastes. A 19th-century French physiologist, Claude Bernard, developed the concept that the body fluids that immediately surround the cells form the *internal environment* (milieu intérieur) of complex organisms. The specialized functions of the various organ systems of the body provide the means of exchange between this internal environment and the external environment. Thus, nutrients from the external environment are absorbed via the gastrointestinal tract; soluble wastes are excreted through the kidneys; and the lungs provide the means of exchange of respiratory gases. The circulatory system serves to transport and distribute substances throughout the internal environment. It is with this internal environment, then, that the body cells interact.

HOMEOSTASIS

Bernard not only developed the concept of the internal environment but also recognized that conditions in the internal environment remain relatively constant. The concentration of nutrients, for example glucose, in the extracellular fluid is fixed within certain limits. Waste products are normally eliminated from the body as rapidly as they are formed, so that their concentration does not exceed limits that would be toxic to the cells. The level of respiratory gases is kept within a limited range. Acidity, salt concentration, osmotic pressure, and temperature are other characteristics of the human internal environment that are kept constant. Bernard realized that for optimum functioning of the cells, these physicochemical properties of the body fluids can fluctuate only within very narrow limits. He explained that the major objective of all the vital mechanisms is to preserve constant conditions of life in the internal environment.

A number of scientists since Claude Bernard have contributed their ideas to the concept that a constant and optimal internal environment is necessary for normal body function. In 1926 an American physiologist, W. B. Cannon, introduced the term *homeostasis* to denote the maintenance of constant conditions in the internal environment. The word is derived from the Greek word roots *homeo*, meaning like or similar, and *stasis*, meaning standing. The term homeostasis encompasses not only the idea of internal constancy or stability but also includes the concept that coordinated body processes are responsible for maintaining the constancy of the internal environment. This constancy should not be viewed as a stagnant thing: it is dynamic. Substances are continually being added to the internal environment and being taken away from it, but the net result is relatively constant. There is variation, but only within narrow limits.

A stable internal environment is necessary for the survival of every cell in the body. In addition to carrying out the basic activities necessary for maintaining its own life, each cell performs some specialized function. This specialized function, together with the activities of other cells, contributes to the constancy of the extracellular fluid. The survival of the total organism, as well as the survival of each cell, depends on the concerted cellular activities that maintain homeostasis. Integration and coordination of these activities is brought about by the nervous system and the endocrine system.

Physiologically, the term *internal environment* refers to the extracellular fluid. The term is also used in a broader context, however, to denote everything inside the skin and mucous membranes. In this context the internal environment is said to consist not only of physiological (or physical) elements but also psychological and sociocultural elements. These elements interact with each other and with their counterparts in the external environment. Similarly, the term homeostasis has been broadened from its original physiological context and is used to denote stability of all aspects of the individual: physiological, psychological, and sociocultural. In other words, homeostasis refers to the stability of the total organism. Sometimes the term homeostasis is used to refer to the self-stabilizing tendency of societies as well as individuals. In this textbook the terms internal environment and homeostasis are used primarily in the physiological sense. It is important to realize, however, that psychological and sociocultural factors influence physiological responses, because an individual is an integrated being.

Maintenance of Homeostasis

Changes in the external environment may produce fluctuations in the internal environment if the organism does not have some means of compensating. Similarly, activities of the individual will produce disturbances in the internal environment. These disturbances must be counteracted in order to maintain homeostasis. For example, fluctuations in the temperature of the external environment and varying degrees of muscular activity, which produce heat within the individual, would tend to alter body temperature if there were no mechanism for temperature regulation.

Maintenance of homeostasis also depends on satisfaction of basic needs. Physiologically these needs include, for example, intake of oxygen, nutrients, and water, and elimination of carbon dioxide and wastes. The amount of oxygen, nutrients, and water required and the quantity of carbon dioxide and wastes to be eliminated will depend on the activity of the individual. Meeting the need for oxygen, nutrients, and water will depend not only on their availability in the external environment but also on the ability of the organism to take them into the internal environment. Therefore, to maintain homeostasis the organism must have mechanisms to compensate for varying demands made on the body. Thus, for example, during exercise the rate of pulmonary ventilation is increased to meet the demand for more oxygen and to eliminate the increased amount of carbon dioxide that is produced. At high altitudes where oxygen availability is decreased, the body responds with increased production of red blood cells, which increases the oxygen-carrying capacity of the blood and facilitates oxygen uptake. The nature of the mechanisms by which the body adjusts to varying demands and counteracts changes is discussed in the section on Homeostatic Mechanisms.

The physical integrity of the organism must be preserved in order to maintain homeostasis. For example, every organism has a surface membrane that forms a barrier between the internal and external environments. In the case of a unicellular organism such as an ameba, the surface membrane is the cell membrane. In human beings the cutaneous membrane on the outside and the mucous membranes lining ducts and body cavities that open to the exterior form the barrier between the internal and external environments. Disruption of the surface membrane will impair the ability of the organism to regulate the exchange of substances between the two environments. Noxious elements from outside may enter the organism, and vital elements from inside may be lost. In order to maintain physical integrity the organism must have mechanisms to protect itself from injury, as well as mechanisms to repair any damage that is done. For example, the body has many protective reflexes, such as blinking if an object comes near the eyes or withdrawing a limb from a painful stimulus. If a blood vessel is damaged, clotting occurs to prevent blood loss. This subject is the topic of Chapter 7. The wound-healing mechanism repairs damage to tissues. This mechanism is described in Chapter 8.

Maintenance of homeostasis involves various forms of adjustment by the organism in response to actual or threatened disturbances in the internal environment. These disturbances may arise from within the individual or may be due to changes in the external environment.

ADAPTATION

The process of adjusting to environmental conditions is called *adaptation*. Adaptability is a characteristic of all living organisms, not only of human beings. Adaptation is necessary for survival. The term adaptation is used in a number of contexts, each with a slightly different meaning.

Adaptation by Species and Groups

Evolutionary Adaptation
Evolutionary adaptation refers to the process of modification of the genetic constitution of popu-

lations through natural selection. In this process, when the external environment of a species is altered over a long period of time, only those individuals most suited to the changed environmental conditions are able to survive and reproduce (and consequently to pass along genetic information to the next generation). The genes that code for the advantageous characteristics become fixed in the population, while genes that code for disadvantageous characteristics are lost. All the inherited anatomical, physiological, and behavioral characteristics of present populations are the result of evolutionary adaptation acting on the ancestral populations of the species. A classic example of evolutionary adaptation is the emergence of a dark form of a particular species of moth in England. Before the industrial revolution, the usual form of the moth was speckled white. Occasionally mutant forms that were much darker would occur. Now in industrialized areas where smoke and soot from factories darken the bark of trees, the dark form of the moth is predominant. The dark moths are hardly visible against the darkened tree trunks and so are not eaten by birds. The light-colored moths stand out against the dark background and are eaten by predators. In nonpolluted areas, however, the light form is still predominant.

Cultural Adaptation

Cultural adaptation denotes the behavioral adjustments of groups of people (societies) to changing conditions of life associated with the processes of civilization. Cultural adaptation occurs almost exclusively in human beings. It depends on the ability of humans to learn from previous experiences, to accumulate knowledge acquired by the members of society, and to transmit this knowledge to other people and to succeeding generations. The processes of cultural adaptation are not genetically transmitted, but they are dependent upon the genetically determined potential of individual members of society to learn and to communicate ideas through language. Changes associated with civilization have occurred so rapidly that there has not been enough time for the genetic constitution of

human beings to be altered significantly through the process of evolutionary adaptation. Therefore, cultural processes that depend on learning are very important in adapting to new conditions. The following situation illustrates cultural adaptation. As a result of technological advances and economic factors the diet of most people today contains large amounts of refined carbohydrates. One effect of this dietary pattern is the development of dental caries. The cultural response to dental caries has been the development of dental technology. Another cultural adaptation in this situation is the addition of fluoride to water supplies.

Individual Adaptation

On another level, adaptation refers to the many processes by which an individual organism adjusts to conditions in its particular environment.

Inherent Adaptive Responses

There are many *inherent*, or *innate*, *adaptive mechanisms* by which an organism spontaneously responds to environmental changes. The term adaptation is primarily used in this context in this book. These innate mechanisms may involve ontogenetic (affecting growth and development), physiological, or behavioral responses. Innate adaptive mechanisms are genetically coded and therefore are the products of evolutionary adaptation. They can help the organism cope only with certain types of environmental changes. Sometimes an unusual environmental situation will trigger an innate adaptive response that is inappropriate to the situation.

An example of an ontogenetic adaptive response is the alteration of growth when nutrition is inadequate. A child's growth slows during periods of food shortage. As a result of this mechanism, food energy is conserved. This slowing of growth is accompanied by delayed maturation, so that if the period of deprivation is not prolonged, it is possible to make up most of the loss when adequate nutrition is available again. Many reports indicate that the growth of children was slowed as a result of food shortages in various countries toward the end of the Second World War. Although the growth of children was retarded at that time, the eventual adult size did not differ significantly from the norm for the population.

An example of a physiological adaptive response is tanning of the skin on exposure to sunlight. This mechanism serves to protect underlying tissues by screening out harmful rays of the sun. Physiologically a person adapts to cold by constriction of blood vessels in the skin to reduce heat loss from the body. Those who live in a cold environment for a long time have a higher rate of metabolism to increase heat production. This response is another example of physiological adaptation.

Shivering and moving around are innate behavioral responses to cold. These activities increase heat production by the body. Another example of an inherent adaptive behavior is reflex withdrawal from a noxious stimulus.

Learned Adaptive Responses

In addition to inherent adaptive mechanisms, learned behavioral responses are very important in human adaptation. Thus, for example, in response to cold a person may put on warmer clothing, or light a fire, or adjust the setting of a thermostat in a house. Through learned behaviors, human beings are able not only to adjust to environmental conditions but also to alter the external environment to suit their needs. Learned behavioral mechanisms are particularly important in adapting to psychological and sociocultural factors in the environment.

Psychological adaptation involves intellectual and emotional adjustments to real or imagined environmental conditions as perceived by the individual. Both conscious and unconscious mental processes are used. Psychological adaptation includes the use of defense mechanisms such as rationalization, projection, reaction-formation, dissociation, repression, and substitution. These mechanisms serve the purposes of protecting a person from excessive anxiety and of maintaining self-esteem.

Sensory Adaptation

In *sensory adaptation* the term adaptation is used in a very restricted context to denote the adjustment of sensory receptors to the intensity or quality of stimulation. This adjustment may occur as a heightened sensitivity (e.g., adaptation of the eye to the dark) or as a decreased response to a constant stimulus (e.g., the gradually diminishing sensation of warmth that occurs when a hand is placed in hot water). Sensory adaptation has two aspects, which are complementary. It involves not only a desensitizing process but also a sensitizing process. For example, adaptation to light makes the eyes more sensitive to dark. As a result of sensory adaptation people become aware of changes in the stimuli impinging upon them.

Adaptive Capacity

Human beings are limited in their ability to adapt to environmental changes. Furthermore, not all people have the same capacity to adapt. A person's adaptive capacity is influenced by several factors.

Genetic constitution, or heredity, determines the *adaptive potential* of an organism. The anatomical, physiological, and biochemical characteristics of an individual are genetically determined. Intelligence is also determined, at least partly, by heredity. (The extent to which heredity determines intelligence and the role of environmental influences is controversial.) These characteristics restrict the ways in which a person can respond to changes. The expression of inherited characteristics is modified to varying degrees by environmental conditions, but the limits of development are determined by genetic constitution. For example, heredity determines that a person has two legs. As a result of environmental conditions, however, a person may have one leg amputated in an industrial accident. Subsequently, he or she is not able to regenerate the lost limb: this inability is genetically determined. One can, however, be provided with an artificial leg (cultural adaptation) and can compensate for the loss of a leg by the use of learned behaviors.

Adaptive capacity is influenced by *age*. A person is generally most adaptable during youth and middle life. During infancy and early childhood, and during old age, adaptive capacity is more limited. The repertoire of learned adaptive behaviors of a young child is necessarily limited by lack of experience. Physiological adaptability during infancy and early childhood is restricted because not all the organs and systems are fully developed. In the neonatal period, regulatory mechanisms are not fully developed due to immaturity of the central nervous system. Regulation of fluid balance is more precarious in infancy than in middle life because the infant's immature kidneys are less efficient at concentrating urine. A very young child is more susceptible to infection than an older child or adult because of incomplete development of the immune system.

The exact reasons for the decline of adaptive capacity in old age are not known. The decreased ability of an elderly person to adapt may be due to altered function of the nervous and endocrine systems, which integrate and coordinate adaptive responses. It has also been suggested by Hans Selye that a person is born with a finite amount of "adaptive energy." Adaptive energy is defined as the capacity to perform adaptive work. When a person reaches old age the supply of adaptive energy is almost exhausted. At the moment Selye's theory is just one among many; it has neither been proven nor disproven. In any event, in the early part of life, a person's adaptive capacity is not fully developed. The capacity to adapt develops as a child grows, and it reaches a maximum in adulthood. After that it gradually declines until death.

Anatomical integrity is a factor in adaptability. Loss of body tissue will generally decrease adaptive capacity. The degree to which a lack of anatomical integrity will alter adaptive capacity, however, will depend on the location and extent of the defect. For example, injury to the hypothalamus will seriously impair a person's ability to maintain homeostasis in the face of environmental change because many control centers are located in the hypothalamus. Damage to the cerebral cortex may reduce the ability of a person to adapt psychologically as well as physiologically, but in this case the amount of brain tissue lost becomes more important than the specific area of the loss. Loss of skin (such as may occur with burns) will impair the ability of a person to maintain fluid balance, to regulate body temperature, or to restrict entry of noxious elements from the external environment into the body. Therefore the person will be extremely vulnerable to environmental changes. In this case, the amount of skin lost is critical in determining the ability to survive.

Past experience alters adaptive capacity in that it "sensitizes" a person to a particular environmental situation. Previous exposure to an environmental situation enables one to develop adaptive mechanisms to deal with that particular situation. This process is particularly operative with learned behavioral adaptations, but also occurs when the adaptive mechanism is an innate physiological response. For example, the first time a person is exposed to a particular microorganism he or she may develop an infection. As the body fights the infection, antibodies against the invading microbe are formed. In subsequent encounters with that microorganism the person will be immune to infection because of the presence of these antibodies. The person has developed a protective adaptive mechanism.

Previous exposure is not, however, always helpful in future attempts at adaptation, especially when the adaptive response to the initial experience was inappropriate or unsuccessful. For example, an inappropriate immune response may produce an allergic reaction when the person is subsequently exposed to a particular antigen.

In addition to the effect of previous exposure to environmental situations, past experience in meeting needs also influences adaptive capacity. If a need has not been adequately met in early life, a person's development can be impaired. In addition, that person will have a decreased ability to respond successfully to environmental challenges in later life. For example, inadequate nutrition during the first two years of life can stunt physical growth and interfere with normal development of the central nervous system.

Characteristics of Adaptation

Adaptation is a dynamic process involving the interaction of an organism with the environment in which it lives. The organism forms part of the total environment, and not only does the environment influence the individual organism but the organism also alters the environment. For example, a bacterium secretes toxins into the surrounding medium; a human being cuts down trees to build a house. It has already been pointed out that a constant exchange of substances occurs between an organism and its environment (e.g., exchange of oxygen and carbon dioxide) in order to satisfy basic needs. According to Claude Bernard, the conditions for life are found neither in the organism nor in the environment, but in both at once.

Adaptation is necessary for survival. The more flexible an organism is in its ability to adapt, the greater will be its capacity to survive. For example, if an organism depends on one type of food, it will be able to survive only in an environment that provides that food. If, however, an organism can use a variety of foodstuffs to satisfy its nutritional requirements, it can survive in a much wider range of environments. If a specific food is not available in a particular environment, the organism can adapt by using a different food instead. As already mentioned in the previous section, the capacity to adapt is limited, and varies from one individual to another.

An organism can adapt more readily to a gradual change in environmental conditions than to a rapid change. In other words, if the body has sufficient time it can adapt to a greater challenge than if it has to adapt quickly. For example, if a blood vessel serving a particular tissue is gradually blocked by a slowly developing process, an alternate blood supply (collateral circulation) to that tissue can develop. When the major blood supply is finally cut off, the tissue is not seriously damaged. When a blood vessel is suddenly blocked, however, the tissue may be damaged as a result of inadequate blood flow because a collateral circulation has not been developed.

Also, if a person is exposed to an environmental situation for a prolonged period of time, that person will gradually achieve a more satisfactory degree of adaptation. For example, if one is exposed to a low partial pressure of oxygen such as occurs at high altitudes, the immediate adaptive response is an increased rate of pulmonary ventilation and increased pulse rate. In spite of this mechanism the person may suffer impaired mental functioning and decreased capacity for muscular work. If the person remains at high altitude for several days, or weeks, or years, he or she gradually becomes better adapted. The low oxygen tension has fewer adverse effects on the body and the person is able to work harder. This increased tolerance to low oxygen tension occurs because the body develops additional adaptive mechanisms: increased production of erythrocytes and hemoglobin; increased blood volume; increased number of capillaries to hypoxic tissues; increased diffusing capacity for oxygen through the pulmonary membrane.

Adaptation requires energy and an organism tends to use adaptive mechanisms that are most economical of energy. It takes less energy to use an old adaptive mechanism than to develop a new one. Therefore, a person usually uses a previously developed technique when confronted with a new situation. The old method may or may not be appropriate or successful in the new situation.

Adaptation involves adjustment to the total environmental situation. An organism does not necessarily respond to one environmental factor in isolation. For example, at high altitude a person must simultaneously adapt to hypoxia and to cold. The response to cold in this situation may be different from the response to cold when oxygen is adequate. One response to cold is to increase activity to produce more heat. But this activity increases the oxygen requirement and so may be impracticable for survival under conditions of hypoxia.

Adaptive responses are not the same for every individual. The nature of an adaptive response depends not only on the evoking stimulus, but also on the internal state of the organism at the time the stimulus is received. The response also depends on the way the individual *perceives* the stimulus, and the *meaning* the stimulus has for that individual. Also, the range of adaptive responses is limited by genetic constitution, and no two people (with the exception of identical twins) are genetically alike. For these reasons, different people may adapt differently in the same situation.

An organism maintains its identity in spite of the use of adaptive mechanisms. Although a person makes adjustments in response to environmental changes, she or he maintains a stability of form and function and a general pattern of behavior that characterizes that person as a unique individual.

Adaptive mechanisms are attempts to maintain homeostasis and preserve the integrity of the organism. Some adaptive responses are elicited by conditions in the external environment. In other cases the stimulus for an adaptive response arises from within the organism as a result of an unsatisfied need.

Homeostasis and adaptation are complementary concepts. For optimum functioning of the body, the internal environment must be kept constant within narrowly defined limits. In other words, a person must maintain homeostasis. In order to maintain homeostasis a person must constantly make rapid adjustments to changes in the environment. That is, she or he must adapt. Ideally, adaptive responses are such that they enable a person to function satisfactorily under the changed conditions.

HOMEOSTATIC MECHANISMS

The body has numerous homeostatic control mechanisms. These mechanisms operate continuously in order to minimize the effects of disturbances and preserve a stable internal environment. In some cases, homeostatic regulation consists of storage of materials when there is excess (e.g., glucose converted to glycogen) and their subsequent release in times of need (e.g., glycogen reconverted to glucose). If the excess cannot all be stored, it may be eliminated from the body. In other cases, homeostatic regulation involves altering the rate of various processes (e.g., altering heat production to maintain constant body temperature). The circulation of the blood is critical in maintaining homeostasis because it is necessary for the distribution of substances (and also heat) throughout the internal environment. Therefore a number of mechanisms exist to maintain blood pressure at the desired level and assure continuous flow of blood through the tissues. All these regulatory mechanisms are controlled by the autonomic nervous system and the endocrine system.

The maintenance of homeostasis requires that any tendency toward change is automatically met by increased effectiveness of the factors that resist the change. This task is accomplished by homeostatic mechanisms operating according to the principle of *negative feedback control.*

In a feedback control system the consequences (output) of an action produced in a system are in some way returned or *fed back* to influence the causes (input) of the action. The concept of a system, as used in this context, refers to a set of components that act together and that can be treated as a whole. The stimuli or disturbances that act on the system are called inputs. The consequence of these inputs is the output or response. In a feedback system, the feedback may be negative or positive. With negative feedback, if the system is disturbed, the disturbance (input) triggers a series of events that counteract the disturbance and restore the system to its original (or desired) state. Negative feedback control mechanisms are therefore negative to any attempt to change the system and they favor stability. Negative feedback control is very common in living organisms. Positive feedback is positive to change. With a positive feedback mechanism, a disturbance to the system triggers a series of events that increases the disturbance and leads the system still further from its original state. Positive feedback mechanisms are uncommon in biological systems because they lead to instability.

Negative Feedback Control

In a negative feedback control system the response (output) is negative to the initiating stimulus (input). Consider, for example, the regulation of carbon dioxide (CO_2) concentration in arterial blood. If the CO_2 concentration is high, pulmonary ventilation is increased, which in turn reduces the CO_2 concentration in the arterial blood. In other words, the response (decreased CO_2 concentration) is negative to the input (high CO_2 concentration).

Components of Negative Feedback Control Systems

A negative feedback control system has several components (Fig. 1-1). First, there are *receptors* (sensors), which detect (sense) the amount or level of the factor to be kept constant (*controlled variable*). In the example just given, the controlled variable is the CO_2 concentration in the arterial blood. The main sensors are chemoreceptor cells in the medulla of the brain. The actual magnitude that is sensed is then compared with a *reference value*. In human beings this comparing function occurs in the central nervous system. The reference value (or set point) is the desired or optimal level of the controlled variable. It is usually determined genetically. In the case of CO_2 concentration the reference value is a partial pressure of CO_2 (PCO_2) equal to 40 mm Hg. The difference between the reference value and the actual level that is sensed is called the *error signal*. This error signal is then fed back to an *effector mechanism* in a negative or inhibitory manner so that the resulting action opposes any change in the desired level. In this way the error is minimized. In the example of CO_2 concentration the effector mechanism is pulmonary ventilation.

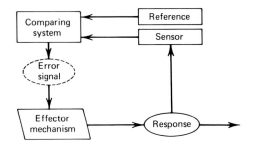

Figure 1-1. *Components of a negative feedback control system. See text for explanation. (Redrawn from Selkurt EE (ed): Physiology, ed 3. Little, Brown, Boston, 1971. By permission.)*

Open-Loop and Closed-Loop Systems

There are two general types of control systems. In an *open-loop system* the sensors (which may be called disturbance detectors) measure the magnitude of the forces tending to disturb the system. The system is then adjusted to compensate for the effect of each disturbing force. This type of control system, in which the response follows the pattern of a variable input, is often called a *servomechanism*. The effectiveness of an open-loop control system depends on precise knowledge not only of the intensity of all the disturbing forces but also of the interactions of all these forces. Open-loop control systems are generally inadequate for accurate control in biological systems.

In a *closed-loop system* the output (response), which is the controlled variable, is kept constant even though there are fluctuating inputs that disturb the system. The sensors in a closed-loop system (often called misalignment detectors) measure the actual value of the controlled variable, which results from the interaction of the forces tending to disturb the system with the factors tending to maintain the desired state. Any discrepancy between this actual value or response and the desired value or response gives rise to the error signal, which is then fed back to the effector mechanism. For example, the chemoreceptors that measure the PCO_2 in arterial blood act as misalignment detectors. Carbon dioxide produced by the cells enters the capillary blood. This blood, with its high CO_2 content, passes through the veins to the right side of the heart and is then pumped to the lungs. As the blood passes through the lungs, CO_2 is normally removed. The blood then returns to the left side of the heart and is pumped out to the systemic arteries. It is at this point that the CO_2 level in the blood is measured. The level of CO_2 measured by the receptors is therefore the result of the interaction between the activity of the cells of peripheral organs in adding CO_2 to the blood and the activity of the lungs in removing it. The rate of ventilation is altered only when there is an imbalance between these two forces.

Knowledge of the source and magnitude of each disturbance is not necessary in the operation of a closed-loop system. This type of control system, in which the response is kept constant, is often called a *regulator*. Biological negative feedback control systems are closed-loop systems. They can provide accurate control even when the components of the system are not particularly stable.

Fluctuations in the Controlled Variable

When an object (or system) fluctuates between one extreme position (or response) and another position around a point of rest (or set point), the object (or system) is said to *oscillate*. (For example, a pendulum swinging back and forth is oscillating.) When an oscillation gradually decreases, it is said to be *lightly damped*. *Heavy damping* causes the oscillations to cease rapidly. A system is said to be *critically damped* when the oscillations stop before a single cycle is completed. In negative feedback control systems, oscillations are usually critically damped. A slight deviation of the controlled variable generates the error signal and the effector mechanism then brings the controlled variable back to the set point. In a good control system the controlled variable never deviates very far from the set point. If the system is disturbed, the factor that changes is the one that counteracts the disturbance (i.e., the effector mechanism). So in the previous example pulmonary ventilation varies in

order to maintain the arterial CO_2 concentration at the desired level.

Oscillations in a control system are usually signs of malfunction. In other words, when a negative feedback control system is unstable the actual value of the controlled variable may deviate quite widely from the set point. When attempts are made to bring the value back to the desired level, an overshoot may occur. Once the oscillations start, they may continue indefinitely.

Cheyne-Stokes breathing is an example of oscillation in a control system. Normally the arterial P_{CO_2} does not deviate far from 40 mm Hg, and the depth of breathing is fairly constant unless a person's activity changes. Cheyne-Stokes breathing is characterized by a cyclic waxing and waning of the depth of respiration. The depth of breathing progressively increases until it is much deeper than usual, then it decreases and breathing stops (apnea) for a few seconds. Breathing is shallow when it starts again, but progressively increases once more. The entire cycle may occur over a period of 45 seconds to 3 minutes. During the phase of very deep breathing the P_{CO_2} in the pulmonary blood falls below normal. When the pulmonary blood reaches the chemoreceptors in the brain, breathing is inhibited as a result of the decreased P_{CO_2}. During the apneic phase the P_{CO_2} of the pulmonary blood increases and may rise above normal. When the blood with the increased P_{CO_2} arrives at the respiratory center in the brain breathing is stimulated; the person overbreathes again and a new cycle is initiated.

Normally the respiratory center prevents involuntary overbreathing; slight changes in the P_{CO_2} bring breathing back toward normal before the P_{CO_2} can decrease enough to cause apnea (i.e., the system is damped). In Cheyne-Stokes breathing the normal damping mechanism is not functioning and the system oscillates between deep breathing and apnea. Cheyne-Stokes breathing usually occurs as a result of either altered responsiveness of the respiratory center or a delay in the circulation time from the lungs to the brain.

As a result of damage to the respiratory center, a slight change in P_{CO_2} may bring about a larger than normal change in ventilation. Thus, an initial slight increase in P_{CO_2} may stimulate breathing more than normal, causing an overshoot that brings the P_{CO_2} below normal. In response to the decreased P_{CO_2} the respiratory center overreacts again and apnea results. As the P_{CO_2} rises again, the overshoot is repeated in the opposite direction, and so on.

When the blood takes longer than usual to flow from the lungs to the brain (e.g., in cardiac failure), the P_{CO_2} may rise significantly above normal before the altered P_{CO_2} is detected by the central chemoreceptors. The high P_{CO_2} then stimulates a great increase in the depth of respiration. The increased ventilation decreases the P_{CO_2}, but now it falls too far because of the delay in circulation time from the lungs to the brain, and apnea results. Thus the system oscillates as a result of a prolonged reaction time.

Use of Disturbance Detectors

As mentioned previously, disturbance detectors, used alone in open-loop systems, cannot provide accurate control in living organisms. Disturbance detectors are sometimes used, however, in conjunction with misalignment detectors; in this way they can reduce the time required for a system to respond to a change in conditions. When both disturbance detectors and misalignment detectors are used, the effect of information (input) from the misalignment detectors predominates. The control system responds only to *changes* in the information provided by the disturbance detectors. When conditions are constant the information from the disturbance detectors is ignored. An example of the use of disturbance detectors is in the control of pulmonary ventilation during exercise. As already mentioned, the rate of ventilation is determined by the level of CO_2 in the arterial blood, as measured by misalignment detectors. This is the case when a person is at rest or is exercising at a steady rate. When a person who has been at rest suddenly begins exercising, however, the rate of ventilation increases sharply before any change in the rate of entry of CO_2 into the blood can be detected. This sudden increase is followed by a further, slower rise. Eventually when the rate of exercise is constant, a steady rate of ventilation is reached. If the only sources of information for the control of ventilation were the misalignment detectors for arterial CO_2 concentration, there would be a definite delay between the start of exercise and the increased rate of ventilation, because it takes time before the increased muscular activity increases the level of CO_2 in the blood. Since the rate of ventilation in fact increases immediately, some other factor must be operating. Experiments have shown that the sharp initial increase in ventilation rate does not depend on chemical changes in the blood but rather on the activation of proprioceptors in the exercising limbs. These proprioceptors are activated by movement and provide the brain with information about when and how rapidly the joints are moving. In the control of ventilation the proprioceptors act as disturbance detectors. When movement occurs at a joint, the proprioceptors notify the control centers in the brain that exercise is taking place. This information is integrated with the knowledge that production of CO_2 by the muscles is likely to increase. In anticipation of this increase in the level of CO_2, the control system produces an increase in the rate of ventilation. During very light exercise the P_{CO_2} increases only a small amount, so that the initial increase in ventilation just about compensates for it and any further increase is slight. During heavy exercise, however, the initial increase in ventilation does not compensate for the large amount of CO_2 produced. Arterial P_{CO_2} rises and this increase stimulates the chemoreceptors (misalignment detectors). As a result of the information from the chemoreceptors, the control center in the brain brings about a further increase in the rate of ventilation. The rate of ventilation continues to increase until the increased rate of removal of CO_2 balances the increased rate of production and the

CO_2 concentration in the arterial blood returns to normal.

Indirect Control

In biological systems many factors are controlled directly, such as arterial CO_2 concentration. Others, however, are controlled indirectly. For example, the amount of oxygen in the arterial blood depends to a great extent on the amount of oxygen in the air and the degree of pulmonary ventilation. Pulmonary ventilation is, in turn, governed by the amount of carbon dioxide in the blood. Thus, oxygen concentration is regulated indirectly under normal conditions.

Ventilation can vary quite widely without having a significant effect on arterial oxygen saturation, because of the nature of oxygen transport in the blood (see Chapter 10). Hemoglobin is normally almost fully saturated with oxygen. Increased ventilation, therefore, has little effect on the amount of oxygen in the arterial blood. Also, ventilation can decrease considerably before oxygen saturation falls below 90%. Arterial carbon dioxide concentration, on the other hand, is very sensitive to slight changes in ventilation. Therefore, it is important that pulmonary ventilation is determined by the arterial P_{CO_2}.

The arterial P_{O_2} (partial pressure of oxygen) can influence ventilation under certain conditions, however, and this influence provides a safety element. As already mentioned, CO_2 exerts its influence on breathing mainly through central chemoreceptors in the medulla. Peripheral chemoreceptors in the carotid and aortic bodies also respond slightly to an increased P_{CO_2}, but normally the influence of these receptors is secondary to the central chemoreceptors. A decreased P_{O_2}, on the other hand, does not activate the central chemoreceptors but rather acts through the chemoreceptors in the carotid and aortic bodies. Whereas slight changes in P_{CO_2} strongly influence ventilation, arterial P_{O_2} must fall below about 70 mm Hg (normally it is about 95 mm Hg) before ventilation is significantly affected.

When the P_{CO_2} rises, ventilation is stimulated; when the P_{CO_2} falls below the desired level, ventilation is depressed. This mechanism maintains the P_{CO_2} at the desired level. The effect of a high P_{CO_2} on stimulating ventilation is greater than the effect of a low P_{CO_2} on depressing ventilation, because when ventilation is depressed by a low P_{CO_2} the arterial P_{O_2} falls to the critical value and stimulates ventilation. In other words, a low P_{O_2} checks the depressant effect of a low P_{CO_2} to maintain a minimum level of breathing. Without this braking effect of a low P_{O_2}, a low P_{CO_2} might cause breathing to stop. Conversely, however, if the P_{CO_2} is normal and the P_{O_2} drops, the increase in ventilation brought about by the low P_{O_2} causes a decrease in the P_{CO_2}, which depresses ventilation and opposes the effect of the low P_{O_2}. Under usual conditions the effect of oxygen lack on ventilation is insignificant compared to the effect of carbon dioxide. Under some abnormal conditions (e.g., lung disease), however, the P_{CO_2} increases at the same time that the P_{O_2} decreases. Under these conditions the effect of the decreased P_{O_2} enhances the effect of the P_{CO_2} in stimulating ventilation. In some cases, the chemoreceptors lose their sensitivity to a high P_{CO_2} and a low P_{O_2} becomes the major stimulus to breathing.

In other words, under normal conditions P_{CO_2} is the directly controlled variable and P_{O_2} the indirectly controlled variable, because one effector mechanism (i.e., pulmonary ventilation) serves both variables and this effector mechanism is primarily activated by changes in the P_{CO_2} (the more sensitive variable). As an added safety factor, however, under some abnormal conditions P_{O_2} may be controlled directly.

Multiple Control Mechanisms Operating on One Factor

Some homeostatic mechanisms have only one effector operating on a particular factor. This situation may occur when the forces disturbing the system always tend to push the system in one direction. Again, the regulation of arterial CO_2 concentration is an example. The body cells always produce CO_2 and with increased activity they produce more CO_2. By altering the rate of pulmonary ventilation, arterial CO_2 concentration is kept within narrow limits. No other effector mechanism operates.

In many homeostatic control systems, however, more than one effector mechanism operates on the same variable. This situation usually exists when there are several forces disturbing the system, some pushing the system in one direction and others pushing it the opposite way. An example is the regulation of body temperature. In order to resist disturbances of temperature in both directions, more than one effector mechanism is employed. If the external temperature is cold, tending to reduce the body temperature, heat production can be increased by muscular activity, and heat loss decreased by reducing the blood flow near the skin surface. These mechanisms will resist a reduction in body temperature. On the other hand, if the external temperature is high the body temperature will tend to increase. This increase can be counteracted by reducing heat production with a decrease in physical activity, and increasing heat loss by active sweating and increased blood flow near the skin surface. Thus in the regulation of body temperature several effector mechanisms operate to resist disturbances in both directions and to maintain body temperature at the desired level.

It is quite common for biological homeostatic mechanisms to have several feedback systems acting on the same variable. In other words, there are several receptors and several effector mechanisms for the control of one factor. This situation provides greater reliability and safety, for if one feedback system fails there are still others operating. An example is the regulation of arterial blood pressure. It is important that arterial blood pressure be maintained within narrow limits. If the blood pressure is too low, blood flow in the peripheral organs may be insufficient. The result may be death of some of the cells and permanent damage to the organs. If the blood pressure is too high, it increases the work load of the heart and may cause damage to the blood vessels.

Baroreceptors for monitoring the blood pressure are located in the walls of many blood vessels. These receptors are actually sensitive to stretch. Since the degree of stretching of the vessel walls is directly related to the blood pressure, these receptors provide information about pressure in the arteries. If the blood pressure increases, there is an increased rate of nerve impulse transmission from the receptors; if the blood pressure decreases, the rate of firing of the receptors decreases. Specialized regions of the carotid arteries, called the carotid sinuses, are baroreceptors that provide information about the blood pressure in the arteries supplying the brain. These seem to be the most important pressure receptors. In addition, receptors of secondary importance are located in the arch of the aorta and in other large arteries. If the nerves that normally convey impulses from the carotid sinuses to the brain are cut or damaged, no impulses can be transmitted from these receptors. The brain interprets the lack of impulses as a drop in blood pressure and initiates actions to raise the blood pressure. The control center soon becomes aware, however, that the information provided by the other baroreceptors does not substantiate the information (or lack of information) provided by the carotid sinuses. Also, there will be no correlation between the attempts to raise blood pressure and the lack of impulses from the carotid sinuses. The brain then ignores the lack of impulses from the carotid sinuses and relies entirely on the information provided by other baroreceptors. The blood pressure then returns to normal and is regulated according to the input from the secondary receptors. If the carotid sinuses are left intact and the secondary baroreceptors are damaged, the blood pressure usually is not altered. This fact does not indicate that the secondary receptors are unimportant, but merely that their significance only becomes apparent if the primary receptors fail.

Not only are several receptors involved in the homeostatic regulation of blood pressure, but several effector mechanisms maintain the pressure at the desired level (Fig. 1-2). Arterial blood pressure depends on cardiac output and total peripheral resistance. If the blood pressure falls, it can be raised

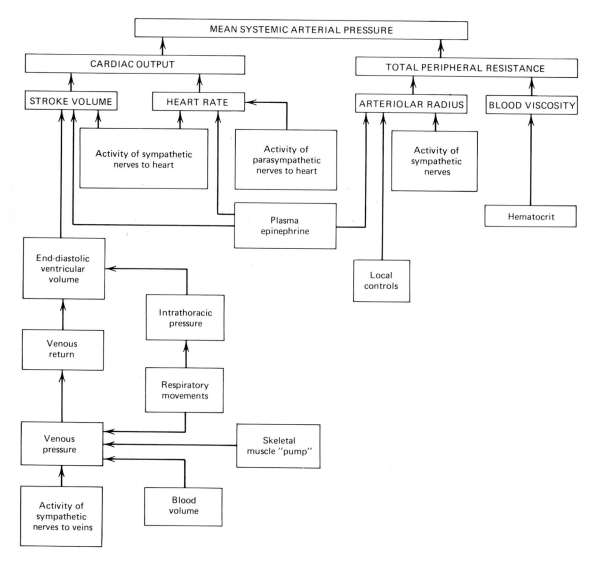

Figure 1-2. *Effector mechanisms involved in the regulation of blood pressure. (Adapted from Vander et al.: Human Physiology. Copyright © 1975 by McGraw-Hill, Inc. Used with permission of McGraw-Hill Book Company.)*

by increasing cardiac output and/or total peripheral resistance. Conversely, an increase in the blood pressure can be counteracted by decreasing cardiac output and/or total peripheral resistance.

Cardiac output can be altered by changing the stroke volume and/or heart rate. Each of these, in turn, can be altered by several different means.

Total peripheral resistance also can be altered by more than one mechanism. The major determinant of total peripheral resistance is the radius of the arterioles. If the arterioles are constricted, total peripheral resistance is increased; if the arterioles are dilated, total peripheral resistance is decreased. Total peripheral resistance is also influenced by blood viscosity. If the viscosity is increased, total peripheral resistance will be increased.

So many effector mechanisms operate on arterial blood pressure that if one of them is impaired or altered it may only produce a slight, temporary effect.

Homeostatic Control Mechanisms Operate at All Levels

Homeostasis is maintained by negative feedback control mechanisms operating at all levels of activity of the organism, from complex behaviors of the individual down to reactions occurring at the molecular level. At the behavioral level, these mechanisms involve observable activity of the total organism. The activity may be a response to a change in the external environment, or may be a response to an internal stimulus, such as an unmet need. At the physiological level, these mechanisms involve internal alterations in the functioning of various tissues or organs in order to counteract disturbances. These alterations are brought about by activity of the nervous and/or endocrine system.

At the molecular level, the activity of metabolic pathways is constantly regulated by negative feedback control to ensure that no metabolic systems are overproducing or underproducing any particular end product. A metabolic pathway involves a series of biochemical reactions, each requiring an enzyme catalyst. Regulation of a metabolic pathway is effected by the action of one or more specific regulatory enzymes. Regulatory enzymes are slightly different from other enzymes. In addition to their catalytic property, their activity is sensitive to some substance that can act as a modulator. Negative modulators inhibit the catalytic activity of the enzyme, whereas positive modulators stimulate enzyme activity. The end product of a biochemical pathway often acts as a negative modulator. The regulatory enzyme is usually the first enzyme of the metabolic pathway; or, if there is a branch in the pathway, it is the first enzyme after the branch. Thus, a negative feedback loop exists for the regulation of the level of end product (Fig. 1-3). A high level of end product inhibits the activity of the first enzyme in the pathway that produces the particular end product. As a result, less end product will be formed and its level will gradually fall as it is used or eliminated. When the amount of end product falls below the desired level, the inhibition on the regulatory enzyme is released and the pathway operates at a faster rate to produce more end product.

As an example of negative feedback control mechanisms operating at all levels of activity, consider the energy requirements of the body. Energy is needed for the activities of an organism and the source of this energy is food. At the behavioral level, the amount of food eaten is regulated by a complex homeostatic mechanism. The control centers for appetite and satiety are located in the hypothalamus. The desired level of food intake varies, depending on physical activity, psychological factors, and a person's general state of health. Receptors (misalignment detectors) in the hypothalamus monitor blood levels of glucose and possibly levels of circulating amino acids and fatty acids as well. If food intake is inadequate, the

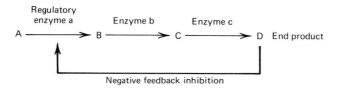

Figure 1-3. *Negative feedback control of a metabolic pathway. The controlled variable is the end product. The effector mechanism is the regulatory enzyme. The set point is determined by the physicochemical properties of the system.*

concentration of these nutrients in the blood will fall below the desired level and the person becomes hungry. Hunger is the error signal. In response to hunger, the person will seek food and eat until food intake reaches the desired level. When food intake is adequate, hunger is absent. Hunger is actually reduced before the ingested food has been digested and absorbed; that is, before the concentration of glucose and other nutrients in the blood rises. Stretch receptors (disturbance detectors) in the stomach and other parts of the gastrointestinal tract provide the brain with information regarding the fullness of the stomach and intestinal tract. Distension of the stomach causes the stretch receptors to send more impulses to the brain. These impulses, in effect, signal the brain that food is on the way and so hunger subsides before the food is absorbed. Information about the taste and texture of the food eaten is relayed to the brain from receptors in the oropharynx. This information also probably influences the amount of food eaten.

Assuming that food intake is adequate, the most important source of energy for cellular activities is glucose. To ensure the availability of glucose to the cells (especially those of the brain) the concentration of glucose in the blood must be maintained within certain limits. Another negative feedback control system with several effector mechanisms regulates blood glucose concentration. After a meal, the blood glucose level rises as the food is absorbed into the body. This high level of glucose stimulates production of the hormone insulin by the pancreas. Insulin facilitates transport of glucose into the cells and promotes its conversion to glycogen and fat for storage. This activity reduces the concentration of glucose in the blood and keeps it within the desired limits. During exercise large amounts of glucose are consumed by the muscle cells. As a result, the blood glucose concentration may fall. This decrease is counteracted by several mechanisms, in addition to a decrease in insulin secretion. The low level of glucose directly stimulates production of the hormone glucagon by the pancreas. Glucagon promotes breakdown of liver glycogen so that glucose is re-

leased into the blood. The nervous system mediates release of epinephrine from the adrenal medulla in response to the low blood glucose level. Epinephrine enhances breakdown of muscle glycogen. Other hormones, the glucocorticoids from the adrenal cortex and growth hormone from the adenohypophysis, also act to raise the blood-glucose level. The glucocorticoids increase the rate of gluconeogenesis (formation of glucose from noncarbohydrate sources, e.g., from amino acids) and slightly decrease the transport of glucose into cells, thus raising blood glucose concentration. Growth hormone affects the blood glucose level by decreasing carbohydrate utilization by cells and promoting catabolism of fat for energy instead. All these mechanisms serve to maintain blood glucose concentration within the desired range.

With the supply of glucose to the cells assured, other negative feedback systems operating at the cellular level control the biochemical reactions that release energy from food molecules. Carbohydrates and fat are stable storage forms of chemical energy. When they are catabolized some of the energy released is used to form adenosine triphosphate (ATP) from adenosine diphosphate (ADP) and inorganic phosphate. ATP might be regarded as the energy "currency" of the cell. When a phosphate group is split off from ATP to form ADP (hydrolysis of ATP), energy is released. By coupling this reaction with a reaction that requires energy, the energy derived from hydrolysis of ATP is used for cell work. When little work is being done and energy is plentiful, the concentration of ATP in the cell is high and ADP concentration is low. Conversely, if energy is being utilized at a faster rate than it is being provided, the level of ATP will fall and the level of ADP will rise.

Release of energy from glucose occurs in several stages (see Chapter 10). In the process of glycolysis, glucose is broken down in a stepwise manner to form pyruvic acid. The pyruvic acid is then converted to acetate, which is not in the free form, but is bound with coenzyme A (CoA) to form acetyl CoA. (Acetyl CoA can also be formed from breakdown of fatty acids.) Acetyl CoA can be used in the synthesis of fats or can enter the Krebs

(TCA) cycle for further oxidation. During the operation of the TCA cycle the coenzymes nicotinamide adenine dinucleotide (NAD) and flavin adenine dinucleotide (FAD) are reduced. These coenzymes are subsequently reoxidized when they pass electrons to the cytochrome chain. The ultimate electron acceptor is oxygen, which then combines with hydrogen ions to form water. During this process of electron transfer along the cytochrome chain, energy is released, which is used to form ATP (oxidative phosphorylation). This process is the major source of ATP for the cell. The reoxidized coenzymes are used again in the TCA cycle.

In the control of breakdown of glucose for energy, ATP acts as a negative modulator and ADP as a positive modulator. When ATP (i.e., energy) is plentiful and the ADP level is low, an enzyme near the beginning of the glycolysis pathway is inhibited. At the same time, an enzyme necessary for conversion of glucose to glycogen is stimulated. A regulatory enzyme near the beginning of the TCA cycle is also inhibited, and conversion of acetyl CoA to fat is enhanced. In other words, when the level of ATP rises in the cell it inhibits further production of ATP and promotes storage of energy as glycogen and fat. As energy is used by the cell, the level of ATP falls and ADP concentration rises, releasing the inhibition on the regulatory enzymes. Glycogen is converted to glucose, fat is broken down to acetyl CoA, and glycolysis and the TCA cycle are stimulated so that more ATP is formed. In this manner the ATP concentration is maintained at an optimum level. Thus, energy balance in the organism is regulated by many homeostatic mechanisms operating at several levels.

These examples are but a few of the many negative feedback control systems operating to maintain homeostasis in the human organism.

Positive Feedback

In a positive feedback system, the error signal is fed back to the effector mechanism in such a way that the error is increased. In other words, the

original error (or change), instead of being corrected, is repeated again and again. For example, a positive feedback situation would exist if a high CO_2 concentration in the arterial blood were to depress ventilation so that the level of CO_2 increased further. This situation does not occur, fortunately, because it would be detrimental to the organism. Unlimited positive feedback causes a progressive change in the response until the system is operating at a maximum or minimum level. This situation is referred to as a *vicious cycle*. Positive feedback sometimes occurs in abnormal situations. In some cases, mild degrees of positive feedback are overcome by the negative feedback control mechanisms of the body, in which case the vicious cycle does not develop and homeostasis is restored. If a vicious cycle does develop, however, it can lead to death. For example, if the heart is damaged so that the contraction of the ventricles is weakened, cardiac output is decreased. This decrease causes the blood pressure to fall, resulting in a decreased supply of blood to the heart itself. As a result, the heart deteriorates further, the cardiac output decreases further, blood pressure falls lower, and so on until death occurs.

Although positive feedback is rare in biological systems, there are a few examples of positive feedback occurring in normal situations. One example is the generation of a nerve impulse. The membrane of a resting nerve fiber (i.e., one in which no impulse is being transmitted) is said to be polarized: the inside is negatively charged relative to the outside. In other words, a potential difference occurs across the membrane. This potential difference, known as the resting membrane potential, has a magnitude of about 70 millivolts (mV). It occurs because the concentration of ions inside the cell is different from that outside the cell. This difference is brought about by the selective permeability of the cell membrane. The resting membrane is effectively impermeable to sodium ions and the concentration of sodium ions outside the cell is much higher than that inside. Therefore a concentration gradient exists, which would tend to force sodium into the cell if the membrane were permeable. When an adequate

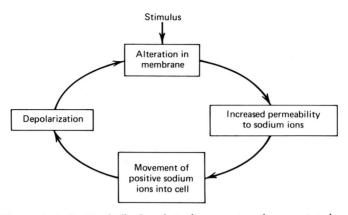

Figure 1-4. *Positive feedback cycle in the generation of a nerve impulse.*

stimulus is applied to a nerve fiber it causes a change in permeability of the cell membrane, allowing sodium ions to rush into the fiber down their concentration gradient. As the positively charged sodium ions move in, the membrane is depolarized (i.e., the membrane potential moves toward zero). This depolarization increases the permeability of the membrane and more sodium ions enter the cell. As more sodium ions enter, the membrane is depolarized further, which in turn causes a still greater increase in permeability to sodium ions (Fig. 1-4). This situation is positive feedback: an increase in the response causes a still further increase in response. When enough sodium ions enter the cell the polarity of the membrane is reversed (i.e., the inside is now positive relative to the outside) and an action potential, or nerve impulse, is generated. If the nerve fiber were to remain positive on the inside relative to the outside, no further impulses could be transmitted. This situation is not the case, however. At the peak of the action potential, some unknown mechanism shuts off the membrane permeability to sodium ions. The resting membrane potential is restored and the sodium ions are pumped out of the nerve fiber.

A second example of positive feedback occurs during the female sexual cycle. Development of ovarian follicles and maturation of the ovum occur under the influence of three hormones: the gonadotropins follicle-stimulating hormone (FSH) and luteinizing hormone (LH) from the adenohypophysis; and estrogen, which is secreted by follicular cells in the ovary. Ovulation is triggered by a sudden surge in the output of LH. Although the precise mechanisms controlling the secretion of the gonadotropins are not yet understood, it appears that a positive feedback mechanism is responsible for the sudden increase in LH secretion. The adenohypophysis secretes FSH and LH in response to stimulation by releasing factor(s) from the hypothalamus. As the ovarian follicles develop, they secrete more and more estrogen and the blood concentration of estrogen becomes quite high. This high level of estrogen inhibits secretion of FSH (negative feedback) and subsequently the level of FSH declines. At the same time, however, the high level of estrogen stimulates secretion of LH-releasing factor and/or increases the sensitivity of the adenohypophysis to LH-releasing factor. As a result, a sudden increase in LH secretion occurs. Thus a positive feedback mechanism is operating as follows: LH stimulates development of the ovarian follicle, which secretes estrogen; a high level of estrogen then stimulates secretion of LH. The outpouring of LH from the adenohypophysis triggers ovulation and induces the subsequent formation of the corpus luteum. The corpus luteum secretes progesterone, which inhibits secretion of LH and breaks the positive feedback cycle.

In both these examples, the positive feedback is limited. When a certain point is reached, the cycle of positive feedback is broken and the system is returned to the initial state. If the positive feedback cycle were not broken, operation of the system would stop after one cycle. Positive feedback systems can be tolerated in living or-ganisms only when the positive feedback is lim-ited.

SUGGESTED ADDITIONAL READING

Koshland DE Jr: Protein shape and biological control. *Sci Am* **229**(4): 52–64, 1973.

Lewontin RC: Adaptation. *Sci Am* **239**(3): 212–230, 1978.

Tustin A: Feedback. *Sci Am* **187**(3): 48–55, 1952.

2

Disease

Health and illness are relative concepts. There is no clear distinction between health and disease, but the varying degrees of wellness and illness form a continuous spectrum. At one end of the spectrum is a high level of wellness: the optimal state of well-being of the human being. At the other extreme is physical death.

THE NATURE OF DISEASE

According to the 25th edition of *Dorland's Illustrated Medical Dictionary*, *health* is "a state of optimal physical, mental and social well-being, and not merely the absence of disease and infirmity." *Disease* is defined as "a definite morbid process having a train of symptoms; it may affect the whole body or any of its parts, and its etiology,

pathology and prognosis may be known or unknown."

Etiology is the study of the factors that cause disease. A condition is said to be *idiopathic* when the cause is unknown. *Patho-* is a combining form derived from the Greek word *pathos*, meaning disease or suffering. Thus, the development of a disease is *pathogenesis*. An agent that causes disease is a *pathogen*. *Pathology* is that branch of medicine that deals with the essential nature of disease, especially of the structural and functional changes in tissues that are associated with disease. The physiology of disordered function is *pathophysiology*. Based on a knowledge of the nature of a given disease and the response of a person to the disease, a forecast of the probable outcome can be made. This forecast is the *prognosis*.

Every abnormal condition of the body is not necessarily disease. For example, a person may have a limb amputated, which is an abnormal situation. Following the amputation, however, the person may function very well and be healthy for the rest of his or her life, even though a limb is missing. Disease represents a struggle taking place in the body, a clash between the forces or agents that tend to disrupt body functioning and the defending forces or mechanisms of the body that attempt to maintain or restore normal function.

Signs and Symptoms

A *sign* is any objective evidence of disease; that is, any evidence that can be perceived by someone examining the person who is ill (e.g., a rapid pulse rate). Any subjective evidence of disease, that is, any evidence perceived by the person who is ill, is called a *symptom* (e.g., palpitations). (In common usage, the term *symptoms* is often used to mean both signs and symptoms.) A *syndrome* is a set of signs and symptoms that occur together.

Some signs and symptoms are characteristic for a given disease. Other signs and symptoms, such as fever, headache, malaise, and anorexia, are commonly associated with many disease conditions. Pain frequently accompanies pathological conditions (see Chapter 9). Some signs and symptoms are produced by the particular agent(s) causing the disease. Many signs and symptoms, however, are manifestations of the body's attempts to combat the agent and maintain homeostasis.

The human body has a limited number of mechanisms for coping with noxious agents and disturbing forces. Therefore, a variety of agents can elicit the same response. For example inflammation occurs in response to irritation by many different physical, chemical, and biological agents (see Chapter 8). The typical manifestations of the inflammatory response are redness, heat, pain, swelling, and limitation of motion or function. Specific signs and symptoms will be determined by the location of the inflammatory process. For example, inflammation of the pleural membranes surrounding the lungs (*pleurisy*) is associated with chest pain on deep breathing; therefore rapid,

shallow respirations are characteristic. On the other hand, inflammation of the meninges of the brain and/or spinal cord (*meningitis*) is accompanied by headache, pain and stiffness in the neck and back, and often an altered level of consciousness. Inflammation of other parts of the body will be accompanied by other specific manifestations, depending on the function of the part and how the inflammation interferes with normal function.

Acute and Chronic Disease

Disease processes are often classified as acute or chronic. An *acute* condition has relatively severe manifestations and runs a short course. A *chronic* condition lasts for a long period of time. Sometimes chronic disease processes begin with an acute phase and become prolonged when the body's defenses are unable to overcome the causative agent or stressor. In other cases chronic conditions develop insidiously and never have an acute phase. An *intercurrent* condition is one that occurs during the course of an already existing disease.

Diseases often progress through several stages. An interval occurring between exposure of a tissue to an injurious agent and the first appearance of signs and symptoms may be called a *latent period*, or in the case of infectious diseases, an *incubation period*. The *prodromal period*, or *prodrome*, refers to the appearance of the first signs and symptoms indicating the onset of a disease. Prodromal symptoms are often nonspecific, such as headache, malaise, anorexia, and nausea. During the *stage of manifest illness*, or *acute phase*, the disease reaches its full intensity and signs and symptoms attain their greatest severity. Sometimes during the course of a disease the signs and symptoms become very mild or disappear for a time. This interval may be called a *silent period*, or *latent period*. For example, in the total body radiation syndrome (see Chapter 23) a latent period may occur between the prodrome and the stage of manifest illness. Another example is syphilis, which may have two latent periods: one occurring between the primary and secondary stage, and another between the secondary and tertiary stage.

Some diseases (e.g., some types of leukemia) follow a course of alternate exacerbations and remissions. An *exacerbation* is a relatively sudden increase in the severity of a disease or any of its signs and symptoms. A *remission* is an abatement or decline in severity of the signs and symptoms of a disease.

Convalescence is the stage of recovery after a disease, injury, or surgical operation. Occasionally a disease process produces aftereffects. A condition caused by and following a disease is called a *sequela*.

Disruption of Homeostasis

It has been repeatedly stated in the previous chapter that maintenance of homeostasis is necessary for optimum functioning of the body. It follows, therefore, that if homeostasis is disrupted, a person cannot function optimally and illness may result. If the demands made on the body are too great, the homeostatic mechanisms may be inadequate to compensate, resulting in disturbances in the internal environment. In other cases there may be failure of the control mechanism; for example, inability to secrete a necessary hormone. As a result, outside intervention may be required in order to maintain homeostasis (e.g., injections of insulin for a person with diabetes mellitus). Sometimes the control mechanism is operating adequately but the set point is altered. As a result the feedback mechanism regulates the variable at an abnormal value. The set point is believed to be altered, for example, in fever. In this case the "thermostat" has been set higher. The control mechanism then maintains the body temperature at an elevated level.

Normal versus Abnormal

The fact that homeostatic mechanisms are operating to maintain constant conditions in the internal environment implies that there is an optimum or normal value for a given factor. This optimum value is the reference level or set point in a negative feedback control system. By means of a variety of clinical and laboratory tests it is possible to measure many characteristics of the internal environment. In a state of health a certain value is consistently obtained for a particular factor. This value is what is considered the normal. Deviations from this particular value are usually considered abnormal.

There is no absolute normal, however. What is usual for one person may be different for another because of genetic variation. For example, a blood pressure of 120/80 mm Hg is the usual value for many people. Others, however, may consistently have a blood pressure of 90/70 mm Hg and yet be in good health. This value represents their normal blood pressure. By sampling a large number of people an "average normal" and a range of normal can be determined. Occasionally, however, a person may consistently show a value outside the usual range for the factor and yet be functioning well. Although she or he may be abnormal for that characteristic in terms of the population as a whole, the unusual value may be considered normal for that person.

Some factors show sexual differences. For example, the normal range of hemoglobin concentration for adult females is 12 to 15 g/100 ml of blood; for males the range is 14 to 17 g/100 ml of blood.

Many factors vary with age. Therefore, what is the normal value for a person at a given age may be abnormal at a different age. For example, a resting heart rate of 120 beats per minute is normal for an infant, but not for an adult.

In some cases a deviation from the usual value may occur as an adaptive mechanism; whether or not the deviation is considered abnormal depends on the situation. For example, the red blood cell count increases when a person moves to a high altitude. This increase is a normal adaptive response to the decreased availability of oxygen at high altitude. A similar increase in the red blood cell count occurring at sea level, however, would be abnormal.

Some factors vary according to the time of day (i.e., they exhibit a *circadian rhythm* or *diurnal variation*). Therefore, in interpreting the result of a particular test it may be necessary to know the time at which the value was determined. For example, plasma concentrations of some hormones exhibit diurnal variation. Reflecting the fluctuation in plasma levels of corticosteroids, urinary excretion of 17-ketosteroids shows a diurnal rhythm. Peak rate of excretion occurs between 0800 h and 1000 h and is about two to three times greater than the lowest value, which occurs between 2400 h and 0200 h.

Some clinical and laboratory measurements may vary according to the method used. For example, prothrombin time is influenced by the procedure used to measure it. To evaluate the significance of the prothrombin time, each laboratory usually draws a graph relating prothrombin concentration in the blood to prothrombin time for the method used.

Disturbances of the internal environment do occur in disease and so a variety of measurable factors can be altered. Therefore, values obtained in clinical and laboratory tests are useful in assessing a person's state of health or disease, in spite of the difficulties just mentioned. Often, however, when assessing a person's health status, a *change* in some measurement is more significant than the actual value of the particular factor. For example, a blood pressure of 90/70 mm Hg may not be significant if that is the usual value for a particular person. If a person usually has a blood pressure of 120/80 mm Hg, however, a reading of 90/70 would be very significant. Deviation from the usual value can be indicative of illness, especially if it is accompanied by other signs and symptoms.

STRESS AND DISEASE

Difficulties in adapting to life situations, disruptions in homeostasis, and disease states are asso-

ciated with *stress*. Everyone is familiar with the feeling we call stress, but what is it? Stress is difficult to define, and different people who have written about stress define it in different ways. Hans Selye, a Canadian endocrinologist, pioneered in the field of stress research and was largely responsible for popularizing the word stress. Yet even Selye had difficulty defining the word. First he defined it as ". . . the rate of all the wear and tear caused by life." (Hans Selye, *The Stress of Life*, McGraw-Hill Book Co., New York, 1956, p. viii). Later Selye defined stress as ". . . the state manifested by a specific syndrome which consists of all the nonspecifically induced changes within a biologic system." (*ibid.*, p. 54). Selye's ideas and his definition were criticized by many people and sparked considerable controversy. Selye now offers the following definition: ". . . stress is the nonspecific response of the body to any demand." (Hans Selye, *Stress in Health and Disease*, Butterworths, Boston, 1976, p. 15). One criticism that Selye received was that his use of the word stress conflicted with the way this word is used in physics. A long-standing principle in physics is that when a force that causes a distortion is applied to a body, internal forces are set up within the body to resist the distortion. The resistance (i.e., response) of the body to the force or to the deformation caused by the force, is called *strain*. Stress is the force that produces the strain. Selye conceded that his concept of biological stress corresponds to the concept of strain in physics. He then introduced the term *stressor* to denote the force or agent that produces the stress. The stressor corresponds to what is called stress in physics.

There is no general agreement on the definition of stress. An American psychiatrist, Harold Wolff, and his colleague, Stewart Wolf, conceived of stress as ". . . a dynamic state within an organism in response to a demand for adaptation" (Stewart Wolf and Helen Goodell, Eds., *Harold G. Wolff's Stress and Disease*, 2nd ed., Charles C Thomas, Publisher, Springfield, Ill., 1968, p. 4) and that stress ". . . is present when the adaptive mechanisms of the living organism . . . are taxed or strained" (*ibid.*, p. 252). According to another American psychiatrist, George Engel, ". . . a stress may be any influence, whether it arises from the internal environment or from the external environment, which interferes with the satisfaction of basic needs or which disturbs or threatens to disturb the stable equilibrium." (In Roy R. Grinker, Ed., *Mid-century Psychiatry*, Charles C Thomas, Publisher, Springfield, Ill., p. 51.) Cedric Mims, a British microbiologist, defines stress as ". . . any disturbance in body homeostasis general enough or severe enough to call into action a co-ordinated bodily response." (In S.V. Boyden, Ed., *The Impact of Civilisation on the Biology of Man*, University of Toronto Press, Toronto, 1970, p. 167.) These are certainly not the only definitions of stress. Other people have other definitions.

Joseph McGrath, an American psychologist, points out that some definitions of stress are based on a particular response of the organism. The occurrence of the response is evidence that the organism is, or has been, under stress. Selye's definition is essentially a response definition. Other definitions of stress are based on the presence of certain types of situations. Still other definitions of stress are based on transaction between an organism and the environment. None of these definitions are perfect. McGrath conceptualizes stress ". . . as a (perceived) substantial imbalance (in either direction) between demand and response capability with resulting adverse consequences." (Joseph E. McGrath, Ed., *Social and Psychological Factors in Stress*, Holt, Rinehart and Winston, Inc., New York, 1970, p. 21.)

Depending on the definition of stress, all stimuli impinging on an organism may be regarded as stressors, or only those stimuli or situations that are noxious to the organism. Selye distinguishes between *eustress*, which is associated with pleasant conditions (e.g., an exhilarating game; a passionate kiss) and has desirable effects, and *distress*, which is associated with unpleasant conditions (e.g., extreme temperatures; pain; anger) and has undesirable effects. Some people consider a noxious stimulus as a stressor only if the stimulus is present for a long time (i.e., for hours or days rather than seconds or minutes).

Since the primary focus of this book is on physiological responses, Selye's definition of stress will be used. The emphasis, however, will be on distress rather than eustress. To reiterate, stress is the nonspecific response of the body to any demand. A stimulus or agent that produces stress is called a stressor.

Characteristics of Stressors and Stress

Stressors may impinge on a person from the external environment (e.g., ionizing radiation) or may arise from within the individual (e.g., low blood-glucose level; an imagined or symbolic threat).

Stressors may be physical (e.g., heat), chemical (e.g., drugs or toxins), biological (e.g., bacteria), sociocultural (e.g., overcrowding; relationships with other people), or psychological (e.g., a threat to self-esteem; lack of love).

The stressor not only produces a nonspecific stress reaction, but also produces specific effects according to the nature of the stressor.

Stress is a state that is associated with feelings, but it manifests itself by physiological (as well as behavioral) changes. Psychological and sociocultural stressors produce physiological changes as well as mental effects, and physiological stressors can give rise to psychological changes.

The degree of stress will depend on the nature of the stressor, the strength or magnitude of the stressor, and the meaning that the stressor has for the individual. The way a person perceives a situation (whether consciously or unconsciously) and the meaning the stressor has for that person are particularly significant in determining not only the degree of stress but also the nature of the response. Many factors influence perception, including genetic constitution, earlier conditioning influences, past life experiences, and cultural pressures.

The same stressor can affect different people in different ways. Different people have different inherent characteristics and will perceive the stressor differently. The same stressor may have quite different meanings to two people and therefore their responses will differ.

A given stressor can affect the same person in different ways at different times. Throughout life a person goes through a number of critical stages in development. At certain critical stages a person may be more vulnerable to a particular stressor than at other times. For example, a high level of bilirubin in the blood can cause brain damage in a newborn because at this stage of development the blood-brain barrier is immature and bilirubin can enter the brain. In an adult, however, the blood-brain barrier is impermeable to bilirubin, and a high concentration of bilirubin in the blood does not have a neurotoxic effect.

A person is also subject to many biological rhythms. These rhythms developed during the course of evolution in response to environmental processes and are now inherent in every organism. Although the environmental periodicity no longer causes the biological rhythm, it acts as a synchronizing agent for the self-sustained cycle within the organism. For example, a powerful synchronizing agent is the light-dark (day-night) cycle. Biological cycles may occur over varying lengths of time. Lunar (28-day) and circadian (about 1-day) cycles are very common. For example, the menstrual cycle follows a lunar cycle. Body temperature, many hormone levels, and periods of rest and activity, for example, exhibit circadian rhythms. As a result of circadian cycles, a person is a different physiological and psychological system at each hour of the day. The phase of the circadian cycle at the time the stressor impinges on the individual, therefore, will partly determine the effects of the stressor and the stress it produces. The effects of long-lasting stress may be influenced by the extent to which the stress interferes with the mechanism for synchronizing the innate cycle with the environmental process.

A person experiencing stress attempts to adapt to it. If adaptation is successful, homeostasis is maintained or restored. Homeostasis will be disrupted if the adaptive response is insufficient or inappropriate or excessive. Consistent faulty adaptation will usually result in illness.

Stress itself can become a source of new stressors. In other words, an attempt to adapt to one stress may lead to other stresses. For example, in response to stress produced by an infection, a person may take an antibiotic. If the person has an allergic reaction to the antibiotic, additional stress is produced.

Everyone experiences some degree of stress all the time. The amount of stress a person can tolerate before being overwhelmed by prolonged severe stress will depend on the adaptive capacity of that person. Everybody has a different adaptive capacity and the limits of adaptability are determined genetically (see Chapter 1).

Stress is not always detrimental. A certain degree of stress is vital and necessary. It increases mental and physical alertness and can enhance productivity. Under conditions of stress many important discoveries have been made and works of art have been produced.

Physiological Responses to Stress

The bodily changes associated with stress are mediated by the central nervous system. Particularly, the part of the brain called the *limbic system*, acting via the hypothalamus, exerts an effect on the autonomic nervous system and on certain endocrine glands (Fig. 2-1).

Impulses from the hypothalamus activate the sympathetic division of the autonomic nervous system to produce the typical fight-or-flight response (see below). Sympathetic stimulation also causes the release of epinephrine and norepinephrine (*catecholamines*) from the adrenal medulla. These substances enhance the sympathetic response.

In addition to stimulating sympathetic nervous activity, the hypothalamus secretes corticotropin-releasing factor (CRF) and thyrotropin-re-

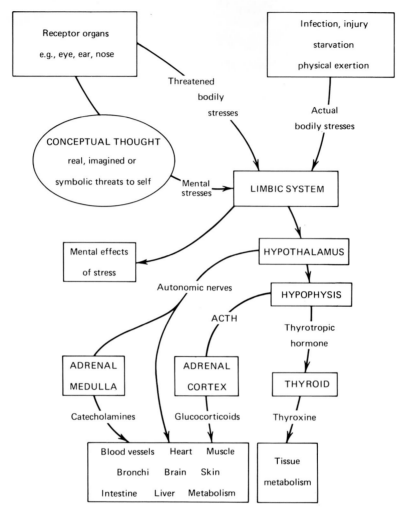

Figure 2-1. *Diagrammatic representation of the human stress response. (Adapted from Mims C: Stress in relation to the processes of civilisation, in Boyden SV (ed):* The Impact of Civilisation on the Biology of Man. *Australian National University Press, 1970, Fig. 7:1, p 168.)*

leasing factor (TRF), both of which act on the adenohypophysis (anterior pituitary). CRF stimulates production and release of adrenocorticotropic hormone (ACTH) by the adenohypophysis. ACTH in turn acts on the adrenal cortex to stimulate production of the glucocorticoid hormones, cortisol and cortisone. ACTH has only a slight effect on secretion of the mineralo-

corticoids, aldosterone and deoxycorticosterone (DOC).

The glucocorticoids are extremely important in the stress response. Local bodily reactions to stress involve vasodilation. If vasodilation were too widespread, as may occur in general stress, it would cause collapse of the circulation in spite of sympathetic nervous activity. The glucocorticoid hormones are essential to permit norepinephrine to bring about vasoconstriction and thus maintain blood pressure. Another effect of the glucocorticoids is to increase protein catabolism, thereby making amino acids available for conversion to glucose (i.e., energy) and also for repair of tissues if injury occurs. The glucocorticoids also stimulate gluconeogenesis and slightly inhibit transport of glucose into cells (except brain cells). This action raises the blood glucose concentration, or helps to maintain it in the case of physical exertion or starvation. In addition, glucocorticoids increase mobilization of fatty acids from adipose tissue.

TRF from the hypothalamus causes the adenohypophysis to secrete more thyrotropic hormone. Thyrotropic hormone stimulates the thyroid gland, thus increasing the amount of circulating thyroxine, which stimulates cellular metabolism.

Secretion of other hormones also increases during stress, although the exact mechanisms of their stimulation are not know. Levels of antidiurectic hormone (ADH) from the neurohypophysis (posterior pituitary) and somatotrophic hormone (STH; growth hormone) from the adenohypophysis are increased, presumably due to stimulation from the hypothalamus. Secretion of mineralocorticoids by the adrenal cortex is also increased. The mineralocorticoids and ADH are responsible for retention of sodium and water in the body. This effect has significance if fluids are lost from the body, for example by hemorrhage or profuse sweating. STH helps to maintain the blood glucose concentration by decreasing carbohydrate utilization and increasing fat catabolism. STH also facilitates transport of amino acids into cells, an effect that is important in the repair of tissue.

The Fight-or-Flight Response

Much of the research on the activity of the autonomic nervous system during stress was done by Walter Cannon. It was Cannon who first described how the bodily changes occurring under certain stress conditions prepared the body for action such as fight or flight.

Cannon noted that fear is associated with the instinct to flee or escape, and anger is associated with the instinct to fight. The physiological responses to these feelings developed through the course of evolution and are inherent in everyone. In prehistoric times our ancestors probably faced primarily physiological stressors. In addition, they had to fight with or run from enemies or wild animals. Therefore, the physiological responses to stress were useful and had a definite adaptive advantage in terms of natural selection. In modern times, however, with the preponderance of sociocultural and psychological stressors, these responses may be inappropriate. (For example, it is not necessarily socially acceptable or always possible to fight with someone when you are angry or to run away from a stressful situation.)

During the fight-or-flight response activity of the sympathetic nervous system is enhanced, while parasympathetic activity is decreased. As a result of this sympathetic stimulation, as well as the increased secretion of epinephrine and norepinephrine by the adrenal medulla, the body is prepared for action. The heart rate and strength of contraction are increased and systemic arterial blood pressure rises. The increased arterial blood pressure increases blood flow through the brain and the lungs. (The direct effect of sympathetic stimulation on blood vessels in the brain and the lungs is negligible.) Blood vessels in the skin and abdominal viscera constrict, while vasodilation occurs in the blood vessels supplying the heart and skeletal muscles. Thus there is decreased blood flow through the skin and abdominal viscera (e.g., kidneys, spleen, and intestines) and increased blood flow through the heart and skeletal muscles, as well as the lungs and brain. In other words, during an emergency situation, blood is shifted from nonvital areas of the body to areas of vital importance. This increased flow of blood is necessary to meet the extra demand for oxygen and glucose and to remove the increased amounts of carbon dioxide and wastes that occur with the increased activity during fighting or running. The oxygen-carrying capacity of the blood is increased by an increase in the number of circulating red blood cells (erythrocytes). This increase is brought about by contraction of the spleen, which releases more erythrocytes into the general circulation. The increased number of red blood cells, together with increased blood flow through the lungs and increased ventilation rate, ensures that more oxygen is delivered to the vital tissues. At the same time, these mechanisms provide for elimination of the extra carbon dioxide produced during activity. Sympathetic nervous stimulation and epinephrine cause the bronchi and bronchioles of the lungs to dilate. This dilation decreases resistance to the flow of air into and out of the lungs and makes breathing easier.

Motility of the gastrointestinal tract and secretion by digestive glands are decreased as a result of the increased sympathetic activity and decreased parasympathetic activity. Since digestive and absorptive functions are temporarily suspended, increased conversion of liver glycogen to glucose and release of glucose into the blood occurs to provide energy for the heart, skeletal muscles, and brain. If muscular activity does not occur, the blood glucose concentration rises.

The activity of the sympathetic nervous system, along with epinephrine and norepinephrine, produces other effects as well. The pupils dilate. The glomerular filtration rate decreases, due to decreased renal blood flow. There is increased coagulability of the blood (i.e., it clots at a faster rate). This effect is important in preventing hemorrhage if wounding should occur. Increased sweating occurs to dissipate the heat generated by muscular exertion.

These changes associated with the fight-or-flight response are automatic and reflex in nature. They cannot be controlled by will.

Cannon was particularly interested in how the body maintains homeostasis. He recognized that while the changes that occur during emotional turmoil appear to be disruptions of homeostasis, they can be explained as preparing the body for extreme muscular exertion. When exertion takes place the changes are useful and are, in fact, counteracted by the effects of physical exertion. It is only when action does not occur (i.e., emotion without motion) that severe disturbances of homeostasis occur.

The General Adaptation Syndrome

Cannon described the importance of the sympathetic nervous system and adrenal medulla in response to stress. Selye later demonstrated the importance of the hormones from the adrenal cortex. Selye observed a number of bodily changes that occur in response to stress and noted that the bodily response changes with time. He called the response the *general adaptation syndrome* (GAS).

Characteristic bodily changes that Selye noted in experimental animals subjected to stress are: enlargement of the adrenal cortex with discharge of its hormones; shrinkage of the thymus and lymphatic structures; reduction in the number of eosinophils and lymphocytes in the blood; and changes in the gastrointestinal mucosa culminating in deep bleeding ulcers in the stomach and duodenum when stress is severe. Similar changes may occur in human beings subjected to stress.

The GAS occurs in three stages. The initial response is the *alarm reaction*. In this stage general mobilization of all the body's defenses occurs. As yet, no one organ system is specially developed to cope with the effects of the stressor. At this time, the body's resistance falls below normal and if the stressor is strong enough (e.g., severe burns) death may occur. During the alarm reaction, there is an outpouring of hormones from the adrenal cortex. In addition, there is increased activity of the sympathetic nervous system and release of catecholamines from the adrenal medulla in the typical fight-or-flight reaction.

The alarm reaction is followed by the *stage of resistance*. By this time the most appropriate specific channel of defense has been developed. In other words, the noxious effects of the stressor are limited to the smallest area of the body capable of dealing with them. The body has adapted to the stressor and resistance is above normal. The signs of acute emergency that characterize the alarm reaction have disappeared. The level of adrenocortical hormones in the blood declines until the level is just slightly above normal.

If the stressor is strong enough and exerts its effect on the body for a long enough time, the *stage of exhaustion* will be reached. Resistance is lost as the most appropriate specific channel of defense wears out. The response becomes general again and the signs of the alarm reaction reappear. The level of adrenocortical hormones in the blood rises once more. Eventually the body's resources are completely exhausted and death occurs.

The hormones of the adrenal cortex play an important role in mediating the body's response to stress. In addition to the important effects mentioned previously, the glucocorticoids inhibit the body's defenses; that is, they have an *antiinflammatory* effect. ACTH from the adenohypophysis also has an antiinflammatory effect because it stimulates production and release of glucocorticoids by the adrenal cortex. The glucocorticoid hormones are responsible for the involution of the thymus and lymphatic structures and for the reduction in the number of eosinophils and lymphocytes mentioned earlier. The exact mechanism for the development of the stress ulcers in the stomach and duodenum is not known, but apparently it involves interaction between the effects of the glucocorticoids and autonomic nervous activity.

The mineralocorticoid hormones have a *proinflammatory* effect; that is, they stimulate the body's defense mechanisms. Somatotropic hormone also has a proinflammatory effect. It is not know whether STH acts directly or whether it stimulates production of mineralocorticoids, or both.

According to Selye, resistance and adaptation depend on a proper balance of three constituents: the direct effect of the stressor on the body; internal responses that stimulate tissue defense; and internal responses that inhibit unnecessary defense and thereby cause tissue surrender.

Adaptation to stress plays a part in every disease. In addition, faulty adaptation can contribute to the development of disease. For example, when the body overdefends itself and produces excess proinflammatory hormones, conditions such as arthritis, allergy, and asthma may develop. On the other hand, when the body overproduces antiinflammatory hormones and inhibits defense mechanisms, the person may develop gastrointestinal ulcers or a severe infection. Selye calls these conditions *diseases of adaptation.*

Stressful Life Events and Illness

It is generally accepted that social environment influences a person's health status. The most healthy people are those who are well adapted to the particular life situation in which they exist. Their life situations satisfy their own particular needs and aspirations, whether these needs and aspirations are the same as those of the general population, or different. On the other hand, when people exist in situations that do not satisfy their needs and aspirations, there is a high probability that they will suffer ill health. Poor health may be indicative of poor adaptive capacity, but not necessarily. A person may be poorly adapted to one particular social environment but would adapt well to many other life situations. Conversely, someone else may be well adapted to his or her own particular life situation but unable to adapt to different social environments.

Regardless of the social environment, it has been noted that episodes of illness tend to be clustered around times when a person has been recently subjected to a large number of *stressful life events.* Stressful life events (or social stressors) are those events that involve a significant change in a person's life pattern. Such events may be negative (i.e., socially undesirable) or positive (i.e., socially desirable), but characteristically they require some adaptive behavior or coping behavior on the part of the person. Examples of social stressors are marriage, divorce, change of home or job, a new family member, or death of a family member or friend.

A person's habits are often altered when a significant change in social or interpersonal relationships occurs. For example, patterns of activity or dietary habits may change. In addition, the person's exposure to potential sources of infection or trauma may change. Alterations in mood are often associated with changes in significant interpersonal relationships. Mood changes can bring about physiological changes mediated by the central nervous system. Any of these factors could influence the frequency or severity of illness.

Exposure to social stressors is in itself not usually sufficient to cause disease. Stressful life events, however, may make a person more vulnerable at a particular period of time and serve as a *precipitating factor*. A precipitating factor is a change in conditions that influences the timing of illness onset. Social stressors influence the timing of the onset of illness but do not determine the nature of the disease.

The nature of the disease will be determined by *predisposing factors* and/or the presence of a specific disease agent. Predisposing factors are personal characteristics that alter one's susceptibility to illness. They include genetic constitution and physiological makeup, as well as long-standing behavior patterns, past experiences, and various psychological characteristics. For example, a person may be predisposed to myocardial infarction if she or he smokes cigarettes, has a high serum cholesterol level, has hypertension, and has a family history of the disease. Stressful life events may then precipitate the occurrence of a myocardial infarction. As another example, during the winter people are constantly exposed to viruses that cause colds or influenza but may not become ill. The occurrence of social stressors, however, may precipitate the onset of influenza in a person.

Presumably, the effect of stressful life events is additive. In other words, the greater the number of stressful life events and the greater the requirement for adaptation, the greater the probability that physical or mental illness or an accident will occur and the more severe the illness will be. Not all social stressors produce the same degree of stress, however. For example, on one commonly used rating scale, death of a spouse is given twice the weight that is assigned to marriage. Other situations are given less weight than marriage. Therefore, the occurrence of a few major stressful life events may have more effect than several minor social stressors.

Not all those who experience major stressful life events become ill. Whether or not a person becomes ill is influenced by a number of *mediating factors*. Mediating factors are characteristics that influence a person's perception of, or sensitivity to, stressors. They include characteristics of the social stressor, personal characteristics, and characteristics of the person's social support system. In general, when the stressor is very severe, the characteristics of the person and his or her social support system are less significant in determining the likelihood of illness onset and the nature of the response. When the stressor is less severe, however, individual characteristics and social supports are important in determining whether or not a person becomes ill.

Several stressor characteristics influence the likelihood and severity of illness. These include magnitude (deviation from baseline conditions), intensity (rate of change), duration, unpredictability, and novelty of the social stressor. The greater the magnitude of the stressor, the greater the degree of physical or psychiatric disability that may result. If a person is unprepared, or lacks previous experience with the stressor, the impact of the event will be greater. Also, the greater the rate of change and the longer the time of exposure, the greater will be the impact of a stressful life event. If the intensity and duration of a stressor are sufficiently great (such as may occur in some wartime situations, for example), it will precipitate physical or mental illness in anyone who is exposed to the stressor, regardless of individual characteristics. Individual differences will be manifested, however, in the length of time before illness onset and in the time required for recovery.

How a person perceives a stressor is critical in determining the impact of a stressful life event and that person's response to it. The perception of social stressors is mediated by internal or personal components and by external or interpersonal components. Personal components include such things as the predisposing factors mentioned previously, physiological and psychological threshold sensitivities, intelligence, verbal skills, psychological defenses, and past experience. In addition, a person's perception of social stressors and his or her response to them is influenced by characteristics such as age, education, income, and occupation.

In general, the more skills, assets, and resources a person has, the more versatile his or her defenses, and the broader his or her experience, the less impact a social stressor will have. Some people do not succumb to illness in spite of major life changes because their psychological constitution apparently "insulates" them from the effects of some of their life experiences. Psychological defenses may prevent recent stressful life events from causing a physiological response. In other words, it appears that if a person has adequate psychological defense mechanisms, then that person will have little or no physiological response to social stressors. On the other hand, if a person's psychological defenses are inadequate, a physiological stress response will occur.

External mediating factors consist of the social supports available to the individual. Social supports are enduring interpersonal ties to a group of people who have the same standards and values, who provide feedback, and who can be depended on to provide emotional support, assistance, and resources when needed. A person may belong to several groups that provide social supports; for example at home, at work, in a religious affiliation, and in recreational settings. Deficiencies in social support systems do not contribute to illness susceptibility if social stressors are lacking. When stressful life events occur, however, someone with weak social supports will have a greater risk of becoming ill than will a person with strong social supports.

SUGGESTED ADDITIONAL READING

Marcinek B: Stress in the surgical patient. Am J Nurs 77(11): 1809–1811, 1977.

Stephenson A: Stress in critically ill patients. Am J Nurs 77(11): 1806–1809, 1977.

UNIT TWO

GENETIC MECHANISMS

3

The Basis of Heredity

Heredity is the transmission from parents to offspring of particular properties, traits, or characteristics that persist from generation to generation. *Genetics* is the branch of science that deals with heredity. The units of heredity, that is, the physical units that are passed on from parents to offspring and that carry the information regarding particular biological attributes, are called *genes*.

Genes are composed of deoxyribonucleic acid (DNA). Most of the DNA in a cell is located in the nucleus in association with protein. (It was once thought that all the genetic material resided in the nucleus of the cell, but it is now known that some cytoplasmic organelles, such as mitochondria, contain a very small amount of DNA. The exact role of this organellar DNA in the func-

37

tioning of the cell has not yet been determined.) After cells are stained with various chemical dyes the DNA-protein complexes within the nucleus can be viewed with a light microscope. In nondividing cells (i.e., during interphase) these complexes form a network of thin threads called *chromatin*. During cell division the chromatin threads condense and become visible as discrete bodies called *chromosomes*. The detailed structure of chromosomes and the exact arrangement of the DNA and protein within them is not yet known. Chromosomes also contain a small amount of ribonucleic acid (RNA).

CHROMOSOMES AND CELL DIVISION

The cells of an organism contain a fixed number of chromosomes. Most cells contain two representatives of each kind of chromosome; that is, they contain a *diploid* set, or the diploid number of chromosomes. The human diploid set consists of 46 chromosomes, or 23 pairs. The two representatives of a particular kind of chromosome (i.e., the members of a chromosome pair) are called *homologous chromosomes*, or *homologues*. Homologous chromosomes are the same in shape and form and contain genetic information about the same traits.

The increase in the number of cells that occurs during growth takes place by mitotic cell division, or *mitosis*. As a result of this process, each daughter cell receives the same number of chromosomes

that was present in the parent cell. During gametogenesis (the formation of gametes, i.e., eggs or sperm), meiotic cell division, or *meiosis,* occurs. As a result of this process the gametes end up with one chromosome of each kind, or the *haploid* number of chromosomes. For human beings the haploid number is 23 chromosomes. With the fusion of an egg and sperm to form a zygote, the diploid number of chromosomes is restored.

Chromosomes

When the chromosomes first become visible they are very long, thin threadlike structures. During the first phase of cell division, however, the chromosomes become shorter and thicker (condensed). This condensation is presumably due to coiling of the chromosomes. Each chromosome contains a specific region called the *centromere* (or *kinetochore*), which usually appears as a localized narrowing or constriction of the chromosome (the *primary constriction*). For any particular chromosome the position of the centromere is constant. The parts of the chromosome on either side of the centromere are called arms.

Some chromosomes contain additional constrictions (*secondary constrictions*), some of which separate off a small chromosomal section, called a *satellite,* from the main body of the chromosome. Often a secondary constriction is associated with the site where a nucleolus is formed or attached.

Chromosomes can be described according to the relative positions of their centromeres (Fig. 3-1).

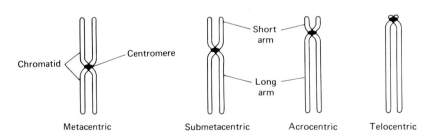

Figure 3-1. *Diagrammatic representation of types of chromosomes.*

When the centromere is approximately in the middle of the chromosome (median), so that the arms are of equal or nearly equal length, the chromosome is said to be *metacentric*. When the centromere is close to one end of the chromosome (subterminal), the chromosome is called *acrocentric*. In this case the arms are of unequal length and are referred to as the long arm and the short arm. In some chromosomes the centromere is located in an intermediate position between median and subterminal (submedian); in this case the chromosome is termed *submetacentric*. When the centromere is at the end of a chromosome (terminal), so that the short arm is barely perceptible, the chromosome is said to be *telocentric*. No telocentric chromosomes are present in human cells.

The Normal Chromosome Complement

The normal set of human chromosomes consists of 22 pairs of *autosomes*, which are alike in both sexes, and two *sex chromosomes*. The sex chromosomes in females are two homologous X chromosomes. Males have one X chromosome and one smaller, nonhomologous chromosome called a Y chromosome. The normal chromosome complement for a human female, therefore, is written as 46,XX. This designation indicates that the total number of chromosomes per somatic cell is 46 and that two of the chromosomes are X chromosomes. For a normal male the chromosome complement is written as 46,XY, indicating a total of 46 chromosomes including one X and one Y chromosome.

Most studies of human chromosomes are done with laboratory cultures of lymphocytes that have been induced to divide. The cells for culture are obtained from a routine blood sample; only a few milliliters of blood are required. The chromosomes are most readily distinguished during the metaphase stage of cell division. Appropriately prepared cells are viewed with a microscope and a photomicrograph is made. Individual chromosomes are cut out and arranged according to size and position of the centromere. This lineup of the chromosome set in a form suitable for analysis is called a *karyotype* (Fig. 3-2).

The chromosomes are divided into seven groups. Group A (chromosomes 1 to 3) consists of large metacentric chromosomes. Group B (chromosomes 4 and 5) are large submetacentric chromosomes. Group C (chromosomes 6 to 12 and the X chromosome) are medium-sized submetacentric chromosomes. Group D (chromosomes 13 to 15) are medium-sized acrocentric chromosomes with satellites on the short arms. Group E (chromosomes 16 to 18) contains rather short submetacentric chromosomes. Group F (chromosomes 19 and 20) are short metacentric chromosomes. Group G (chromosomes 21 and 22 and the Y chromosome) are very short acrocentric chromosomes.

Mitosis

Mitosis is essentially a mechanism for ensuring that when a cell divides each progeny, or daughter cell, receives a complete complement of chromosomes (i.e., genetic information). It is the process by which the nuclear contents of a cell reproduce and divide. Subsequent division of the cytoplasm (*cytokinesis*) produces two daughter cells.

Many mitotic cell divisions occur following fertilization of an egg to produce a multicellular organism from a single–celled zygote. Mitosis also occurs in the somatic cells of the body as a person is growing. After full growth is attained, some somatic cells continue to divide by mitosis to replace worn-out cells as they die and are broken down or shed from the body. For example, mitosis occurs in hematopoietic tissue, and in the epithelial tissue of the skin and of the gastrointestinal mucosa. Mitosis also occurs in the processes of regeneration and repair following the wounding of tissues (see Chapter 8).

Mitosis is really continuous, but for convenience in describing the process it is arbitrarily divided into several stages, or phases (Fig. 3-3). These stages are called prophase, metaphase, anaphase, and telophase. The normal functioning state of the cell between divisions is called *interphase*, or the intermitotic period. During inter-

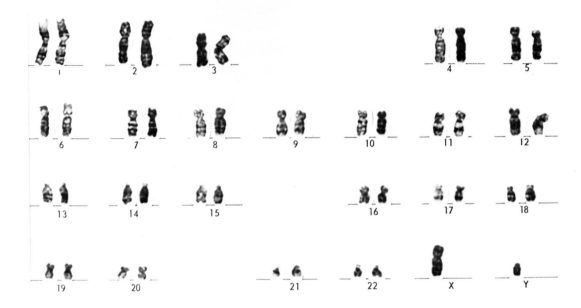

Figure 3-2. *A normal karyotype of a human male. (Courtesy of Dr. F. J. Dill, Department of Medical Genetics, University of British Columbia, Vancouver, B.C., Canada.)*

phase the DNA in the chromosomes is replicated and certain proteins needed during mitosis are synthesized. The process of mitosis usually takes about one hour, although this time may vary. The length of time in interphase varies greatly from one cell type to another. It may be minutes, hours, days, months, or even years. Some highly differentiated cells (e.g., neurons) are no longer capable of dividing. These cells are referred to as fixed postmitotic cells.

Prophase

In prophase the chromatin threads condense to form distinct chromosomes. At first they are long and thin, but gradually they become shorter and thicker. Each chromosome appears to be split longitudinally (i.e., it is double) for most of its length, but the duplicate strands are joined at the centromere. Each strand is called a *chromatid,* as long as it is still joined to its "sister" chromatid.

The two chromatids making up a chromosome are identical.

When the chromosomes are condensing, the centrioles, two rodlike structures lying just outside the nucleus, separate and move to opposite sides of the nucleus. A series of protein fibers formed in the cytoplasm extend between the centrioles, forming a structure called the *spindle.* The two ends of the spindle, near the centrioles, are called poles; the region midway between the poles is called the equator.

The nucleoli disappear by late prophase. The nuclear membrane breaks down, marking the end of prophase.

Metaphase

As the nuclear membrane breaks down the centromere of each chromosome becomes attached to a spindle fiber. The chromosomes move toward the equator and become arranged in a flat plane

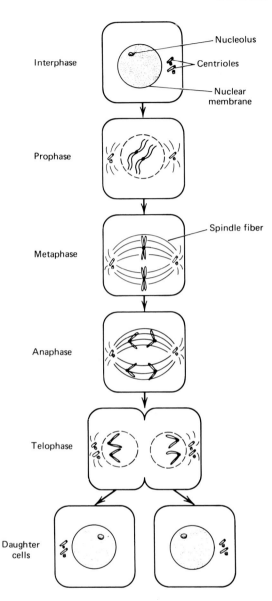

Interphase — Nucleolus, Centrioles, Nuclear membrane

Prophase

Metaphase — Spindle fiber

Anaphase

Telophase

Daughter cells

Figure 3-3. *Schematic representation of mitosis. See text for explanation. Only two chromosomes are shown.*

(the metaphase plate) through the equator. Viewed from the side they form a line across the middle of the spindle.

Anaphase

In anaphase the centromeres divide. The sister chromatids (now considered separate chromosomes because each has its own centromere) separate and move to opposite poles of the spindle.

Telophase

Telophase begins when the daughter chromosomes (i.e., the former sister chromatids) have reached the poles. The chromosomes begin to uncoil. The spindle breaks down and a nuclear membrane forms around each group of chromosomes at the opposite poles. The cell membrane indents at the equatorial plate and the cytoplasmic portion of the cell divides. The end result is two daughter cells, each with an identical chromosome complement and genetic constitution.

Meiosis

Meiosis is a special type of nuclear division that occurs in germ cells to produce haploid gametes. The fact that the gametes contain the haploid number of chromosomes is important. If the gametes contained the diploid number, fusion of an egg and sperm to form a zygote would result in an offspring with twice as many chromosomes as the parents (i.e., four members of each particular chromosome).

Meiosis actually involves two successive divisions. Only one replication of the chromosomes is involved, however, so that the two divisions result in a reduction in the number of chromosomes per cell. (For this reason meiosis is sometimes referred to as *reduction division.*) As with mitosis, meiosis is divided into several stages. The stages are given the same names as in mitosis, but the names are followed by I or II to indicate whether the stage is part of the first meiotic division (meiosis I) or the second meiotic division (meiosis II). Meiosis is illustrated in Figure 3-4.

Prophase I

The first prophase is a long and varied process, which is further divided into several stages. During the first stage, called *leptotene*, the chromosomes become evident as long thin threads. At this time the chromosomes appear as single strands. There is evidence that the DNA of each chromosome has replicated by this time, but the whole chromosome has not yet doubled.

During the next stage, called *zygotene*, homologous chromosomes appear to attract each other and come to lie side by side in a very close pairing arrangement called *synapsis*. The X and Y chromosomes in the male are an exception to this arrangement. Instead of lying side by side, the X and Y chromosomes are associated end to end.

The third stage of prophase I is called *pachytene*. In this stage the chromosomes become shorter and thicker. Each chromosome has duplicated and appears as two chromatids attached at the centromere. The homologous chromosomes are still paired, so that the two sister chromatids of one chromosome are associated with the two sister chromatids of its homologue, forming a group of four chromatids called a *bivalent*, or a *tetrad*. Thus, in human cells there are 92 chromatids in 46 chromosomes, forming 23 tetrads. (The number of chromosome entities is determined by the number of centromeres. So long as the chromatids are joined at the centromere they are considered as one chromosome.)

The next stage is called *diplotene*. Now the homologues appear to repel each other and begin to separate, especially near the centromere. At some points, however, the chromatids of homologous chromosomes remain in contact, forming X-shaped attachments between the chromosomes. These crossed areas are called *chiasmata* (singular: chiasma). During this crossing over, different chromatids in the tetrad may exchange pieces. This process can bring about a rearrangement of groups of genes on the chromatids involved.

The last stage of prophase I is called *diakinesis*. The chromosomes continue to condense and become very short and thick. The chiasmata move

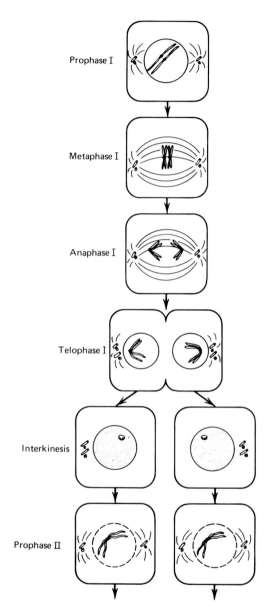

Figure 3-4. *Schematic representation of meiosis. See text for explanation. Only one pair of chromosomes is shown.*

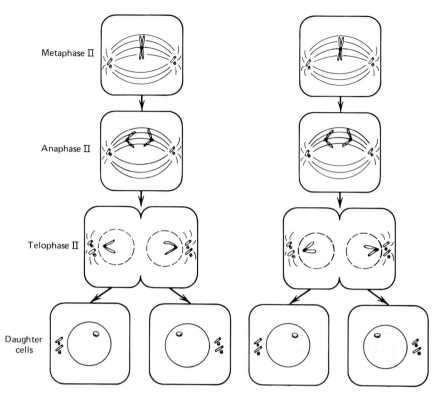

Figure 3-4. *Continued.*

toward the ends of the chromosomes. The nucleoli disappear, the nuclear membrane breaks down, and spindle fibers form. The chromosomes become attached to the spindle and move toward the equator.

Metaphase I
The chromosomes appear in their most condensed state in this stage. The tetrads are lined up at the equatorial plate. The chiasmata are now at the ends of each chromosome (chiasma terminalization).

Anaphase I
Members of each homologous pair separate and move to opposite poles of the spindle. This separation of homologous chromosomes is called *disjunction.* In human cells the result is that 23 chro-

mosomes are at one pole and 23 chromosomes are at the opposite pole. Each chromosome is still double; that is, it consists of two chromatids joined at the centromere. These double chromosomes are called *dyads*.

Telophase I
Nuclear membranes form around each group of dyads at the opposite poles and the chromosomes uncoil, so that they are no longer visible as discrete entities. Cytokinesis occurs, producing two daughter cells with the haploid number of chromosomes.

Interkinesis
The period between the two meiotic divisions is called interkinesis. It is similar to interphase between two mitotic divisions, except that duplica-

tion of the chromosomes is not necessary because they are already double.

Prophase II
The dyads reappear as thin threads. The nuclear membrane disappears and the spindle forms.

Metaphase II
The dyads (23 in human cells) are lined up at the equatorial plate.

Anaphase II
The centromeres divide. The sister chromatids separate and move to opposite poles. Each chromatid is now a separate chromosome.

Telophase II
Nuclear membranes form around each group of chromosomes at the opposite poles. The chromosomes uncoil. The spindle breaks down and cytokinesis occurs. The result is four haploid cells from each diploid cell that entered meiosis.

Differences Between Meiosis and Mitosis
In meiosis I, pairing of homologous chromosomes occurs; this pairing does not occur in mitosis. In mitosis the centromeres duplicate and the chromatids separate. In meiosis I the centromeres do not duplicate; duplication of the centromeres and separation of the chromatids does not occur until meiosis II. Following mitosis each daughter cell has the same number of chromosomes and the same genetic composition as the parent cell. Meiosis, however, results in a reduction in the chromosome number. Each daughter cell has half as many chromosomes as the original parent cell.

Gametogenesis

The development of gametes (sex cells) from undifferentiated germ cells is called *gametogenesis*. In the female this process is called *oogenesis* and the gametes are called *ova* (singular: ovum), or eggs. The development of gametes in the male is called *spermatogenesis* and the male gametes are called *spermatozoa* (singular: spermatozoon) or simply sperm.

Spermatogenesis
The epithelial cells next to the basement membrane of the seminiferous tubules of the testis are called *spermatogonia*. These cells are diploid and divide many times by mitosis. As a result of these successive cell divisions, some of the daughter cells are pushed toward the tubule lumen and form a second layer. The cells in the second layer grow and develop into large round cells called *primary spermatocytes*. With the onset of puberty, meiosis begins in the primary spermatocytes. Each primary spermatocyte goes through the first meiotic division to produce two *secondary spermatocytes,* each containing the haploid number of dyads. The spermatogonia of the first layer continue to divide by mitosis, producing more spermatogonia and more primary spermatocytes. Therefore the secondary spermatocytes are pushed closer to the lumen.

Each secondary spermatocyte undergoes the second meiotic division to produce two *spermatids.* Thus, four spermatids are derived from each primary spermatocyte. Each spermatid contains the haploid number of chromosomes; that is, 22 autosomes plus an X or a Y chromosome. The spermatids differentiate into mature *spermatozoa* without further cell division. The spermatozoa are pushed into the lumen of the tubule as underlying cells continue to divide. They move through the ducts of the testis to the epididymis, where they are stored until ejaculation occurs.

Spermatogenesis is outlined in Figure 3-5.

Oogenesis
Oogenesis is outlined in Figure 3-6. In the human female, oogenesis begins before birth. During fetal development, diploid cells derived from the germinal epithelium on the surface of the ovaries divide by mitosis to form *oogonia*. Clusters of cells from the germinal epithelium invaginate into the stroma. At the center of each cluster is an

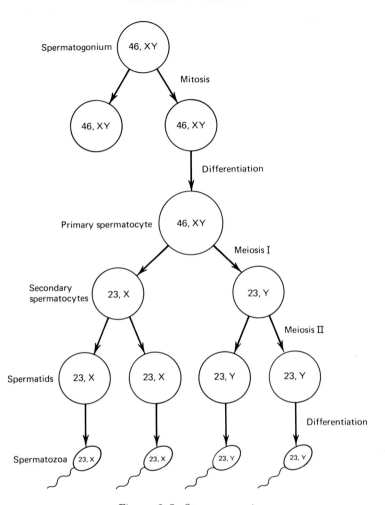

Figure 3-5. *Spermatogenesis.*

oogonium; the surrounding cells develop into follicle cells. The follicle cells protect the developing ovum and help it accumulate nutritional materials.

The oogonia develop into *primary oocytes.* These cells are diploid. By the fourth month of gestation primary oocytes begin to undergo meiosis. They progress only to diakinesis (the last stage of prophase I), however, and then meiosis is suspended. The primary oocytes remain in this state until after sexual maturity. This prolonged

prophase I is called the *dictyotene* stage. It may last 30 to 40 years for some cells.

The primary oocyte surrounded by follicle cells is called a primary follicle. At birth each ovary contains more than 200,000 primary follicles, but only about 400 follicles reach maturity. Following menarche, usually one primary follicle reaches maturity each month. As the follicle develops, the primary oocyte completes the first meiotic division.

The nucleus of the primary oocyte is not at the

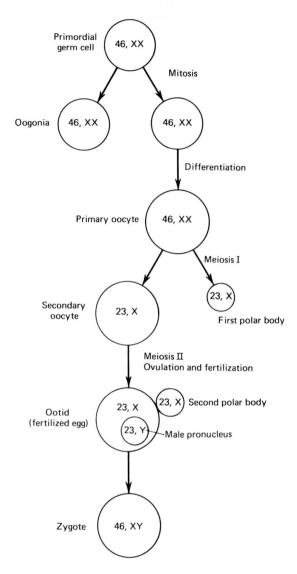

Figure 3-6. *Oogenesis.*

generates, but occasionally it persists and undergoes meiosis II.

The secondary oocyte begins meiosis II, but ovulation occurs before this process is completed. At ovulation the secondary oocyte is released into the peritoneal cavity and drawn into the fallopian tube. It is still surrounded by some of the follicle cells, which form the corona radiata. If the discharged egg (i.e., secondary oocyte) is penetrated by a sperm, the sperm tail and midpiece disintegrate and the sperm head swells to form the male pronucleus. The male pronucleus, which contains 23 chromosomes, rests in the cytoplasm of the oocyte while meiosis II is completed. The second meiotic division produces a large cell, which may be considered an ootid, and a small cell called the second polar body. Each of these cells contain 22 autosomes plus one X chromosome (i.e., the haploid number). The ootid is actually a mature ovum, which has already been fertilized. The male pronucleus moves toward the pronucleus of the ovum and the two fuse, producing a zygote that has 46 chromosomes, or 23 pairs of chromosomes (i.e., the diploid number). One member of each pair is contributed by the father, and its homologue comes from the mother. If the sperm pronucleus contains a Y chromosome, the zygote will have one X chromosome (from the mother) and one Y chromosome and will give rise to a male offspring. If the sperm pronucleus contains an X chromosome, the zygote will have two X chromosomes and give rise to a female.

THE MOLECULAR BASIS OF INHERITANCE

center of the cell, but is closer to one end. Therefore, when cytokinesis occurs at the end of meiosis I, the cytoplasm is not equally divided. The cell that contains most of the cytoplasm is the *secondary oocyte*; the smaller cell is called the *first polar body*. Each of these two cells contains the haploid number of dyads. Usually the first polar body degenerates.

As stated earlier, the genes are composed of DNA, most of which resides in the nucleus of each cell. The genetic code is determined by the structure of the DNA molecule. Many cell functions are carried out in the cytoplasm of the cell; therefore some means must exist to take the information present in the nuclear DNA out to the cytoplasm.

This function is served by RNA. The DNA provides a pattern, or *template,* from which working copies of RNA are made; this process is called *transcription.* The RNA moves from the nucleus to the cytoplasm and directs the synthesis of protein molecules. The synthesis of proteins according to the genetic message is called *translation.* In other words, the message carried by the genes is translated into protein.

Two kinds of proteins are made by cells: *structural proteins* and *enzymes.* Examples of structural proteins are collagen, hemoglobin, and myosin. Enzymes are proteins that act as biochemical catalysts; they speed up the chemical reactions that occur in the body. Under the conditions of temperature, pressure, and concentration of reactants that exist in the body, biochemical reactions could not proceed without enzymes. Therefore enzymes are required for every metabolic process and determine the functions of a cell.

DNA and RNA

DNA and RNA belong to a class of compounds called *nucleic acids.* They are long chains made up of repeating subunits called *nucleotides.* A nucleotide consists of a 5-carbon sugar (pentose) that has a nitrogenous base attached to one side of it and a phosphate group attached to the other side (Fig. 3-7). In RNA the sugar is ribose; in DNA the sugar is deoxyribose. Two classes of nitrogenous bases are found in nucleic acids: the pyrimidines and the purines. DNA contains the pyrimidine bases cytosine (C) and thymine (T). RNA also contains cytosine, but in place of thymine it contains uracil (U). Both DNA and RNA contain the purine bases adenine (A) and guanine (G).

Many nucleotides linked together form a *polynucleotide* chain, or strand. The sugar portion of one nucleotide is linked to the sugar portion of the next nucleotide by a phosphate group. The backbone of the polynucleotide chain is therefore made up of alternating sugar-phosphate-sugar-phosphate groups. The bases stick out perpendicular to the backbone (Fig. 3-8). A DNA molecule consists of two polynucleotide chains; an RNA molecule is made up of a single strand.

DNA Structure:
The Double Helix

The two long polynucleotide strands of a DNA molecule are arranged parallel to each other. The bases on each strand point in toward each other and are linked by hydrogen bonds. (A hydrogen bond is formed when two very electronegative atoms, such as nitrogen or oxygen, share one hydrogen atom between them. Hydrogen bonds are weak chemical bonds, but so many of them link the two polynucleotide strands together that the entire structure is quite stable.) Pairs of bases therefore span the gap between the two parallel polynucleotide backbones. The backbones of the two polynucleotide strands are twisted around each other to form a *double helix* (Fig. 3-9). The structure may be envisaged as a spiral staircase, with the base pairs forming the steps.

The pairing of the bases on the opposite strands is very specific. The distance between the backbones of the two polynucleotides is such that only a purine on one strand and a pyrimidine opposite it will fit. Because of the chemical structures of the bases, the only possible base-pair combinations are adenine with thymine and guanine with cytosine. As a result of this base-pairing arrangement, the two polynucleotide strands in a DNA molecule are not identical but are *complementary* to each other. The sequence of bases in one strand determines the sequence of bases in the opposite strand.

It is not yet known whether a single human

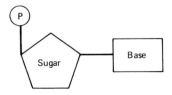

Figure 3-7. *Schematic representation of the structure of a nucleotide. P represents a phosphate group.*

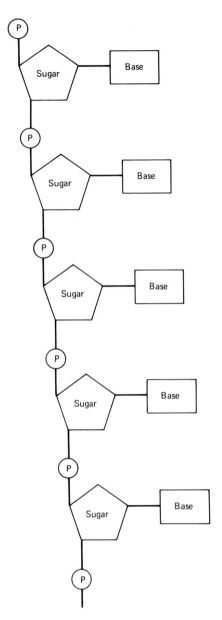

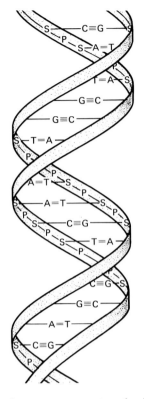

Figure 3-9. *Schematic representation of a short portion of a DNA molecule. The sugar-phosphate backbones of two polynucleotide strands twist around each other to form a double helix. The two strands are linked by hydrogen bonds between the base pairs.*

Figure 3-8. *Schematic representation of a portion of a polynucleotide chain. P represents a phosphate group.*

chromosome contains one DNA molecule or more.

Replication of DNA

The complementary nature of the two strands in the DNA molecule provides the basis for replication of the DNA before cell division. Each strand serves as a template for the synthesis of a new complementary strand (Fig. 3-10). First the double helix unwinds. The hydrogen bonds between the complementary base pairs are broken, and the polynucleotide strands separate. The bases on each strand are thus exposed. The bases of free deoxyribonucleotides (i.e., nucleotides containing

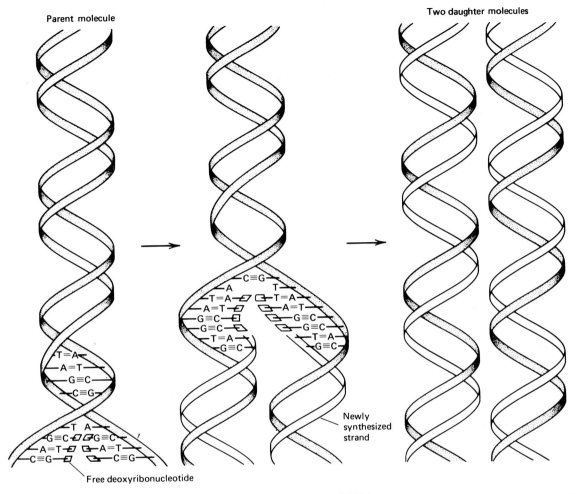

Figure 3-10. *Replication of DNA.*

deoxyribose as the sugar) pair with the exposed bases on the polynucleotide strands. Sugar-phosphate bonds then form between adjacent free nucleotides, producing a new polynucleotide strand opposite each original parent strand. The formation of the sugar-phosphate bonds is catalyzed by the enzyme DNA polymerase.

The whole DNA molecule does not unwind and separate all at once. A small portion unwinds, and as new complementary strands are formed the parent molecule gradually unwinds further. As the new polynucleotide strands are formed, each par-

ent strand and its newly synthesized complementary strand twist into another double helix. The result is two daughter molecules that are identical to each other and identical to the original parent molecule. Each daughter molecule contains one polynucleotide strand from the original molecule and one newly synthesized strand.

Transcription of RNA

Complementary base pairing also provides the mechanism by which RNA is transcribed from the DNA template (Fig. 3-11). A section of the DNA

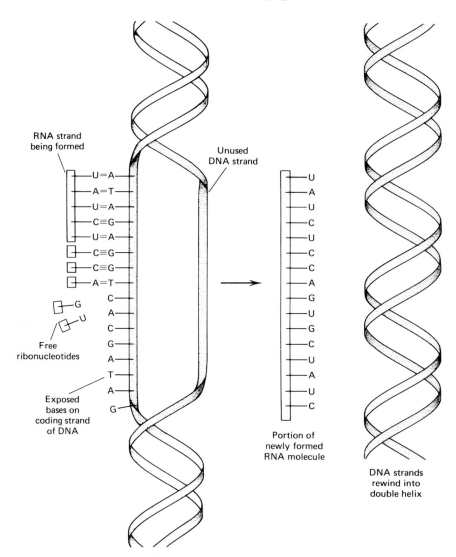

Figure 3-11. *Transcription of RNA.*

molecule unwinds and the two strands separate, exposing the bases. Complementary bases on free ribonucleotides (i.e., nucleotides containing ribose as the sugar) then pair with the exposed bases on one of the DNA strands. As stated previously, RNA does not contain thymine, but has uracil instead. Therefore uracil on a ribonucleotide pairs with an exposed adenine base on the

DNA strand. Sugar-phosphate linkages are then formed between adjacent ribonucleotides, catalyzed by the enzyme RNA polymerase. The newly synthesized single-stranded RNA molecule detaches from the DNA template and the two DNA strands reunite.

Three types of RNA are transcribed from different regions of DNA: messenger RNA (mRNA), ribosomal RNA (rRNA), and transfer RNA (tRNA). *Messenger RNA* carries the instructions for making specific protein molecules. *Ribosomal RNA* forms part of the structure of the ribosomes, cytoplasmic organelles that are involved with protein synthesis. *Transfer RNA* molecules pick up amino acids that are present in the cytoplasm and bring them to the ribosomes for assembly into protein molecules (see below).

Translation

The RNA molecules that are transcribed from the DNA template move from the nucleus to the cytoplasm, where they direct the translation of the genetic message into protein.

A protein is a large molecule made up of one or more *polypeptide chains.* The subunits of polypeptides are *amino acids;* the amino acids are linked together by peptide bonds (Fig. 3-12). Twenty different amino acids occur in proteins. The sequence, type, and number of amino acids in a particular polypeptide chain determine the structure and function of the protein molecule that is formed. Many combinations of the 20 amino acids are possible, therefore many different proteins can be made.

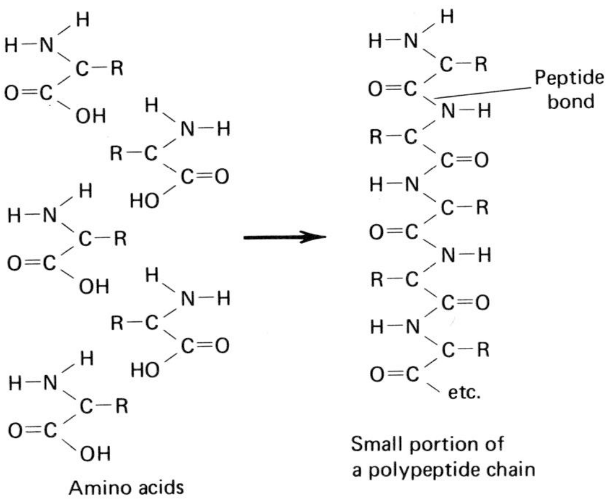

Figure 3-12. *Polypeptide chains are made up of many amino acids linked together by peptide bonds. R represents a side chain of variable structure.*

The Genetic Code

The genetic code lies in the sequence of the nitrogenous bases in DNA. Each base is like a letter in an alphabet. A code word, or *codon,* consists of a sequence of three letters (i.e., a base triplet) that specifies a particular amino acid. The sequence of codons (i.e., bases) in the DNA determines the sequence of the amino acids in a polypeptide chain. Since there are four different bases (letters) and each code word consists of three bases, 64 codons are possible, but there are only 20 amino acids. It has been found that more than one base triplet can code for the same amino acid. In addition, three of the codons act as "punctuation" codons for terminating protein synthesis.

The "master copy" of the genetic code is in the sequence of the bases in the DNA, which resides in the nucleus. The "working copies" are in the base sequences of the messenger RNA molecules. (The base sequence of the mRNA is complementary to the DNA strand that is transcribed, but the same as the DNA strand that is not transcribed, except that the mRNA contains U instead of T.) When scientists were decoding the genetic message, they determined the mRNA codons. Some examples of mRNA codons and the amino acids they code for are: UUU or UUC, phenylalanine; UAU or UAC, tyrosine; GGU, GGA, GGC, or GGG, glycine; AAA or AAG, lysine; and CCU, CCA, CCC, or CCG, proline.

What, then, is a gene? In most cases a gene is conceptualized as being a particular sequence of nucleotides (each base is part of a nucleotide) in DNA that codes for a single polypeptide chain. Messenger RNA is transcribed from such sequences, which are sometimes referred to as *structural genes.* The portions of DNA that code for ribosomal RNA are referred to as rRNA genes, and the parts that code for transfer RNA are referred to as tRNA genes.

Protein Synthesis

Protein synthesis involves all three types of RNA. Transfer RNA molecules act as "adaptors" that line up appropriate amino acids with corresponding codons on the mRNA. One end of a tRNA molecule binds with a specific amino acid. The other end of the molecule contains an exposed triplet of bases, called the *anticodon,* that is complementary to the mRNA codon for the specific amino acid bound to the tRNA. (Although the tRNA molecule is made up of a single polynucleotide chain, the molecule folds on itself and bases in some regions of the molecule pair with complementary bases in other regions of the molecule. Therefore most of the bases are not exposed.) Many types of tRNA exist to accommodate the 20 amino acids and various codons.

As stated earlier, rRNA forms part of the structure of the ribosomes. Ribosomes also contain protein. A ribosome serves to line up the anticodon on the tRNA with the codon on the mRNA and to facilitate the formation of peptide bonds between adjacent amino acids. Each ribosome is made up of two subunits, a small subunit that associates with the mRNA and a large subunit that binds tRNA molecules.

The mechanism of protein synthesis is shown in Figure 3-13. A ribosome threads onto a messenger RNA strand and moves along it, triplet by triplet, "reading" the codons. Two tRNA molecules, each carrying a specific amino acid, temporarily bind to two sites on the large subunit of a ribosome. (The sites are designated I and II in Fig. 3-13.) The anticodons on the tRNA molecules pair with the codons on a portion of the mRNA molecule that is temporarily attached to the small subunit. An enzyme present in the large ribosomal subunit then catalyzes the formation of a peptide bond between the amino acids carried by the two tRNA molecules. The linked amino acids (i.e., the growing polypeptide chain) are released from the tRNA at site I but remain attached to the tRNA at site II.

The tRNA at site I is ejected from the ribosome and is free to pick up another amino acid. The second tRNA, with the growing polypeptide chain attached, shifts from site II to site I and the ribosome moves one triplet further along the mRNA

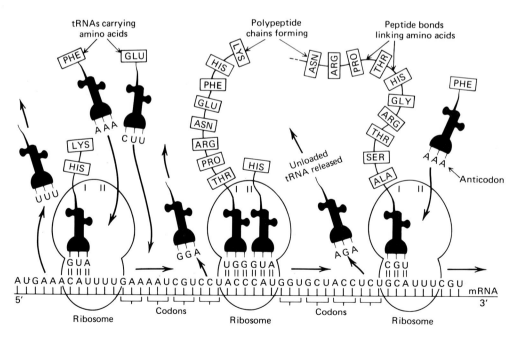

Figure 3-13. *Translation of the genetic message into protein. See text for explanation. (From Cohen A:* Handbook of cellular chemistry, *ed 2. St. Louis, The C. V. Mosby Co., 1979.)*

molecule. Another tRNA molecule carrying a specific amino acid enters site II and another peptide bond is formed. This process is repeated many times, adding one amino acid at a time to form a complete polypeptide chain. When the ribosome reaches the termination codon on the mRNA, the completed polypeptide is released. One or more polypeptide chains then fold into a specific three-dimensional structure to form a functional protein. The way the polypeptides fold depends on the amino acid sequence and the properties of the particular amino acids making up each polypeptide chain.

As one ribosome moves from the starting point to a point farther along the mRNA strand, another ribosome moves on to the mRNA molecule. Thus, many polypeptide chains are simultaneously formed on one mRNA strand. Ribosomes farther along the mRNA molecule have longer polypeptide chains than ribosomes near the beginning. A group of ribosomes attached to an mRNA molecule is referred to as a polyribosome, or polysome.

Control of Gene Expression

Each person is made up of millions of cells, all of which were derived from one cell, the zygote. Every cell in the body (with the exception of the sex cells) normally contains the same number of chromosomes and presumably the same genetic information. Yet it is obvious that many different cell types, with varying structures and functions, are present in the human body. How is it that cells containing the same genetic information can be so different?

It appears that different genetic information is expressed (i.e., different proteins are made) at different times during embryological development and in different types of cells. In other words, not all the genes in a cell are functioning at the same time. What it is that tells which genes to function when is not known, although it appears that the chemical environment of the cell has an influence. It is possible that information regarding which genes are to be transcribed at a particular time is somehow programmed into the DNA molecule.

According to one theory, certain genes are linked together in a linear group called an *operon,* which contains one or more structural genes and nucleotide sequences (i.e., genes) that control the functioning of the structural gene(s). Controlling genes are of two types. *Operator genes* turn the structural genes of their own operon on and off (i.e., determine whether RNA will be transcribed from the structural genes). *Regulator genes,* through their RNA or polypeptide products, modulate the activity of the operator genes. A regulator gene can influence the activity of more than one operator gene and is not necessarily located within the operon it regulates.

In some cases certain enzymes are not made by a particular cell all of the time, but only when the substrate for the enzyme is present. (The substrate is the molecule that the enzyme acts upon; i.e., the reactant in the reaction catalyzed by the enzyme.) The synthesis of a protein (enzyme) in response to the presence of its substrate is referred to as *enzyme induction,* and the enzyme is said to be an inducible enzyme. For example, some drugs can induce certain enzymes in liver cells (see Chapter 25 under Metabolism of Foreign Chemicals).

Heterochromatin
and Euchromatin

When chromosomes are stained with chemical dyes they do not take up the stain evenly. Some regions stain darkly and are called *heterochromatin;* other areas stain relatively lightly and are referred to as *euchromatin.* Heterochromatin represents regions of chromosome material that are compactly coiled; this chromatin remains visible during interphase. Euchromatin is less coiled and is not usually visible during interphase. Genetic experiments have shown that RNA is not transcribed from the DNA in heterochromatic regions (i.e., the genes are not active). Euchromatin, however, contains active genes that are transcribed into RNA.

Some regions of heterochromatin remain constant, but other regions are heterochromatic during some stages of development and euchromatic at other stages. For example, some regions appear as euchromatin during early embryological development and presumably contain genes that are active at that stage, but later in life the same regions appear as heterochromatin. Also, some regions of heterochromatin may differ from one cell type to another.

In females, only one of the X chromosomes in each cell appears to be genetically active. The other chromosome is highly condensed (heterochromatinized) and appears as a dark-staining spot near the nuclear membrane (Fig. 3-14). This spot is referred to as a *Barr body*, after the man who first discovered it, or simply as sex chromatin. Cells containing a Barr body are said to be "chromatin positive." Normal male cells have only one X chromosome and do not contain a Barr body; these cells are said to be "chromatin negative." The inactivation of one X chromosome appears to be random. In other words, in some cells the paternally derived X chromosome is inactive, while in other cells the maternally derived X chromosome is inactive.

Mutations

Occasionally a change occurs in the genetic material of a cell; this change is called a *mutation*. A mutation that occurs in a germ cell (*germinal mu-*

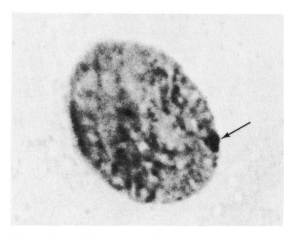

Figure 3-14. *Photomicrograph of a human cell. The dark spot near the nuclear membrane is a Barr body. (Courtesy of Dr. F. J. Dill, Department of Medical Genetics, University of British Columbia, Vancouver, B.C., Canada.)*

tation) can be transmitted from parent to offspring. A change in the genetic material of a somatic cell (*somatic mutation*) cannot be transmitted from parent to offspring, but it can be expressed in the cells or tissues derived from the cell in which the mutation took place. Most mutations are harmful. In some cases, called *lethal mutations*, the genetic change leads to early death.

Some mutations involve an alteration in the base sequence of part of a DNA molecule. This type of change, called a *gene mutation*, is not visible under a microscope but may be expressed as an unusual characteristic in the person carrying the mutation. Other changes involve alterations in the gross structure of chromosomes and are visible under the microscope. These changes are sometimes referred to as *chromosome mutations*. Some people, however, prefer to restrict the term mutation to mean a gene mutation and prefer to call chromosomal changes *chromosome aberrations*. In addition to changes in chromosome structure, variations in chromosome number can occur. Chromosome aberrations are discussed in Chapter 5.

Genetic changes that occur under ordinary environmental conditions are called *spontaneous mutations*, and are relatively rare. A variety of environmental agents can produce changes in the genetic material and increase the mutation rate. These agents are called *mutagens*, or mutagenic agents. Genetic changes caused by exposing an organism to a known mutagen are called *induced mutations*. Known mutagens include ionizing radiation and ultraviolet radiation (see Chapter 23), as well as many chemicals. Examples of chemical mutagens are acridine dyes, hydroxylamine, nitrous acid, and nitrogen mustard.

Gene Mutations

Gene mutation involves a change in the nucleotide (base) sequence in a part of a DNA molecule corresponding to a single gene. Often only one base is changed (a *point mutation*). As a result of this base-sequence change, one or more codons are altered.

Several types of gene mutations can occur. An

incorrect nucleotide (base) might replace the correct one; this is called a *substitution*. One or more extra nucleotides might be added; this is called an *insertion*. Or a nucleotide or nucleotides might be left out; the result is called a *deletion*. Another possibility is that two nucleotides might be put in backwards, producing an *inversion*. Sometimes an inversion involves more than two nucleotides. As an analogy to the various kinds of gene mutations that can occur, consider how the following misprints in a line of type convey the wrong information.

Intended:	Please sign here.
Substitution:	Please sigh here.
Insertion:	Please sign there.
Deletion:	Please sin here.
Inversion:	Please sing here.

A mutation in a structural gene can cause a change in the sequence of amino acids in a polypeptide chain. As a result the structure and function of the protein product is altered; the protein may be nonfunctional. The consequences of such changes are described in Chapter 6. Since more than one codon can specify a particular amino acid, a single base change in the DNA does not always alter the protein product (i.e., the change may be to a "synonymous" codon). Theoretically, mutations can also occur in operator genes and regulator genes. For example, thalassemia is believed to be due to a mutation in an operator gene (see Chapter 10).

SUGGESTED ADDITIONAL READING

Changeaux J-P: The control of biochemical reactions. *Sci Am* 212(4): 36–45, 1965.

Crick FHC: The genetic code: III. *Sci Am* 215(4): 55–62, 1966.

Edwards RG, Fowler RE: Human embryos in the laboratory. *Sci Am* 223(6): 44–54, 1970.

Miller OL Jr: The visualization of genes in action. *Sci Am* 228(3): 34–42, 1973.

Rich A, Kim SH: The three-dimensional structure of transfer RNA. *Sci Am* 238(1): 52–62, 1978.

4

Principles
of Genetics

Inheritance is based on the transmission of genes, but it is frequently described according to observable features of organisms. An observable feature of an individual is called a *character*, or *trait;* it may be a biochemical property, an anatomical structure, a function of a cell or organ, or a mental characteristic. Characters are derived from the action of genes, but they are not the same as genes. *Genotype* is the term used to denote the actual genetic constitution. The term *phenotype* refers to an organism's appearance and functional characteristics; that is, the way the genetic information is expressed as particular characters or traits. The phenotype is influenced by environment as well as by genotype.

Differences in phenotype between two individuals may be such that the trait manifested by one may be regarded as normal (e.g., normal color vision) and the trait manifested by the other as abnormal (e.g., color blindness). Alternatively, two different phenotypes may be variants of normal traits (e.g., brown eyes or blue eyes). Variants of abnormal phenotypes may also occur (e.g., hemoglobin S and hemoglobin C; see Chapter 6 under Sickle Cell Anemia).

As stated in Chapter 3, the genes are composed

of DNA. They appear to be linearly arranged in the chromosomes. The specific site of a gene in a chromosome is called the *locus* (plural: loci) of the gene. Genes occupying corresponding loci on homologous chromosomes affect the same character, although not necessarily in exactly the same way. Alternative forms of genes (i.e., genes that affect the same character in different ways) that occupy corresponding loci on homologous chromosomes are called *alleles*.

When an individual possesses identical alleles at a given locus on both members of a pair of homologous chromosomes the condition is said to be *homozygous* and the individual may be called a *homozygote*. When two different alleles are present the condition is said to be *heterozygous* and the individual may be called a *heterozygote*. In the heterozygous state, one allele may be expressed over the other. The allele that is expressed is said to be *dominant;* the one that is not expressed is said to be *recessive*. In other words, a dominant trait is capable of expression when the responsible allele is carried by only one member of a pair of homologous chromosomes. A recessive trait is capable of expression only when the responsible allele is carried by both members of a pair of homologous chromosomes.

For example, in human beings albinism is determined by a recessive allele, which can be designated *a*. The normal pigmented condition is dominant and the responsible allele can be designated *A*. A person may be homozygous *AA*, homozygous *aa*, or heterozygous *Aa*. Since *A* is the dominant allele, both a heterozygote and a homozygous *AA* person will have pigmented skin. In other words, *AA* and *Aa* are different genotypes, but they give rise to the same phenotype. A homozygous *aa* person will exhibit albinism (i.e., will not have pigment in the skin).

Knowledge of the genetic code provides insight into the mechanism by which a particular genotype can give rise to a certain phenotype. For example, in albinism the normal allele *A* codes for an enzyme that is necessary to catalyze a biochemical reaction by which pigment is produced in the skin. The product of allele *a* is nonfunctional; therefore, no pigment is produced. Whether *A* is present in the homozygous or heterozygous condition, functional enzyme is produced and the skin will be pigmented.

MENDELIAN PRINCIPLES

Over a century ago, before the existence of chromosomes and genes was known, an Austrian monk named Gregor Mendel carried out hundreds of genetic experiments with pea plants. He traced the transmission of certain biological characteristics and enunciated two fundamental principles of inheritance. Although Mendel worked with pea plants, these principles are also true for other organisms, including human beings. Mendel also proposed the concepts of dominance and recessiveness on the basis of his work with pea plants. Therefore, conditions that have a simple autosomal dominant or autosomal recessive pattern of inheritance (see below) are often referred to as mendelian traits.

The Principle of Segregation

From the results of his experiments, Mendel concluded that each pea plant contains two hereditary factors for each character, and that during the formation of gametes the two factors separate cleanly from one another (i.e., segregate) and pass into separate gametes. Thus, each gamete contains only one factor for each character. When a new plant is formed it receives one factor for each character from the female parent (gamete) and one factor for each character from the male parent (gamete).

Mendel's principle of segregation can be restated as follows: the members of a pair of alleles separate cleanly from one another during gametogenesis. Using the previous example, if an individual is heterozygous *Aa*, half of the gametes

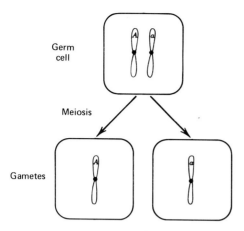

Figure 4-1. *The principle of segregation. Genes A and a are on different members of a pair of homologous chromosomes. During meiosis homologous chromosomes separate; therefore half of the gametes contain A and half contain a.*

that are formed will contain A and half of the gametes will contain *a*. The basis for the segregation of alleles during gametogenesis is the separation of homologous chromosomes during meiosis. One chromosome carries *A* and its homologue carries *a* (Fig. 4-1).

The Principle of Independent Assortment

Mendel studied seven different characters in pea plants (e.g., seed color, seed shape, stem length). He observed not only the transmission of single characters but also the patterns of inheritance of two or more characters. For example, he cross-pollinated plants from a pure-breeding stock that produced wrinkled green seeds with plants from a pure-breeding stock that produced round yellow seeds. The resultant seeds were collected and planted, and gave rise to plants that produced round yellow seeds (round is dominant over wrinkled; yellow is dominant over green). These plants, which belong to what is called the first filial (F_1) generation, were self-pollinated. The seeds were sown to give rise to plants that belong to what is called the second filial (F_2) generation.

Among these plants, Mendel found some with wrinkled yellow seeds and some with round green seeds, as well as plants with the original parental phenotypes (i.e., round yellow and wrinkled green seeds). On the basis of such experiments he concluded that the factors for one character segregate independently of those for another character when gametes are formed, and that each member of a pair of factors for one character may be associated with either member of another pair.

Mendel's principle of independent assortment can be restated as follows: the members of different pairs of alleles assort independently of each other during gametogenesis, and each member of a pair of alleles may occur randomly with either member of another pair of alleles. For example, consider an individual who is heterozygous *Aa* at one locus and heterozygous for a different allelic pair, *Bb*, at another locus (genotype *AaBb*). When the gametes are formed, half of them will contain A and the other half will contain *a*. Since the *Bb* allelic pair segregates independently of the *Aa* allelic pair, the probability is that half of the gametes with A will contain B and half will contain *b*. Similarly, half of the gametes with *a* will contain B and half will contain *b*. Therefore, one-fourth of the gametes will contain AB, one-fourth will contain Ab, one-fourth will contain aB, and one-fourth will contain *ab*. If this individual mates with another individual who is heterozygous for the same two characteristics, the offspring could have any of the following genotypes: AABB, AABb, AAbb, AaBB, AaBb, Aabb, aaBB, aaBb, or aabb (Fig. 4-2).

Since Mendel first stated the principle of independent assortment it has been modified as scientists learned more about the nature of genes and chromosomes. Members of different pairs of homologous chromosomes assort independently of each other (i.e., randomly), but each chromosome contains many genes. Therefore, members of different pairs of alleles that are in different chromosomes assort independently, but genes located in the same chromosome do not. (The genes that governed the characters studied by Mendel happened to be located in different chromosomes.)

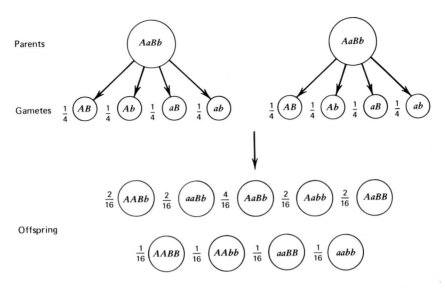

Figure 4-2. *Results of a mating between two individuals who are heterozygous for the same two characteristics (i.e., a dihybrid cross). The numbers represent the ratio of each genotype expected by chance.*

When the parental combinations of characters tend to be transmitted together (i.e., the genes responsible for the characters do not assort independently), the genes are said to be *linked* and the phenomenon is known as *linkage*. Linked genes are located in the same chromosome. The principle of independent assortment and the phenomenon of linkage are illustrated in Figure 4-3.

New combinations of linked genes occasionally occur and are called *recombinations*. Recombination of linked genes occurs through the process of *crossing over*, in which homologous chromosomes exchange parts. Crossing over takes place during meiosis I.

PATTERNS OF INHERITANCE

The *mode of inheritance* of a particular character or condition refers to the way the character is transmitted. When a character is due to a recessive allele at a particular locus on an autosome, the mode of inheritance is *autosomal recessive*. *Autosomal dominant* means that a particular trait is governed by a dominant allele located on an autosome. Characters that are governed by genes located on autosomes usually occur with equal frequency in males and females. The frequency of occurrence of some characters differs between males and females because the gene responsible for the character is located on a sex chromosome. The mode of inheritance is then said to be *sex-linked*. Some characters have a *polygenic* mode of inheritance; that is, they are governed by two or more genes that occur at separate loci and have an additive effect.

Autosomal Inheritance

This section describes the inheritance of characters dependent on differences between the alleles at a single locus on an autosome pair. In the inheritance of autosomal genes it makes no difference which parent carries a particular genotype, since the autosomes are equivalent in both sexes.

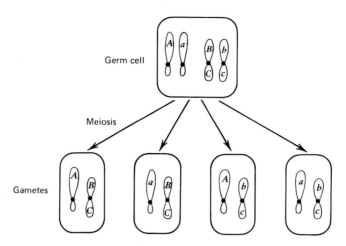

Germn cell

Meiosis

Gametes

Figure 4-3. *The principle of independent assortment and the phenomenon of linkage. Genes* A *and* B *assort independently of each other because they are located on different chromosomes. Genes* B *and* C *do not assort independently because they are located on the same chromosome (i.e., they are linked).*

Dominant Inheritance

Consider a trait governed by a dominant allele D; let d represent the recessive allele. The trait will be apparent if the dominant allele is present in the heterozygous *(Dd)* or homozygous *(DD)* state, and the phenotype will not indicate the genotype. If the dominant gene is rare, however, most people will be carrying it in the heterozygous state. On the other hand, if the dominant allele is common, both heterozygous and homozygous *DD* genotypes will be common in the population. All children affected by a dominant trait have at least one affected parent (unless the dominant allele arose as a result of a new mutation in the germ cells of one of the parents). In other words, dominant traits are manifested in every generation.

If a person who is heterozygous for the dominant gene marries a person who is not carrying the dominant allele (i.e., is homozygous *dd*), the probability is that half of their children will be heterozygous and will be affected by the trait. Half of their children will not exhibit the trait. Half of the gametes produced by the heterozygous parent will contain the allele D and half will contain d. The gametes of the homozygous *dd* parent will all

contain d. One of these gametes from the homozygous *dd* parent can unite with either a gamete carrying D to produce a heterozygous *Dd* individual or with a gamete carrying d to produce a homozygous *dd* child. This situation is outlined in Figure 4-4.

In marriages between heterozygotes, the probability is that one-quarter of the children will be homozygous *DD*, one-half of the children will be heterozygous *Dd*, and one-quarter of the children will be homozygous *dd* (Fig. 4-5). Since the dominant allele is expressed in both the heterozygous and homozygous state, the probability is that three-quarters of the children will be affected by the trait and one-quarter (those who are *dd*) will not be affected.

If a person who is homozygous *DD* marries a person who is homozygous *dd*, all their children will receive the D allele from one parent and the d allele from the other parent (Fig. 4-6). Therefore all children of this couple will be heterozygous *(Dd)* and will exhibit the trait.

An example of a human trait that has an autosomal dominant mode of inheritance is a white forelock. This condition is characterized by

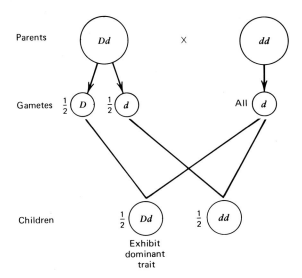

Figure 4-4. *A marriage between a person who is heterozygous for a dominant gene (genotype Dd) and a person who is not carrying the dominant gene (genotype dd).*

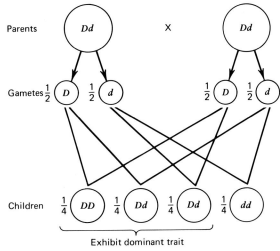

Figure 4-5. *A marriage between two people who are heterozygous for a dominant gene.*

an unpigmented patch of skin above the forehead with white hair growing from it. Brachydactyly, or short-fingeredness, is another trait that shows autosomal dominant inheritance.

Recessive Inheritance

A trait governed by a recessive allele will be manifested only when the allele is present in the homozygous condition (genotype rr, if r represents the recessive allele and R the corresponding dominant allele). When both parents manifest the trait (i.e., both have the genotype rr), then all their children will exhibit the trait.

If an affected person (rr) marries someone who is homozygous RR, all their children will be heterozygous Rr (Fig. 4-7). None of the children will manifest the trait, but all will be *carriers* of the recessive allele. If an affected person (rr) marries a carrier (Rr), the probability is that half of their children will be affected and half will be carriers (Fig. 4-8).

If two carriers (i.e., two heterozygous Rr individuals) marry, the probability is that one-quarter

of their children will be affected, one-half will be carriers, and one-quarter will be homozygous RR (Fig 4-9). Phenotypically, the carriers and the homozygous RR offspring will appear the same. If a carrier marries a person with the genotype RR, the

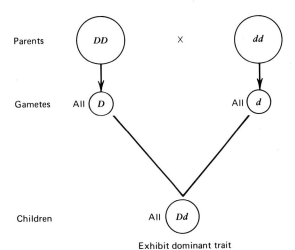

Figure 4-6. *A marriage between a person who is homozygous for a dominant allele (genotype DD) and a person who is homozygous for the corresponding recessive allele (genotype dd).*

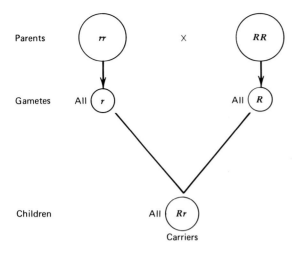

Figure 4-7. *A marriage between a person who exhibits a recessive trait (genotype rr) and a person who is homozygous for the corresponding dominant allele (genotype RR).*

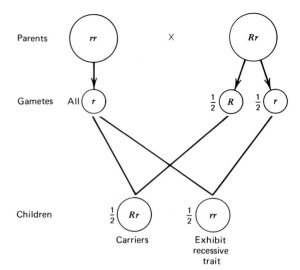

Figure 4-8. *A marriage between a person who exhibits a recessive trait (genotype rr) and a carrier of the recessive allele (genotype Rr).*

probability is that half of their children will be carriers *(Rr)* and half will have the genotype *RR* (Fig. 4-10). None will manifest the trait.

If the *r* allele for a particular condition is rare, affected *(rr)* people will be very rare and even those who are heterozygous *(Rr)* for the trait will be uncommon. Marriages between two affected people or between an affected person and a heterozygous person will be rare. Most likely an affected *(rr)* person will marry a person with the genotype *RR*, and all their children will be heterozygous. They, in turn, will probably marry homozygous normals *(RR)*, and all their children will have the normal phenotype. Therefore the allele *r* may be carried for many generations without the trait being manifested.

Albinism is an example of a condition that has an autosomal recessive mode of inheritance.

The Role of Chance

In the preceding discussion it was stated that a certain fraction of the children would have a particular genotype, while a certain fraction would have a different one. These fractions, or ratios, represent probabilities and are valid only for a large population. Since human families tend to be small, these ideal ratios are not usually seen.

For example, it was stated that in a marriage between two heterozygotes for a dominant trait, one-quarter of the children would have the genotype *dd*. Another way of expressing this situation would be to say that if a child from such a marriage is selected at random, there is one chance in four that it will have the genotype *dd*. It does not mean that in any one family one out of four children has the genotype *dd*. All the children of one pair of heterozygous parents may have the genotype *dd*; in another marriage of heterozygotes none of the children may have the *dd* genotype. If all the children from a large number of marriages between heterozygotes are considered, however, the probability is that one-quarter of them have the genotype *dd*.

The actual genotypes of the children in a particular marriage are a matter of chance. Although the alleles *D* and *d* separate from each other during gametogenesis, not all the potential gametes become mature sperm or ova. Therefore inequalities in the number of *D* gametes and *d* gametes can

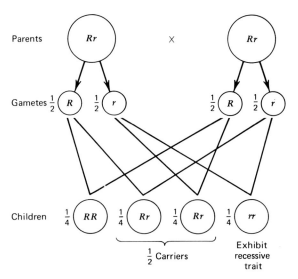

Figure 4-9. *A marriage between two people who are carriers of a recessive allele (genotype* Rr).

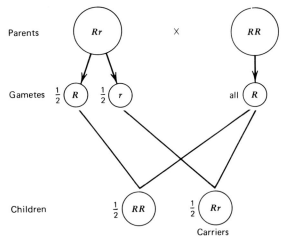

Figure 4-10. *A marriage between a person who is a carrier of a recessive allele (genotype* Rr) *and a person who is homozygous for the corresponding dominant allele (genotype* RR).

result from chance elimination. Since only one functional ovum and three polar bodies are produced from one primary oocyte each month, whether the ovum contains the allele *D* or *d* is a matter of chance. In addition, whether a *D* or *d* sperm unites with the egg is a completely random event. Whether or not a *d* sperm fertilizes a *d* egg in the first pregnancy, a subsequent fertilization will not be influenced by this event. In a later fertilization the chance is still one in four that a *dd* embryo will result.

Incomplete Dominance and Codominance

In the discussion of dominance and recessiveness, it was stated that the heterozygous genotype produces the same phenotype as the homozygous condition for the dominant allele. In other words, *Dd* produces the same phenotype as *DD*. This situation is known as *simple,* or *complete,* dominance. The heterozygous genotype does not always produce the same phenotype as one of the homozygous genotypes, however; other types of phenotypic expression can occur in the heterozygous state.

In some cases, the heterozygous genotype gives rise to a phenotype intermediate between the phenotypes manifested by those with either of the homozygous genotypes. This situation is called *partial,* or *incomplete,* dominance. For example, when the allele responsible for thalassemia is present in the homozygous state, a severe anemia (thalassemia major) occurs, but in the heterozygous state the condition is much milder (thalassemia minor).

When the two alleles in a gene pair are each responsible for the production of different substances, both substances may occur in the heterozygous state. This situation is called *codominance.* In other words, with the homozygous genotype A^1A^1, only substance one is produced; with the homozygous genotype A^2A^2, substance two is produced. In the heterozygous state (A^1A^2), both substances one and two are produced. The AB blood type and the MN blood type are examples of codominance.

Some rare genetic disorders are considered to have a simple dominant mode of inheritance because the condition is manifested when the responsible allele is present in the heterozygous state. In some cases, however, the condition is so rare that the homozygous genotype for the abnormal allele has not been observed. It is possible that the condition expressed in heterozygotes is intermediate between the phenotypes of the two homozygotes (i.e., the abnormal homozygote may be more abnormal than the heterozygote).

Many genetic disorders are considered to have a recessive mode of inheritance because the disease is manifested only when the abnormal allele is present in the homozygous state. In some cases, however, differences in homozygotes and heterozygotes may be discernible at the biochemical level. For example, when the normal allele is present in the homozygous state, an enzyme with a certain level of activity may be produced. When the abnormal allele is present in the homozygous state, enzyme activity may be lacking. In the heterozygous condition the activity of the enzyme may be less than the enzyme activity in the homozygous normal state. In other words, the heterozygous condition may be intermediate between the two homozygous states at the biochemical level, but in distinguishing between health and illness the abnormal allele may be considered recessive because the level of enzyme activity in the heterozygote is adequate for normal health. This situation emphasizes the fact that dominance and recessiveness are relative terms. Classification of the heterozygote depends on the level of phenotypic expression under consideration.

Multiple Alleles

A gene is said to possess *multiple alleles* when more than two alleles (i.e., more than two alternative forms of the gene) are present in the population. Only two of the possible alleles can be present in a given individual, because the cells contain only one pair of each type of chromosome. For example, the ABO blood group system consists of three alleles: I^A, I^B, and i. I^A and I^B show codominance; i is recessive to both I^A and I^B. Six genotypes and four phenotypes are possible. The genotypes I^AI^A and iI^A produce type A blood; genotypes I^BI^B and

iI^B produce type B blood; genotype I^AI^B produces type AB blood; and genotype ii produces type O blood. The Rh blood group system is also governed by multiple alleles and genetically it is very complex. At least eight different Rh alleles are known.

Sex-Linked Inheritance

As stated in Chapter 3, females have two homologous X chromosomes, whereas males have one X chromosome and one smaller nonhomologous Y chromosome. Therefore, males and females are not equivalent with respect to genes located in the sex chromosomes. Genes located in the X chromosome are said to be X-linked; many such genes are known. Genes located in the Y chromosome are said to be Y-linked. Except for genes that determine maleness, evidence for Y-linked genes is limited. Therefore the term sex-linked usually refers to X-linked genes; unless otherwise specified.

Males cannot transmit X-linked genes to their sons, but only to their daughters. Conversely, males can only receive X-linked genes from their mothers. This situation follows from the fact that if a sperm carrying an X chromosome fertilizes an egg, which can only have an X chromosome, a female offspring is produced. Males result from the fertilization of an egg by a sperm carrying a Y chromosome.

Females may be homozygous or heterozygous for the alleles of X-linked genes, because they have two X chromosomes. Males have only one allele for each X-linked gene, because they have only one X chromosome. Therefore males are said to be *hemizygous* for X-linked genes.

X-Linked Recessive Inheritance

Regardless of whether an X-linked allele shows recessiveness in females, it will be manifested in males because the Y chromosome does not carry a corresponding gene. In other words, in males no homologous locus exists that could carry an alternative allele to "cover up" the effects of the X-linked recessive allele.

Usually an X-linked recessive allele will be expressed in females only when the allele is present in the homozygous state. Occasionally, however, a heterozygous female carrier of an X-linked allele will manifest the trait, because of the random inactivation of one X chromosome in each cell (see Chapter 3 under Heterochromatin and Euchromatin). Whether or not a heterozygous female manifests the trait and the degree to which the trait is manifested, will depend on the proportion of cells that contain the dominant allele in the inactivated X chromosome. When the dominant allele is present in the inactivated chromosome in a large proportion of cells, the recessive trait may be manifested in heterozygous females.

Let X^r represent an X-linked recessive allele; X^R the corresponding X-linked dominant allele; and Y the Y chromosome, which is lacking the homologous locus. If a woman is homozygous for the recessive allele (X^rX^r), she will manifest the trait. All her sons will manifest the trait because all males receive their X chromosome from their mother. The sons will have the genotype X^rY. Her daughters will all be heterozygous carriers (X^rX^R) if their father carries the dominant allele (Fig. 4-11).

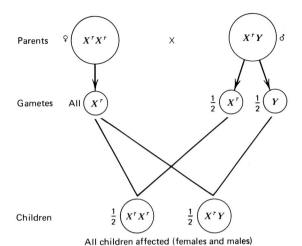

Figure 4-12. *A marriage between a woman who manifests a sex-linked trait* (X^rX^r) *and a man who is also affected* (X^rY).

If the father carries the recessive allele (i.e., also exhibits the trait) all the woman's daughters will be homozygous recessive (X^rX^r) and will manifest the trait (Fig. 4-12).

In a marriage between a heterozygous female (X^rX^R) and a man possessing the dominant allele (X^RY), the probability is that half of the sons will exhibit the recessive trait (i.e., will have the genotype X^rY) and half of the daughters will be carriers (Fig. 4-13). If a heterozygous woman marries a man who possesses the recessive allele (i.e., manifests the trait), the probability is that half of their sons will manifest the trait, half of their daughters will manifest the trait, and half of their daughters will be carriers (Fig. 4-14).

If a man who manifests the trait (X^rY) marries a woman who is homozygous for the dominant allele (X^RX^R), none of their sons will exhibit the trait. All their daughters will be carriers (Fig. 4-15).

Some types of color blindness and hemophilia are examples of human conditions that have an X-linked recessive mode of inheritance.

X-Linked Dominant Inheritance

Traits due to X-linked dominant alleles will be manifested in heterozygous females as well as those

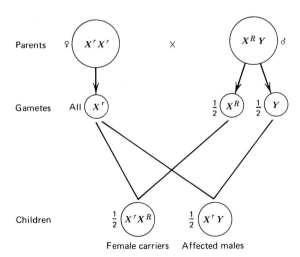

Figure 4-11. *A marriage between a woman who manifests a sex-linked recessive trait* (X^rX^r) *and a man who is not affected* (X^RY).

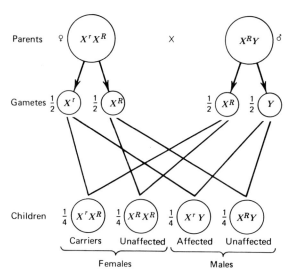

Figure 4-13. *A marriage between a woman who is a carrier of a sex-linked recessive allele* (X^rX^R) *and a man who is not affected* (X^RY).

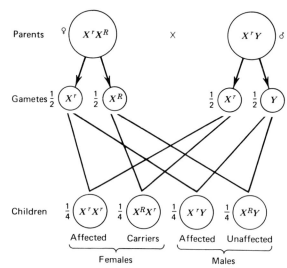

Figure 4-14. *A marriage between a woman who is a carrier of a sex-linked recessive allele* (X^rX^R) *and a man who manifests the trait* (X^rY).

who are homozygous for the dominant allele. Since females receive one of their X chromosomes from their fathers, all the daughters of an affected man will exhibit the trait. An affected man cannot pass the gene on to his sons.

Let X^D represent the X-linked dominant allele and X^d the corresponding recessive allele. If a heterozygous (affected) female marries an affected male, all their daughters will be affected and the probability is that half of their sons will be affected (Fig. 4-16). If a heterozygous woman marries a man who is not affected, the probability is that half of their children will manifest the trait, regardless of sex (Fig. 4-17).

All the children of a homozygous affected female (X^DX^D) will exhibit the trait, regardless of whether the father is affected. If the father is also affected (X^DY), all of the daughters will be homozygous X^DX^D. If the father is not affected (X^dY), the probability is that half of the daughters will be homozygous X^DX^D and half will be heterozygous.

Hypophosphatemic vitamin D–resistant rick-

ets (see Chapter 16) is a condition that appears to have an X-linked dominant mode of inheritance.

Y-Linked Inheritance

Traits governed by Y-linked genes will occur only in males, since only males possess a Y chromosome. A man transmits a Y chromosome to all his sons but to none of his daughters; therefore traits with a Y-linked mode of inheritance should appear in all the males of each generation in a family but in none of the females.

In human beings, no traits showing Y-linked inheritance have been demonstrated with certainty. Hairiness of the pinna of the ear (hypertrichosis) is possibly due to a Y-linked gene. This trait is characterized by the growth of long stiff hairs on the surface of the pinna and along the rim of the ear.

Polygenic Inheritance

Many inherited traits are not manifested as sharply defined alternative phenotypes, but show a con-

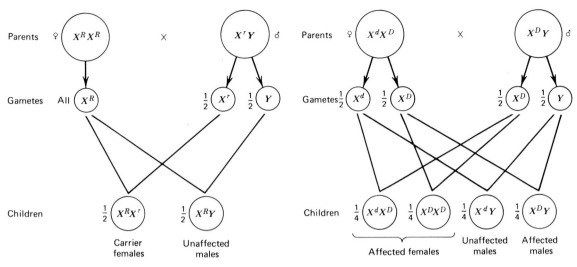

Figure 4-15. *A marriage between a woman who is homozygous for the dominant allele of a sex-linked character* (X^RX^R) *and a man who exhibits the recessive trait* (X^rY).

Figure 4-16. *A marriage between a woman who is heterozygous for a sex-linked dominant trait* (X^dX^D) *and an affected man* (X^DY).

tinuous gradation in a population (e.g., height, skin color). Such *quantitative* characteristics appear to be determined by the cumulative effects of two or more genes at separate loci. Each gene contributes more or less equally in the production of the final phenotype. This mode of inheritance is called *polygenic*, or *multifactorial*, inheritance. The term polygenic emphasizes the genetic component, whereas the term multifactorial implies that many factors, including environmental ones, are important in determining the phenotype.

Quantitative characters can be classified on a numerical scale that extends over a range of values. The largest number of individuals have a phenotype that is close to the mean measure of the range; few individuals fall at the extremes of the range. Graphically, the frequency of individuals of each phenotype approximates a bell-shaped normal distribution curve. The greater the number of segregating gene pairs involved, the greater the number of phenotypic classes there will be and the more closely they will grade into each other. In addition, individual variation due to different environmental effects on those with the same

genotype will cause one class to merge into the next and "smooth" the normal distribution curve.

Consider a hypothetical quantitative character determined by four genes at separate loci. The phenotypic classes range from 4 to 36 units on a numerical scale. Suppose the genotype *aabbccdd* produces the phenotype of 4 units and the genotype *AABBCCDD* produces the phenotype of 36 units. The presence of each allele represented by a capital letter results in an increase of 4 units over the basic phenotype of 4 units. Thus, for example, the genotype *AaBbCcDd* would produce a phenotype of 20 units. A mating between an *AABBCCDD* individual and an *aabbccdd* individual will produce offspring that are heterozygous for all four gene pairs (i.e., *AaBbCcDd*). Matings between individuals that are heterozygous for all four gene pairs will produce nine phenotypic classes, and the probable number of individuals in each class will fit a normal distribution curve (Fig. 4-18). Independent assortment will produce 16 kinds of gametes from an *AaBbCcDd* individual; 256 different combinations of gametes are possible from matings between *AaBbCcDd* individuals. Of

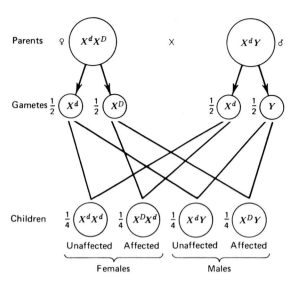

Figure 4-17. *A marriage between a woman who is heterozygous for a sex-linked dominant trait* (X^dX^D) *and a man who is not affected* (X^dY).

this number, the probability is that one would have the genotype *aabbccdd* and produce a phenotype of 4 units and one would have the genotype *AABBCCDD* and produce a phenotype of 36 units. Eight would have seven small letters and one capital letter (8 units); 28 would have six small letters and two capital letters (12 units); 56 would have five small letters and three capital letters (16 units); 70 would have four small letters and four capital letters (20 units); 56 would have three small letters and five capital letters (24 units); 28 would have two small letters and six capital letters (28 units); and eight would have one small letter and seven capital letters (32 units).

GENE EXPRESSION

The relationship between genotype and phenotype is complex. The way that a gene is expressed depends on interactions with other genes and with the environment. These interactions occur at

many levels of development throughout a person's lifetime.

Gene Interaction

As discussed in Chapter 3, the genes contain coded information for the production of proteins. Complex interactions occur among the products of different genes. For example, the product of one gene may be an enzyme that catalyzes the conversion of substance S to product P; P may then enter one or more biochemical pathways catalyzed by various enzymes that are coded by other genes. Two generalizations can be drawn from this example: first, a single gene can affect more than one trait; second, most characters are not determined by a single gene.

The quality of a gene having multiple phenotypic effects is called *pleiotropy*. The multiple effects of the gene can arise in several ways. The gene may code for an enzyme that catalyzes one reaction in a network of biochemical pathways, as in the example just given. Or the effects may be further removed from the primary effects. For example, in sickle cell disease an alteration in a gene results in the formation of abnormal hemoglobin (see Chapter 6). Consequently the red blood cells become sickle-shaped. This basic effect causes several other effects. The abnormal red blood cells have a decreased survival time, which results in anemia; the anemia in turn causes several effects (see Chapter 10). Accumulation of the sickled red blood cells in the spleen causes splenic enlargement. In addition, sickled red blood cells may block small blood vessels, thus impeding blood flow and impairing the functions of many organs.

Most traits are not determined solely by one gene, but result from the interaction of many genes. Often, however, a single gene may have a major effect on a character. For example, several protein factors, each coded by a different gene, are necessary for normal blood clotting. A change in a single gene, causing a defect in any one of these proteins, can produce a bleeding tendency (i.e.,

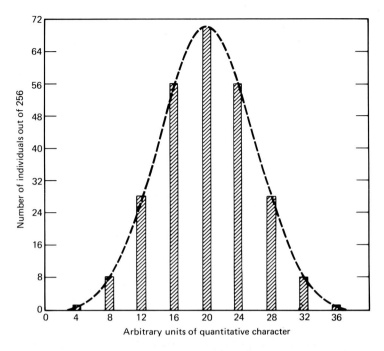

Figure 4-18. *Probable frequency distribution for nine phenotypic classes of a quantitative character determined by four pairs of genes at different loci.*

the phenotype hemophilia). This example points up another fact: different individuals who have the same phenotype may have genotypically distinct conditions. For example, hemophilia A is practically indistinguishable from hemophilia B (see Chapter 7), but hemophilia A is due to an abnormality of clotting factor VIII, whereas hemophilia B is due to an abnormality of clotting factor IX, which is coded by a gene at a different locus.

The gene that is primarily responsible for the appearance of a given character is referred to as the *main* gene and all the other genes as its *genetic background*. Genes at different loci that influence the expression of a main gene are called *modifier genes*. The mode of action of a modifier gene is not always known. In some cases a modifier may enhance the effect of a particular allele (i.e., main gene) and in other cases it may suppress the phenotypic expression of the main gene.

Penetrance and Expressivity

Some individuals that have a particular genotype may not show the expected phenotype. Whether or not a particular gene is expressed is referred to as the *penetrance* of the gene. If a gene is expressed, it is said to be penetrant; if it is not expressed it is said to be nonpenetrant. A dominant allele is said to be fully penetrant when the trait it controls is always manifest in an individual possessing the allele. A recessive allele is said to be fully penetrant when the trait it controls is always evident in an individual who is homozygous for the allele. When a particular genotype produces a given trait in some individuals but not in others, the gene is said to be incompletely penetrant, or to show partial penetrance. The term penetrance also refers to the proportion of individuals with a particular genotype who show the expected phenotype. For example, if only 75% of the individuals carrying a particular dominant allele in the heterozygous state express the expected phenotype, the gene is said to have 75% penetrance.

Among those who express the effects of a particular gene, the phenotype may be variable; in some the effects may be more severe than in others. For example, some people with the dominant gene for hypophosphatemic rickets may have severe rickets, while others with the gene may have only a low blood phosphorus level and no clinical signs of rickets. The term *expressivity* refers to the degree or extent to which an individual expresses the effects of a gene. Expressivity and penetrance are related concepts. Nonpenetrance may be viewed as one extreme of a range of variable expressivity.

Differences in penetrance and expressivity result from environmental differences and from the interaction of a particular gene with other genes. Gene interactions have already been discussed. Although two persons may have the same genotypes at some loci, no two people, except monozygotic (identical) twins, have completely identical genotypes at all loci. Therefore variations in phenotypic expression can occur due to differences in the genetic background.

Effects of Environment

The phenotype results from the interaction of the genotype with the environment. Each person arises from a single cell, the zygote. For growth and development to occur, materials from the external environment must be assimilated into the internal environment. Then, through a complex network of metabolic reactions directed by messages in the genes, constituents of the internal environment are organized to form the phenotype. In many cases, although it is apparent that the development of a particular phenotype is influenced by environment, the exact nature of the environmental agent(s) is not known.

In some cases, specific environmental factors may modify the development of an organism to produce a phenotype that mimics the phenotype usually produced by a specific genotype, even though the individual does not possess that genotype. A nongenetic (i.e., environmentally induced) trait or disorder that simulates the phenotype usually produced by a specific genotype, or an individual exhibiting such a phenotype, is called a *phenocopy*. For example, exposure to the drug thalidomide during embryonic development produces limb abnormalities that resemble those caused by rare mutant genes.

Nutrition and Availability of Substrates

Not only the materials that are needed to form bodily structures, but also the energy to carry out metabolic processes, come from food. The quality and quantity of food that a person eats influences the development of the phenotype from the genotype.

A *substrate* is a substance on which an enzyme acts; that is, a reactant in a reaction catalyzed by an enzyme. Some substrates must be provided in the diet; in other words they come from the external environment. Other substrates are derived from metabolic reactions within the cells. The product of one reaction may be the substrate for a subsequent reaction. For example, consider a hypothetical metabolic pathway in which substrate A is converted to product B; B is then the substrate for a subsequent reaction and is converted to C. The reaction A to B is catalyzed by the enzyme a, which is coded by the gene alpha. The reaction B to C is catalyzed by the enzyme b, which is coded by the gene beta. For gene beta to be expressed (i.e., for product C to be formed and to give rise to a certain phenotype), substance B must be available in the internal environment of the cells. The availability of B depends on two factors: the presence of active enzyme a, which is coded by gene alpha (an example of gene interaction, as discussed earlier); and the availability of substrate A, which is provided in the diet (i.e., comes from the external environment). Thus, a person's nutritional status has an important effect on gene expression.

In addition to substrates that come from the diet (e.g., essential amino acids, essential fatty acids, and carbohydrates), vitamins, which act as coenzymes, and minerals, many of which act as cofactors for enzymes, must be provided by the diet. The influence of diet on gene expression is particularly apparent in the case of inborn errors of metabolism (see Chapter 6). For example, in phenylketonuria (PKU), a genetic defect results in decreased activity of an enzyme that is necessary for the conversion of phenylalanine to tyrosine. The substrate phenylalanine comes from the diet. When people with the appropriate genotype eat foods containing phenylalanine, the severe phenotypic manifestations of the disease PKU occur. On the other hand, by restricting phenylalanine in the diet the severe manifestations of PKU do not occur; instead the phenotype may be normal. In this case the genotype has not been altered, but by changing the environment the phenotype has been altered.

Other External Environmental Factors

Temperature and light are important external environmental factors in the development of certain phenotypes in some organisms. For example, fur color in some animals is influenced by temperature. No specific temperature effects on the development of human phenotypes have been demonstrated, unless one counts the sterility in males with undescended testes as an example. In this case, if the testes remain in the abdomen after the onset of puberty, sterility occurs because the higher temperature in the abdomen as compared with the scrotum interferes with normal spermatogenesis.

Light has an influence on some human phenotypes. For example, freckling of the skin occurs when people with certain genotypes are exposed to sunlight. Exposure to sunlight also influences the phenotypic expression of an inherited condition called xeroderma pigmentosum (see Chapter 23 under Effects of Ultraviolet Radiation).

Internal Environmental Factors

External environmental factors can influence the internal environment and thereby influence gene expression. In addition, certain changes within an organism can lead to phenotypic changes. Age and sex influence the composition of the internal environment, and thus gene expression. Hormones are other internal environmental constituents that influence gene expression.

Much still has to be learned about the mechanism of action of hormones, but in many cases hormones bring about increased synthesis of specific enzymes or other proteins in target tissues. For example, estrogens influence protein synthesis in the uterus. It appears that at least some hormones may act, either directly or indirectly, by turning certain genes "on." Therefore varying hormone levels can influence the phenotypic expression of some genes.

Not all traits are fixed at birth; some change with age. For example, some people have light hair when they are young, but as they grow older their hair becomes dark. Some inherited disorders are not evident at birth, although the genes responsible for the conditions are present from the time of fertilization. For example, diabetes mellitus and Huntington's chorea often are not manifested until adulthood.

The fact that the phenotype depends on the age of an individual may be due to changes in gene action and/or changes in the internal environment. As mentioned in Chapter 3 (see under Control of Gene Expression), not all the genes are active at the same time. Different genes appear to be turned on or off (i.e., are active or inactive) at different times. It is not well understood what determines when particular genes are to be active. In some cases phenotypic effects at one age cause changes in the internal environment that permit other genes to be expressed. For example, changes in hormone secretion at puberty permit the expression of secondary sexual characteristics. Possibly in other cases a certain phenotypic effect that becomes evident at a later age is due to the cumulative effects of continuous action of a certain gene or genes.

Some sexual phenotypic differences are due to differences in the sex chromosome constitution. In addition, however, some traits are influenced by sex even though the responsible genes are not located in the sex chromosomes. A trait that is expressed in one sex only, although the responsible gene is present in both sexes and is not located in a sex chromosome, is called a *sex-limited trait.* An example is beard growth. Certain traits, although they occur in both sexes, are much more common in one sex than the other. These traits are said to be *sex-controlled,* or *sex-influenced.* Examples are

baldness and gout, which occur much more frequently in males than females, and congenital dislocation of the hip, which occurs more frequently in females than in males. Penetrance of the genotype for hip dislocation is apparently influenced by the normal sexual difference in the shape of the pelvis. Many sex-limited and sex-controlled traits are influenced by sex hormone levels.

SUGGESTED ADDITIONAL READING

Davidson EH: Hormones and genes. Sci Am 212(6): 36–45, 1965.

McKusick VA: The mapping of human chromosomes. Sci Am 224(4): 104–113, 1971.

5

Genetics and Disease

Human diseases can be classified as having a genetic, possibly genetic, or nongenetic etiology. *Nongenetic disorders* are caused by environmental agents, although the specific environmental factors are not always known. In some cases nongenetic disorders are of a developmental nature; that is, they result from abnormal embryonic development, but no specific genetic or environmental factor is know to be responsible. Diseases are classified as *possibly genetic* when the family history suggests a genetic component but the exact genetic basis of the condition is not known. In other cases a condition may be classified as possibly genetic when the diagnosis is uncertain. In some cases a particular condition may be caused either by genetic or environmental influences, but in the specific case in question the exact etiology has not been determined. Again, the disorder would be classified as possibly genetic.

Genetic disorders fall into three main categories: chromosomal disorders, single gene disorders, and polygenic disorders. Chromosome aberrations and polygenic disorders are discussed in this chapter; single gene disorders are discussed in Chapter 6. In addition to genetic disorders that can be categorized in this manner, there are some cases in which it appears clear that the condition has a genetic basis, but the exact genetic mechanism is not known. For example, it is not always clear whether an inherited condition has a polygenic mode of inheritance or whether it is due to a single mutant gene. Also, some inherited conditions show genetic heterogeneity. That is, in some families the condition may have one mode of inheritance, while in other families it may have a different mode of inheritance. For example, diabetes mellitus appears to be genetically heterogeneous.

No disease or condition is purely genetic. As discussed in the last chapter, genotype and environment interact to produce the phenotype. Some disorders (e.g., accidental trauma) are purely environmental. In many cases varying combinations of genetic and environmental factors interact to produce the condition (e.g., spina bifida, diabetes mellitus). In some disorders, however, the genetic component is predominant (e.g., Down's syndrome), in which case optimal environmental conditions cannot overcome the adverse effects of the genetic factor (although environment can still influence the phenotype).

A *familial* condition is one that occurs in more members of a family than would be expected by chance (i.e., the condition "runs in families"). Familial disorders may be, but are not always, genetic. In many cases they result from some common environmental factor that is affecting all or many of the members of the family.

Some, but not all, genetic disorders are apparent at birth or shortly thereafter. Not all disorders that are apparent at birth have a genetic etiology, however. The term *congenital* refers to conditions that are present at birth, regardless of their cause. Some congenital conditions are genetic, some result from an interaction of genetic and environmental influences, and some are caused by environmental influences. As mentioned previously, sometimes it is not known whether an environmental or a genetic factor is responsible for a particular congenital malformation and the condition is simply referred to as a developmental anomaly. Some congenital disorders are due to incompatibilities between mother and fetus, for example erythroblastosis fetalis (see Chapter 30 under Isoimmune Reactions).

Environmental factors can act during embryological development to cause congenital malformations. Alternatively, environmentally caused congenital conditions can be due to injury during the birth process. Environmental agents that cause physical defects in developing embryos are called *teratogens*. Known teratogens include ionizing radiation (see Chapter 23), infectious agents (particularly viruses, e.g., rubella virus; see Chapter 28), and chemicals and drugs (e.g., organic mercurials, thalidomide, amethopterin, possibly diphenylhydantoin).

CHROMOSOME ABERRATIONS

The normal human chromosome complement is described in Chapter 3. Chromosome aberrations may be numerical or structural abnormalities. Too much or too little chromosomal material usually disrupts normal development, but the exact mechanisms by which chromosomal abnormalities produce their effects are not known. Some chromosome aberrations are incompatible with life and are only seen in spontaneously aborted embryos and fetuses.

The normal chromosome complement of the gametes, in which there is one of each kind of chromosome, is called a *haploid* set, or the haploid (n) number of chromosomes. The human haploid set consists of 23 chromosomes. When two of each kind of chromosome are present (i.e., each chromosome is paired), as in somatic cells, the cells are said to possess the *diploid* (2n) number of chromosomes. Cells that have a balanced set of chromosomes, in any number (i.e., any exact multiple of the haploid number of chromosomes), are said to be *euploid*. Thus, cells containing the haploid or diploid number of chromosomes are euploid.

Types of Chromosomal Abnormalities

Numerical Abnormalities
An increase in the number of chromosomes above the diploid number in exact multiples of the haploid number is called *polyploidy*. For example, three times the haploid number (69 in human

cells) is the *triploid* (3n) number; four times the haploid number (92 in human cells) is the *tetraploid* (4n) number. These polyploid states are also euploid because the cells contain an exact multiple of the haploid number of chromosomes.

Polyploidy occurs normally in some cells of the body. Many liver cells are tetraploid. Such cells arise when duplication of the chromosomes is not followed by cell division. Polyploidy also occurs in the megakaryocytes of the red bone marrow. Polyploidy of an entire human being does not appear to be compatible with life; it is one of the most common types of chromosome abnormality found in spontaneously aborted fetuses.

Aneuploidy is a deviation from an exact multiple of the haploid number of chromosomes. In other words, it is an abnormal increase or decrease in the number of chromosomes involving less than a haploid set. *Trisomy* is an aneuploid state in which an additional (i.e., third) chromosome of one kind is present in an otherwise diploid cell. That is, the chromosome number is 2n plus 1, or 47 chromosomes in human cells. The presence of an extra chromosome in the karyotype is indicated by a plus sign followed by the number of the extra chromosome. For example, the karyotype of a male with trisomy for chromosome 21 is written as 47,XY,+21. Previously in some cases the exact chromosome could not be identified and the letter of the group was used instead of the chromosome number.

Monosomy is an aneuploid state in which one chromosome is absent from an otherwise diploid cell. In other words, the chromosome complement is 2n minus 1, or 45 chromosomes in human cells. Cells lacking an autosome are usually not viable, but cells lacking an X chromosome are often viable. The chromosome constitution 45,X produces Turner's syndrome (see below, under Sex Chromosome Abnormalities).

Three mechanisms can produce aneuploid cells. Recall from Chapter 3 that normally during meiosis I homologous chromosomes pair and then separate from each other (disjoin), with one member of each chromosome pair going to one

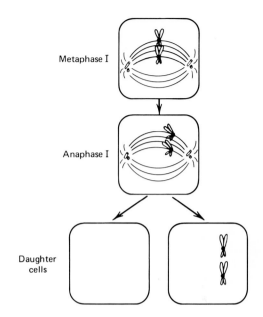

Metaphase I

Anaphase I

Daughter cells

Figure 5-1. *Failure of homologous chromosomes to pair during meiosis I produces aneuploidy.*

daughter cell and its homologue going to the other daughter cell. If two *homologous chromosomes fail to pair* during meiosis I, then by chance both chromosomes might go to one daughter cell (Fig. 5-1). As a result, one daughter cell will contain 24 chromosomes, the other 22 chromosomes. If a gamete containing 24 chromosomes unites with a normal gamete, the result will be a zygote with 47 chromosomes (i.e., trisomy). If a gamete containing 22 chromosomes unites with a normal gamete, the result will be a zygote with 45 chromosomes (i.e., monosomy).

Aneuploidy can also result from *nondisjunction*. A pair of homologous chromosomes may fail to disjoin in meiosis I, so that both members of the homologous pair go to one daughter cell and neither member of the pair goes to the other daughter cell (Fig. 5-2). Alternatively, sister chromatids may fail to separate during meiosis II (Fig. 5-3). In either case the result is one daughter cell with 24 chromosomes and one with 22 chromsomes. Failure of sister chromatids to sepa-

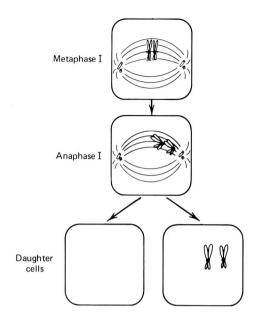

Metaphase I

Anaphase I

Daughter
cells

Figure 5-2. *Nondisjunction during meiosis I produces aneuploidy.*

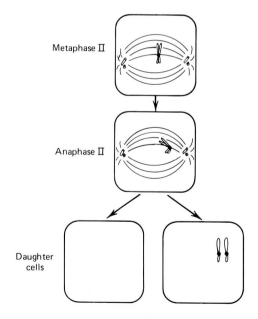

Metaphase II

Anaphase II

Daughter
cells

Figure 5-3. *Nondisjunction during meiosis II produces aneuploidy.*

rate during anaphase of mitosis is another form of nondisjunction. In this case the result will be one daughter cell with 47 chromosomes and one with 45 chromosomes. If mitotic nondisjunction occurs during the first cell division of a zygote, two aneuploid cells result, of which usually only the trisomic one is viable. The viable cell develops into an aneuploid individual. Mitotic nondisjunction occurring at the second or a later cell division may result in two viable cell lines, one having the normal diploid number of chromosomes and the other having an aneuploid number (Fig. 5-4). The presence in an individual of two or more cell lines that are karyotypically distinct and are derived from a single zygote is called *mosaicism,* and the individual is referred to as a mosaic.

Anaphase lag is the third mechanism that can produce aneuploid cells. In this case, one chromosome may not move quickly enough toward one of the poles during anaphase (i.e., it lags behing the other chromosomes). As a result, it does not get incorporated into one of the daughter cells but is simply lost. Consequently, one daughter cell will have the normal number of chromosomes, but the other will be lacking one.

Structural Abnormalities

Five types of structural abnormalities occur: isochromosomes, deletions, translocations, inversions, and duplications. The first three abnormalities are the ones most commonly seen clinically. In the karyotype nomenclature, the short arm of a chromosome is designated by "p" and the long arm by "q". An increase in length of a chromosome is indicated by a plus sign after a symbol; a decrease in chromosome length is indicated by a minus sign after a symbol. For example, a deletion from the long arm of chromosome 18 is designated 18q−.

Isochromosomes result from abnormal division of the centromere. Recall that when a chromosome duplicates, the two sister chromatids are joined at the centromere. Subsequently, during anaphase of mitosis or anaphase II of meiosis, the centromere divides longitudinally and the two sister

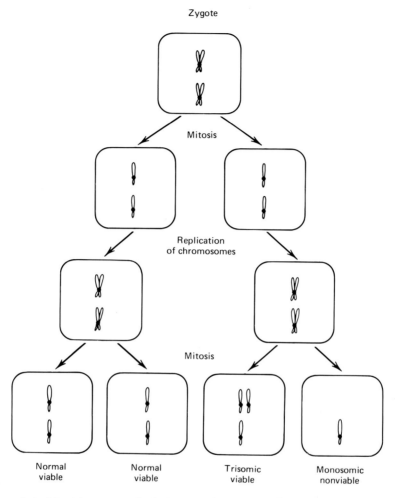

Zygote

Mitosis

Replication
of chromosomes

Mitosis

Normal
viable

Normal
viable

Trisomic
viable

Monosomic
nonviable

Figure 5-4. *Mosaicism as a result of mitotic nondisjunction at the second cell division producing two viable cell lines, one euploid and one aneuploid.*

chromatids separate. Occasionally, however, the centromere divides transversely by mistake. The resulting chromosomes are called isochromosomes; one has two long arms but no short arm, and the other has two short arms but no long arm (Fig. 5-5). Each isochromosome is equivalent to a simultaneous deletion and duplication. Thus, the presence of an isochromosome in a diploid cell results in three copies of one arm (i.e., trisomy for that arm) and one copy of the other arm (i.e.,

monosomy of one arm). In the karyotype nomenclature an isochromosome is abbreviated "i." For example, the karyotype of a male having an isochromosome of the long arm of chromosome 21 is designated 46,XY,i(21q).

Deletions result from chromosome breakage with subsequent loss of part of a chromosome. As a result, the chromosome is shorter than normal and some of the genetic material is lost. Following chromosome breakage, the ends of the fragments

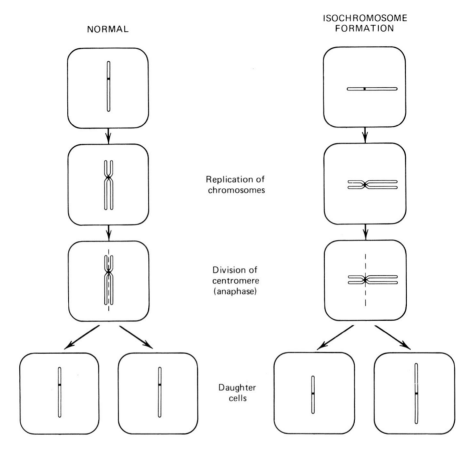

Figure 5-5. *Isochromosomes are produced when the centromere divides transversely instead of longitudinally.*

are "sticky" and tend to reunite if they remain in close proximity. If cell division occurs before the broken ends have reunited, however, the fragment without the centromere is left behind and lost when the chromosomes move to the poles, because the centromere is necessary for attachment to the spindle. Deletions are illustrated in Figure 5-6. Loss of a fragment from the end of a chromosome produces a *terminal deletion*. An *interstitial deletion* is produced when two breaks occur within an arm and the middle fragment is lost. If breaks occur near the ends of both arms of a chromosome and the terminal fragments are lost, the two arms may loop around and unite with each other to

form a *ring chromosome*. In the karyotype nomenclature a ring chromosome is indicated by "r." For example, the karyotype of a female having a deletion in the form of a ring for chromosome 5 is designated 46,XX,r(5).

A *translocation* occurs when a piece of one chromosome becomes attached to a nonhomologous chromosome. When two chromosomes break and exchange fragments, the result is a *reciprocal*, or *balanced, translocation*. This type of translocation is not harmful to the person who carries it, since the full complement of genetic material is present. When the chromosomes segregate during gametogenesis, however, the genetic material may be un-

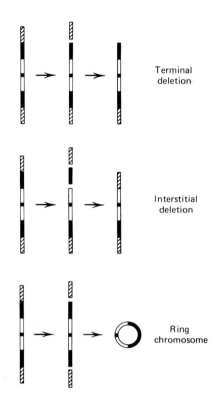

Terminal deletion

Interstitial deletion

Ring chromosome

Figure 5-6. *A deletion occurs when a chromosome breaks and a fragment is lost.*

equally distributed. As shown in Figure 5-7, six types of gametes are possible. After fertilization by a normal gamete, one of these will result in a normal zygote and one will produce another carrier. The other four will produce abnormal zygotes that have some duplication and some deficiency of chromosomal material.

In a *centric-fusion translocation,* two almost complete chromosomes fuse. This type of translocation, which mainly affects acrocentric chromosomes, is believed to result from breakage of two chromosomes near their centromeres, with subsequent joining of the two long arms at a common centromere. Presumably the short fragments are lost. Again, six types of gametes are possible, depending on how the chromosomes segregate during meiosis (Fig. 5-8). After fertilization by a nor-

mal gamete, one of these will produce a normal zygote, one will produce another carrier, two will result in monosomic zygotes, and two will result in trisomic zygotes. In the karyotype nomenclature, a translocation is indicated by "t" followed by symbols in parentheses to indicate which chromosomes and which arms are involved. For example, a centric-fusion type of translocation involving chromosomes 14 and 21 is designated t(14q21q).

An *inversion* occurs when one piece of a fragmented chromosome is put in backwards when the pieces recombine. A *duplication* is produced when a fragment of a broken chromosome attaches to the homologous chromosome. The chromosome is then longer than normal and has a section that is repeated.

Ionizing radiation, viruses, and a number of chemicals and drugs have been implicated as causes of chromosome breakage. It is believed that in most cases broken chromosomes reunite normally. Sometimes, however, deletions, translocations, inversions, and duplications occur.

Autosomal Abnormalities

Many autosomal abnormalities that produce clinical disorders are now known. As cytological techniques improve, undoubtedly more structural defects of chromosomes will become apparent and possibly some currently unexplained congenital malformations will be found to be due to chromosomal abnormalities. A description of all the known chromosome defects is beyond the scope of this book; only the more frequently encountered disorders will be presented.

Down's Syndrome
This syndrome is relatively common. Affected people usually have the karyotype 47,+21 (i.e., trisomy 21), but Down's syndrome can also result from a translocation of the long arm of chromosome 21 with a D group chromosome (usually chromosome 14). In this case the karyotype is 46,−D,+t(Dq21q). That is, the person has 46 chromosomes but is lacking one of the D group

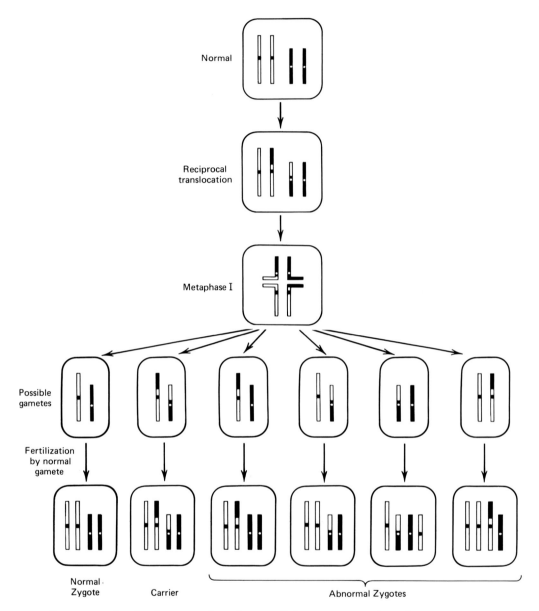

Figure 5-7. *Results of a reciprocal translocation. Following a reciprocal translocation, pairing of the translocated homologous segments produces a cross-shaped arrangement of the chromosomes at metaphase I. Depending on the way the chromosomes segregate during meiosis, six different types of gamete are possible.*

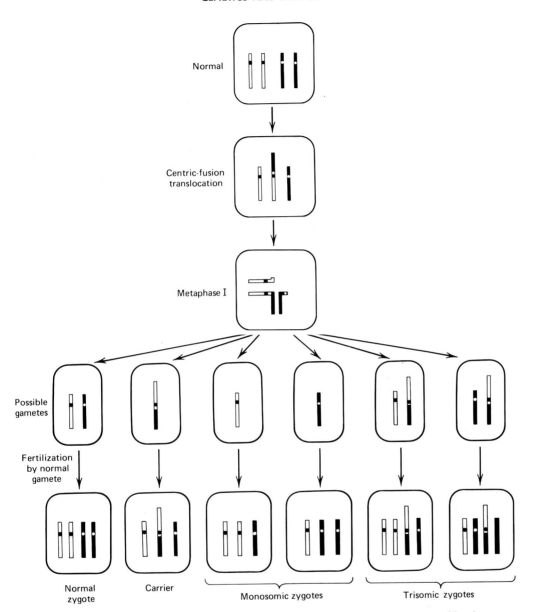

Figure 5-8. *Results of a centric-fusion translocation. Six types of gamete are possible, depending on the way the chromosomes segregate during meiosis.*

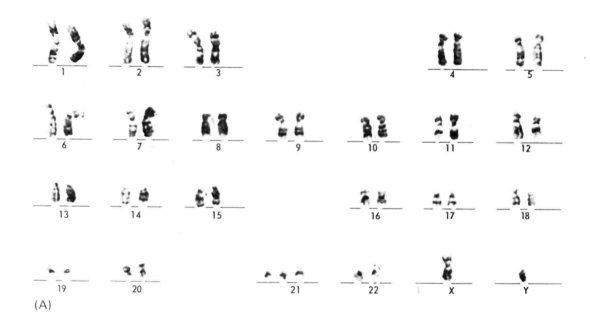

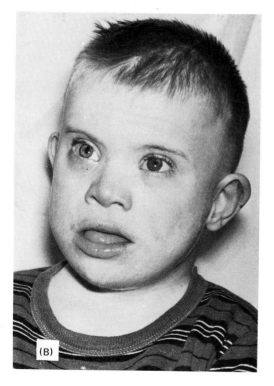

Figure 5-9. *(A) A karyotype showing trisomy 21. (Courtesy of Dr. F. J. Dill, Department of Medical Genetics, University of British Columbia, Vancouver, B.C., Canada.) (B) A child with Down's syndrome. (From Gardner EJ: Principles of Genetics, ed 5. New York, John Wiley & Sons, 1975. Courtesy of Irene A. Uchida.)*

chromosomes; in its place is a chromosome made up of the long arm of a D chromosome and the long arm of chromosome 21. The karyotype and appearance of a child with trisomy 21 are shown in Figure 5-9.

A few children have trisomy 21 mosaicism; that is, some of their cells are normal and some are trisomic. Such children may appear normal or may exhibit the classic features of Down's syndrome, presumably depending on the proportion of their cells that are trisomic.

Down's syndrome affects males and females equally and is usually recognizable at birth. The facial appearance is characteristic: the eyes have an epicanthic fold and the palpebral fissures slant slightly upward at the lateral borders. Frequently small white spots (Brushfield's spots) are apparent on the periphery of the iris. The oral cavity is small because the maxilla is small and the palate is narrow; therefore the tongue usually protrudes. The bridge of the nose is flat. The occiput is also somewhat flat. The ears are small and may be malformed.

The hands may have a simian crease (a single transverse line across the palm, formed by fusion of the proximal and distal palmar creases). The fifth finger is curved inward and the fingers are short. The first and second toes have a wide space between them and a furrow extends down the plantar surface from this gap. Congenital heart defects occur in about half the cases.

Infants with Down's syndrome have poor muscle tone and appear "floppy." Growth and development are slow and affected children are mentally retarded. Thyroid dysfunction occurs in many cases. Cryptorchism (undescended testes) is common, and adult males with Down's syndrome (except those with mosaicism) are sterile. Adult females are not sterile, however, and in cases where women with Down's syndrome have had children, about half of the offspring are also affected. This result is to be expected: since the mother's cells contain three number 21 chromosomes, when gametes are formed the chromosomes are of necessity divided unequally. Half of the gametes will receive one chromosome 21 and give rise to normal offspring, and half of the gametes will receive two number 21 chromosomes (a situation referred to as obligatory nondisjunction). When these ova are fertilized by a normal sperm, which contains one chromosome 21, trisomy 21 will result.

Trisomy 21 can result from nondisjunction occurring in the father or the mother. It is believed that trisomy 21 is due to meiotic nondisjunction in the oocyte in many cases, however, because the incidence of Down's syndrome shows a strong correlation with maternal age, but not with paternal age. Down's syndrome due to a translocation is not correlated with maternal age, but mothers over the age of 35 years have a much greater risk than younger women of having a child with trisomy 21.

One explanation for the maternal age effect is that the primary oocytes, which remain in a state of suspended meiosis for many years (see Chapter 3 under Oogenesis), are particularly vulnerable to damage by environmental agents such as viruses, x-rays, and certain chemicals that can damage the spindle or interfere with cell division in other ways. Obviously, the older a woman is, the more she will have been exposed to these harmful environmental agents. Another theory suggests that aging processes within the ovaries cause the increased incidence of nondisjunction in the ova of older women. A third possible reason for the maternal age effect is delayed fertilization, presumably due to decreased frequency of intercourse with increased age. The ovum begins to break down within about a day after it is ovulated, and it is known that fertilization occurring toward the end of this period often leads to abnormal development in animals.

Trisomy 18

This condition, which is also referred to as E trisomy (for chromosome group E) or Edward's syndrome, is the second most common disorder due to autosomal trisomy. Hypertonicity, flexion deformity of the fingers, low-set malformed ears, small chin, and prominent occiput are characteristic in this syndrome. Most affected infants have congenital heart defects. Growth and development are retarded. Affected children often die within six months, although some live for several years. A majority of the known cases of trisomy 18 are female infants. A reason for this sexual bias is not known; perhaps it reflects increased survival of affected females over affected males.

Trisomy 13 (D_1 Trisomy)

This condition, which is also called Patau's syndrome, is rare. Affected infants have multiple congenital malformations, including cleft lip, cleft palate, eye abnormalities, defects of the midface and forebrain, heart defects, urogenital defects, and polydactyly (extra fingers and toes). Development is retarded and affected infants fail to thrive. Death usually occurs during the first year.

Cri-Du-Chat (5p−) Syndrome

This syndrome is due to a deletion from the short arm of chromosome 5. It affects females more often than males. The name cri-du-chat (cat-cry) syndrome is based on the fact that affected infants have a plaintive mewing cry that sounds like a kitten in distress. The physical features of this syndrome are not as striking as those of the autosomal trisomies. The head is small and the eyes are widely spaced. About half of the affected infants have congenital heart defects. Mental retardation occurs in all cases.

Trisomy 8 Mosaicism

Most cases of trisomy 8 are mosaics, having one normal cell line and one aneuploid cell line. The karyotype is designated 46/47,+8. The trisomy presumably results from mitotic nondisjunction during early embryonic development.

Trisomy 8 mosaics usually have a variety of skeletal abnormalities involving the vertebrae and the joints. The patellae are frequently absent and the chest is long and narrow. Deep skin furrows are evident on the soles of the newborn. Deep-set eyes and strabismus are common. The ears are abnormal and the neck is webbed. Renal abnormalities also occur. Affected children are mildly to moderately mentally retarded.

In Chapter 3 it was stated that lymphocytes are usually used for karyotype analysis. With trisomy 8 mosaicism, however, the proportion of aneuploid lymphocytes may be low and often more than one tissue is examined for karyotype. The cells most commonly studied are skin fibroblasts obtained by skin biopsy.

Sex Chromosome Abnormalities

Numerical aberrations of the sex chromosomes are relatively common; and many types have been observed, including XO, XXX, XXXX, XXXXX, XXY, XXXY, XXXXY, XXYY, and XXXYY. Some structural aberrations of the X chromosome have also been observed. The most common sex chromosome disorders are Klinefelter's syndrome, which is due to the 47,XXY karyotype; and Turner's syndrome, which is due to the 45,X karyotype.

The sex chromosome constitution is determined quite simply. Cells are scraped from the buccal mucosa, spread on a slide, fixed, and stained appropriately. This "buccal smear" is then viewed with a microscope to reveal the presence or absence of Barr bodies in the nuclei of the cells. (Barr bodies are discussed in Chapter 3 under Heterochromatin and Euchromatin.) All but one of the X chromosomes in each cell are heterochromatinized. Therefore, the number of X chromosomes equals the number of Barr bodies plus one. Thus, a normal female has one Barr body; a person with the karyotype 45,X has no Barr body, nor does a normal male. Two Barr bodies indicate three X chromosomes.

In Chapter 3 it was stated that heterochromatinization of one X chromosome occurs randomly. That is, either X chromosome in a normal female has an equal chance of being inactivated. Thus, in some cells the maternally derived X chromosome is heterochromatinized, while in other cells the paternally derived X chromosome is heterochromatinized. When a structural abnormality of one X chromosome is present, however, it has been observed that the abnormal X chromosome is always the one that is heterochromatinized.

The number of Y chromosomes is determined by staining the cells with a fluorescent dye such as quinacrine and observing the number of "fluorescent Y bodies" in the nucleus of each cell. The number of Y chromosomes is equal to the number of fluorescent Y bodies.

Klinefelter's Syndrome

Klinefelter's syndrome is due to a 47,XXY chromosome complement. Occasionally, however, individuals with the apparent karyotype 46,XX show signs of Klinefelter's syndrome. This unusual situation may be due to a translocation between the X and Y chromosome occurring in the germ cells of the father.

People with Klinefelter's syndrome are phenotypically male and appear normal during childhood. The condition is rarely detected in infancy or childhood unless survey studies of karyotype are done. Klinefelter's syndrome becomes evident in adolescence and young adulthood due to inadequate sexual development. The testes remain small and an affected individual is sterile. Body hair is sparse. Enlargement of the breasts (gynecomastia) occurs in about 25% of cases. Intellectual development is usually fairly good, although less than that of siblings.

Turner's Syndrome

Turner's syndrome, or ovarian dysgenesis as it is sometimes called, is due to the 45,X karyotype. Affected people are phenotypically female, but the cells do not show a Barr body. The ovaries are abnormal, affected people are sterile, and secondary sexual characteristics fail to develop. Intelligence is usually within the normal range, although less than that of siblings.

People with Turner's syndrome have a short stature and a shield-shaped chest with widely spaced nipples. These people often have epicanthic folds, a narrow maxilla, a small chin, and a "sharklike" mouth with curved upper lip and straight lower lip. The ears are usually low-set and prominent. Webbing of the neck occurs in about 50% of the cases.

Short fourth and fifth metacarpals, cubitus valgus (a deformity in which the elbow deviates away from the midline of the body when the arm is extended with the palms facing forward), and tibial exostosis (a benign bony growth projecting outward from the surface of the tibia) are other features that may be exhibited in Turner's syndrome. Lymphedema of the hands and feet is common during infancy but disappears later. About 35% of affected people have cardiovascular abnormalities, of which coarctation of the aorta is the most common.

Another condition, called the Ullrich-Noonan syndrome, is phenotypically similar to Turner's syndrome but affected people have normal female (46,XX) or normal male (46,XY) karyotypes. Some affected females are fertile. Affected males usually have cryptorchism and most are infertile. People with Ullrich-Noonan syndrome frequently have ptosis (drooping of the upper eyelid) and hypertelorism (a wide space between the eyes); these signs only rarely occur in Turner's syndrome. Another difference between the two syndromes is the type of cardiovascular anomaly. In Ullrich-Noonan syndrome the most common cardiovascular abnormality is pulmonary valve stenosis; coarctation of the aorta is uncommon. The opposite is true for Turner's syndrome. Ullrich-Noonan syndrome is believed to be due to an autosomal dominant gene.

X Chromosome Inactivation

In Chapter 3 it was stated that the condensed (i.e., heterochromatinized) X chromosome in each cell, as represented by the Barr body, is genetically inactive. If only one X chromosome is active in each cell, why do people with the karyotypes 47,XXY and 45,X have abnormal phenotypes? Two hypotheses have been put forward. Heterochromatinization of all but one X chromosome in each cell takes place at about the 16th day of gestation. Even though ovarian differentiation takes place after this time, it is possible that some effect is produced during the first 16 days that persists after X chromosome inactivation takes place. The second possibility is that the heterochromatinized X chromosome is not completely inactive; portions of it may remain genetically active.

POLYGENIC DISORDERS

Many disorders have a polygenic hereditary component. That is, the condition is determined by the cumulative effects of many genes. Each gene has a small positive or negative influence and the exact number of genes involved is not known. Development of a polygenic disorder depends on interaction between hereditary and environmental factors (i.e., the disorder is multifactorial), but the adverse environmental influences that contribute to the development of the abnormal phenotype are not always known.

The sum of the genetic and the environmental constituents that make a person more or less likely to develop a given condition is called the *liability* of the person. If a person's liability exceeds a critical value, called the *threshold,* the pathological condition is manifested. The liabilities of the individuals in a population have a normal distribution pattern. Affected people represent a small fraction of the population at one end of the distribution curve in whom the total number of "risk" genes plus environmental influences exceeds the threshold liability (Fig. 5-10).

It is not possible to tell where a person is on the liability-distribution curve. If a couple has an affected child, however, it is probable that they are carrying more than the average number of risk genes, since they must have passed on to the child a relatively large number of genes for liability.

Therefore, the risk will be greater than average that future children of this couple will also be affected.

A person with a small number of risk genes is unlikely to manifest the disorder unless exposed to very adverse environmental conditions. For a person with a large number of risk genes, however, few adverse environmental factors will be necessary to put him or her over the threshold liability. Also, the greater the number of risk genes a person has, the more severe the manifestations of the condition will be. Many polygenic disorders occur more frequently in one sex than the other. Presumably the sex with the lower incidence of the condition has a higher threshold and requires more risk genes before the condition is manifested.

Polygenic Congenital Malformations

A variety of congenital malformations involving a single organ system or tissue are inherited as polygenic traits. Not all cases of these malformations are due to polygenic inheritance; in some cases the disorder may be part of a syndrome caused by a chromosomal aberration, a single gene defect, or a teratogen.

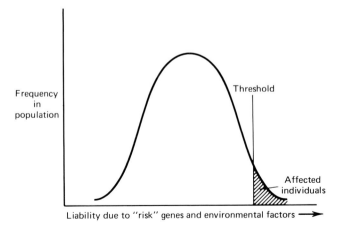

Figure 5-10. *With polygenic disorders, affected people represent a small fraction of the population at one end of the distribution curve in whom the total number of "risk" genes plus environmental factors exceeds the threshold liability.*

Specific disorders that can have a polygenic mode of inheritance include *cleft palate* and/or *cleft lip*. Cleft palate as a polygenic disorder affects females more often than males. Conversely, cleft lip occurs more frequently in males than females.

Anencephaly, encephaloceles, myelomeningoceles, and certain forms of spina bifida can be polygenic traits. These conditions are different manifestations of the same basic genetic disorder and can be collectively referred to as *neural tube defects*.

Congenital heart disease can be inherited as a polygenic disorder, although it can also occur as a component of many other disorders due to other causes. Polygenic congenital heart disease is about equally common in males and females.

Pyloric stenosis is a fairly common congenital disorder that occurs more frequently in males than females. In this condition hypertrophy of the muscular layer of the pylorus obstructs passage of food from the stomach to the duodenum. The hypertrophied pyloric muscle may be detected at birth by palpation of an epigastric mass, but often the condition is not recognized until the infant continually vomits after feedings.

Congenital hip dysplasia, or congenital dislocation of the hip, affects females more often than males. Two genetic effects, acetabular dysplasia and laxity of the joint capsule, predispose to hip dislocation. Acetabular dysplasia seems to have a polygenic mode of inheritance. Two specific environmental influences associated with hip dislocation are breech birth and tight swaddling after birth. Swaddling of the infant with legs extended and adducted favors hip dislocation, whereas carrying the infant in a sling with hips flexed and abducted decreases the likelihood of dislocation. *Clubfoot* (talipes equinovarus) is another type of polygenic congenital malformation. This condition affects males about twice as often as females.

Other Polygenic Traits

A number of conditions that are manifested later in life appear to have a polygenic mode of inheritance. Arteriosclerotic heart disease, atopic allergies (see Chapter 30), and schizophrenia are believed to be polygenic inherited disorders. Many researchers consider essential hypertension (high blood pressure; see Chapter 13) to have a polygenic mode of inheritance, although some researchers contend that this condition is due to a single dominant gene. Diabetes mellitus probably has more than one mode of inheritance, including a polygenic one (see Chapter 18).

SUGGESTED ADDITIONAL READING

Friedmann T: Prenatal diagnosis of genetic disease. *Sci Am* **225**(5): 34–42, 1971.

Mittwock U: Sex differences in cells. *Sci Am* **209**(1): 54–62, 1963.

Taussig HB: The thalidomide syndrome. *Sci Am* **207**(2): 29–35, 1962.

6

Single Gene Defects

This chapter is concerned with hereditary disorders due to an alteration in a single gene. As discussed in Chapter 3, the sequence of bases in the DNA determines the sequence of amino acids in a polypeptide chain. According to the properties of the particular amino acids in the polypeptide, one or more polypeptides then fold into a three-dimensional structure to become a functional protein. A change of even one amino acid may alter the structure and function of the protein. By changing the bases in the DNA the code words are altered and a polypeptide with a different sequence of amino acids may be produced. The result is often a defective protein that either has an altered function or is nonfunctional. In other words, if the gene is defective or altered, the gene product (protein) will also be altered. If an entire gene has been deleted the body cells will not be able to produce the protein normally coded by that gene.

SICKLE CELL ANEMIA: DISEASE RESULTING FROM A SINGLE BASE CHANGE

One of the best-understood changes caused by mutation is the alteration in the structure of hemoglobin that causes sickle cell anemia. The hemoglobin molecule consists of a protein attached to the iron-containing pigment heme. The protein portion of normal adult hemoglobin (Hb A) is made up of four polypeptide chains: two alpha (α) and two beta (β) chains. The α chains contain a known characteristic sequence of 141 amino acids, the β chains a known sequence of 146 amino acids. People with sickle cell anemia have an abnormal hemoglobin (Hb S). The difference between Hb A and Hb S is a change of one amino acid. Hb A contains glutamic acid in position 6 of the β chain, whereas in Hb S this position is occupied by valine. The sequence of the other 145 amino acids is identical. Glutamic acid is coded by the messenger RNA triplet GAA and its complementary DNA codon CTT. A single base change in the DNA produces the codon CAT and its complementary messenger RNA triplet GUA, which codes for valine and produces Hb S (Fig. 6-1). By changing this one amino acid, the properties of the hemoglobin molecule are altered. The Hb S molecules are less water soluble than normal

hemoglobin and interact with each other in such a way that they form linear aggregates and become stacked up. This stacking of the Hb S molecules occurs especially if the oxygen concentration is low, as in venous blood, and causes the red blood cells to become elongated and sickle-shaped (Fig. 6-2). Sickled red blood cells cause an increase in the blood viscosity, impede blood flow in the venules, and may block small blood vessels. Impaired blood flow in turn leads to thrombus formation and tissue infarction (see Chapter 7). The abnormal shape of the sickled red blood cells causes them to be broken down more rapidly than normal red blood cells, resulting in hemolytic anemia (see Chapter 10). People with the homozygous genotype for Hb S have a severe anemia; this condition is called sickle cell disease. Heterozygous individuals have some abnormal Hb S and some normal Hb A. Therefore their anemia is not as severe and the condition is referred to as sickle cell trait.

Sickle cell disease usually manifests itself when a child is 2 to 3 years old, as Hb S gradually replaces

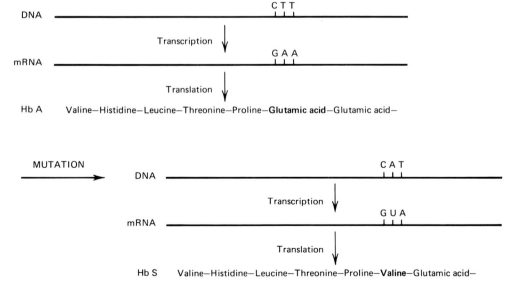

Figure 6-1. *A single base change in the DNA causes a change of one amino acid in the β chain of the hemoglobin molecule and produces hemoglobin S.*

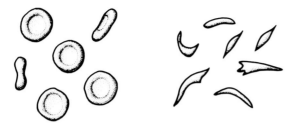

Normal red blood cells   Sickled red blood cells

Figure 6-2. *Normal red blood cells are biconcave discs. In sickle cell anemia the red blood cells are elongated and deformed.*

the fetal hemoglobin (Hb F). In addition to the usual symptoms of severe anemia (see Chapter 10), the person may be jaundiced. "Sickle cell crises" occur periodically, during which there is sudden exacerbation of the anemia accompanied by pain, usually in the abdomen. Splenomegaly (enlargement of the spleen) is common in children with the disease. In adults splenomegaly is not found because congestion of splenic tissue by sickled red blood cells causes hypoxic tissue damage and eventually causes the spleen to become fibrotic and shrunken. Hepatomegaly (liver enlargement) is characteristic. Other clinical manifestations depend on which areas are most severely affected by thromboses and hypoxia. Damage to the heart, liver, and kidneys is common. There is an inability to concentrate urine normally, presumably due to altered circulation in the renal medulla. Leg ulcers often occur, due to hypoxia of the subcutaneous tissues. The prognosis is poor: many victims die in childhood and few people with sickle cell disease live beyond 30 years of age. Those with sickle cell trait, however, usually do not manifest symptoms unless they are exposed to abnormally low oxygen tensions, such as may occur at high altitudes or in unpressurized aircraft. Sickle cell anemia is a dramatic example of how a single base substitution in the DNA can cause systemic manifestations of a disease.

People with Hb S appear to be resistant to malaria. A fairly high incidence of sickle cell anemia occurs in areas such as Africa, where malaria is common. Evidently, the protection against malaria offered by the heterozygous condition (trait) more than counterbalances the severe effects of the less frequently occurring homozygous condition, so that the abnormal gene persists in the population with a relatively high frequency. In North America, where malaria is not a problem and sickle cell trait has no adaptive advantage, sickle cell anemia occurs much less frequently.

Another abnormal hemoglobin, hemoglobin C (Hb C), is the result of a different mutation in the same codon as the mutation that produces Hb S. In people with Hb C, the DNA codon is altered to TTT, which corresponds to the messenger RNA base triplet AAA and codes for the amino acid lysine. Therefore Hb C has lysine instead of glutamic acid at position 6 of the β chain. Hb C does not cause sickling of the red blood cells; it produces only a mild hemolytic anemia in the homozygous condition. The genes for Hb S and Hb C are allelic with each other, however, and double heterozygotes can occur (i.e., the genotype SC). People with hemoglobin SC disease have a hemolytic anemia that is almost indistinguishable from sickle cell disease because the second abnormal hemoglobin interacts with the Hb S, producing sickling of the red blood cells.

INBORN ERRORS OF METABOLISM

Many metabolic pathways, each consisting of a series of biochemical reactions occurring in a particular sequence, are involved in the functioning of cells. Each reaction is catalyzed by an enzyme. Under the conditions of temperature, pressure, and concentrations of reactants that exists in cells, these reactions are unable to proceed without the enzyme catalyst. Therefore, the enzymes that are present in a cell will determine the functions of the cell. All enzymes are proteins, which means they are produced according to the message in the

DNA of the genes. Other proteins are vital to metabolism because they are necessary for transporting substances across cell membranes. Many proteins circulate in the blood, serving various functions and influencing metabolism. All these proteins are gene products. As stated previously, if a gene is altered, the gene product will also be altered. When the altered gene product interferes with normal metabolic functioning the resulting condition is called an *inborn error of metabolism*.

Inborn Errors Due to Blocked Metabolic Pathways

Many inborn errors occur because the defective gene product is an enzyme that normally catalyzes one step in a major metabolic pathway. When an enzyme is lacking or nonfunctional, the particular reaction normally catalyzed by that enzyme is effectively stopped. The result is a block in the metabolic pathway. These blockages can produce pathophysiological manifestations by several mechanisms (Figs. 6-3 and 6-4). It should be pointed out that while the major manifestations of a blocked metabolic pathway may be due to one particular mechanism, in many cases more than one of these mechanisms are involved in the production of the signs and symptoms of an inborn error of metabolism.

Conditions Caused by Accumulation of Toxic Precursor

Suppose a metabolic reaction that involves the conversion of a precursor substance A to a product B is catalyzed by an enzyme *a*. Because of a genetic defect, enzyme *a* is nonfunctional or lacking.

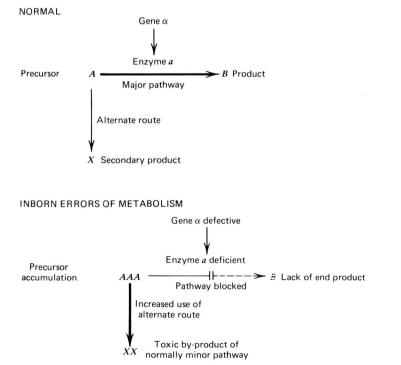

Figure 6-3. *Mechanisms by which a block in a metabolic pathway can produce the manifestations of an inborn error of metabolism.*

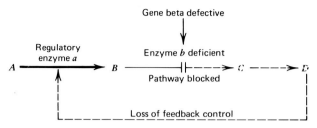

Figure 6-4. *A block in a metabolic pathway can result in a loss of feedback inhibition of a metabolic pathway. (See also Figure 1-3.)*

Substance A then cannot be converted to B and so it accumulates in the tissues. Substance A may be toxic in large quantities and a pathological condition results when this precursor accumulates. Examples of this mechanism are alkaptonuria and galactosemia, two autosomal recessive inherited disorders.

In *alkaptonuria*, the defect involves a pathway for the breakdown of the amino acid tyrosine (Fig. 6-5). In the normal reaction sequence tyrosine is converted to hydroxyphenylpyruvic acid, which in turn is converted to a substance called homogentisic acid. Homogentisic acid is converted to maleylacetoacetic acid, which is then further ca-

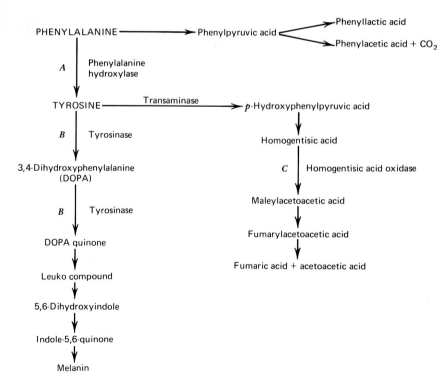

Figure 6-5. *Pathways for the metabolism of phenylalanine and tyrosine, showing the sites of enzyme defects in various inborn errors of metabolism. A. Phenylketonuria. B. Albinism. C. Alkaptonuria.*

tabolized. In alkaptonuria the enzyme that normally catalyzes the conversion of homogentisic acid to maleylacetoacetic acid (homogentisic acid oxidase) is absent. As a result, homogentisic acid accumulates in the tissues, particularly cartilage, and is excreted in the urine. Oxidation of homogentisic acid causes it to turn black, so that cartilaginous tissues acquire a characteristic dark tinge and the urine turns black on standing. Accumulation of homogentisic acid in cartilaginous tissues is associated with the development of arthritis in people with alkaptonuria. The manifestations of this condition usually are not apparent before 30 years of age.

Galactosemia results from a block in the major pathway for metabolism of the sugar galactose. Galactose is a monosaccharide that can be converted to glucose in a three-step process:

1. Galactose + ATP $\xrightarrow{\text{galactokinase}}$ Gal-1-P + ADP
2. Gal-1-P +
   UDPG $\xleftarrow{\text{Gal-1-P uridyl transferase}}$ UDPGal + G-1-P
3. UDPGal $\xrightarrow{\text{UDPGal-4-epimerase}}$ UDPG

In the first step, galactose receives a phosphate group from adenosine triphosphate (ATP); that is, the galactose is phosphorylated, to form galactose-1-phosphate (Gal-1-P). Normally in the second step, Gal-1-P and uridine diphosphate glucose (UDPG) react to form uridine diphosphate galactose (UDPGal) and release glucose-1-phosphate (G-1-P). The UDPGal is then converted to UDPG. The enzymes necessary to carry out these reactions are normally present in the liver, brain, and blood cells. In people with galactosemia, however, the enzyme that is necessary to catalyze the reaction in the second step (Gal-1-P uridyl transferase) is inactive or absent. As a result, galactose and galactose-1-phosphate accumulate in the tissues. In an untreated person, the amount of Gal-1-P in the erythrocytes may be as high as 20 to 100 mg/100 ml, as compared with 0 to 3 mg/100 ml in a treated person. A major source of galactose is the breakdown of the disaccharide lactose, which is in milk. Therefore, signs and symptoms of galactosemia usually develop two to three days after an affected infant starts milk feedings. Presenting signs and symptoms vary, but vomiting and/or diarrhea, with subsequent failure to thrive, occurs commonly. Signs of abnormal liver function, such as jaundice and an enlarged liver (hepatomegaly), are frequent because accumulation of Gal-1-P interferes with normal function of the liver. As galactose levels increase in the blood (galactosemia), hypoglycemia may occur because a reciprocal relationship exists between the levels of glucose and galactose in the blood. Excessive galactose may be excreted in the urine (galactosuria). Protein may also appear in the urine because the accumulation of Gal-1-P in the kidneys interferes with normal renal function. Excessive galactose is metabolized by an alternate route to form galactitol, which is trapped in the lens of the eye. This excess galactitol leads to degeneration of the lens fibers and development of cataracts several weeks after birth. If galactosemia is not treated promptly by a galactose-free diet, accumulation of Gal-1-P in the brain may interfere with normal metabolism in the brain and cause mental retardation.

Conditions Caused by Toxic By-Product(s) of Normally Minor Pathway(s)

Usually more than one pathway is available for the metabolism of a substance: a major metabolic pathway and one or more minor secondary routes. Therefore, if the major pathway is blocked, some of the precursor substance may accumulate, but most of it may take an alternate route instead. So, for example, if substance A cannot be converted to B it might be converted to substance X. Normally only small amounts of X are formed, but now large quantities of this compound are produced. These excessive amounts of substance X are toxic and are responsible for the manifestations of the disease. An example is the development of cataracts in galactosemia, as just described. Phenylketonuria (PKU) is another example.

Phenylketonuria, which is inherited as an autosomal recessive trait, is caused by a deficiency of an enzyme that is necessary for metabolism of the amino acid phenylalanine. PKU is associated with abnormal development of the central nervous system and destruction of myelin, which becomes manifest three to six months after birth. Neurological symptoms such as hyperactivity, muscular hypertonicity, hyperactive reflexes, speech difficulties, problems with control of voluntary muscles, tremors, and seizures commonly develop. Abnormal electroencephalograms (EEGs) occur in most cases. Mental retardation usually results.

Normally in the body most of the phenylalanine, if it is not incorporated into protein, is converted to tyrosine for further metabolism. In PKU there is decreased activity of the enzyme phenylalanine hydroxylase, which catalyzes this reaction, and so this pathway is blocked (Fig. 6-5). Serum phenylalanine levels may rise to 20 mg/100 ml or higher (normally there is less than 3 mg/100 ml). Moderately elevated levels of phenylalanine alone, however, do not necessarily cause permanent brain damage. Alternative pathways for metabolism of phenylalanine exist, which are now utilized to a greater extent than normal. Much of the phenylalanine is deaminated to form phenylpyruvic acid. Normally only small amounts of phenylpyruvic acid are formed, but in PKU there are large amounts. Some of the phenylpyruvic acid is further metabolized to phenyllactic acid and phenylacetic acid. Although the exact mechanism(s) for the abnormal neurological development and mental retardation in PKU is not known, these compounds could interfere with metabolism in the brain by many possible ways. In addition, the high concentrations of these acids in the body fluids cause metabolic acidosis and result in their excretion in the urine. The presence of phenylacetic acid causes the urine to have a characteristic "mousy" odor. When ferric chloride is added to the urine it reacts with the phenylpyruvic acid, giving a green color. This reaction is the basis of an early diagnostic test used in screening infants for PKU. (Current screening methods usually involve determination of blood levels of phenylalanine). Children with PKU often have blond hair and a fair complexion, because tyrosine is necessary for formation of the pigment melanin.

The blockage in the conversion of phenylalanine to tryosine decreases the amount of tyrosine that is available.

Conditions Caused by Lack of End Product

When a metabolic pathway is blocked, obviously the end product of that reaction sequence will be lacking unless it can be obtained from another source. In other words, if A cannot be converted to B, there will be no B unless it can be obtained from another metabolic pathway or from the diet. The consequences of the lack will depend on the function of the end product. Albinism and cretinism are examples of conditions caused by the deficiency of an end product of a blocked metabolic pathway.

Albinism is caused by impaired production of melanin from tyrosine (Fig. 6-5). The first two steps in the production of melanin involve the conversion of tyrosine to dihydroxyphenylalanine (DOPA) and its subsequent oxidation to form DOPA-quinone. Both reactions are catalyzed by the same enzyme, tyrosinase. Although there are several forms of albinism with different genetic patterns of inheritance, classic albinism (type I) is inherited as an autosomal recessive trait and is presumably due to a deficiency of the enzyme tyrosinase. The condition is expressed as hypopigmentation of the skin, hair, and eyes due to a lack of the end product melanin. Exposure to light results in burning instead of tanning in people with albinism. Photophobia and visual impairment occur because of the melanin deficiency in the eye.

Cretinism results from a congenital lack of thyroid hormone (thyroxine), which can have a number of causes (see Chapter 19). In some cases, a defective enzyme in the pathway for the synthesis of thyroid hormone results in a deficiency of this end product.

Conditions Caused by Loss of Feedback Inhibition

In many metabolic reaction sequences the end product of the pathway regulates its own produc-

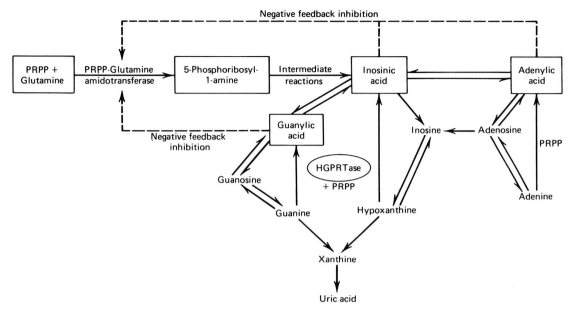

Figure 6-6. *Purine metabolism. In Lesch-Nyhan syndrome the enzyme HGPRTase is defective; therefore, conversion of guanine to guanylic acid and hypoxanthine to inosinic acid is blocked.*

tion by a negative feedback control mechanism (see Chapter 1). Take, for example, a series of reactions in which A is converted to B, which subsequently forms C; C is then converted to D. High concentrations of D then inhibit the enzyme that converts A to B. As a result, less end product is formed and gradually the concentration of D falls. With the decreased amount of D, inhibition on the first step is released, so that more A can be converted to B and consequently more D can be formed again. If there is a block in the pathway at step B to C, there will be a lack of the end product D and therefore nothing to inhibit the reaction A to B. As a result, B will accumulate and may or may not be metabolized by an alternative pathway. An example of this mechanism is a defect in the pathway of purine metabolism (Fig. 6-6), which results in the bizarre manifestations of Lesch-Nyhan syndrome.

The purine ribonucleotides guanylic acid, adenylic acid, and inosinic acid are necessary for the formation of nucleic acids. The purine ribonucleotides can be formed in two ways. The nucleotides can be synthesized de novo from small precursor molecules through a series of steps. The first complete purine ribonucleotide to be formed is inosinic acid, which can then be converted to adenylic acid and guanylic acid. Alternatively, in the presence of 5-phosphoribosyl-1-pyrophosphate (PRPP), preformed purine bases from the diet or from cellular catabolism can be converted to their respective nucleotides. This process requires the enzyme hypoxanthine-guanine phosphoribosyl transferase (HGPRTase) to catalyze the transfer of ribose-5-phosphate from PRPP to the free bases in the formation of guanylic acid and inosinic acid. (A different enzyme catalyzes the conversion of adenine to adenylic acid.) Both this process and the pathway for de novo synthesis are inhibited by the same purine nucleotide end products.

In *Lesch-Nyhan syndrome* there is an absence of HGPRTase, an increased de novo synthesis of purines, and overproduction of uric acid. As a result of the HGPRTase deficiency, less guanylic acid and inosinic acid will be formed. The increased de novo synthesis of purines may result from decreased feedback inhibition of the first reaction in the sequence, due to decreased production of guanylic acid. (This mechanism is only one of several that have been postulated to account for the increase in de novo purine synthesis. Some controversy exists as to which of the possible mechanisms is in fact operating in this case). Hypoxanthine and guanine can also be converted to uric acid. Therefore, when the pathway for formation of mononucleotides from these substances is blocked, as occurs in HGPRTase deficiency, large amounts of uric acid are formed from the hypoxanthine and guanine.

As a result of this increased production of uric acid, high levels of uric acid in the blood (hyperuricemia) and increased urinary excretion of uric acid occur. The high concentration of uric acid in the urine leads to formation of urate crystals and calculi (stones). In an affected infant the initial manifestations of this condition are often increasing irritability and colic due to the passage of urate gravel and stones. The calculi may cause obstruction. Microscopic or gross hematuria often occurs. The increased load of uric acid to be excreted may lead to polyuria, which is accompanied by polydipsia (excessive thirst) to compensate for the excessive fluid loss. These clinical manifestations may occur by 2 months of age. Dehydration and metabolic acidosis may also occur. Gout may eventually develop due to the excess of uric acid.

Neurological and behavioral manifestations are also characteristic of Lesch-Nyhan syndrome. The neurological abnormalities develop progressively from birth and include choreoathetosis (involuntary irregular movements and repetitive slow gross movements), spastic cerebral palsy, and developmental retardation. Striking behavioral features of this syndrome are aggressiveness and compulsive self-mutilation. Affected children tend to mutilate themselves by biting the lips, tongue, and hands. These children welcome restraints that protect them against self-destruction and will sometimes ask for them. The mechanism by which a deficiency of HGPRTase interferes with normal brain

functioning is not known. Possibly a deficiency of an important purine nucleotide or overproduction of an intermediate compound is responsible.

Another mechanism of regulation of the end product does not involve feedback inhibition of the first step in the reaction sequence, but involves inhibition of a substance that stimulates that metabolic pathway. This type of feedback inhibition is involved in the control of hormone production. For example, tropic hormones from the adenohypophysis such as thyrotropin and adrenocorticotropin (ACTH) stimulate production of thyroid hormone and hormones of the adrenal cortex, respectively. High levels of these hormones will, in turn, inhibit production of the tropic hormones. As a result there will be less stimulation of the target glands and less production of thyroid hormone and adrenocortical hormones. If the target gland is unable to produce its hormone because of a defective enzyme in the necessary metabolic pathway, there will be nothing to inhibit production of the tropic hormone. Examples of conditions caused by this mechanism are the goiter of familial hypothyroidism (see Chapter 19) and adrenogenital syndrome.

As mentioned previously, an inherited defect in the pathway for synthesis of thyroxine will result in a deficiency of that end product and produce cretinism (familial hypothyroidism). Associated with this condition is enlargement of the thyroid gland (goiter). The goiter results from the loss of end product (thyroxine) inhibition of thyrotropin production by the adenohypophysis. In other words, there is no thyroxine available to inhibit production of thyrotropin by the adenohypophysis and consequently large quantities of thyrotropin are released. Thyrotropin stimulates all the activities of the thyroid gland. The thyroid gland is unable to produce thyroxine, but it is able to secrete large amounts of thyroglobulin (colloid) into the follicles; thus the gland grows larger and larger.

In *adrenogenital syndrome* there is a genetic lack or decrease of the enzyme 11-hydroxylase, which is necessary for the production of the hormone cortisol by the adrenal cortex. Cortisol normally inhibits the release of ACTH by the adenohypophysis. When the level of cortisol is decreased, as occurs in 11-hydroxylase deficiency, the normal negative feedback control is lost. As a result excessive ACTH is produced and continues to stimulate the adrenal cortex. The adrenal cortex produces many hormones and the pathways for their syntheses are interrelated (see Chapter 19). Therefore, excessive amounts of other adrenocortical hormones, particularly androgens, are produced due to this loss of feedback inhibition. The excessive production of androgens causes masculinization. If this condition occurs in a female infant the clitoris is enlarged and there may be posterior labial fusion at birth, so that the child is mistakenly thought to be male (pseudohermaphroditism). Progressive virilization occurs but may not become obvious until the child is about 2 years of age.

In male infants at birth the external genitalia usually appear normal, although there may be enlargement of the penis or increased pigmentation of the genitals. Starting between 1 and 2 years of age progressive virilization occurs, but the testes retain their infantile size. This condition is sometimes referred to as pseudosexual precocity.

In untreated children of both sexes increased muscular development and rapid linear growth occur due to the excessive androgens. The accelerated growth is associated with an increased rate of skeletal maturation, leading to early closure of the epiphyses. Therefore, although the person may be taller than average for his or her age during early childhood, the final height achieved may be less than normal for an adult.

Hypoglycemia may occur because of the deficiency of cortisol. Surprisingly it does not occur very often, presumably because of the ability of other homeostatic mechanisms to control the blood glucose level.

Inborn Errors Due to Defective Membrane Transport

Many substances cannot simply diffuse across cell membranes, but require a protein-carrier molecule to transport them from the exterior of a cell to the inside. Epithelial cells lining the small intestine and the proximal convoluted tubules of the kidney nephrons, in particular, have the ability to transport essential substances across the cell membrane. This ability is important in the absorption of nutrients by the intestine and in the selective reabsorption of essential substances by the kidneys in the process of urine formation. A number of inherited disorders involve malabsorption of various substances. These disorders are presumably due to a defect in the protein-carrier molecule, which results in impairment of the membrane transport function.

One example is a condition called *cystinuria*, which has an autosomal recessive mode of inheritance. In this case, there is a defect in the transport mechanism for the amino acid cystine in the proximal renal tubules. Thus large amounts of cystine are excreted in the urine instead of being reabsorbed. When the concentration of cystine is greater than 30 mg/100 ml of urine, the cystine crystallizes and forms stones. The usual manifestations of renal lithiasis result (see Chapter 21). The condition is often complicated by urinary tract infections. Some people with cystinuria never manifest symptoms, while others have multiple stone formation starting in early childhood. These individual differences seem to reflect differences in dietary patterns and fluid intake. The peak age of onset of symptoms is the third decade of life.

Not only cystine, but also lysine, arginine, and ornithine are excreted in excessive quantities in cystinuria. Apparently these amino acids share a common transport mechanism. Lysine, arginine, and ornithine are much more soluble than cystine, however, and their presence in the urine does not appear to cause pathological manifestations.

Another example of an inborn error caused by defective membrane transport is *glucose-galactose malabsorption*. This condition is also inherited as an autosomal recessive trait and involves faulty transport of glucose and galactose by the intestinal cells. As a result, these sugars cannot be absorbed into the body, but are lost in the stool. The presence of these sugars in the intestinal lumen creates an osmotic effect that interferes with the absorption of water and results in severe diarrhea. The diarrhea begins shortly after birth and is accompanied by signs of irritability, abdominal distension, and crampy abdominal pain. Vomiting frequently occurs, as do the usual fluid and electrolyte disturbances that result from vomiting and diarrhea. Hypoglycemia occurs due to the inability to absorb glucose and galactose. Generally there is failure to thrive. When sources of glucose, galactose, and lactose (a disaccharide that yields glucose and galactose on digestion) are removed from the diet the diarrhea subsides. The infant thrives when fructose is substituted as the dietary carbohydrate.

Inborn Errors Due to Deficient or Abnormal Circulating Proteins

Many proteins circulate in the blood. These plasma proteins are genetically determined and have many functions. Alteration of some of these proteins may have no significant effect on a person as a whole. In other cases, depending on their functions, alteration of circulating proteins can have serious results. A few examples are given below.

A genetic deficiency of thyroxine-binding globulin causes a reduction in the serum protein-bound iodide but has no apparent effect on metabolic function. This trait is governed by a gene on the X chromosome.

Blood clotting requires several protein clotting factors that are genetically determined. An inherited defect of one or more of these factors causes hemophilia and results in a tendency to bleed. (See Chapter 7 for a discussion of blood clotting and hemophilia.) Classic hemophilia (type A) is a sex-linked recessive trait characterized by defective clotting factor VIII. Hemophilia B (Christmas disease) also has a sex-linked recessive pattern of inheritance. In this condition the defect is in clotting factor IX. Another condition, vascular hemophilia (von Willebrand's disease), has an autosomal dominant mode of inheritance. Like classic hemophilia it involves factor VIII. In von Willebrand's disease this clotting factor is absent, whereas in hemophilia A an altered, nonfunctional form of factor VIII is present. Following transfusions of plasma or factor VIII, synthesis of factor VIII is stimulated in people with von Willebrand's disease, but not in those with hemophilia A. The structural gene that codes for the factor VIII protein appears to be located on the X chromosome, but possibly a regulator gene that controls synthesis of factor VIII is located on an autosome. The differences between hemophilia A and von Willebrand's disease might be explained on this basis. In hemophilia A the defect is in the structural gene, whereas in von Willebrand's disease the defect could be in the regulator gene. (See Chapter 3 for a discussion of structural and regulator genes.)

A number of blood lipid disorders are described in Chapter 18. One of these, β-lipoprotein deficiency (a-β-lipoproteinemia), is inherited as an autosomal recessive trait and characterized by reduced amounts of circulating β-lipoprotein. β-Lipoprotein is involved in the transport of triglycerides in the blood. Therefore, when it is lacking, transport of triglycerides from the liver and the intestinal tract is impaired. Chylomicron formation by the intestinal mucosal cells is decreased. Triglycerides accumulate in the intestinal mucosa and interfere with further absorption of lipids. Plasma concentrations of cholesterol, phospholipid, and triglyceride are decreased.

The earliest manifestations of this condition begin in infancy and result from malabsorption of lipids. Following ingestion of increased amounts of fat, steatorrhea occurs. Steatorrhea is commonly accompanied by abdominal discomfort, and vomiting may occur. Secondary deficiencies of minerals and vitamins, particularly A and E, may result (see Chapter 17). Symptoms of fat malabsorption often subside as the child becomes older and learns to avoid excessive fat in the diet.

Lipids are major components of myelin. Thus, degenerative and demyelinating changes in the spinocerebellar tracts, posterior columns, and peripheral nerves result from the disturbed lipid metabolism in β-lipoprotein deficiency. The first manifestation of these degenerative changes is weakness, especially of the legs, during childhood. Eventually ataxia and marked disability occur. Proprioceptive functions are affected and sensitivity to pain and thermal stimuli is decreased. In late adolescence visual complications occur, manifested by blurred vision, scotomas, impaired dark adaptation, and possibly loss of sight.

Another characteristic of a-β-lipoproteinemia is an abnormality of red blood cell structure called acanthocytosis, which is caused by a disturbance in the lipid component of the cell membrane. As a result of the abnormal structure, increased breakdown of red blood cells occurs and the sedimentation rate is low.

Vitamin-Dependent Inborn Errors

Many vitamins are used by the body to form coenzymes. A coenzyme is an organic molecule that acts as a cofactor in an enzymatic reaction and is necessary for the enzyme to function. Some genetically determined metabolic disorders affect a reaction involving a vitamin as a coenzyme. Often these conditions can be overcome by administering large doses of the particular vitamin. When this is the case, the condition is called a vitamin-dependent inborn error of metabolism. Several possible mechanisms underlie these conditions. The vitamin may not be transported into a specialized cell. Or perhaps an enzyme necessary for conversion of the vitamin to its active coenzyme is defective or lacking. In other cases the coenzyme may not be able to bind properly to the enzyme with which it works.

An example of a vitamin-dependent inborn error of metabolism is cystathioninuria; this disorder is believed to have an autosomal recessive mode of inheritance. In this condition there is an alteration in the specific portion of the enzyme cystathionase where binding of the active coenzyme, pyridoxal phosphate, normally occurs. Cystathionase, with its coenzyme, catalyzes the conversion of the amino acid cystathionine to cystine. In cystathioninuria this reaction cannot proceed normally, and large amounts of cystathionine are excreted in the urine. The active coenzyme, pyridoxal phosphate, is derived from vitamin B_6. Administration of large amounts of this vitamin partially overcomes the metabolic block in this condition. A consistent clinical picture of cystathioninuria has not yet evolved. It is a rare defect, and the clinical manifestations of the few reported cases are varied.

Inborn Errors of Drug Metabolism

After a drug is absorbed into the body it may be excreted unchanged, but often it undergoes structural alteration before being excreted (see Chapter 25). This structural alteration changes the pharmacological activity of the drug and may affect its rate of excretion from the body. The metabolism of drugs in this manner depends on biochemical reactions catalyzed by enzymes. If an enzyme involved in the metabolism of a drug is defective or lacking due to a genetic defect, the result will be an inborn error of drug metabolism (pharmacogenetic disorder). Such a condition will be manifested only if the person is stressed by administration of the particular drug.

An example of an inherited disorder of drug metabolism is the inability to hydrolyze (break down) succinyldicholine, a muscle relaxant often used during general anesthesia. The condition is due to an abnormality of serum pseudocholinesterase. Three abnormal variants of this enzyme are known, which appear to have an autosomal recessive mode of inheritance. The three mutant genes are allelic with one another and with the normal allele, therefore several genotypes are possible. One mutant, referred to as the "silent" allele, is responsible for complete or almost complete absence of pseudocholinesterase activity. If this mutant occurs in the homozygous state (a rare occurrence) or in combination with one of the other mutant alleles, the person has extreme sensitivity to succinyldicholine. Normally the drug is inactivated very rapidly in the liver, but affected people may experience prolonged muscle relaxation, or paralysis or respiratory arrest for several hours, following succinyldicholine administration. There are no apparent manifestations of this condition when the drug is not administered.

Another genetic condition involves the metabolism of isoniazid (INH), a drug used in the treatment of tuberculosis. In some people ("rapid inactivators"), INH is quickly removed from the blood and excreted in the urine in an acetylated form. Other people ("slow inactivators") excrete the drug unchanged and it remains in the blood for a prolonged period of time. Slow inactivators have decreased activity of the enzyme acetyl-coA transferase in the liver. This condition is inherited as an autosomal recessive trait. Acetyl-coA transferase is involved not only with transferring the acetyl group onto INH but also in acetylation of drugs such as sulfamethazine and sulfadiazine.

Isoniazid is an antagonist for pyridoxine (vitamin B_6). Therefore, slow inactivators of INH are more likely than rapid inactivators to develop neurotoxic side effects following prolonged administration of the drug. Concurrent administration of large doses of pyridoxine with INH will prevent the development of peripheral neuropathy.

SUGGESTED ADDITIONAL READING

Allison AC: Sickle cells and evolution. *Sci Am* **195**(2): 87–94, 1956.

Linehan MS: Sickle cell anemia—the painful crisis. *J Emerg Nurs* **4**(6): 12–19, 1978.

Reyzer N: Diagnosis: PKU. *Am J Nurs* **78**(11): 1895–1898, 1978.

UNIT THREE

PHYSICAL RESPONSE TO TISSUE INJURY

7

Hemostasis

The integrity of the circulatory system is critical in maintaining homeostasis. Any breaks that occur in the blood vessels must be quickly sealed to prevent excessive loss of blood. The body has three mechanisms working together to halt the flow of blood from a damaged blood vessel: constriction of the blood vessel; formation of a platelet plug; and formation of a blood clot (coagulation). The arrest of bleeding by these physiological means (or by surgical means) is called *hemostasis*.

The blood contains not only factors that bring about clotting but also factors that prevent blood from clotting (anticoagulants). These factors are necessary to ensure that the blood does not solidify within the blood vessels. Normal hemostasis represents a balance between the factors that promote coagulation of the blood and those that prevent coagulation. If this balance is upset, excessive bleeding (hemorrhage) or excessive, inappropriate platelet aggregation and clotting (thrombosis) may occur.

NORMAL HEMOSTASIS

Many factors are required for normal hemostasis. A smooth endothelial lining and adequacy of the supporting structures within and around the blood vessels are necessary. A rough endothelium contributes to the formation of abnormal intravascular clots. Abnormal or inadequate connective tissue support of blood vessels leads to a bleeding tendency.

Platelets (thrombocytes) are essential for hemostasis and have several functions. They form a plug that immediately fills the gap in a blood vessel until a clot can be formed; they release vasoactive substances that cause constriction of the injured blood vessel; and they release factors that contribute to the clotting process. In addition, platelets may contribute to the support and maintenance of the endothelial lining of blood vessels. Platelets are small cytoplasmic fragments formed from large multinucleated cells called megakaryocytes. In an adult, megakaryocytes are found mainly in the red bone marrow. Not all the platelets circulate; about one-third are stored in the spleen. The platelet count in peripheral blood normally is about 150,000 to 350,000/mm³. It is believed that old or damaged platelets are removed from the blood by the reticuloendothelial system.

Calcium ions are required for hemostasis. They are necessary for platelet aggregation and also participate in several stages of the clotting process. The addition of citrate to blood collected for laboratory tests or for transfusion prevents clotting because citrate binds calcium ions so they are not available for clotting reactions (i.e., citrate is a chelating agent). Oxalate is another chelating agent sometimes used to prevent blood samples from clotting, but it is not used in blood for transfusion because of its toxicity.

Many protein (or glycoprotein) clotting factors are essential for the clotting process. These substances circulate in the blood plasma in an inactive form and become activated with the initiation of the clotting process. Some of the activated factors act as enzymes, which then activate other factors. Researchers working in different parts of the world assigned different names to the various plasma clotting factors. Now by international agreement, however, the clotting factors are designated by Roman numerals (Table 7-1). The Roman numerals are usually used for factors V through XIII but factors I through IV are still most

Table 7-1. Blood Clotting Factors

Factor	Alternative Names
I	Fibrinogen
II	Prothrombin
III	Tissue factor, thromboplastin
IV	Calcium ions
V	Proaccelerin, accelerator globulin, Ac-globulin, labile factor
VII	Proconvertin, autoprothrombin I, serum prothrombin conversion accelerator (SPCA), stable factor
VIII	Antihemophilic factor (AHF), antihemophilic globulin (AHG), platelet cofactor I, antihemophilic factor A
IX	Christmas factor, antihemophilic factor B, plasma thromboplastin component (PTC), platelet cofactor II, autoprothrombin II
X	Stuart-Prower factor
Xa	Activated factor X, thrombokinase, autoprothrombin C
XI	Plasma thromboplastin antecedent (PTA), antihemophilic factor C
XII	Hageman factor, surface factor
XIII	Fibrin stabilizing factor

often called by their common names. There is no factor designated VI. Factor I is fibrinogen; factor II, prothrombin; factor III is called thromboplastin or tissue factor; and number IV is assigned to calcium ions.

Fibrinogen, prothrombin, factors V, VII, IX, and X, and possibly factors XI and XIII are synthesized in the liver. The synthesis of prothrombin and factors VII, IX, and X requires vitamin K. The site of synthesis of factor XII is not known. Factor VIII synthesis appears to be associated with macrophages of the spleen, but lymphocytes and bone marrow may also be involved.

Phospholipid substances also take part in the clotting process. These are derived from platelets and from damaged tissue.

In addition to the clotting factors present in the blood, a number of substances present in the blood and other tissues inhibit blood clotting. These substances may neutralize or destroy various clotting factors or they may interfere with some clotting reaction without actually destroying any clotting factor. The plasma anticoagulants include several antithrombins as well as inhibitors of other clotting factors. A substance called plasminogen (profibrinolysin) is present not only in plasma but also in smaller amounts in all body fluids and secretions. Plasminogen can be activated to form plasmin (fibrinolysin), which breaks down both circulating fibrinogen and the fibrin of clots. Another naturally occurring anticoagulant is heparin. Most body tissues contain heparin, but the highest concentrations are in the liver and the lungs. Heparin inhibits the conversion of prothrombin to thrombin and also interferes with the thrombin-fibrinogen reaction.

Blood normally does not clot within the blood vessels for several reasons. As just mentioned, many anticoagulants are naturally present. In addition, the flow of blood dilutes the concentration of any clotting factor that may become activated. Also, as the blood passes through the liver any activated clotting factors are removed by liver cells. Another contributing factor may be the net negative charge present on the surface of blood cells, platelets, and blood vessel endothelium. Since like charges repel one another, this surface charge inhibits platelets from adhering to the endothelium and forming clumps. Some substances that have anticoagulant effects apparently increase the net negative charge on platelets and endothelium. Other substances, which promote clotting, tend to decrease the repelling force.

When a blood vessel is torn or cut, platelets stick to the exposed subendothelial surface and simultaneously a series of events designed to arrest the flow of blood is initiated: (1) vasoconstriction; (2) formation of a platelet plug; and (3) clot formation.

Blood Vessel Contraction

Damage to the wall of an artery or vein initiates a vasoconstrictive reflex. Afferent nerve impulses travel to the spinal cord and efferent impulses in sympathetic nerve fibers bring about contraction of the blood vessel wall extending several centimeters on either side of the injury. The spasm is strong enough to completely stop blood flow for several minutes. This neurogenic vasospasm is followed by vasoconstriction due to humoral factors (i.e., factors present in the blood or other body fluids). The exact cause of this humoral vasoconstrictive effect is not known, but it is possibly mediated by epinephrine, which is released by the platelets; or it could be that norepinephrine is released from the damaged tissues. In any case, this humoral vasospastic effect may last as long as an hour, which provides ample time for the formation of a clot to check the flow of blood.

The walls of capillaries have no muscle fibers. Following damage, however, contraction of the precapillary sphincters occurs and temporarily arrests bleeding from the capillary beds.

Formation of a Platelet Plug

The cohesion or sticking of platelets to surfaces other than platelets or endothelium is called *platelet adhesion.* When a blood vessel is injured a layer of platelets adheres to exposed subendothelial tissue components, particularly collagen and a collagenlike material in the vascular basement membrane. This reaction does not require calcium ions. After platelet adhesion to subendothelial surfaces, other circulating platelets stick to the already adhered platelets. This sticking of platelets to each other is called *platelet aggregation.* Platelet aggregation requires fibrinogen, calcium ions, and adenosine diphosphate (ADP). Several substances, including collagen, thrombin, serotonin, epinephrine, and some fatty acids will cause platelet aggregation. These agents either induce the local accumulation of ADP and/or bring about the release of endogenous ADP from the platelets. ADP causes the platelets to change their shape from smooth discs to spheres with extending pseudopodia of various lengths. The exact significance of the change in shape is not known, but presumably it facilitates platelet aggregation in some way. If the ADP concentration is low, disaggregation may occur; if it is high enough, aggregation continues and is enhanced by the release of endogenous platelet ADP. Aggregation continues until large clumps of platelets plug the opening in the blood vessel. Sometimes, if the opening in the blood vessel is small, the formation of a platelet plug is sufficient to stop bleeding and a clot does not form.

When platelet aggregation occurs a number of substances are released from the platelets. In addition to the ADP already mentioned, several factors that influence coagulation are released, including a phospholipid substance (platelet factor 3) and a substance that antagonizes the effect of heparin.

Several drugs inhibit aggregation and the concomitant release of substances from the platelets. They are phenothiazine and imipramine derivatives and nonsteroid antiinflammatory drugs such as phenylbutazone and acetylsalicylic acid (aspirin). The mechanism of this inhibition is not known.

Clot Formation

The coagulation process involves several factors that interact with one another. According to the present conception of coagulation, the process involves a cascade effect. In this scheme, initiation of the clotting process is brought about by activation of one of the clotting factors. This activation triggers a stepwise series of reactions in which one activated factor activates the next factor in the series, which in turn activates another factor, and so on. Ultimately this process leads to the conversion of prothrombin to thrombin. As a result of this cascade effect, activation of a few molecules of the initiating factor can quickly lead to the formation of large amounts of thrombin because each molecule of active factor acts on many molecules of the next factor in the series. Thrombin then catalyzes the conversion of soluble fibrinogen to insoluble fibrin. Strands of fibrin form a network around the platelets and trap red blood cells (Fig. 7-1). The result is a solid clot.

Two important interrelated mechanisms can lead to the formation of a fibrin clot; they appear to function simultaneously in the coagulation of blood in the body, although they can be separated in laboratory tests and experiments. The *intrinsic clotting mechanism* (or system or pathway) uses only factors present in the plasma. The *extrinsic clotting mechanism* involves tissue factors as well as plasma components. Clot formation occurs more quickly with the extrinsic mechanism because it bypasses several of the reactions found in the intrinsic pathway. The pathways for intrinsic and extrinsic clotting are summarized in Figure 7-2.

Intrinsic Clotting

The intrinsic clotting mechanism is apparently initiated when factor XII comes in contact with a surface such as collagen or vascular basement membrane (or outside the body with a surface such as glass). Somehow this contact triggers the activation of factor XII to form XIIa. Factor XIIa converts a substance called prekallikrein to kallikrein.

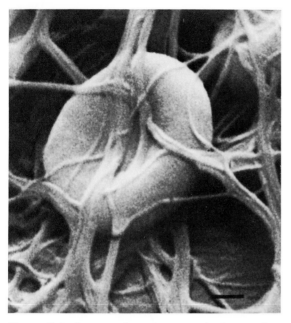

Figure 7-1. *Scanning electron micrograph of an erythrocyte enmeshed in fibrin. (Courtesy of Emil Bernstein and Eila Kairinen, Gillette Company Research Institute, Rockville, Maryland. Cover photo, Science **173**, August 27, 1971. Copyright 1971 by the American Association for the Advancement of Science.)*

Kallikrein is important in activating the kinin system, which is involved in inflammation (see Chapter 8). In addition, however, kallikrein will activate more factor XII. Thus a positive feedback cycle occurs in which activation of small amounts of factor XII cause formation of kallikrein, which in turn activates more factor XII. Activated factor XII (XIIa) then converts factor XI to its active form (XIa). Factor XIa in turn activates factor IX to form IXa. This reaction requires calcium ions. Activation of factor IX may also be brought about by a factor present in the platelets. Factor IXa interacts with factor VIII in some way to form a complex, which activates factor X in the presence of platelet phospholipids and calcium ions. Active factor X (Xa) forms a complex with factor V. This complex, in the presence of calcium ions and

phospholipid, catalyzes the conversion of prothrombin to thrombin. Thrombin increases the clotting activity of factor VIII and also apparently activates factor V. Primarily, however, thrombin acts as an enzyme that converts fibrinogen to fibrin and also activates factor XIII to form XIIIa. Both these reactions require calcium ions. Thrombin also triggers the release of substances from the platelets.

In the formation of fibrin, small pieces (fibrinopeptides) are split off the end of the fibrinogen molecule. The remaining portion of the molecule is called the fibrin monomer. Many fibrin monomers immediately form fibrin polymers by hydrogen bonding; these polymers are weak and are easily dissolved. The fibrin polymer strands are strengthened, however, by the action of factor XIIIa, which catalyzes the formation of peptide bonds between adjacent fibrin strands, resulting in a strong cross-linkage. This cross-linkage stabilizes the clot.

Extrinsic Clotting

When injury occurs, a lipoprotein called tissue factor (factor II) is released from the damaged tissue. Tissue factor interacts with factor VII in some way to activate factor X. The process from this point is the same as intrinsic clotting. Activated X, together with factor V and in the presence of phospholipid and calcium ions, converts prothrombin to thrombin. Thrombin then causes the conversion of fibrinogen to fibrin.

It seems that both the intrinsic and the extrinsic clotting systems are necessary for normal hemostasis. The nature of the interaction between the extrinsic and intrinsic mechanisms, however, is not known at this time.

Clot Retraction

Soon after the clot is formed it begins to shrink, expressing clear serum as it does so. This process, called *clot retraction,* is brought about by the platelets. Platelets contain a contractile protein, thrombasthenin, which is similar to the acto-

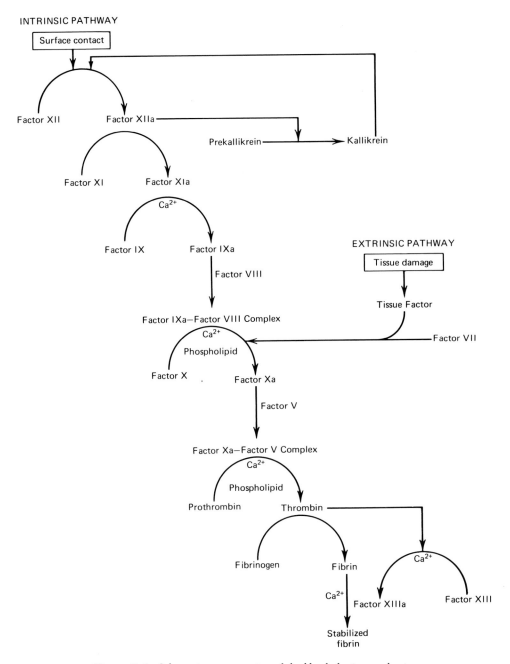

Figure 7-2. *Schematic representation of the blood clotting mechanism.*

myosin of muscles. During clot formation the platelet pseudopodia become attached to the fibrin strands. Subsequently the platelet pseudopodia contract, drawing the fibrin threads together and making a more compact clot. Presumably the function of clot retraction is to pull the edges of an injured blood vessel closer together and thus promote hemostasis.

Fibrinolysis

In addition to the clotting components present in blood there are substances that promote dissolution of clots. Dissolution, or breakdown, of clots is called *fibrinolysis*. It is brought about by plasmin (fibrinolysin), an enzyme present in plasma. Plasmin not only breaks down fibrin but also fibrinogen, clotting factors V and VIII, and several other substances. Plasmin is present in the blood mainly in an inactive precursor form called plasminogen (profibrinolysin).

Several plasminogen activators are present in the body fluids and tissues. The plasminogen activator present in plasma is believed to be released from vascular endothelial cells. Plasminogen activator is also present in red blood cells. The tissue plasminogen activators are probably concentrated in the lysosomes of cells. Plasminogen activators are not found in the liver or the placenta, but occur in other tissues. The prostate, uterus, thyroid, lungs, heart, ovaries, adrenal glands, and lymph nodes contain especially high amounts of plasminogen activator. A plasminogen activator called urokinase is secreted by the kidneys and is present in urine. Presumably its function is to prevent fibrinous deposits from accumulating in the urinary tract and occluding the ducts. Milk, tears, saliva, bile, and seminal fluid also contain plasminogen activator. Perhaps this plasminogen activator functions in keeping small excretory ducts patent. Some bacteria secrete plasminogen activators. The best known of these is streptokinase, which is secreted by streptococci.

Plasma contains antiplasmins that inhibit plasmin activity. Platelets also contain antiplasmin. In addition, there are substances in plasma that inhibit the activation of plasminogen. Many factors influence fibrinolysis. At the present time the regulation of this process is not completely known.

Plasminogen has an affinity for fibrin and during clot formation plasminogen adheres to the fibrin as it is laid down. When plasminogen activator is released into the circulation it diffuses slowly into the clot and converts plasminogen to plasmin, which then breaks down the fibrin. If activator is present as well as plasminogen when the clot is formed, fibrinolysis occurs much more rapidly. For some unknown reason, clots usually become quite resistant to fibrinolysis after about five to seven days. Presumably the action of clotting factor XIIIa in stabilizing the fibrin is a major reason.

Breakdown of circulating fibrinogen or dissolution of fibrin clots by plasmin releases fibrinogen and fibrin degradation products (FDP) into the circulation. These FDP have an anticoagulant effect. The FDP form complexes with fibrin monomers and thus interfere with the polymerization of fibrin monomers into a fibrin strand. Clots that do form in the presence of FDP have an abnormal structure and are weak. FDP also interfere with platelet function and thrombin activity.

It has been hypothesized that a dynamic equilibrium exists between blood clotting and fibrinolysis not only to maintain an intact vascular system but also to maintain the patency of the blood vessels. In this case the clotting mechanism may be constantly operating to seal any gaps that occur in the endothelium. At the same time the fibrinolytic system is constantly operating to remove deposits of fibrin after they have served their function. Interactions occur between the clotting mechanism and fibrinolysis. Activated clotting factor XII activates plasminogen in addition to initiating intrinsic clotting. Stress and exercise increase fibrinolytic activity; they also increase the plasma level of clotting factor VIII and the number of circulating platelets.

Many factors influence fibrinolytic activity. As just mentioned, stress and exercise increase fibrinolysis. Exercise in the evening causes a greater increase in fibrinolytic activity than does exercise in the morning. Fibrinolytic activity exhibits a circadian rhythm, being higher during the day than at night. This rhythm is not just a consequence of greater activity during the day because the effect is also noticed in people immobilized in bed. Fibrinolytic activity appears to be greater in elderly people than in the young, and greater in females than in males. Fibrinolytic activity is decreased in obese people. Increased body temperature promotes fibrinolysis.

During normal pregnancy fibrinolytic activity decreases and the amount of many plasma clotting factors increases, particularly toward the end of pregnancy. This alteration may be a protective mechanism to prevent excessive bleeding when the placenta separates at the time of delivery. Fibrinolytic activity returns to normal 15 to 60 minutes after placental separation. The cause of the reduced fibrinolytic activity during pregnancy and its subsequent return to normal is not known. A strong possibility, however, is that the placenta produces substances that inhibit fibrinolysis.

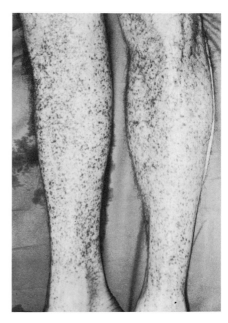

Figure 7-3. *Petechiae. (Photograph courtesy of Dr. J. Burton, Vancouver General Hospital, Vancouver, British Columbia, Canada.)*

BLEEDING DISORDERS

Hemorrhage is the escape of blood from the blood vessels. It may be the result of rupture of a blood vessel or abnormal permeability of the capillaries allowing the passage of red blood cells through intact vessels in the absence of visible injury. Rupture of blood vessels may be caused by mechanical trauma or may occur spontaneously due to disease of the blood vessel walls.

Very small hemorrhages into intradermal or submucous tissues give rise to *petechiae*: perfectly round, pinpoint, nonraised purplish red spots. Slightly larger (up to 1 cm) brownish-red discolorations of the skin caused by hemorrhage into the tissues are called *purpura*. The term purpura also refers to a group of disorders characterized by these hemorrhages. Larger hemorrhagic spots in the skin or mucous membranes are called *ecchymoses*. They

appear as nonelevated, rounded or irregular blue or purplish patches. Petechiae are shown in Figure 7-3. A massive localized collection of blood within a tissue is called a *hematoma*.

An increased tendency to bleed occurs if platelets are defective or lacking, if clotting factors are deficient, or if vascular structural components are abnormal. Conditions characterized by excessive bleeding may be inherited or may be acquired secondarily to other disorders.

The hemostatic mechanism can be considered to have two phases: (1) vasoconstriction and platelet adhesion and aggregation; (2) the clotting process and formation of a fibrin network. Defects of the first phase are usually characterized by excessive bleeding immediately after an injury, but once bleeding is controlled it usually does not restart. Defects of the second phase of hemostasis are not usually associated with abnormal bleeding immediately after injury but are characterized by delayed bleeding. In these cases bleeding tends to recur hours or even days after the initial injury and may persist for weeks.

Platelet Abnormalities

Thrombocytopenia

The most common platelet disorder is *thrombocytopenia,* a decrease in the number of circulating platelets. Thrombocytopenia may be due to decreased production of platelets, decreased survival time of platelets, sequestering of platelets in the spleen, or dilution with platelet-poor blood.

Platelets are destroyed during storage of blood. Therefore if a person receives massive blood transfusions, the existing platelets in that person's blood will be diluted.

A number of diseases are associated with splenomegaly (enlargement of the spleen): for example, Gaucher's disease, miliary tuberculosis, and Hodgkin's disease. In these conditions the enlarged spleen is congested with blood and fewer platelets are available in the general circulation.

Decreased platelet survival may occur if there is excessive consumption of platelets, such as occurs in disseminated intravascular coagulation (see below). More often, however, it is associated with immune mechanisms. *Idiopathic thrombocytopenic purpura* (ITP) is the most common form of thrombocytopenia due to overdestruction of platelets. ITP occurs mainly in children and young women, and is generally believed to be due to the occurrence of antibodies against the platelets, probably as a result of an autoimmune reaction. (Autoimmunity is discussed in Chapter 30.) Other autoimmune diseases (e.g., systemic lupus erythematosus) are also associated with thrombocytopenia. In addition, thrombocytopenia due to immune reactions may occur following acute infections or as a result of drug sensitivity. Quinine, quinidine, and digitoxin are among the drugs that have been implicated.

Decreased production of platelets can be due to failure of development of the megakaryocytes. This failure is sometimes congenital but is more often acquired as a result of bone marrow depression by drugs, chemicals, or ionizing radiation. It may also occur secondarily to chronic renal disease. Malignant disease of the bone marrow (e.g., leukemia) also causes failure of platelet production. Platelet production is also impaired by deficiency of vitamin B_{12} or folic acid.

When the platelet count falls below about 100,000/mm³, a person may manifest a bleeding tendency roughly proportional to the degree of thrombocytopenia. It appears that platelets normally function constantly to seal any small gaps that may occur in the capillary wall. Therefore, in thrombocytopenia, bleeding is usually from the capillaries rather than from large vessels. An affected person bruises readily and commonly has petechiae and purpura on the skin and mucous membranes. Spontaneous bleeding from the nose, the gingiva, the gastrointestinal tract, or the genitourinary tract may occur. Menorrhagia is a common problem in women with thrombocytopenia.

Abnormal Platelet Function

Bleeding disorders due to abnormalities of platelet function are not as common as thrombocytopenia, but do occur. *Thrombasthenia* (Glanzmann's disease) is a rare hereditary disorder in which the platelet count is normal but the platelets do not aggregate normally, resulting in a long bleeding time. This condition is also associated with impaired clot retraction. Thrombasthenia becomes manifest in early childhood. Trivial injuries lead to the development of bruises and ecchymoses. Superficial cuts and abrasions have a tendency to bleed excessively and epistaxes (nosebleeds) are common. Menorrhagia is a serious problem for women with this condition.

The term *thrombopathia* is applied to another group of rare hereditary bleeding disorders in which platelet adhesion and aggregation are defective due to a failure of release of substances from the platelets. Affected people usually have only a minor bleeding tendency characterized mainly by superficial bruising and ecchymoses.

Impaired platelet function occurs secondarily to a wide variety of diseases (e.g., liver disease) and after ingestion of various drugs (e.g., aspirin). In uremia there is often a bleeding tendency due to impaired platelet adhesion and aggregation and nonavailability of platelet phospholipids. Presumably a retained metabolite causes these abnormalities, since the bleeding tendency in uremia can be corrected by dialysis.

Deficient Clotting Factors

Hemophilia

Hemophilia is the name given to a group of inherited disorders characterized by a bleeding tendency due to lack of a plasma clotting factor. Classic hemophilia (type A) is the most common and is due to a defect of factor VIII. Hemophilia B (Christmas disease) is due to a deficiency of factor IX and occurs about one-fifth as frequently as hemophilia A. Both hemophilia A and B are inherited as sex-linked recessive disorders and so affect males primarily. Females are rarely affected but can be carriers of the gene. (For a discussion of sex-linked inheritance see Chapter 4.) The severity of the bleeding tendency in hemophilia varies. Not only the condition, but also the degree of severity, is inherited. Hemophilia C is a much more rarely diagnosed condition caused by a deficiency of factor XI; it is transmitted as an autosomal trait and so occurs equally in males and females. Although probably more common than hemophilia A, it often goes unrecognized.

It was once thought that people with hemophilia A were lacking factor VIII, but it is now known that they have normal amounts of a structurally abnormal factor VIII. As a result of the structural abnormality of this protein it has less functional activity. Factor VIII is associated with the intrinsic clotting mechanism, therefore bleeding in hemophilia A occurs primarily in the joints, muscles, kidneys, and subcutaneous tissues, which do not have the tissue thromboplastin of the extrinsic system.

Hemophilia A usually does not become manifest during the first three to six months of life, although the condition is present at birth. If an affected infant is circumcised, however, the bleeding tendency may become apparent at that time. Usually the first signs of hemophilia are bruises about the head or buttocks when the child begins to crawl. When the teeth erupt the child may bite his tongue or lips, with subsequent persistent bleeding from these sites.

Hemarthroses (hemorrhages into joints) are the most common clinical manifestation of hemophilia and may occur following exercise or physical exertion. Severely affected people may have spontaneous hemorrhages into deep muscles and joints, whereas those who are mildly affected do not bleed into joints and muscles although they still bleed after trauma. Hemorrhages into the joints of a moderately or severely affected child with hemophilia usually occur first when the child begins to walk. The knees and ankles are affected most, and later the elbows become involved. Hemarthroses are extremely painful and are damaging to the joint structure. Joint deformity and crippling may result. In addition, atrophy of bones and muscles occurs due to the immobilization that is necessitated by the hemarthroses.

Hemorrhages into muscles also occur and can be very painful. Large hematomas in the muscles may cause pressure on nerves, resulting in transient motor or sensory loss. Crippling may occur due to fibrosis and contractures if muscle tissue is damaged by the hemorrhages. Intramuscular injections can cause hemorrhage and therefore cannot be given unless the person is receiving treatment with antihemophilic globulin.

Both midly and severely affected people with hemophilia may manifest hematuria. It apparently occurs spontaneously, without prior infection or injury, and may continue for days or weeks. The next most common clinical manifestation is gastrointestinal bleeding. In many cases such bleeding occurs without any evidence of ulceration.

Hemorrhage into the central nervous system is

rare in hemophilia, but is extremely serious when it does occur. It usually results from some trauma.

Many people with hemophilia have noticed that their bleeding tendency shows seasonal fluctuations, being worse at one time of the year than at another. The reason for this fluctuation is not known. It has also been observed that people with hemophilia tend to bleed less as they become older.

Clotting factor IX is also involved in the intrinsic pathway and the clinical picture of hemophilia B is the same as that of hemophilia A. In a few cases, female carriers of the genetic defect for hemophilia B have manifested a bleeding tendency. Some people with hemophilia B do not appear to have any factor IX protein, whereas other afflicted people apparently synthesize a functionally abnormal protein.

Deficiency of factor XI (hemophilia C) is a much milder bleeding disorder. Spontaneous bleeding usually does not occur in this condition, although bruising, nosebleeds, and retinal hemorrhages have been reported. Many affected women suffer from menorrhagia, and postpartum hemorrhage may be a problem. Bleeding into the joints is rare with hemophilia C. Excessive bleeding in people with hemophilia C usually only occurs after severe injury or surgery. The tendency to bleed postoperatively is most likely to occur when the surgery involves the nose and throat, teeth, bones, female genital tract, mucous membranes, or cataracts of the eye. Postsurgical bleeding is uncommon following operations in which vessels are ligated to control blood loss (e.g., appendectomy). Liver disease of any type aggravates the bleeding tendency in people with factor XI deficiency.

Von Willebrand's Disease

Von Willebrand's disease (vascular hemophilia) is another inherited disorder that differs from hemophilia A but also involves clotting factor VIII. Von Willebrand's disease is not sex-linked but shows an autosomal dominant mode of inheritance. Theoretically the condition should af-

fect men and women equally, but the disease seems to be more common among women, probably because women with von Willebrand's disease are more likely to be diagnosed than are affected men due to the menorrhagia suffered by the women.

Whereas those with hemophilia A synthesize a structurally abnormal factor VIII protein, people with von Willebrand's disease actually lack factor VIII. There may be total absence of factor VIII or a reduced amount of a structurally normal protein (see Chapter 6). After transfusions of plasma or factor VIII, people with von Willebrand's disease show an increase in the level of circulating factor VIII that is greater than can be due to the amount of transfused material. Presumably factor VIII synthesis is somehow being stimulated.

Another defect that occurs in people with von Willebrand's disease, but not in those with hemophilia A, is decreased platelet aggregation. There is some evidence that another factor (von Willebrand's factor; VWF) exists that influences platelet aggregation. VWF is very closely associated with factor VIII and difficult to separate from it. Presumably people with von Willebrand's disease are lacking VWF as well as factor VIII.

As with hemophilia A and B, von Willebrand's disease has varying degrees of severity. In contrast to hemophilia, hemarthroses are uncommon in von Willebrand's disease but do occur in severely affected people. Deep subcutaneous and intramuscular hematomas are also uncommon. Prolonged bleedings from trivial injuries are common in von Willebrand's disease. Nosebleeds occur frequently. Another fairly common manifestation is bleeding from the oral cavity. Prolonged serious bleeding postoperatively is a frequent problem, especially following surgery of the ear, nose, or throat. Bleeding may increase or recur several days or even weeks postoperatively. The most common bleeding problem in women with von Willebrand's disease is menorrhagia. Bleeding from the ruptured ovarian follicle at the time of ovulation may also occur. This bleeding is characterized by intermenstrual abdominal pain that may be quite severe.

Gastrointestinal bleeding is not very common in von Willebrand's disease, but is usually severe when it does occur. Hematuria is very rare and is not usually severe.

Inherited Deficiencies of Other Clotting Factors

Inherited deficiencies of other clotting factors occur rarely. They seem to have an autosomal recessive mode of inheritance and so affect males and females equally. *Congenital afibrinogenemia* is a condition in which there is no detectable fibrinogen in the blood. As a result, the blood is not able to clot, but platelet adhesion and aggregation can occur normally. Spontaneous bleeding does not occur in people with congenital afibrinogenemia but excessive bleeding occurs following injury and there is a tendency to easy and excessive bruising. The condition is usually manifested at birth by prolonged bleeding from the umbilicus.

Epistaxes, easy bruising, and excessive postoperative bleeding are the major clinical manifestations of *congenital prothrombin deficiency*. Menorrhagia and hemorrhage at childbirth are common problems in affected women. The usual manifestations of *factor V deficiency* are epistaxes, easy bruising, and menorrhagia. Bleeding manifestations in *factor VII deficiency* are generally mild, although hemarthroses do occur. Epistaxes, excessive bruising, and menorrhagia are problems, but postoperative bleeding is rarely serious. Bleeding following surgery and dental extractions is characteristic of *factor X deficiency*. Menorrhagia and excessive bleeding at childbirth occur in affected women. People with *factor XII deficiency* are usually asymptomatic, but occasionally a person with this condition may bleed excessively.

People with an inherited *deficiency of factor XIII* may have a serious bleeding tendency. In this condition the blood clots, but the fibrin is unstable and breaks down easily. Factor XIII deficiency becomes manifest at birth with bleeding from the umbilical stump. Excessive bleeding does not necessarily occur at the time of injuries but usually occurs 24 to 36 hours later. Wound healing is delayed and excessive scar formation may occur.

Acquired Deficiencies of Clotting Factors

The most common causes of acquired clotting-factor deficiencies are liver disease and lack of vitamin K. Vitamin K is necessary for the normal synthesis of prothrombin and factors VII, IX, and X. Deficiencies of these factors, with a resultant tendency to bleed, will occur if vitamin K is not available in sufficient amounts. The major source of vitamin K is the production of this material by intestinal bacteria. When normal flora are absent from the intestine, as is the case in newborns and following oral administration of broad-spectrum antibiotics to sterilize the bowel, deficiency of vitamin K may result. Newborns may also have clotting-factor deficiencies due to immaturity of the liver and lack of stored vitamin K. Vitamin K is a fat-soluble vitamin; therefore whenever absorption of fat is impaired vitamin K deficiency may occur. Bile salts are necessary for absorption of fat and vitamin K, so a bleeding tendency commonly accompanies biliary obstruction.

People with cirrhosis of the liver or severe hepatitis often have a severe tendency to bleed. The causes of this bleeding tendency are multiple and complex. The liver plays a vital role in normal hemostasis: not only does it synthesize many clotting factors but it also removes activated clotting factors and fibrinogen/fibrin degradation products (FDP). In addition, the liver influences platelet numbers and platelet function. With liver disease these functions are impaired: not only will there be deficiencies of clotting factors but also a buildup of FDP, which have an anticoagulant effect. Thrombocytopenia may occur due to excessive destruction of platelets. Failure of the diseased liver to clear bilirubin from the blood leads to an elevated level of bilirubin, which interferes with platelet aggregation. If the liver disease is secondary to alcoholism, suppression of platelet production may be caused by the alcohol. As a result of these multiple abnormalities in liver disease, life-threatening hemorrhages may occur. Often the hemorrhagic sites are peptic ulcers or esophageal varices, which may occur concurrently with liver disease such as cirrhosis.

Disseminated Intravascular Coagulation

Disseminated intravascular coagulation (DIC) is a paradoxical condition in which excessive clotting leads to severe bleeding. This condition is also referred to as consumption coagulopathy and acute defibrination syndrome. DIC can be initiated secondarily to many conditions due to the release of thromboplastinlike material into the blood. This material triggers intravascular clotting and causes excessive deposition of fibrin in the capillaries of many organs. Fibrin deposition evokes a fibrinolytic response to maintain the patency of the blood vessels. As a result, large amounts of fibrin degradation products are released into the general circulation. Severe hemorrhage can then occur for two reasons: (*1*) the excessive clotting consumes platelets and various clotting factors faster than they can be produced and so deficiencies of platelets and clotting factors (primarily fibrinogen and factors V and VIII) result; (*2*) the excessive amounts of FDP have a powerful anticoagulant effect.

DIC can be associated with complications of pregnancy such as abruptio placentae, amniotic fluid embolism, toxemia, and retained dead fetus. The resultant hemorrhage may be fatal. DIC can also be initiated by bacterial septicemia and some rickettsial and viral diseases; by anaphylactic and massive transfusion reactions; by massive trauma (including burns); and by a number of other conditions. A less acute form of DIC may occur secondarily to carcinoma.

Vascular Abnormalities

Spontaneous hemorrhage or bleeding after minor trauma may occur if structural abnormalities of vessel walls exist. Faulty connective tissue leads to fragility of blood vessels; initiation of intrinsic clotting may also be impaired if collagen is defective.

Several hereditary disorders of connective tissue result in inadequate vascular support. An example is *Meekrin-Ehlers-Danlos syndrome*, an autosomal dominant inherited condition characterized by abnormal collagen structure. Affected people bruise easily and may have subcutaneous hematomas. Sometimes spontaneous rupture of a large artery occurs, with fatal results. Other manifestations that may occur in this condition are hypermobility of joints, hyperelasticity of skin, diaphragmatic hernia, and dislocation of the lens of the eye.

Scurvy is a condition caused by prolonged deficiency of vitamin C. Vitamin C is necessary for the formation of collagen and has other metabolic functions as well. In scurvy synthesis of connective tissue is impaired, with a resultant loss of structural support in and around blood vessels, and capillary fragility. Platelets may also be defective. Bone and joint hemorrhages, gingival bleeding, petechiae, and ecchymoses commonly occur.

Senile purpura is thought to be due to the structural changes that occur in connective tissue with aging. In this condition dark purple spots due to cutaneous hemorrhage occur, primarily on the forearms and in the region where eyeglasses exert pressure on the face.

Weakening of the vascular wall can occur due to excessive amounts of glucocortiocoid hormones. Thus purpura and ecchymoses are frequently associated with Cushing's syndrome (see Chapter 19).

Allergic purpura is believed to be the result of immunological damage to blood vessels. Petechiae and purpura occur, particularly on dependent portions of the body such as the buttocks and flexor surfaces of the legs. When allergic purpura is associated with gastrointestinal hemorrhage and arthritis, the condition is called *Schönlein-Henoch purpura*. It occurs primarily in children and usually follows an infection. When it occurs in adults it is usually triggered by a drug reaction.

THROMBOSIS

Thrombosis is the development or formation of a blood clot in the blood vessels or the heart during life. The intravascular clot that is formed is called a *thrombus*. A thrombus is slightly different from the usual clot that forms outside the body, or when a blood vessel is severed, or within the vessels after death. A thrombus is composed primarily of platelets, fibrin, and leukocytes and so appears paler than the usual blood clot, which has many red blood cells trapped in the fibrin mesh.

A thrombus starts to form when platelets stick to the endothelial lining of a blood vessel and aggregate there. Fibrin then forms around the mass of platelets, trapping leukocytes and a few red blood cells, as well as more platelets. As more platelets aggregate, the process is repeated and the thrombus increases in size, layer by layer. This buildup of a thrombus "head" slows the flow of blood enough that red blood cells settle out behind it and become trapped in fibrin. The resultant clot forms a red "tail" on the thrombus that may extend for a considerable distance along the length of the blood vessel.

Dissolution of a thrombus may occur spontaneously within a few days due to activation of the fibrinolytic system. If dissolution does not occur, the presence of the thrombus initiates an inflammatory response at the site where the thrombus is attached to the blood vessel wall. The thrombus is then gradually transformed into a connective-tissue scar. New channels for blood flow may develop through the thrombus, in a process called canalization. Eventually the exposed surfaces of the thrombus are covered by endothelium and the thrombus becomes incorporated into the blood vessel wall, resulting in narrowing of the lumen of the blood vessel.

Thrombosis most commonly occurs in the veins, particularly those of the legs. Thrombus formation may also occur in the heart, particularly in the auricular appendages of the atria or around damaged valves. Arterial thrombosis occurs primarily in the coronary ateries and the cerebral arteries; the iliac and femoral arteries may also be affected.

Factors Predisposing to Thrombosis

Three basic factors lead to the development of a thrombus: (1) slowing of blood flow; (2) changes in the wall of the blood vessel; and (3) changes in the blood itself.

Slowing of Blood Flow

Normally, when blood is flowing rapidly through a large vessel, the blood cells and platelets travel in a column in the center of the vessel lumen, surrounded by a clear zone of plasma. Therefore, normally only the plasma makes contact with the blood vessel endothelium. For thrombus formation to occur, platelets must stick to the endothelium. If blood flow is rapid, any platelets that do stick are quickly swept off before a large mass can aggregate. When blood flow is slow or stasis of blood occurs, however, there is more likelihood of platelets coming into contact with the endothelium and aggregating.

In addition, small amounts of clotting factors are continually being activated. If blood flow is rapid these activated factors are diluted and quickly carried to the liver where they are removed from the blood. If stasis of blood occurs, however, the local concentration of activated factors may become high enough to initiate clotting.

Slow blood flow and stasis occur mainly in the venous circulation. Venous blood flow is particularly slowed in people with heart disease and those immobilized in bed. Stasis commonly accompanies varicose veins. During pregnancy, pressure on abdominal veins impedes venous return from the legs. Pressure behind the knees, such as may occur from prolonged sitting or lying in bed with pillows under the knees, impedes blood flow and causes stasis in the leg veins. All these factors can contribute to thrombus formation.

Changes in the Blood Vessel Wall

Normal smooth endothelium does not attract platelets. Whenever there is damage to the blood vessel wall or roughening of the endothelium, however, platelets aggregate at the site of damage. Thrombi may develop at sites of damage due to trauma or inflammation. Venous thrombi often develop at the valves, especially if they are damaged, as in varicose veins. Arteriosclerosis is a common cause of roughening of the arterial endothelium and a major predisposing factor in the development of arterial thrombi.

The term *arteriosclerosis* is applied to a group of conditions characterized by thickening, hardening, and loss of elasticity of the walls of arteries and arterioles. It occurs almost universally with aging. The most common form of arteriosclerosis is *atherosclerosis*. Atherosclerosis is characterized by the development of lipid-containing plaques or thickenings (atheromas) within the tunica intima and later the tunica media of large and medium-sized arteries. Fibrosis of the plaque occurs, and eventually calcium may be deposited in the atheroma. Atherosclerosis narrows the lumen of the artery, thus reducing blood flow. The roughening of the arterial lining provides sites for the development of thrombi. In addition, atheromas weaken the arterial wall. Atherosclerosis is a major predisposing factor in coronary thrombosis and cerebral thrombosis.

Changes in the Blood

Increased viscosity of the blood slows blood flow and may contribute to thrombosis. Increased numbers of erythrocytes or dehydration will increase blood viscosity.

The importance of increased coagulability (hypercoagulability) of the blood in the development of thrombi has been difficult to establish, but undoubtedly it does play a role, especially if combined with slow blood flow and changes in the vessel wall.

An increased level of clotting factors alone does not increase the tendency to thrombosis. Increased concentrations of clotting factors in the blood produce a *potentially* hypercoagulable state. To precipitate thrombosis, however, the factors have to become activated.

A deficiency of one of the naturally occurring antithrombins (antithrombin III) can lead to a hypercoagulable state. This antithrombin normally binds any circulating thrombin as quickly as it is formed from the activation of prothrombin. When antithrombin is deficient a buildup of thrombin can occur.

An increased number of circulating platelets does not necessarily cause hypercoagulability. A hypercoagulable state may exist, however, as a result of changes that make the platelets stickier and increase platelet aggregation.

Many factors contribute to the development of hypercoagulability. Release of epinephrine from the adrenal medulla during stress causes increased platelet adhesiveness as well as an increased number of circulating platelets. In addition, epinephrine causes the release of a substance with thromboplastin activity from the aortic endothelium, particularly when atherosclerosis is present.

Increased levels of free fatty acids in the blood (especially long-chain saturated fatty acids) have a coagulant effect. They bring about platelet aggregation and can activate clotting factor XII. Stress causes an elevation in the level of free fatty acids in the blood.

Increased incidence of thrombosis is associated with the long-term use of oral contraceptives that contain high doses of estrogen. Increased levels of clotting factors, decreased antithrombin III activity, and increased platelet aggregation are associated with the high estrogen levels.

Cigarette smoking is associated with hypercoagulability. Platelet aggregation is increased after a person smokes a cigarette. Cigarette smoking also increases the blood lipid concentration, which contributes to hypercoagulability.

People with blood group A have a greater risk of thrombosis than people with other blood groups.

All the reasons for this risk are not known, but it has been found that people with group A blood have higher levels of clotting factors II, VII, VIII, and X and lower levels of antithrombin III.

Effects of Thrombosis

A thrombus presents two hazards: it may obstruct blood flow (occlusion) or a portion of the thrombus may break away and form an embolus. Pulmonary embolism is the most serious effect likely to occur from a venous thrombus. On the arterial side, the most serious problem is obstruction of blood flow with subsequent infarction.

Embolism

An *embolus* is a mass of undissolved material traveling in the blood; it may be solid, liquid, or gaseous. The most common form of embolus is a freely floating blood clot that has become detached from a thrombus. Emboli are more likely to arise from venous thrombi than from arterial thrombi. Emboli are carried in the blood until they reach a narrow point in the circulation where they become impacted and cause obstruction. The process of occlusion of a blood vessel by an impacted embolus is called *embolism.*

Arterial emboli usually arise from thrombi within the heart or large arteries and eventually become lodged in smaller arteries or arterioles. The effect of arterial embolism depends on where the clot lodges and whether or not the tissue has an alternate blood supply.

Venous blood flows from smaller vessels to larger vessels. Therefore, an embolus originating in the venous system usually does not become impacted until it reaches the pulmonary circulation, where it causes *pulmonary embolism.* If the embolus is large enough to block the main pulmonary artery death occurs instantly, without any warning signs and symptoms. A large embolus may lodge astride the bifurcation of the pulmonary artery. In this case immediate death may occur, or the person may die within 24 hours due to acute hypoxia or due to acute dilation of the right side of the heart

(cor pulmonale). Signs and symptoms vary but usually include dyspnea, a feeling of substernal pressure, cardiac arrhythmias, and anxiety. Sometimes an embolus does not cause complete occlusion immediately, but once it becomes lodged the clot may grow, causing further obstruction and possibly death several days later.

Small emboli occur more commonly than large ones. These small emboli become lodged in a small branch of the pulmonary artery or in an arteriole. The usual signs and symptoms are dyspnea, rapid breathing, and fever. Chest pain may occur and there may be coughing with hemoptysis (blood in the sputum). Although a small pulmonary embolus may not have serious results, it is often followed by a second, large embolus, which may be fatal.

Occlusion

Occlusion may be caused by a thrombus or by an embolus that becomes lodged in a blood vessel. Occlusion is usually accompanied by pain. Occlusion of a vein will result in edema due to an increase in capillary hydrostatic pressure. (See Chapter 11 for a discussion of edema.) Most venous thrombi occur in leg veins, in which case the leg swells. Venous thrombi do not always cause complete occlusion, however, and often are asymptomatic.

A far more serious effect of occlusion is ischemia. *Ischemia* is a deficiency of blood in a part. It may be due to actual obstruction of a blood vessel, as occurs with thrombosis, or it may be due to constriction of a blood vessel. As a result of ischemia, necrosis (death) of the tissue may occur. An area of necrosis in a tissue due to ischemia is called an *infarct.* The process of formation of an infarct is called *infarction.* Arterial occlusion is more likely than venous occlusion to cause infarction.

Infarction does not necessarily occur after occlusion. If the area has an alternative blood supply (collateral circulation), occlusion of one vessel may have no significant effect. Other factors influencing the development of an infarct are the duration of the obstruction and how well the tissue can withstand anoxia. As a result of clot retraction a small amount of blood may flow through the tissue and prevent immediate cell death. Due to fibrinolysis blood flow to the area may then improve enough over the next few days that death does not occur. Infarction is very likely to occur in tissues that are vulnerable to anoxia. Cells of the nervous system, myocardial cells, and epithelial cells of the proximal tubules of the kidney nephrons are very vulnerable. On the other hand, fibroblasts (connective tissue cells) can tolerate anoxia for a much longer period of time. In some instances, such as massive pulmonary embolism or coronary occlusion, normal functioning is so disrupted by vascular occlusion that the person may die before an infarct can develop.

Cerebral occlusion and coronary occlusion are two serious consequences of arterial thrombosis.

Cerebral thrombosis. Cerebral thrombosis, with resulting occlusion and necrosis of brain tissue, is the most frequent cause of cerebrovascular accident. A *cerebrovascular accident* (stroke) is a focal disturbance of cerebral function of more than 24 hours' duration due to a vascular lesion. It may be caused by occlusion as a consequence of thrombosis or embolism, or it may be due to intracranial hemorrhage. Strokes due to cerebral thrombosis are sometimes preceded by transient ischemic attacks. A *transient ischemic attack* is a short period of impaired neurological function due to a focal disturbance of the cerebral circulation. Recovery occurs within 24 hours, with no residual effects.

Signs and symptoms of cerebrovascular accident develop suddenly, and an affected person may lose consciousness. Often the blood pressure is elevated. If the person remains conscious, temperature, pulse, and respiratory rate are usually normal. If the person is unconscious, however, an elevated temperature, altered pulse rate, and irregular, labored respirations may occur. Specific signs and symptoms will vary depending on the site of tissue damage. Hemiplegia, with loss of sensation in the paralyzed side, is common. If the infarction occurs in the dominant hemisphere of the brain, aphasia (loss of speech or loss of comprehension of written or spoken language) and/or apraxia (inability to carry out purposeful movements) may result.

Coronary thrombosis. The effects of coronary thrombosis will largely be determined by the rate at which occlusion occurs. When occlusion develops slowly, the collateral circulation usually enlarges enough to provide sufficient blood to the area normally served by the occluded vessel. The collateral circulation in the heart is comprised of numerous minute anastomoses between the small arteries; there are relatively few anastomoses between the large coronary arteries.

Following sudden occlusion of a large coronary artery, the diameters of the anastomoses increase to their maximum within a few seconds. Blood flow through these minute collateral vessels is insufficient, however, and ischemia results. The ischemic cardiac muscle becomes nonfunctional, and if the blood flow is reduced beyond a critical level, myocardial cells begin to die within about an hour. The result is *myocardial infarction.* The amount of necrosis is determined by the degree of ischemia and the metabolic requirements of the heart muscle. Increased activity of the heart, such as occurs during physical exertion, increases cardiac muscle metabolism and therefore increases the need for oxygen and nutrients. When cardiac activity is increased, however, the collateral vessels are unable to supply the ischemic areas as well as the areas of the heart that they normally supply. Under these circumstances, a greater degree of cellular death occurs.

If the ischemic area is small, infarction may not occur but part of the myocardium is temporarily nonfunctional because the amount of oxygen and nutrients reaching the cells is not enough to support muscle contraction. If the ischemic area is large, myocardial cells in the center of the area die rapidly. The tissue immediately around the necrotic area is nonfunctional. The nonfunctional area is surrounded by an area of cardiac muscle that is still contracting, but only weakly. During the next few days the area of the infarct enlarges as many of the marginal myocardial cells succumb to the prolonged ischemia.

The most characteristic symptom of myocardial infarction is a feeling of substernal pressure or constriction, which may persist for several hours. This feeling is commonly accompanied by dyspnea. The person usually appears ashen, and the skin is cool as a result of decreased blood flow. Sympathetic nervous stimulation causes the person to sweat. The pulse may be weak and thready, and is usually rapid and irregular.

Decreased cardiac output is a serious consequence of coronary occlusion. Ventricular pumping ability is decreased when some of the myocardial cells are nonfunctional and others are only contracting weakly. In addition, the pressure that develops inside the ventricle when the undamaged portions of the myocardium contract actually forces the ischemic area outward. This outward bulging, which is called *systolic stretch*, dissipates some of the pressure developed by the contracting ventricle. The inability to develop sufficient force

from the ventricular contraction causes a decreased cardiac output, which can lead to shock (see Chapter 14) and death.

Another cause of death due to coronary occlusion is rupture of the ischemic area. Dead myocardial tissue begins to degenerate a few days after infarction. As a result, the necrotic muscle may become very thin. The degree of systolic stretch increases until the heart actually ruptures, causing death.

Ventricular fibrillation (rapid repetitive excitation of myocardial fibers without coordinated contraction of the ventricle) is another serious consequence of coronary occlusion (Fig. 7-4) and is a frequent cause of death. Fibrillation is most likely to occur in the first 10 minutes after occlusion or in the period from about 3 to 10 hours later. Several factors cause increased irritability of cardiac muscle following coronary occlusion and contribute to the tendency for fibrillation to occur. Acute ischemia causes a loss of potassium from the myocardial cells and consequently an increase in the potassium concentration of the extracellular

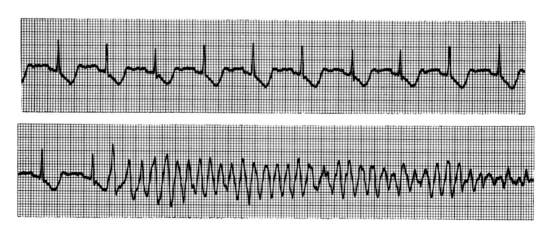

Figure 7-4. *Recording of a continuous monitor lead (similar to V_5) in a patient with myocardial infarction. The upper strip shows a regular sinus rhythm with a rate of 80 beats/min, and ST depression and T wave inversion indicative of ischemia. Following the second sinus beat in the lower strip, a ventricular ectopic beat occurs within the T wave of the previous beat (i.e., in the vulnerable period during repolarization of the ventricles) and initiates ventricular fibrillation. (Reproduced, with permission, from Goldman MJ: Principles of Clinical Electrocardiography, ed 10. Copyright 1979 by Lange Medical Publications, Los Altos, California.)*

fluid in the cardiac muscle. The elevated level of potassium in the extracellular fluid interferes with normal conductivity and causes increased cardiac irritability. In addition, the ischemic myocardial cells cannot repolarize, so that the ischemic area of myocardium is negative outside, whereas the normal polarized myocardium is relatively positive on the outside of the cell membrane. As a result, electrical current flows from the ischemic area to the normal area of the cardiac muscle. This current can cause abnormal impulses and initiate fibrillation. A third element that increases the irritability of the cardiac muscle is sympathetic stimulation. Following coronary occlusion sympathetic nervous activity is increased, mainly because the decreased cardiac output elicits reflex sympathetic responses.

Pulmonary edema is another cause of death following coronary occlusion; it occurs several days after the occlusion. Pulmonary edema is discussed in Chapter 11.

If death does not occur due to acute coronary thrombosis, gradual recovery occurs. During the period from 8 to 24 hours after occlusion the collateral blood vessels enlarge further and so blood flow to the affected area increases. As a result, the area of nonfunctional myocardium diminishes in size. Most of the nonfunctional area of cardiac muscle becomes functional again after two to three weeks. At the same time, fibrous tissue develops among the dead myocardial cells at the center of the ischemic area. Gradually the necrotic myocardial tissue is replaced by a strong fibrous scar. This scar stops the systolic stretch and the entire force generated by contraction of the functional myocardium pumps blood from the ventricles rather than stretching the nonfunctional area of the heart. In addition, hypertrophy of the normal myocardium occurs, which partially compensates for the loss of functional tissue.

The recovered heart is able to maintain a normal cardiac output, and the affected person can still engage in normal activities of a nonstrenuous type. The cardiac reserve is decreased, however, and the person cannot perform strenuous exercise (see Chapter 22).

SUGGESTED ADDITIONAL READING

Benditt EP: The origin of atherosclerosis. Sci Am 236(2): 74–85, 1977.

Fein JM: Microvascular surgery for stroke. Sci Am 238(4): 58–67, 1978.

O'Brian BS, Woods S: The paradox of DIC. Am J Nurs 78(11): 1878–1880, 1978.

8

Inflammatory-Reparative Response

Inflammation is the local response of living tissues to damage. Many agents can cause tissue damage and thus incite an inflammatory reaction. *Physical agents* may be mechanical agents that cause trauma, such as bullets, knives, and various blunt or sharp-edged objects; extremes of temperature; or various forms of electromagnetic radiation. Many *chemical agents,* for example, strong acids and strong alkalis, are irritating to body tissues and produce an inflammatory reaction. *Biological,* or *living, inflammatory agents* are viruses, bacteria, rickettsia, protozoa, and sometimes higher plants and animals. Bacteria are perhaps the most common living inflammatory agents. *Immunological agents* are antigen-antibody reactions that cause tissue injury, as, for example, in allergy or autoimmunity.

The initial response to injury involves vascular and cellular changes and is known as *acute inflammation*. Acute inflammation persists as long as tissue damage continues. When the irritating agent is removed or withdrawn, phagocytic cells remove the debris, in what might be called the *demolition phase*. If there has been no loss of tissue, the area may return to normal, that is, *resolution* may occur. Sometimes, however, *fibrosis* results. If tissue loss occurs, integrity of the part will be restored by *repair* and/or *regeneration* (Fig. 8-1).

When the inflammatory agent produces extensive tissue damage resolution may be impossible and *suppuration* occurs. When the injurious agent

cannot be removed or destroyed the acute inflammation may progress to a state of *chronic inflammation*.

INFLAMMATION

Acute Inflammatory Response

Immediately after tissue damage small blood vessels in the area of injury constrict. The vasoconstriction is brief, however, and is followed by *vasodilation*. The vasodilation is partly due to a neural axon reflex and partly mediated by chemicals. As a result of dilation of the arteries and arterioles, blood flow to the area increases, which in turn increases the hydrostatic pressure (blood pressure) in the capillaries. Therefore an increased amount of

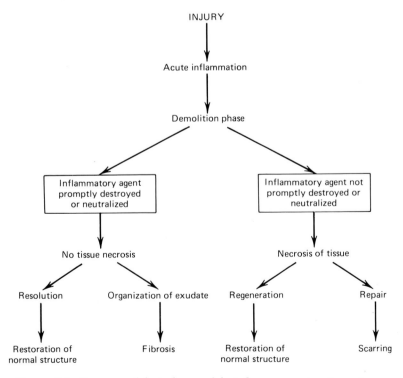

Figure 8-1. *Summary of the pathways of the inflammatory-reparative response.*

fluid leaves the vessels and enters the tissue spaces. (The amount of fluid leaving the capillaries depends on the difference between the hydrostatic pressure, which tends to force fluid out, and the osmotic pressure created by the plasma proteins, which tends to hold fluid in the capillaries. See Chapter 11.) As a result, lymph flow increases during the initial stages of inflammation. Later, however, lymph flow from the area may decrease as lymphatic vessels become plugged by fibrin clots.

Concurrently with the vasodilation, *vascular permeability increases*, primarily in the venules but later in the capillaries as well. Normal blood vessel endothelium is composed of a single layer of thin, flat nucleated cells that are tightly attached to each other. During inflammation the endothelial cells become swollen and rounded and gaps appear between them. These gaps allow the passage of plasma proteins, as well as fluid, from the venules into the tissue space. As a result, the blood remaining in the venules becomes concentrated and blood flow slows as the viscosity increases. If the damage is great enough, blood flow may actually stop; that is, *stasis* occurs. Thrombosis may occasionally occur at this time. With the slowing of blood flow the red blood cells begin to clump together (rouleau formation), and the leukocytes adhere to the endothelium. Within 30 to 60 minutes the leukocytes form a layer covering the entire endothelium of the venules. This layering is referred to as *pavementing*, or *margination*.

Shortly after pavementing occurs the leukocytes leave the blood vessels and enter the tissue spaces in a process called emigration. *Emigration* is an active process in which the leukocytes extend pseudopodia and pass between the endothelial cells by ameboid movement. Subsequently they force their way through the basement membrane. Varying numbers of red blood cells may also leave the blood vessels. Red blood cells are not capable of ameboid motion, but hydrostatic pressure sometimes forces red cells through the gaps in the endothelium in the paths of leukocytes. This passive process is called *diapedesis*. (Some people also refer to the passage of the leukocytes through the vessel wall as diapedesis.)

The leukocytes that leave the venules travel through the tissue toward the site of injury by chemotactic attraction. *Chemotaxis* is the movement of an organism in response to a chemical concentration gradient. When they arrive at the site of injury the leukocytes become actively phagocytic and ingest cellular debris, particulate foreign material, and any microorganisms that may be present (Fig. 8-2). The leukocytes participating in the inflammatory response initially are primarily polymorphonuclear neutrophils. Later monocytes predominate; the monocytes are transformed into macrophages.

When injury occurs, damage to lymphatic vessels is usually greater than damage to blood vessels because the lymphatic vessels are more fragile. Fibrinogen and other clotting factors are present in the fluid that escapes from the venules, and the damaged lymphatics become plugged by fibrin clots. The clots prevent drainage of fluid from the injured area and the inflammatory reaction remains localized. Later the fibrin plugs are removed by fibrinolysis and drainage once again takes place. If the lymphatic vessels are not blocked by fibrin, lymph flow is increased.

Signs of Inflammation

The cardinal signs of inflammation have been known for many centuries. These are *redness, heat, swelling, pain,* and *loss of function* (or motion). The redness and heat are due to the local vasodilation and increased volume of blood in the area. The leakage of fluid from the blood vessels and blockage of lymphatic drainage produce swelling. The cause of the pain is not known, but is believed to be due to pressure and possibly the action of chemicals on nerve endings. Neither is the exact reason for loss of function known, though it may be partly due to inhibition of muscle movements in response to pain. Destruction of tissue is also a contributing factor.

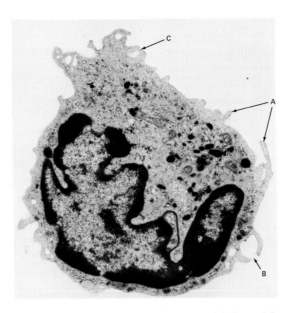

Figure 8-2. *Electron micrograph section of a whole neutrophil obtained from arachnoid space of a guinea pig. Phagocytic response was initiated by injecting bacteria into the arachnoid space. (A) Early stage of phagocytosis in which pseudopodia are extending outwardly. (B) Pseudopods are forming a cuplike vesicle. (C) Pseudopodia have fused to form a phagocytic vesicle. (From Brown WV, Bertke EM: Textbook of cytology, ed 2. St. Louis, The C.V. Mosby Co. 1974. Courtesy J. Beggs, Laboratory of Neuropathology, Barrow's Neurological Institute, Phoenix, Arizona.)*

Chemical Mediators of Inflammation

Many chemical substances are released or activated when tissue is damaged. Some of these chemicals are responsible for the vasodilation and increased permeability that occur during inflammation. The exact role of other chemical substances is not known. Cells such as mast cells, neutrophils, and macrophages are one source of these chemicals. Other chemical mediators of inflammation are present in the plasma.

Histamine is present in most tissues, mainly in the granules of mast cells. When injury occurs histamine is released, producing vasodilation and increased permeability during the early part of the inflammatory response.

Epinephrine and norepinephrine, which are normally present extracellularly, have a vasoconstrictive and antipermeability effect. When injury occurs some of the intracellular enzymes that are released can destroy epinephrine and norepinephrine. As a result, the action of other chemicals that cause vasodilation and increased permeability may be potentiated.

Kinins are small polypeptides that are released from a plasma globulin (kininogen) due to the action of proteolytic enzymes, particularly kallikrein. The most important kinins are *bradykinin* and *kallidin*. Active clotting factor XII causes the formation of kallikrein from prekallikrein (see Chapter 7). Kallikrein then catalyzes the formation of bradykinin and kallidin from kininogen. The kinins cause increased vascular permeability and are also potent vasodilators. In addition, bradykinin causes pain.

Some of the components of the *complement system* are also mediators of the inflammatory response. (Complement is involved in immune reactions. See Chapter 29.) Following activation of complement several polypeptide products are released. Certain of these cause increased vascular permeability and chemotaxis of neutrophils.

The Inflammatory Exudate

The fluid that escapes from the blood vessels, together with the leukocytes and cellular debris that accumulate at the site of injury, form the *inflammatory exudate,* which has several functions. As already mentioned, the leukocytes are actively phagocytic and clear away foreign material and cellular debris. The fluid of the exudate dilutes any toxins or irriting substances that are present. In addition, the plasma fluid contains antibacterial substances and specific antibodies that provide defense against microbial invasion. Some antibodies (antitoxins) neutralize specific toxins. The fibrinogen in the fluid exudate may form a fibrin clot. This fibrin may protect against bacterial invasion by forming a barrier; it also aids phagocytosis by providing a framework in which the neutrophils may trap microorganisms. If the tissue has been severed, as in a cut, the fibrin fills the gap between the cut edges.

The nature and amount of exudate is influenced by the severity of injury and to some extent by the specific injurious agent. A watery exudate containing little protein and few cells is called a *serous* exudate. This type is usually seen when tissue damage is mild. When a greater degree of injury occurs there is increasing vascular permeability. As a result more protein molecules, including fibrinogen, are able to escape from the venules. The fibrinogen is converted to fibrin. When large amounts of fibrin are present in the exudate it is described as *fibrinous.* A *purulent* exudate is one that contains large numbers of leukocytes, particularly polymorphonuclear neutrophils. The

exudate is then called pus. (See the section on Suppuration.) Purulent exudates are associated with relatively severe inflammatory responses. A *hemorrhagic* or *sanguinous* exudate is characterized by the presence of many red blood cells. This type of exudate occurs particularly when there is rupture or necrosis of blood vessel walls.

Systemic Manifestations

Severe acute inflammation is usually accompanied by systemic manifestations. Leukocytosis and fever are common, especially if the inflammation is caused by bacteria. In addition there is increased synthesis of certain proteins by the liver.

Leukocytosis is an increase in the number of circulating white blood cells (leukocytes). It is believed to be mediated by a chemical substance (leukocytosis-promoting factor) that is released by the inflamed tissue. This chemical mediator causes release of granulocytes, particularly neutrophils, from the bone marrow. In addition the marrow is stimulated to produce more granulocytes.

Fever is an increase in body temperature above the normal range. During inflammation a protein substance (pyrogen) is liberated from the neutrophils and monocytes. This pyrogen is carried by the circulation to the temperature-regulating center in the hypothalamus, where it somehow increases the setting of the thermostat. (Fever is discussed more fully in Chapter 24.) Some bacterial toxins cause the release of pyrogen from neutrophils and monocytes. Pyrogen can also be released when neutrophils are lysed at the site of inflammation.

Various factors that are released from inflamed tissues stimulate the synthesis of a number of proteins by the liver. These proteins include fibrinogen and some other clotting factors, and some complement components. As a result of the increased concentration of fibrinogen in the blood the *erythrocyte sedimentation rate (ESR) is increased.* The size of red blood cells determines the rate at which they settle out of plasma. Normally the negative charges on the surface of red blood cells keep them separated. When there is increased fibrinogen in the blood, however, it coats the red blood cells and reduces their surface charge. As a result the red blood cells clump together and settle faster.

Demolition Phase

The debris at the site of inflammation has to be removed before resolution or healing can take place. This process is accomplished by the phagocytic activity of the macrophages. Neutrophils have a short life span and are easily lysed at the acid pH of the exudate. Macrophages, however, have a long life span and are resistant to lysis; they accumulate at the site of inflammation and ingest fibrin, red blood cells, dead neutrophils, cellular debris, foreign material, and bacteria. Sometimes fusion of macrophages occurs, producing giant cells. These continue the scavenging process until resolution or healing is accomplished.

Resolution

Resolution is the complete return to normal after acute inflammation. It can only occur when injury to the tissues is slight and necrosis does not occur. The chemical mediators of inflammation are neutralized, destroyed, or removed. Normal vascular permeability and vasomotor tone are restored, and normal blood flow resumes. Fibrinous deposits are broken down and absorbed. Some of the fluid of the exudate reenters the capillaries, but most of the exudate is drained from the area by the lymphatics. Debris in the exudate is removed by phagocytic cells in the regional lymph nodes. Thus the tissue returns to normal.

Sometimes, when an excessive amount of fibrin has been laid down, removal of the exudate is delayed. New connective tissue is formed (fibrosis) is a manner similar to wound healing and resolution does not occur. This process occurs most often in fibrinous exudates in serous cavities. The result is the formation of *fibrous adhesions*, which cause the visceral and parietal surfaces of the serous membrane to be joined together.

Suppuration

Resolution is impossible when the inflammatory agent produces extensive damage, with necrosis of tissue. In this case, *suppuration* occurs. Suppuration is the process of pus formation due to destruction and digestion of tissue. It is typically caused by *pyogenic* (pus-producing) bacteria, such as staphylococci, but can also be caused by chemical agents, for example, turpentine.

Large numbers of neutrophils migrate to the site of inflammation when tissue damage is severe. Many of the neutrophils are killed by the inflammatory agent and others die because of the acid pH of the exudate. (Stasis of blood leads to anoxia in the inflamed tissue. Therefore aerobic respiration cannot proceed and anaerobic glycolysis occurs, which produces lactic acid.) Enzymes released from the dead leukocytes digest connective tissue as well as the necrotic tissue, causing further destruction. Digestion of the tissue makes it soluble.

The fluid material that results from suppuration is called pus. Pus consists of dead and dying leukocytes, protein-rich fluid that has escaped from the blood vessels, fibrin, and cellular debris such as lipids and nucleic acids, as well as dead and living microorganisms if the inflammation was caused by a living agent. The pus is usually contained in a cavity, forming an *abscess*. The abscess is initially surrounded by a wall of acutely inflamed tissue containing many neutrophils. As the pus accumulates it is forced along the path of least resistance until it reaches a free surface. Spontaneous rupture of the abscess with discharge of the pus may then occur (or an abscess may be surgically incised and drained). Following drainage the abscess heals by repair, unless viable microorganisms persist at the site. The continued presence of the inflammatory agent results in development of a chronic abscess. Pus continues to be produced and may drain to the surface or into a hollow organ by way of a narrow tract called a *sinus*. In the case of a chronic suppurative process, fibrous tissue is laid down around the abscess, walling it off. Many macrophages, lymphocytes, and plasma cells infiltrate the area, in addition to neutrophils.

Sometimes an abscess does not drain but remains walled off in the tissue. Healing may still occur once the inflammatory agent is destroyed or neutralized. If the abscess is small the pus may be digested by enzymes and absorbed, and a fibrous scar formed. With larger abscesses the liquid portion of the pus may be absorbed, leaving behind the granular debris (inspissation). Eventually calcium may be deposited in the mass.

An ulcer is formed when an epithelial surface is destroyed by acute suppurative inflammation (Fig. 8-3). The floor of the ulcer is composed of inflammatory exudate and an adherent layer of dead tissue. This necrotic tissue resists digestion and forms a *slough*, which eventually becomes detached. The ulcer then heals by repair and regeneration.

Chronic Inflammation

Chronic inflammation is a prolonged process in which attempts at healing occur simultaneously with destruction and inflammation. It occurs when the body is unable to remove or destroy the inflammatory agent. Chronic inflammation may result from progression of an acute response or it may begin as a low-grade response without an acute phase.

Chronic inflammation can be caused by insoluble foreign bodies such as silica or asbestos particles. Biological inflammatory agents against which the body has limited resistance are another cause: for example, the tubercle bacillus, the agent of syphilis, and actinomyces. When a person's resistance is low due to general conditions she or he may not be able to overcome a living agent that would usually cause an acute inflammation of short duration; the result may be chronic inflammation. Chronic inflammation is also associated with

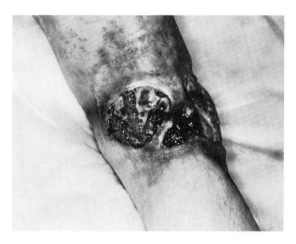

Figure 8-3. *Extensive ulceration about the ankle. (From Braverman IM: Skin Signs of Systemic Disease. Philadelphia, W.B. Saunders Co., 1970.)*

hypersensitivity and autoimmunity (see Chapter 30).

Macrophages are the characteristic cells of chronic inflammation. They are derived from emigrating monocytes and tissue histiocytes. Large numbers are present at the site of inflammation, engulfing foreign agents and cellular debris. Often the macrophages fuse to form giant cells. Usually there are very few neutrophils present at the site of chronic inflammation, except in the case of chronic suppuration. Lymphocytes and plasma cells (small round cells) are typically found in the inflammatory lesion. The exact role of the lymphocytes is not know, although they may give rise to other cell types. Plasma cells are involved in the production of immunoglobulins (see Chapter 29). Large numbers of eosinophils are sometimes present at the site of chronic inflammation. These cells seem to be associated with hypersensitivity reactions.

Formation of new connective tissue is characteristic of chronic inflammation. In the early stages this tissue is very vascular and contains many fibroblast cells (granulation tissue). The fibroblasts lay down collagen. Gradually the blood vessels are absorbed and as more collagen is deposited dense bundles of fibers are formed. Newly formed connective tissue has a tendency to contract, and this contraction may have serious results. For example, it may narrow the lumen of a duct of hollow organ (stenosis). Chronic inflammation of internal organs results in a loss of parenchymal cells and their replacement with nonfunctional fibrous tissue.

Granuloma Formation

A *granuloma* is a tumorlike mass or nodule of granulation tissue produced in some cases of chronic inflammation. The inflammatory agent may be a living organism or a nonliving foreign particle. Granuloma formation is typical of some chronic infectious diseases such as tuberculosis, brucellosis, and actinomycosis. Insoluble foreign bodies such as silica particles and talc are also associated with the formation of granulomas.

Macrophages persist at the site of chronic inflammation when they are unable to kill living agents or solubilize particulate foreign material. This persistence of macrophages is the basis of granuloma formation; somehow it attracts fibroblasts to the area. The fibroblasts deposit collagen fibers around clusters of macrophages; each cluster then is a granuloma. Frequently the center of the granuloma contains multinucleated giant cells formed by the fusion of macrophages. These giant cells may be surrounded by epithelial-like cells (epithelioid cells), which possibly arise from the transformation of macrophages. The outer zone contains lymphocytes, fibroblasts, and sometimes plasma cells. Eventually the mass is enclosed in connective tissue. When the inflammatory agent is a living organism, necrosis may occur at the center of the granuloma. This necrosis is typical for example in tubercles, the granulomas of tuberculosis.

Systemic Manifestations

Depending on the nature and amount of the inflammatory agent, chronic inflammation may be accompanied by a number of general effects. A localized reaction to a foreign body usually does not produce systemic manifestations, but chronic infectious processes such as tuberculosis may be accompanied by widespread effects.

The *production of antibodies* is a common feature of chronic inflammation. *Hyperplasia of the reticuloendothelial system* is also frequently associated with chronic inflammation. Hyperplasia is an abnormal increase in the number of normal cells in a normal arrangement in a tissue. In this case the hyperplasia is probably caused by stimulation of phagocytic and immunological functions of the reticuloendothelial cells.

During chronic inflammation a number of changes may occur in the blood. *Leukocytosis* usually occurs, with changes in the relative numbers of specific white blood cells depending on the inflammatory agent. The ESR is usually increased. There is usually an *elevated level of gamma globulins* due to increased antibody production. At the same time there is a *reduction in plasma albumin* due to dcreased synthesis by the liver. *Anemia* is also associated with chronic inflammation. For some unknown reason the ability to use iron for hemoglobin sythesis is impaired.

General malaise, headache, anorexia, and *weight loss* are common. The cause of these manifestations is unknown, although they may be due to the release of toxic substances from the site of inflammation.

As with acute inflammation, *fever* may also accompany chronic inflammation.

HEALING

In the pathological context, *healing* means the restoration of integrity to injured tissue. In other words, lost or destroyed tissue is replaced by living tissue. Loss or destruction of tissue can occur in several ways: by traumatic excision, either accidental or surgical; due to physical or chemical agents, for example, burns; due to ischemia, which leads to infarction; or due to severe inflammation, which leads to tissue necrosis.

Replacement of lost tissue can be accomplished by regeneration or repair. *Repair* is the replacement of lost tissue by granulation tissue that matures to form a fibrous connective-tissue scar. Scar tissue cannot restore the function of the lost tissue, but it fills the anatomical defect and restores tissue integrity. *Regeneration* is the replacement of lost tissue by tissue of the same type. It is accomplished by multiplication of undamaged cells of the same kind as those that were destroyed or by multiplication and differentiation of primitive stem cells. When regeneration is complete, normal function is usually restored.

Restoration of normal structure as well as restoration of tissue mass by regeneration requires the survival of the basic structural framework of the tissue. If the framework is lost, surviving cells may proliferate and restore normal tissue mass, but the mass will be structurally disorganized, so that normal function will not be restored.

Not all body tissues are capable of regeneration: tissues can regenerate only if their cells retain the ability to divide. Cells can be classified into three groups according to their regenerative capacity.

Labile cells normally continue to multiply throughout life and therefore are capable of regeneration. This category includes epithelial cells of the skin and of the mucous membranes lining the oral cavity, the gastrointestinal tract, the respiratory tract, the urinary tract, and the male and female genital tracts. Hematopoietic bone marrow cells and lymphoid cells are also labile.

Stable cells normally stop dividing when growth ceases, but are still capable of mitosis during adult life; therefore they can regenerate. This group includes parenchymal cells of glands such as the liver, pancreas, and endocrine glands; skin glands; and renal tubular epithelium. Connective tissue cells are also included in this category. Some researchers consider muscle cells to be stable cells, but the evidence is inconclusive.

Permanent cells lose their mitotic activity in infancy and so regeneration is impossible. This group includes neurons, and possibly striated, cardiac, and smooth muscle cells. If the neuron cell body is not destroyed, however, a severed axon can be regrown.

Formation of Granulation Tissue

Granulation tissue is composed mainly of capillaries and fibroblasts and has a reddish granular appearance.

After wounding, an acute inflammatory reaction ensues and then the debris is cleared away by macrophages, as previously described. Migration and proliferation of fibroblasts and vascular buds from the surrounding connective tissue then form the granulation tissue.

Capillary sprouts grow out from blood vessels at the edges of the wound by rearrangement, migration, and proliferation of existing endothelial cells. These capillary buds are usually solid at first but later develop a lumen. The vascular sprouts form loops by uniting with one another or with capillaries already carrying blood. The newly formed capillaries are more permeable than normal and allow the leakage of protein-rich fluid into the tissue. Some of the vessels acquire a muscular coat and differentiate into arterioles and venules. The origin of the muscle cells is not known. They may arise by differentiation from mesenchymal cells or by migration from existing blood vessels.

Simultaneously with the development of new capillaries, fibroblasts secrete soluble collagen molecules that aggregate into fibrils. Fibroblasts are also believed to produce the mucopolysaccharide ground substance of the tissue. After about two weeks collagen production decreases, but a process of remodeling takes place. The randomly oriented small collagen fibrils are rearranged into thick bundles, giving the tissue greater strength.

While the collagen is being remodeled a gradual process of devascularization occurs. Some of the newly formed blood vessels atrophy and others become obliterated. They are gradually absorbed and a pale, avascular scar remains.

Formation of granulation tissue occurs under a number of conditions in addition to wound healing and is called organization. *Organization* is the replacement of necrotic tissue (e.g., an infarct), inflammatory exudate (e.g., fibrinous exudates in serous cavities), thrombus, or hematoma by granulation tissue.

Healing of Surface Wounds

Healing of a wounded surface, whether the skin or a mucous membrane such as the lining of the gastrointestinal or respiratory tract, involves closure of the subepithelial defect with connective tissue as well as regeneration of the surface epithelium.

Specialized epithelial structures of the skin, such as hair follicles, sweat glands, and sebaceous glands cannot be replaced if they are completely destroyed. If part of the original structure remains, however, they can regenerate.

Healing of a clean incised wound in which the edges are in close apposition is referred to as *healing by primary union* (first intention). An example of this process is the healing of a surgical incision that has been sutured. When the edges of the wound are widely separated or extensive loss of tissue has occurred, the process is referred to as *healing by secondary union* (second intention). Examples of this situation would be a gaping laceration which has not been sutured or an ulcer. The two processes are basically the same but healing by secondary union takes much longer and leaves a large scar.

Healing by Primary Union

When wounding occurs, blood escapes from cut vessels and clots. The blood clot, with its fibrin strands, fills the narrow gap and unites the edges of the wound. A mild inflammatory reaction ensues: a fluid exudate forms and neutrophils and later monocytes migrate into the wound.

Within 24 hours, cells from epithelium close to the cut edges begin to migrate into the wound area. At the same time other epithelial cells adjacent to the wound undergo mitosis to replace the migrating cells. The migrating epithelial cells travel beneath the surface clot and bridge the gap between the cut edges within two or three days.

When the wound is on the external surface of the body the surface clot may dry to form a hard scab. Initially the new epithelial surface is composed of a single layer of cells. Proliferation of cells then restores a multilayered (stratified) epithelium if one was originally present. As the new layers of epithelium are forming, differentiation (formation of specialized cells) occurs. For example, epidermal cells begin producing keratin. In the trachea some cells differentiate into ciliated columnar cells while others develop into goblet cells and begin secreting mucus. In areas where a single layer of epithelial cells is normally found, such as in some parts of the gastrointestinal tract, differentiation occurs after the cells have covered the defect.

Meanwhile, by about the third day, granulation tissue starts to form under the new epithelium. Fibroblasts migrate into the wound and are closely followed by the ingrowth of new capillary buds. The process proceeds as described previously, with the fibroblasts laying down collagen fibers. As the granulation tissue is formed, fibrin is removed. The capillary endothelial cells contain a plasminogen activator and thus fibrinolysis occurs as the capillaries grow into the area. By the seventh day the subepithelial gap is filled in with granulation tissue and the surface of the wound is covered by epithelium of normal thickness.

The healing of a skin incision by primary union is illustrated on the end paper at the front of the book.

In a newly healed wound the scar is raised above the surface. It is red due to the vascularity of the underlying granulation tissue. Gradually, as the blood vessels disappear, the scar changes from red to white and decreases in size. The final result is usually a pale scar that is level with the adjacent surface.

Although the edges of a surgically incised wound may be united after a week, several weeks or months are required for the wound to regain tensile strength. Wound strength never returns completely to the strength of the original tissue. Until the fourth to sixth day the wound edges are held together only by fibrin and by the surface layer of epithelial cells. Therefore, the wound edges can be easily broken apart. From about the fourth to sixth day until the fifteenth day the fibroblasts are synthesizing collagen and the strength of the wound quickly increases. The strength of the wound continues to increase even after this time, however, as remodeling and cross-linking of collagen fibers occur. Six months to a year may be required for completion of this process, especially for healing of fibrous tissues such as fascia. A number of factors can influence the rate of healing and strength of the wound, as discussed in a later section of this chapter.

Healing by Secondary Union

As with a wound in which the edges are closely approximated, bleeding occurs from the injured surface and a clot forms. The clot is unable to completely close the gap but covers the surface of the wound. An inflammatory reaction follows. As with healing by first intention, epithelial cells from the edges of the wound begin to migrate and proliferate. The epithelial cells move across the wound in a series of tonguelike projections underneath any remaining blood clot or exudate. Since the wound area is large, stratification of cells at the margin of the wound occurs before a single layer of epithelial cells has covered the center of the wound.

Granulation tissue starts to fill in the base of the wound before the epithelium has completely covered the surface. The granulation tissue grows upward from the base and inward from the edges until the defect is gradually filled. The capillary buds unite with each other and form loops filled with blood, giving the wound a red, granular appearance. The newly formed granulation tissue is very fragile and bleeds easily if the wound is not treated gently. Despite its fragility, the granulation tissue provides temporary protection of the wound, particularly against infection, until the epithelium covers the surface.

With skin wounds in which there has been an actual loss of tissue, there is a rapid reduction in the size of the defect by a process known as *wound contraction*. This process occurs while the wound is filling in with granulation tissue. The cause of wound contraction is not known but is believed to be due to contraction of fibroblasts in the granulation tissue. Contraction reduces the time required for healing and results in a scar that is much smaller than the original size of the wound. Unfortunately, deformity and loss of function may occur due to wound contraction, depending on the location and original size of the wound. On areas of the body where the skin is very mobile there will be no deformity and little scarring, for example, over the back, the buttocks, and the abdomen. Distortion and possibly impaired function result, however, in areas where the skin is attached to underlying structures, for example, in the extremities and over the anterior chest.

Complications of Healing

Occasionally an excessive amount of collagen is formed during repair, resulting in a large, irregularly shaped, raised area of scar tissue called a *keloid* (Fig. 8-4). Keloids frequently occur after burns and are most common in the neck region. They are more common in blacks than in whites.

If there is a delay in the covering of the wound with epithelium, granulation tissue may protrude

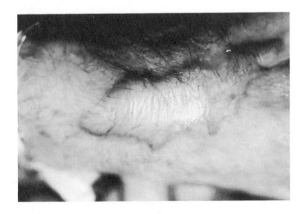

Figure 8-4. *A keloid on the back of the hand following a burn. (Photograph courtesy of Drs. J. Burton and W. S. Wood, Vancouver General Hospital, Vancouver, B.C., Canada.)*

above the surface of the wound. This situation is called *"proud flesh,"* or *exuberant granulation*, and it may in fact interfere with epithelialization. Exuberant granulation is more likely to occur during healing by second intention than healing by first intention.

Scar tissue may stretch if it is continuously strained. The result will be a *weak scar* and possibly an incisional hernia.

Occasionally *dehiscence*, or splitting open of a wound, may occur. Most cases of dehiscence involve upper abdominal incisions. General conditions that interfere with wound healing, for example, poor nutrition, or local factors such as infection or excessive tension on the wound contribute to dehiscence. Dehiscence of abdominal wounds is most likely to occur between the fifth and eighth postoperative days but has been known to happen as late as 25 days postoperatively. Dehiscence is usually preceded by a brown serosanguinous discharge from the wound and is sometimes, but not always, accompanied by *evisceration* (the extrusion of internal organs from the wound).

Healing of Fractures

Since bone is a type of connective tissue, healing of a fracture is similar to repair of soft tissue, except that it also involves osteogenesis to reunite the bone ends. Bone healing is regeneration because the characteristic structure of the bone is restored. The regenerative capacity of bone is limited, however, in that if half of a long bone is removed, the missing part will not be restored.

Composition of Bone

Bone tissue is composed of a mucoprotein ground substance (osseomucin) in which collagen fibers are embedded. This matrix is called *osteoid*. Bone salts crystallize on the collagen, making the tissue hard. The major bone mineral belongs to a group of calcium phosphate substances called hydroxyapatites, which have the approximate composition $Ca_{10}(PO_4)_6(OH)_2$. Small amounts of calcium carbonate and other minerals are also present. The exact mechanism by which calcification of bone collagen occurs is not known. The reason bone collagen calcifies but the collagen of soft tissues does not is also not clearly understood.

There are three types of bone cells. *Osteoblasts* are the bone-forming cells. They synthesize collagen and osseomucin. As bone is formed some cells become trapped in spaces called lacunae. These cells, called *osteocytes*, appear to regulate bone metabolism. Multinucleated cells called *osteoclasts* resorb, or break down, bone.

When the collagen bundles are irregularly arranged, *woven*, or *nonlamellar, bone* is formed. This type is immature and contains less osseomucin and calcium than mature bone. Woven bone is formed by intramembranous ossification during embryonic development of skull bones, the mandible, and the clavicle. Woven bone is also formed from granulation tissue during fracture healing.

Lamellar bone consists of collagen bundles arranged in parallel sheets. The sheets may be arranged either as flat plates or in concentric rings to form haversian systems. Lamellar bone is formed during the process of endochondral bone formation. In this process a cartilage model is replaced by bone. As the bone is laid down by osteoblasts the cartilage cells die and the cartilage is removed by osteoclasts. Lamellar bone is also formed during growth and by remodeling of woven bone. The normal adult skeleton is completely formed of lamellar bone, regardless whether the bone was formed by intramembranous or endochondral ossification during embryonic development.

According to its gross appearance, bone is divided into two types. *Cancellous* (spongy) bone consists of bony plates or columns, called trabeculae, which form a latticework around large spaces filled with marrow. Cancellous bone forms the central part of bones and the ends of long bones. The outer part of a bone is composed of dense *cortical* (compact) bone. Haversian systems are characteristic of compact bone. The outer surface of a bone is covered by a fibrous sheath called the *periosteum*. The *endosteum* is a similar sheet of fibrous tissue that lines the marrow spaces.

Bone Healing

When a bone is fractured, bleeding occurs from ruptured vessels in the haversian canals, marrow, and periosteum. As a result, a blood clot (fracture hematoma) forms between the broken bone ends. Damage to surrounding soft tissues may occur and contribute to the bleeding and clot formation. A typical inflammatory response follows, causing the periosteum to be lifted away from the surface of the bone.

Within a day or two necrosis of bone adjacent to the fracture occurs due to the disruption of the blood supply. Macrophages enter the wound and remove fibrin, red blood cells, inflammatory exudate, and debris in the usual demolition phase. Osteoclasts also develop in the area and resorb necrotic bone.

This phase is followed by the formation of granulation tissue. Capillaries grow into the wound from blood vessels of the periosteum, endosteum, and marrow. Undifferentiated osteogenic cells from undamaged periosteum and endosteum near the fracture site migrate into the area and proliferate. This granulation tissue is sometimes called a *soft callus*, or *procallus*.

The osteogenic cells then differentiate into osteoblasts or chondroblasts (cartilage-forming cells). Where the blood supply is good and there is adequate oxygen, osteogenic cells are transformed into osteoblasts. The osteoblasts lay down osteoid, which quickly becomes calcified to form woven bone. Bone starts to be formed at the fracture site after about two weeks. Where the blood supply is less adequate, however, the osteogenic cells differentiate into chondroblasts and hyaline cartilage is formed first. Later, as capillaries grow into the tissue, the cartilage is replaced by bone. Cartilage formation also occurs in inadequately immobilized fractures. Therefore, depending on conditions, varying amounts of woven bone and cartilage are formed to unite the bone ends. This mixture of woven bone and cartilage is called the *callus*.

Callus formed by endosteal cells fills the marrow cavity and is called the *internal callus*. The marrow cavity has a relatively good blood supply, so cartilage is rarely formed here. Cells from the periosteum form a sleeve of tissue called the *external callus*, which surrounds the bone fragments. The osteogenic cells closest to the bone surface usually differentiate into osteoblasts, but as the migrating and proliferating osteogenic cells move away from the blood supply they transform into chondroblasts. The external callus is therefore initially composed of three merging layers: an innermost layer of woven bone; a middle layer of cartilage; and an outer layer of osteogenic cells covered by fibrous tissue. Gradually direct union across the fracture surfaces is achieved by migration of osteogenic cells from the endosteum and periosteum and extension of the internal and external callus. This callus that is formed across the fracture gap in line with the cortex of the bone is called the *intermediate callus*.

The cartilage and woven bone are eventually invaded by capillaries, osteoclasts, and osteoblasts. The callus is replaced by lamellar bone. A final stage of remodeling then occurs, and bone is laid down according to the lines of stress. The internal callus is resorbed, thus restoring the marrow cavity. The intermediate callus is converted to compact bone, and the excess bone of the external callus is removed. Eventually the bone is restored to normal, and there may be little or no remaining sign of the injury. Bone healing is illustrated in Figure 8-5.

Healing of Articular Cartilage

The articular surfaces of bones are covered by hyaline cartilage. This cartilage has limited ability to regenerate and heals by repair with fibrocartilage.

Complications of Fracture Healing

Occasionally the undifferentiated cells from the periosteum and endosteum transform into fibroblasts. These cells lay down large amounts of collagen and the bone ends become united by fibrous connective tissue, similar to the scar that forms in soft tissue. This situation is called *fibrous union*; it occurs when the bone ends are not immobilized.

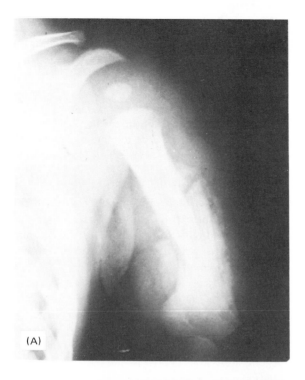

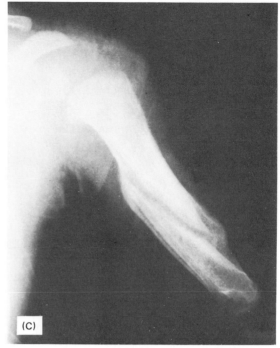

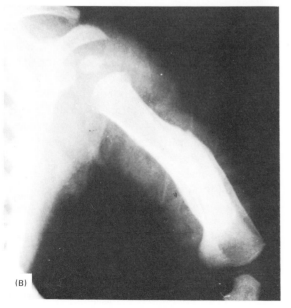

Figure 8-5. *X-ray photographs of bone healing in a child. (A) Fracture of the left humerus, one month postinjury, showing good callus formation bridging the fracture site. (B) Seven weeks postinjury. There is bony bridging at fracture site and early remolding of bone configuration. (C) Seven weeks postinjury. Oblique view showing bony bridging at fracture line and new bone.*

According to some authorities the fibrous tissue can sometimes be replaced by bone, but the process is very slow.

Nonunion is the complete failure of the bone to heal; it occurs if soft tissues such as muscle or fascia become interposed between the fracture ends.

Slow healing of a fracture is called *delayed union*. Excessive hemorrhage delays healing because a large hematoma requires more time to be removed. A large hematoma also leads to formation of a larger callus, which requires more time to be remodeled and removed. Inadequate immobilization delays healing because movement damages the granulation tissue and prolongs the inflammatory response. If movement is excessive, there may be fibrous union rather than eventual union with bone. Infection prolongs inflammation and may lead to extensive necrosis of bone, thus delaying union. A poor blood supply will delay union by slowing the formation of granulation tissue.

Healing of Nervous Tissue

Neurons cannot divide and so regeneration of lost nervous tissue is not possible. Healing in the central nervous system (CNS) is therefore a process of repair, similar to that in other parts of the body. Fibroblasts are not found in the CNS, but their counterparts are glial cells called astrocytes. Repair in the CNS thus involves scar formation with neuroglia rather than fibrous tissue.

If a neuron process is damaged but the cell body remains intact, the process may be restored. This restoration is most often seen in the peripheral nervous system. There is some controversy as to whether it occurs in the CNS.

Structure of a Peripheral Nerve

A peripheral nerve is made up of bundles of axons (nerve fibers) held together by connective tissue. Most axons are covered with a myelin sheath. Small gaps in the myelin sheath, called nodes of Ranvier, occur at regular intervals along the length of the axon. Surrounding an axon, whether it is myelinated or not, is a thin membrane called the neurilemma, or sheath of Schwann. With an electron microscope it can be seen that the myelin is formed by a Schwann cell that wraps itself around and around the axon. The nodes of Ranvier are the junctions between the Schwann cells. Unmyelinated fibers are also enveloped by Schwann cells, but in this case the Schwann cells do not spiral many times around the axon. The neurilemma is actually the cell membrane of the Schwann cell.

Outside the neurilemma each nerve fiber is enclosed in a connective-tissue sheath called the endoneurium. The perineurium surrounds a group of nerve fibers to form a bundle. The outermost layer of connective tissue is called the epineurium. It is located between and around the many bundles of nerve fibers that make up the whole nerve. Small blood vessels are also enclosed in the epineurium.

Regeneration of Perpheral Nerve Fibers

After injury to a nerve, if the fibers have been cut through, the severed ends retract. Characteristic changes occur in the neuron cell body after an axon has been damaged. The Nissl bodies disappear (chromatolysis), the nucleus is displaced from its usual central position to the periphery of the cell body, and the cell body swells. If an axon has been damaged close to the cell body, the cell may die. Otherwise the cell body returns to normal after a few weeks.

There is little or no change in the proximal portion of the damaged axon, but the distal fragment degenerates. Nonmyelinated fibers degenerate faster than myelinated fibers. After about 48 hours the myelin sheath (if present) also begins to degenerate. The debris is removed by macrophages.

Schwann cells close to the site of injury enlarge and proliferate. They also appear to ingest debris from the degenerating axon and myelin by phagocytosis. The proliferated Schwann cells fill the space formerly occupied by the axon, forming a pathway for its regrowth.

Within two days after injury, neurofibrils sprout out from the proximal portion of the severed axon and push their way through the Schwann cells. They grow at a rate of about 1 to 3 mm/day. Some of the fibrils make contact with an appropriate end-organ and form the new axon; it is very thin, but gradually increases in diameter. The fibrils that do not reach the end-organ degenerate. About six or seven days after injury a myelin sheath starts to form around the axon. Complete remyelinization takes about a year.

Restoration of function is a slow process and may never be completely achieved. The degree of restoration after nerve injury depends on several factors. Functional recovery is often poor when a mixed nerve is severed, because fibrils from a motor neuron may reach a sensory end-organ and vice versa. Recovery of a pure motor or pure sensory nerve is better. Functional recovery is best if the nerve trunk itself is not severed when the axons are damaged. For example, if a nerve is crushed axons may be severed while the endoneurium and perineurium remain intact. In this case regrowth of the axons occurs more easily because the structural framework of the nerve has been preserved. Functional recovery occurs more readily if the cut ends of the nerve are in close apposition than if there is a large gap.

Sometimes proliferation of axon sprouts and Schwann cells gives rise to a tangled mass of fibers. The result is a nonfunctional bulbous swelling called an *amputation neuroma* at the end of the proximal segment of a severed nerve. This complication is most likely to occur when a large gap exists between the cut ends of the nerve.

Healing of Liver

The liver has excellent regenerative capacity. Regeneration by division of existing hepatic cells occurs when a mass of liver is resected or undergoes necrosis, providing the person survives. Small surgically produced wounds such as result from biopsies, however, are repaired with fibrous tissue. The stimulus for hepatic regeneration is apparently a metobolic one that acts on the liver as a whole. The nature of the metabolic stimulus is not known. Presumably small surgical wounds do not provide an adequate stimulus.

Liver Regeneration

The success of regeneration depends on the adequacy of the blood supply and on the maintenance of the basic structural framework of the tissue. The outcome following hepatic necrosis depends on the extent and distribution of the necrotic lesions.

When microscopic foci of necrosis are scattered throughout the liver the condition is called *focal necrosis*. This condition accompanies many acute infections and is typical of viral hepatitis. Healing occurs by regeneration (i.e., division of surviving adjacent liver cells) with restoration of normal structure and function.

Zonal necrosis is the term applied when necrosis occurs in a particular part of each lobule throughout the liver. Central zonal necrosis is caused by many poisons, for example, carbon tetrachloride and chloroform. Midzonal necrosis is uncommon, but typically occurs with yellow fever. Peripheral zonal necrosis is also uncommon but is characteristic of phosphorus poisoning. It may also occur in eclampsia. In zonal necrosis the reticulin framework of each lobule is not destroyed and so healing by regeneration restores the normal liver architecture. If repeated zonal necrosis occurs, however, regeneration is not complete and fibrous scarring results.

Massive necrosis consists of large areas of necrosis throughout the liver. The condition may be idiopathic (i.e., the cause is unknown), or it may result from severe hepatitis or chemical poisoning. Death usually results from acute liver failure, but the person may survive long enough for some regeneration to occur. The architectural framework of the liver is destroyed, however, so that normal structure and function are not restored. Islands of surviving cells proliferate and form irregular lobules, but these are not normally oriented around blood vessels and bile ducts. A considerable amount of fibrous tissue scarring also occurs. The fibrous tissue forms bands that separate nodules of parenchymal tissue.

Cirrhosis

Cirrhosis is a chronic liver disease characterized by destruction of parenchymal cells and by loss of the normal lobular architecture due to the formation of bands of fibrous connective tissue and nodules of regenerating liver cells. In some cases the regenerating nodules are large (macronodular); in other cases they are small (micronodular). Sometimes large amounts of fat are present in the liver. The liver may be enlarged in the early stages of cirrhosis, but later it becomes smaller.

Many factors that cause liver damage can lead to cirrhosis: nutritional deficiencies, alcohol, viral hepatitis, and poisons are common causes. Cirrhosis may also occur secondary to prolonged biliary obstruction. Often the cause is not known.

In the early stages, cirrhosis of the liver may be asymptomatic. Generalized weakness, easy fatigability, and dependent edema are usually the earliest manifestations. The edema is due to hypoalbuminemia (a decreased amount of albumin in the blood) and retention of salt and water by the kidneys. (See Chapter 11 for a discussion of the mechanisms of edema formation.) Albumin is one of the major plasma proteins responsible for the colloid osmotic pressure, which holds fluid in the capillaries. Plasma albumin is synthesized only by the liver; therefore impaired liver function leads to a decrease in the plasma albumin concentration and thus a decrease in the colloid osmotic pressure. The salt and water retention is due to excess aldosterone. Aldosterone excess occurs because the diseased liver fails to inactivate aldosterone and because failure of the liver to inactivate renin leads to an increase in aldosterone production.

The disruption of the normal hepatic lobular architecture distorts the channels for blood flow. As a result, resistance to blood flow in the portal system is increased and portal hypertension develops. Blood from the spleen, stomach, intestine, and peritoneum flows into the portal vein; backpressure due to portal hypertension therefore has several consequences. The spleen enlarges and leukopenia, thrombocytopenia, and anemia occur as a result of sequestering of blood cells in the spleen. Hemorrhoids and esophageal varices (dilated, tortuous veins) develop. As mentioned in Chapter 7, life-threatening hemorrhage may occur from esophageal varices. Another consequence of portal hypertension is the development of ascites, an abnormal accumulation of fluid in the abdominal cavity. Backpressure due to portal hypertension causes increased capillary hydrostatic pressure, which results in an excessive loss of fluid from the capillaries. (See Chapter 11 for a discussion of the forces that influence movement of fluid across the capillary membrane.) Hypoalbuminemia and excess aldosterone are contributing factors in the development of ascites.

Cirrhosis impairs liver function, with several consequences. As already mentioned, plasma albumin is decreased. In addition, decreased synthesis of clotting factors and failure to remove FDP result in a bleeding tendency, as discussed in Chapter 7. Synthesis and/or secretion of bile salts may be decreased, resulting in impaired fat absorption and steatorrhea. Failure to excrete bilirubin in the bile results in increased levels of both conjugated and unconjugated bilirubin in the blood and development of jaundice (yellow or orange discoloration of the skin and sclera).

Many hormones are normally modified and inactivated by the liver. As already mentioned, failure to inactivate aldosterone leads to salt and water retention. In addition, sex-hormone metabolism is disturbed. In men with cirrhosis this disturbance may be manifested by atrophy of the testes and prostate, loss of hair on the chest, and gynecomastia (enlargement of the breasts).

The liver normally detoxifies many drugs and other substances (see Chapter 25). In cirrhosis, this function is impaired. Consequently, people with cirrhosis have a decreased tolerance for nitrogenous substances and for drugs, especially sedatives, narcotics, tranquilizers, and alcohol.

Healing of Other Tissues

Muscles
Damage to *cardiac muscle*, such as an infarct, is repaired by fibrous scar tissue. Apparently regeneration of myocardial cells occurs in children, however, after certain infections where there is damage to individual fibers without destruction of the endomysium.

Healing of visceral *smooth muscle* is usually by repair with fibrous scar tissue. There is evidence, however, that smooth muscle of the gastrointestinal tract may regenerate, especially if damage is not extensive.

Lost or damaged *striated muscle* tissue is usually replaced with fibrous tissue, but regeneration can occur under some circumstances. If the supporting structural framework of the muscle has not been damaged, new sarcoplasm can form within it. This process occurs in a condition called Zenker's degeneration, which may accompany severe infections (e.g., typhoid fever). If cut ends of skeletal muscles are carefully brought together, new growth may occur from the ends of the cut fibers to bridge the gap. This process does not involve cell division, but extension of existing cells. It is a slow process and may be stopped by the ingrowth of fibrous tissue.

Kidney

Nephrons cannot be regenerated if they are destroyed. Healing is by fibrous tissue repair when there is loss of kidney parenchyma, for example due to infarction. Regeneration of the renal tubular epithelium can occur, however, if the tubular basement membrane is intact.

Factors Influencing Healing

The general health status of a person, as well as local factors at the wound site, can influence inflammation and healing.

Local Factors

An adequate *blood supply* is probably the most critical factor in wound healing. Oxygen and nutrients, which are essential for restoring lost tissue, are brought to the wound site by the blood. Therefore, anything that impairs blood flow to the area will interfere with wound healing.

Although healing begins shortly after injury, while the acute inflammatory phase is in progress, repair or regeneration cannot be completed until acute inflammation subsides and debris is removed from the wound. Therefore, any factor that incites inflammation, such as the presence of *infection* or *foreign bodies*, will delay healing. Sutures are foreign bodies, and too many sutures can interfere with healing.

Excessive *hemorrhage* into the wound site not only stimulates inflammation but the clot also must be removed before healing can be completed. Therefore, excessive bleeding slows wound healing.

Immobilization of the wound is critical in the healing of fractures. It may also promote healing of soft-tissue wounds, especially if they are large. Movement may separate the wound edges and disrupt the fragile granulation tissue, causing bleeding.

General Factors

Age may influence wound healing. It is generally thought that healing is better in the young than in old people. The young do heal fast and healing may be slower in the elderly, but it has not been proven that this difference is directly due to age. Healing is normal in old age unless the blood supply to the wound is impaired or some debilitating disease is present. Impaired healing in the elderly is most often associated with inadequate circulation due to atherosclerosis.

Nutrition is an important factor in wound healing. Protein deficiency impairs the formation of granulation tissue and collagen and decreases wound strength. The sulfur-containing amino acids, methionine and cystine, are essential for synthesis of the mucopolysaccharides of the ground substance, as well as collagen. The lack of these components is the critical factor responsible for impaired healing during protein deficiency. Sufficient amounts of other amino acids necessary for wound healing are usually available from mobilization and breakdown of tissue proteins.

Vitamin C (ascorbic acid) is necessary for the formation of collagen. Deficiency of vitamin C results in delayed wound healing and decreased wound strength. The tissue levels of ascorbic acid are rapidly decreased in people with severe burns and multiple injuries, due to increased use of the vitamin. Therefore, the usual intake of vitamin C may be inadequate in these circumstances.

Adequate calcium and vitamin D are necessary

for healing of fractures. Vitamin D is required for calcification of bone.

Zinc may be necessary for wound healing. Experiments in animals have shown that zinc promotes healing, but a definite requirement in humans has not been established. The exact role of zinc in wound healing is not known, but zinc is a cofactor for several enzymes and so its beneficial effect in wound healing may be related to this function.

Adequate *oxygen* is critical for wound healing. It would be expected that *anemia* interferes with wound healing because it impairs oxygen transport in the blood. Experimental results are conflicting, however, and there is no agreement that anemia significantly impairs healing. Severe anemia may interfere with healing. Also, it has been shown that the incidence of complications is definitely lowered if anemia is corrected before surgery is performed.

Hormones, particularly the adrenocorticosteroids, influence the inflammatory-reparative response. The glucocorticoids, especially cortisol, inhibit inflammation and wound healing if they are present in large amounts, but the amount normally secreted has no significant effect. On the other hand, deoxycorticosterone, a mineralocorticoid, stimulates fibroblast proliferation and collagen formation.

Large doses of glucocorticoids decrease vascular permeability and thus prevent the leakage of fluid and protein in acute inflammation. Pavementing and emigration of leukocytes is apparently impaired by high levels of cortisol. Glucocorticoids also have a stabilizing effect on lysosomal membranes and thus prevent release of cellular enzymes that destroy tissues. Glucocorticoids also interfere with the formation of granulation tissue. ACTH produces similar effects because it stimulates glucocorticoid production. Increased quantities of these hormones are produced during stress (see Chapter 2). Acute stress apparently does not interfere with wound healing, but chronic stress may retard healing and decrease wound strength. Similarly, administration of large doses of glucocorticoids may inhibit healing, particularly if they are given just before or at the time of wounding. Mild starvation and protein deficiency enhance the effect of glucocorticoids. Under these conditions relatively low doses of cortisone inhibit the formation of granulation tissue.

There is little evidence that other hormones have any direct effect on wound healing, but severe metabolic disturbances caused by hormone imbalances do influence the healing process. Normal hormone levels, therefore, are probably a contributing factor in providing optimum conditions for healing. Healing tends to be impaired in people with diabetes mellitus, which may be related to poor blood supply to the wound, since people with diabetes are prone to atherosclerosis. If the diabetes is not well controlled, dehydration or ketoacidosis may interfere with healing. Parathyroid hormone and calcitonin regulate calcium metabolism and influence bone formation and resorption. Therefore, imbalances of these hormones, particularly hyperparathyroidism, can interfere with fracture healing. Estrogens and androgens stimulate protein synthesis and thus may be beneficial to healing.

SUGGESTED ADDITIONAL READING

Ross R: Wound healing. *Sci Am* **220**(6): 40–50, 1969.

9

Nervous System Responses

The nervous system performs vital functions in integrating and controlling bodily processes. Not only does it regulate activity of the internal environment but the nervous system also perceives stimuli impinging on a person from the external environment and directs responses to those stimuli. Therefore, any disturbance of homeostasis calls forth a response from the nervous system. Whenever wounding or tissue damage occurs, it is reflected by activity in the nervous system, usually in the form of increased sympathetic activity and perception of pain. In addition, alterations in the internal environment that disrupt homeostasis can interfere with brain function. Therefore, conditions such as hypoxia or hypoglycemia can alter a person's level of consciousness. Convulsive seizures may result from local irritation or damage to brain structures or as a response to systemic conditions such as fever or hypoglycemia. Damage to the nervous system can result in an altered state of consciousness and can also interfere with functioning of other parts of the body.

PAIN

From the physiological point of view, *pain* is a sensation of discomfort produced when tissue is damaged. The innate behavioral response to pain is to withdraw from or avoid the source of the pain. In this way pain serves as a protective mechanism to prevent further tissue damage.

Pain is accompanied by increased sympathetic nervous activity. Sympathetic stimulation causes an increased heart rate, which may increase cardiac output. It also causes vasoconstriction, which increases peripheral resistance. Therefore, blood pressure may rise during pain. In addition, pain is usually accompanied by a general stress response (see Chapter 2). Severe pain can produce shock by a neurogenic mechanism (see Chapter 14).

Pain causes reflex skeletal muscle responses. An external noxious stimulus impinging on an extremity (e.g., pricking a finger with a pin) elicits a flexor-withdrawal reflex, which is mediated at the spinal cord level. Pain arising from an internal source (i.e., visceral or deep pain) causes reflex contraction of muscles over the affected part. For example, abdominal muscle tension occurs with the pain of appendicitis. The increased muscle tension that accompanies pain can itself contribute to increased pain. In cases of prolonged severe pain particularly, a vicious cycle may be established in which the pain causes muscle tension and the muscle tension causes more pain.

The increased muscle tension that occurs with pain may be manifested in voluntary muscle activity as well as in involuntary responses. For example, a person in pain may respond with restlessness, writhing, pacing, or fist clenching. Such manifestations may occur particularly when it is impossible to avoid or withdraw from the source of the pain, for example, when the cause of the pain is internal.

Pain is much more than a physiological response to a noxious stimulus, however. It is a subjective psychological experience that varies from one person to another according to past experience and the meaning that the pain has for the person.

Types of Pain

Many words are used to describe pain, but three major types of pain are pricking, burning, and aching pain. *Pricking pain* is a stinging or piercing sensation. It is felt when the skin is pierced with a sharp point such as a needle or is cut with a knife. Strong irritation of a large area of the skin may also produce pricking pain. *Burning pain* is an intense sensation felt when a body surface is burned. It is caused not only by thermal burns but also by chemical irritation. For example, hot spices may cause a burning sensation on the tongue (which may be regarded as pain or pleasure, depending on the person). Another example is the sensation of burning on voiding that may occur when a person has a urinary tract infection. Burning pain can be excruciating. *Aching pain* usually has a dull quality, not sharp, although it can cause considerable discomfort. Aching pain is associated with deep structures rather than the surface of the body.

Referred Pain

Pain felt in a part of the body that is different from the tissue being stimulated is called *referred pain*. Pain is often referred from a visceral organ to an area on the surface of the body (Fig. 9-1). For example, damage to the heart may give rise to a pain sensation in the neck and shoulders or the left upper arm or radiating down the left arm and hand. Pain is occasionally referred from one surface area to another or from one deep part of the body to another.

The exact mechanism of referred pain is not known. One explanation is that primary afferent neurons from different sources converge on some of the same second-order neurons in the CNS. Stimulation of afferent neurons from one source

may then cause a "spillover" of activity to neurons that are usually excited by the afferent neurons from the other source. The sensation is then projected to the wrong source.

Phantom Pain

Phantom pain is a sensation of pain in a part of the body that has been amputated. In this case, activity of a nervous pathway arising either through stimulation at the site of amputation or due to some central abnormality gives rise to a sensation of pain that is projected to the once-present origin (i.e., receptor) of that pathway.

Causes of Pain

Anything that causes tissue damage can cause pain. *Noxious stimuli* that can produce pain include pressure, heat or cold, electric shock, and chemicals, as well as mechanical trauma. Activation of sensory receptors appears to result either from mechanical distortion or from the action of chemicals. Regardless of the original noxious stimulus, when tissues are damaged various chemical substances are formed or released (e.g., bradykinin and histamine), which may cause pain.

Ischemia can give rise to pain, although the exact reason for this is not known. One suggestion is that the accumulation of lactic acid in ischemic tissues is the stimulus for pain. During ischemia anaerobic glycolysis occurs in the tissue, producing large amounts of lactic acid. Ischemic pain is relieved by supplying oxygen to the affected tissue. Another possibility is that tissue damage due to ischemia liberates histamine and bradykinin, which then stimulate sensory nerve endings.

Muscle contractions can generate pain. Prolonged or repeated contraction of a skeletal muscle against an unaccustomed load results in fatigue or an ache that may become quite severe. For example, carrying a heavy suitcase can cause discomfort in the arm and shoulder muscles that eventually becomes so severe that the suitcase must be set down.

Acute muscle pain also occurs in people with

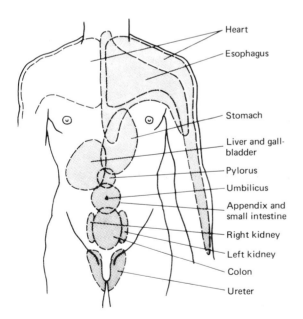

Figure 9-1. *Surface areas of referred pain from different visceral organs. (From Guyton AC: Textbook of Medical Physiology, ed 5, Philadelphia, W.B. Saunders Co., 1976.)*

Heart

Esophagus

Stomach

Liver and gallbladder

Pylorus

Umbilicus

Appendix and small intestine

Right kidney

Left kidney

Colon

Ureter

arterial disease. For example, when the femoral arteries are narrowed due to arteriosclerosis, *intermittent claudication* occurs. In this condition the person experiences discomfort in the leg muscles after walking a short distance. The pain is relieved when the person stops and rests, but returns when she or he walks a short distance again. When coronary blood supply is diminished, as in atherosclerosis, the flow of blood to the myocardium may become inadequate in relation to the load on the heart during exercise or stress. The resulting discomfort is known as *angina pectoris*.

Muscle spasms frequently cause pain. A spasm is an involuntary, sudden contraction of a muscle or group of muscles. The pain produced by muscle spasm is called a *cramp*.

In all these cases there is some degree of ischemia in the muscle because prolonged contraction interferes with blood flow. It has been suggested, however, that a toxic metabolic product other than lactic acid is responsible for the pain, since people with a deficiency of the enzyme that converts muscle glycogen to lactic acid can experience severe muscle pain. Whatever the toxic substance is, it is produced by the contracting muscle, it is not directly related to oxygen deficiency, and it apparently requires flowing blood to wash it out of the tissue. The discomfort is relieved when adequate blood flow through the tissue is resumed.

Another type of muscle pain is the dull aching pain that follows unaccustomed exercise and lasts for several days. This pain is presumably due to overload and damage to the muscles and their tendons. Regular exercise causes hypertrophy of the muscles and lessens the chance of injury.

Although pain is primarily associated with tissue damage, it may also be produced by psychological factors. Sometimes a person may have pain although there is no evidence of tissue damage or irritation of nerves. This condition is called *psychogenic pain*. Most, if not all pain, has a psychological component, but when the causes of pain are mainly or wholly psychological the term psychogenic pain is used. When the pain is primarily due to physical causes it is called *organic pain*.

Three main mechanisms give rise to psychogenic pain. On rare occasions pain may be a hallucination; this mechanism is usually associated with schizophrenia or endogenous depression. The second mechanism of psychogenic pain is muscle spasm due to tension caused by psychological factors. Tension headaches are believed to arise this way. Conversion hysteria is the third mechanism of psychogenic pain. In this case pain is believed to occur as the result of an unconscious emotional conflict. The "labor pains" suffered by some men while their wives are in childbirth are an example.

Pain Mechanisms

Exactly how and where pain is perceived is not known. The most prominent theories for a pain mechanism are the specificity theory and the gate-control theory.

Specificity Theory

According to the specificity theory, pain is a sensory modality like any other sense. There are specific pain receptors and pathways that carry impulses directly to a pain center in the brain (Fig. 9-2). The pain receptors are free nerve endings that are abundantly distributed in the skin and in some internal tissues such as the periosteum, arterial walls, joint surfaces, and meninges. Free nerve endings are not as numerous in other deep tissues but are diffusely distributed.

Impulses are carried from the receptors to the spinal cord via two types of fibers in the peripheral nerves: unmyelinated C fibers, which have a slow conduction velocity; and myelinated fibers of the A-delta class, which have a faster conduction velocity. The A-delta fibers are believed to carry impulses responsible for the pricking pain sensation, while the type C fibers transmit signals for burning and aching pain. The viscera are mainly supplied with C fibers, which travel with the sympathetic nerves.

Fibers of the pain pathway enter the spinal cord through the dorsal roots and ascend or descend one to three segments before synapsing with second-order neurons in the posterior horns. Fi-

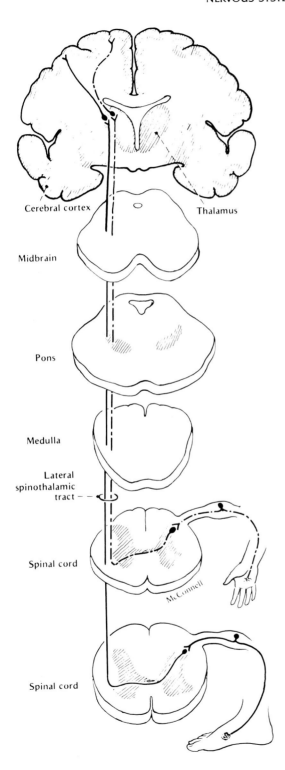

Cerebral cortex

Thalamus

Midbrain

Pons

Medulla

Lateral spinothalamic tract - -

Spinal cord

Spinal cord

bers from the second-order neurons immediately cross to the opposite side of the cord and ascend to the brain in the lateral spinothalamic tract. These fibers terminate in the thalamus.

A pain center in the thalamus is believed to be responsible for pain perception. Fibers from the thalamus then carry impulses to the cerebral cortex. At this level psychic influences modulate the appreciation of the pain and the response to it. According to the specificity theory, pain perception is the same for everyone, but people react differently to pain.

Gate-Control Theory

According to the gate-control theory, not only do people react differently to pain but they also perceive pain differently. This theory proposes that incoming impulses can be modulated in the spinal cord, as well as at higher levels. Inhibition by certain cells in the spinal cord can block transmission of impulses to the brain and thus prevent pain perception. In other words, incoming impulses are modulated by a gating mechanism. When the gate is open, impulses are transmitted to the brain. When the gate is closed, transmission is blocked. Cells of the substantia gelatinosa in the dorsal horns of the spinal cord are postulated to act as the gate.

When the skin is stimulated, nerve impulses are transmitted to three systems in the spinal cord: substantia gelatinosa (SG) cells; fibers of the dorsal column that send impulses to the brain; and central transmission (T) cells in the dorsal horn. The SG cells modulate afferent impulse patterns before they influence the T cells. Afferent impulses in the dorsal column system act, at least partly, as a central control trigger that activates selective brain processes. Impulses in descending fibers from the central control can then modulate properties of the gate-control mechanism. (Thus

Figure 9-2. *The sensory pathway for pain. (From Landau BR: Essential Human Anatomy and Physiology. Copyright © 1976 by Scott, Foresman and Company. Reprinted by permission.)*

psychological factors could influence sensory input.) The T cells transmit impulses to the brain and activate the neural mechanisms of the action system responsible for pain perception and response. There is no "pain center" responsible for perception and response. The action system involves neurons in many parts of the brain, including the brainstem reticular formation, thalamus, hypothalamus, limbic system, and cerebral cortex. The output of the T cells must reach or exceed a preset, critical level before the action system is triggered. In other words, there is temporal summation of incoming impulses by central cells of the action system.

Two types of afferent fibers can excite the T cells if they are not blocked by the gating mechanism: large-diameter, rapidly conducting fibers; and small-diameter, slowly conducting fibers. Activity of the SG cells can block transmission of impulses from the peripheral fibers to the T cells by presynaptic inhibition. This activity, in effect, closes the gate. The peripheral fibers synapse not only with the T cells, but also with the SG cells. Impulses from the large fibers excite the SG cells (close the gate), while impulses from the small fibers inhibit the SG cells (open the gate). Therefore, whether or not the gate is open is determined by the balance of activity in the large and small fibers (as well as by modulating factors, in either direction, from the central control). The gating mechanism is shown in Figure 9-3. In the absence of any obvious stimulation the gate is usually partially open.

Perception of pain would then occur in the following manner. Impulses would be generated in both the large and small fibers by stimulation of the skin. Impulses in the large fibers would rapidly reach the T cells and initially excite them. Almost simultaneously, however, impulses from the large fibers would also reach the SG cells and excite them. This stimulation of SG cells would close the gate and prevent transmission of impulses to the T cells from both large and small fibers. Impulses would still reach the SG cells from the peripheral fibers, however, and as more impulses arrive the SG cells are influenced by opposing effects

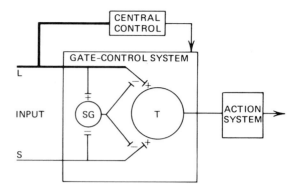

Figure 9-3. *Schematic diagram of the gate-control theory of pain. L indicates the large diameter fibers; S, the small diameter fibers; SG, the substantia gelatinosa cells; T, the T cells; +, excitation; −, inhibition. See text for explanation. (From Melzack R, Wall PD: Pain mechanisms: a new theory. Science* **150:** *971–979, November 19, 1965. Copyright 1965 by the American Association for the Advancement of Science.)*

from the large and small fibers. If there are more impulses coming in over the small fibers than over the large fibers, the SG cells are inhibited, presynaptic inhibitory activity of the SG cells stops, and the gate is opened. The T cells are then activated and send impulses to the brain. When a critical level of T-cell firing is reached the action system is triggered and pain is perceived.

The gate-control theory suggests that by selectively increasing the afferent input in the large fibers the gate can be closed and pain controlled. The relief of pain by acupuncture is possibly mediated in this manner. The large-diameter fibers can be stimulated by pressure, vibration, scratching, and massage. Clinically, electrical stimulation of the large fibers has been used to relieve chronic pain.

Sensitivity to Pain

Excessive sensitivity to pain is called *hyperalgesia.* Primary hyperalgesia is due to increased sensitivity of the receptors, such as occurs in sunburned skin. Secondary hyperalgesia results from an abnormality in the CNS. *Hypalgesia* is a decreased sensitivity to pain. The absence of pain is *analgesia*; this term is used particularly to denote the relief of pain without loss of consciousness.

Pain Threshold and Pain Tolerance

The *pain threshold* is the lowest intensity of stimulus that evokes a sensation of pain when the stimulus is applied continuously. Measurements of the pain threshold under laboratory conditions using a thermal stimulus indicate that there is no significant difference in the pain thresholds of different people. Most people feel pain when the skin temperature reaches 45°C (113°F). At this temperature heat begins to cause tissue damage. Using electrical stimulation, however, other researchers find that the pain threshold varies from one person to another.

The pain threshold is affected in several ways. If the threshold is increased, a greater stimulus is required to evoke pain. Distraction—that is, diverting attention away from the noxious stimulus—raises the threshold. The pain threshold is also increased by simultaneous stimulation of another part of the body. Fear tends to lower the pain threshold; in other words, a smaller stimulus will produce pain. A slight decrease in the threshold may occur with fatigue.

Pain tolerance is the degree of stimulus intensity a person will endure before requesting that the stimulus be withdrawn. It appears that tolerance to cutaneous pain increases with age, whereas tolerance to deep pain decreases with increasing age. There also appear to be racial and ethnic differences in pain tolerance. Some studies indicate there is no sexual difference in pain tolerance, but other researchers report that men have a higher pain tolerance than women. Pain tolerance is apparently more dependent on psychological factors, whereas pain threshold is more dependent on physiological factors.

As stated previously, pain is a subjective experience. It has been argued that pain produced in a laboratory setting is not the same as pain in a clinical setting. Clinical pain is often accompanied by fear and anxiety, which enhance pain perception. In addition, anticipation of pain and anxiety about pain increase the subjective pain experience. Some people tolerate pain well if they know it will not last very long or if the prognosis of the disease or injury is favorable. On the other hand, if the prognosis is poor, pain tolerance may be low.

Inherited Lack of Pain

Some people have an inherited lack of sensitivity to pain. Lack of pain is due to two major types of disorders. With *congenital indifference to pain*, affected people appear to have normal nerve-impulse transmission. They are believed to perceive pain physiologically, but appreciation of pain at the cerebral level is lacking and these people do not react to pain. Those with *congenital insensitivity to pain* usually have a defect in the peripheral nerves so that impulse transmission is impaired and affected people are unable to perceive pain. Although lack of pain might seem delightful, it can be a problem because those affected are lacking a protective mechanism. Affected people can experience tissue damage due to trauma, burns, or frostbite and be unaware that anything is wrong. As a result, tissue damage may be extensive and severe before some other factor draws their attention to the injury.

Reaction to Pain

Whether or not everyone has the same pain threshold and whether or not everyone perceives pain the same way, it can definitely be said that people react differently to pain. In addition to the physiological responses mentioned previously, many different psychically induced behaviors are manifested during pain. Some people become quiet and withdrawn, whereas other people react noisily and strike out at those around them. Some people want to be left alone, while others want familiar people with them. Some people become nauseated when they are in pain.

Past experience with pain, cultural attitudes, and religious beliefs can influence the way a person reacts to pain. Religious beliefs can also influence the meaning that pain has for a particular person. The meaning that pain has for the person experiencing it is very significant in determining the degree of suffering engendered by the pain. For example, a study of soldiers wounded in battle showed that they requested fewer analgesics than civilians with surgical wounds of similar magnitude. The explanation given for this behavioral difference is that the meaning of the painful experience was different in the two cases. For soldiers the wounds represented an honorable release from danger; they were still alive and did not have to continue fighting. For the civilians, on the other hand, surgery represented an unwelcome disruption of their normal lives; it was a disaster.

STATES OF CONSCIOUSNESS

Consciousness is a state of awareness of oneself and one's environment, consisting of two aspects: content and arousal. The *content* of consciousness refers to all the mental functions of a person, such as reasoning, thinking, and feeling. *Arousal* refers to the state of wakefulness or responsiveness of an individual. It is difficult to define consciousness precisely, because it can only be inferred from a person's appearance and behavior.

Brain Activity and Consciousness

Very little is known about the neural mechanisms involved in consciousness. Certainly, consciousness involves the integrated activity of many parts of the brain. The content of consciousness is largely a function of the cerebrum, but physiologists and psychologists do not know the mechanisms involved. Mental processes appear to be not only influenced by external stimuli but also generated by spontaneous activity of brain cells.

Arousal is largely a function of parts of the reticular formation. The reticular formation is a diffuse network of fibers and gray matter in the core of the brainstem, extending from the lower medulla to the thalamus. The functional component of the reticular formation responsible for arousal is called the *reticular activating system* (RAS).

The RAS involves parts of the reticular formation in the upper pons and midbrain and has synaptic connections with many parts of the brain. It receives branches (collaterals) from every major sensory pathway and therefore is stimulated by all major afferent input. An alert, responsive, conscious state apparently depends on interactions between the RAS and the cerebral cortex. The RAS stimulates thalamic reticular nuclei, which then activate the cerebral cortex and alert it to incoming sensory information. The cerebral cortex in turn restimulates the RAS and modulates its activity. This feedback mechanism may be the basis of selective arousal, which depends on the meaning of incoming sensory information. (For example, a mother may be aroused when her child cries, but not by other sounds of equal or greater intensity.) There are also connections between the reticular formation and the rhinencephalon, a part of the brain believed to be involved with emotions and memory.

The Electroencephalogram (EEG)

The electroencephalogram is a recording of the electrical activity of the cerebral cortex determined by placing electrodes on the skull. Although the EEG records cortical activity, stimuli from deeper brain structures to the cortex determine the form of the normal EEG. The EEG records the activity of many neurons, which are not necessarily firing in phase with one another. When neuronal activity is synchronized, large slow waves are produced on the EEG, but unsynchronized activity results in smaller, higher-frequency waves. The different types of waves seen on an EEG are shown in Figure 9-4.

In a normal adult who is awake but relaxed, with eyes closed, the predominant EEG pattern is the *alpha rhythm*. Alpha waves have a frequency of 8 to 13 cycles per second, or hertz (Hz), and an average amplitude of 25 to 50 microvolts (μV). Alpha rhythm differs from one person to another but is generally quite constant for a given individual. Metabolic changes, such as are produced by anoxia or hypoglycemia, decrease the frequency

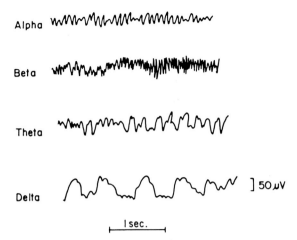

Alpha

Beta

Theta

Delta] 50 μV

|— 1 sec. —|

Figure 9-4. *Different types of normal electroencephalographic waves. (From Guyton AC: Textbook of Medical Physiology, ed 5, Philadelphia, W.B. Saunders Co., 1976.)*

of the alpha rhythm. During mental effort or when a person is alert to external stimuli, the EEG pattern changes and the alpha rhythm is replaced by lower-amplitude, higher-frequency waves.

Beta waves are also present in all normal adult EEGs. They have a frequency greater than 13 Hz and a low amplitude (less than 20μV). Beta rhythm tends to predominate and may replace the alpha rhythm in people who are tense and anxious.

Theta waves have a frequency of 4 to 7 Hz and an amplitude less than 20μV. In awake adults they do not usually form more than 5% of the EEG. Theta rhythm is the predominant EEG pattern, however, in children from 2 to 5 years of age. The pattern changes and gradually becomes intermingled with alpha waves as a child gets older.

Delta waves have a frequency of 1 to 4 Hz. This pattern is predominant in the EEG of infants up to 1 year of age. Delta rhythm is not normally present in the EEG of an awake adult.

The EEG pattern changes during sleep. Four different EEG patterns are recognized, and during sleep, a person normally passes sequentially through these stages several times.

In stage 1 there is first a slight slowing of the alpha rhythm. Shortly afterward the alpha waves are replaced by low-amplitude theta waves, but brief periods of alpha rhythm recur from time to time. The first episode of stage 1 EEG activity is associated with drowsiness and very light sleep, but later episodes are associated with deeper sleep and are accompanied by rapid eye movements (REM). This deep sleep accompanied by an EEG pattern suggesting wakefulness is sometimes called paradoxical sleep; dreaming occurs at this time.

The stage 2 EEG is associated with light sleep. The low-amplitude theta waves are interrupted from time to time by brief bursts of activity called sleep spindles. These spindles have a high amplitude and a frequency of 12 to 14 Hz.

The stage 3 EEG is characterized by the appearance of high-amplitude delta waves with a frequency of 1 to 2 Hz. Some sleep spindles still occur. This stage represents moderate sleep.

The stage 4 EEG is associated with deep sleep. High-amplitude slow waves (delta waves) predominate. These waves have an amplitude of 100 μV or more and a frequency of 1 to 2 Hz. No sleep spindles occur in this stage.

Disorders of Consciousness

A functionally intact brain is necessary for normal conscious behavior. Impaired consciousness indicates severe brain dysfunction. The content of consciousness may be reduced by localized cerebral defects without affecting arousal (e.g., aphasia). This condition is not usually considered an altered state of consciousness. People with acute global aphasia, however, are unable to communicate, and therefore it may be difficult to determine their responsiveness.

Clouding of Consciousness

In *clouding of consciousness* the content of consciousness is altered and arousal is reduced. Periods of drowsiness alternate with episodes of excitability and irritability. Perception is altered and the person is easily startled. In addition, the person cannot think clearly and is easily distracted.

A greater degree of clouding produces a *confusional state*. A confused person is often drowsy during the day and agitated at night. She or he misinterprets sensory stimuli, has a short attention span, and is often unable to follow commands. Memory is impaired. Disorientation for time and possibly for person or place may occur. Confusion is associated with reduced cerebral metabolism.

Delirium

Delirium is characterized by mental dysfunctioning; that is, altered content of consciousness. A delirious person is disoriented, has illusions, and frequently has visual hallucinations. Loud incoherent speech and physical restlessness are common. Delusions, during which the person is completely out of contact with the environment, are also common. Sometimes delirium is interspersed with lucid periods, during which the person may be terrified of his or her mental disturbance. The frequency of the EEG waves is slowed during delirium.

Delirium is usually associated with toxic states and metabolic disturbances. It was once commonly associated with severe systematic infections (e.g., typhoid fever) but rarely occurs with infections now that antibiotics are available. Delirium often occurs just before a person goes into stupor or coma or as she or he is coming out of coma.

Stupor and Coma

In stupor and coma the defect in arousal is so severe that it is not possible to determine potential mental content.

Stupor is a state of unresponsiveness from which a person can be aroused only with difficulty. That is, repeated intense stimulation is required to rouse a stuporous person. Stupor is usually associated with diffuse organic cerebral dysfunction, but can sometimes occur during deep physiological sleep. Stupor may also occur in catatonic schizophrenia.

Coma is a state of unconsciousness from which a person cannot be aroused; that is, he or she is to-tally unresponsive. A person in coma does not respond to external stimuli or internal needs. During the first few days or weeks of unconsciousness, people in coma do not show behavioral signs of sleep-wake cycles. With prolonged severely impaired consciousness, however, many people later have periods of quietness and restlessness that suggest the occurrence of sleep-wake cycles.

Coma was once regarded to be the same as sleep; certainly both are characterized by an absence of conscious behavior. The two are quite different, however. A person can be aroused from sleep but not from coma. In coma the EEG is characterized by slow waves. Slow waves also occur during sleep, but in coma the EEG does not show the changes characteristic of REM sleep. Decreased oxygen uptake by the cerebrum occurs during coma but not during sleep.

Brief States of Altered Consciousness

Two other conditions of altered consciousness occur frequently: syncope and concussion. *Syncope* is a sudden transient loss of consciousness due to cerebral ischemia.

Concussion is a brief period of unconsciousness after a closed head injury (e.g., being struck on the head with a blunt object). The mechanism of concussion is unknown. It apparently is not associated with any organic brain damage but represents suspended functioning in the cerebrum and/or the brainstem reticular formation. Concussion may last from a few minutes to several hours and is followed by a brief period of confusion.

Causes of Coma

Conditions that cause coma can be classified into four groups: (1) supratentorial mass lesions; (2) subtentorial lesions; (3) metabolic and diffuse cerebral disorders; and (4) psychiatric disorders.

Supratentorial and Subtentorial Lesions

The *tentorium cerebelli* is a part of the dura mater that extends transversely between the cerebrum and the cerebellum. The external border of the tentorium is attached to the skull. The internal aspect of the tentorium forms the border of an opening called the *tentorial notch*. The brainstem passes from the undersurface of the cerebrum through the tentorial notch into the posterior cranial fossa. *Supratentorial lesions* affect the structures of the anterior cranial fossa (i.e., above the tentorium). *Subtentorial lesions* affect structures in the posterior fossa (i.e., below the tentorium).

Supratentorial and subtentorial lesions can be due to traumatic injuries, hematomas, hemorrhage, infarction, tumors, or abscesses. Supratentorial lesions can cause coma if they produce diffuse bilateral abnormalities of the cerebral cortex or underlying white matter without brainstem damage. Localized lesions of the cerebral hemispheres can cause coma if they impinge on or compress deep medial structures of the diencephalon (thalamus and hypothalamus).

Subtentorial lesions located within the brainstem can cause coma if they destroy the reticular formation of the pons and midbrain. Lesions outside the brainstem (e.g., in the cerebellum) that compress the reticular formation can also produce coma.

Metabolic Disorders

Brain dysfunction caused by intrinsic metabolic disorders of neurons or glial cells is called *primary metabolic encephalopathy*. This category includes several degenerative brain diseases that develop insidiously, are usually irreversible, and ultimately cause coma. When brain metabolism is impaired by some condition arising outside the brain, the term *secondary metabolic encephalopathy* is used. Secondary metabolic encephalopathy is much more common than the primary disorders.

The brain requires a constant supply of energy for three major functions: to maintain neuron membrane potentials and restore them following nerve-impulse transmission by actively transporting potassium into and sodium out of cells; to synthesize acetylcholine and other substances necessary for synaptic transmission; and to synthesize enzymes and structural cellular components to re-

place those that have been catabolized. Energy for these purposes comes from the oxidation of glucose. Under normal physiological conditions glucose is the brain's only energy source. Glucose is also used for the synthesis of other compounds required by the brain. The brain depends on glucose because other substances, such as fatty acids, are unable to cross the blood-brain barrier. (Experiments have shown that isolated brain tissue can metabolize other substances.) Betahydroxybutyrate and other ketone bodies derived from fat catabolism can cross the blood-brain barrier and are used for energy during starvation. This condition is discussed in Chapter 17.

Glucose enters the brain by a process called *facilitated diffusion*. Facilitated diffusion is mediated by a carrier molecule that assists in the transfer of a given substance across the cell membrane. Unlike active transport, which also involves a carrier molecule, facilitated diffusion does not require energy expenditure by the cell. As with ordinary diffusion, facilitated diffusion involves movement of a substance from a region of high concentration to a region of lower concentration. Therefore, the amount of glucose entering the brain cells depends on the concentration of glucose in the blood. Insulin does not directly affect uptake of glucose by brain cells, but influences the availability of glucose by its effect on the blood glucose level.

The energy released by the oxidation of glucose is used to form ATP, which is then used to drive other energy-requiring processes. When oxygen is not available in sufficient amounts, glucose is catabolized by the process of anaerobic glycolysis, which yields only two molecules of ATP per molecule of glucose. In contrast, when adequate oxygen is available 36 ATP molecules are produced per molecule of glucose. A constant supply of oxygen is therefore essential to provide enough ATP for normal brain functioning.

Coma due to secondary metabolic encephalopathy, therefore, can be caused by any factor that interferes with the supply of glucose and/or oxygen to the brain or interferes with the functioning of the enzymes involved in glucose metabolism.

Thus, hypoxia and hypoglycemia can cause coma. Lack of blood flow deprives the brain of both oxygen and glucose; therefore, ischemia can cause coma. Deficiencies of vitamins required as cofactors for enzymes can cause secondary encephalopathy. In particular, the B vitamins thiamine, niacin, pyridoxine, and cyanocobalamin are necessary for glucose metabolism. Electrolyte and acid-base imbalances (see Chapters 15 and 16) can also interfere with enzyme activity and cause coma.

Many toxins can interfere with activities of enzymes. A buildup of toxins in the internal environment due to organic diseases outside the nervous system can interfere with brain metabolism and cause coma. Examples are hepatic coma due to liver disease and uremic coma due to kidney disease (see Chapter 26). Secondary metabolic encephalopathy can also result from drug overdoses (e.g., barbiturates, salicylates) or ingestion of poisons (e.g., methanol, cyanide), and from diseases producing toxins in the CNS (e.g., meningitis, encephalitis). Thermal imbalance, such as hypothermia and heat stroke, can also interfere with brain metabolism and cause coma (see Chapter 24).

Psychiatric Disorders

People in states of psychic withdrawal or psychogenic unresponsiveness may appear to be in stupor or coma in the absence of organic disease. In psychogenic disturbances, however, the EEG is usually that of a normal awake person rather than someone in coma. People with catatonic schizophrenia may have abnormal EEG patterns, but the patterns differ from the EEG pattern seen in those with coma due to organic disease.

EPILEPTIC SEIZURES

An *epileptic seizure* is an abrupt disturbance of cerebral functioning resulting from excessive discharge by a group of hyperexcitable neurons. An individual epileptic seizure is not the same thing as epilepsy. The term *epilepsy* refers to a chronic condition characterized by recurrent epileptic seizures. An individual epileptic seizure may represent one episode of a chronic condition or may occur as an isolated incident in conjunction with an acute illness. An *epileptic prodrome* may occur several hours or days before an epileptic seizure takes place. The prodrome may be manifested as a change in mood or behavior, or occasionally as a headache. It is usually due to an increase in neuronal excitability. An *aura* is a strange sensory experience that occurs at the onset of some epileptic seizures.

A *convulsion* is an involuntary contraction or series of contractions of skeletal muscles. A convulsion may be a manifestation of an epileptic seizure, in which case it is due to a cerebral disturbance. Not all convulsions have an epileptic origin, however. Some convulsions are due to disturbances in the spinal cord or peripheral nerves.

Types of Epileptic Seizures

There are many forms of epileptic seizures, and a description of all of them is beyond the scope of this book. The various types of seizures, however, have been grouped into four main categories: generalized seizures; unilateral (hemigeneralized) seizures; partial (focal, local) seizures; and seizures that cannot be classified because of incomplete data.

Generalized Seizures

Generalized seizures involve the entire cerebral cortex. Synchronous firing of neurons throughout most, if not all, the gray matter occurs simultaneously in both hemispheres. Generalized seizures are characterized by impaired consciousness, massive autonomic discharge, and often bilateral generalized motor changes. The motor changes may be manifested as either convulsions or hypotonia (decreased muscle tone).

The aura that occurs at the start of some seizures

is actually a partial (localized) seizure that precedes the generalized seizure. Some people therefore distinguish between seizures as partial with secondary generalization (i.e., those with an aura), or generalized from the onset (i.e., those without an aura).

Tonic-clonic (grand mal) seizures present a classic picture of a convulsive generalized epileptic seizure. Grand mal is the most common type of epileptic seizure, except during the first six months of life. The synchronous repetitive firing of neurons that is necessary to produce a grand mal seizure is not possible during early infancy because of incomplete myelination of cerebral neuron fibers.

Usually a series of massive bilateral muscular contractions lasting several seconds immediately precedes the seizure. The muscular contractions tend to cause flexion and as a result the person falls. This phase is often accompanied by a spasmodic cry.

An affected person is in coma throughout a grand mal seizure. The attack starts with a tonic phase of 10 to 20 seconds in duration, which is characterized by sustained tetanic contractions of all skeletal muscles in succession. The tonic contractions start with flexor muscles. Muscles that elevate and depress the jaw are equally involved, so that the mouth is rigidly held half open at this time. The period in flexion is brief and is followed by a longer period in extension. Contraction of muscles that depress the jaw is followed by contraction of muscles that elevate the jaw. As a result, the mouth opens wide and then snaps closed. The tongue may be bitten at this time. Contraction of thoracic and abdominal muscles causes a prolonged expiration. Air is forced across a spasmodic glottis, producing a typical cry.

Recurrent decreases in muscle tone cause the tonic contractions to be replaced by tremors. The person then enters the clonic phase, which lasts about 30 seconds. This phase consists of alternate muscular contractions and relaxations in rapid succession. The entire body is involved in a series of violent flexor spasms. Each spasm may be accompanied by an explosive cry and the tongue is often bitten. The periods of relaxation gradually become longer, and the seizure ends with a final massive contraction.

Massive discharge by autonomic neurons causes a number of functional changes during a grand mal seizure. The autonomic manifestations reach a maximum at the end of the tonic phase and then decline at the beginning of the clonic phase. Heart rate and blood pressure increase. Bladder muscles contract and cause a great increase in pressure inside the bladder. Urinary incontinence does not occur at this time, however, because the sphincter muscles are also in spasm. Dilation of the pupils occurs during the tonic phase and is followed by alternate dilation and constriction during the clonic phase. Increased perspiration and salivation occur, as well as an increase in tracheobronchial secretions. Following the prolonged expiration in the tonic phase, a period of apnea occurs, which continues throughout the clonic phase and results in hypoxia. The sustained muscle contractions interfere with venous return of blood and cause vascular congestion. As a result of the impaired circulation and hypoxia, the skin color changes from pallor to flushing to cyanosis.

The EEG pattern during a generalized tonic-clonic seizure is shown in Figure 9-5. The EEG activity indicates an end to the epileptic seizure at the end of the clonic phase, but a complete return to normal functioning does not occur immediately. A period of muscular flaccidity (lack of muscle tone) lasting five to eight seconds follows the clonic phase. Relaxation of the urinary sphincters at this time allows passive emission of urine, although the bladder pressure is low. Fecal incontinence rarely occurs. The flaccidity is followed by another phase of tonic muscular contraction, primarily affecting the facial muscles, which may last a few seconds or several minutes. Pupillary dilation, tachycardia, and rapid breathing occur at this time. A period of recuperation follows, which is characterized by muscular flaccidity. Autonomic functions return to normal. Consciousness is

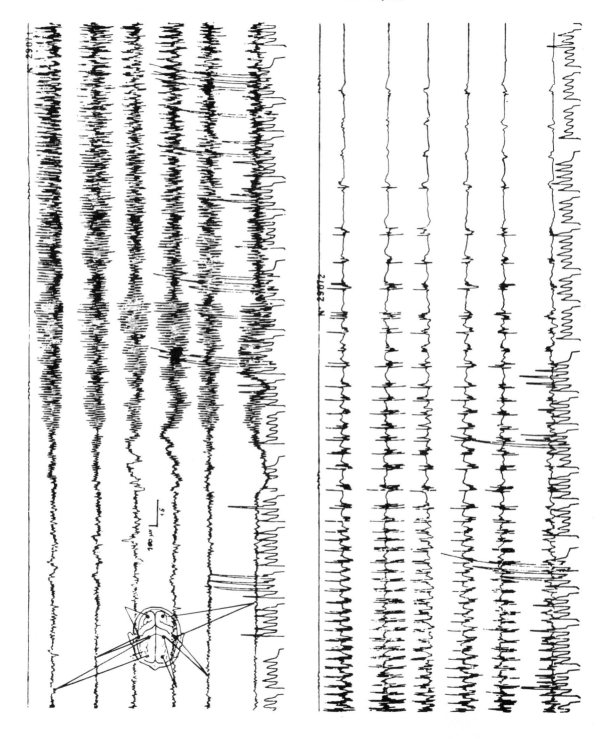

gradually regained, with a state of confusion occurring before full consciousness is reached. The person has no memory of the events occuring during the seizure or immediately preceding it (retrograde amnesia).

A nonconvulsive type of generalized epileptic seizure is the *typical absence (petit mal seizure)*. The term absence came from the French and in the original context meant "absence of mind." Petit mal seizures occur most commonly in children between the ages of 4 and 16 years.

The typical absence begins with an abrupt loss of consciousness and lasts 5 to 30 seconds. All mental functions are suspended, and the person does not usually see, hear, or feel. Activity stops and the person becomes motionless, staring blankly. The only motor manifestations are flickering of the eyelids or possibly twitching of some facial muscles. The seizure usually ends with a smile, and the person resumes activity where she or he left off. Although complete retrograde amnesia usually occurs, the person may realize the seizure has occurred because of an awareness of time-related changes in the environment.

Occasionally a petit mal seizure does not involve complete suspension of mental functions, but only mild confusion. This type of attack occurs particularly with very brief (three to four seconds or less) absences and the affected person is able to carry on simple behavior that is more or less automatic (e.g., walking).

Unilateral Seizures

Unilateral seizures are similar to generalized seizures except that they occur on only one side of the body or are more predominant on one side than the other. These seizures result from diffuse neuronal discharge in one cerebral hemisphere and its subcortical connections. Unilateral seizures do not always occur on the same side in a particular individual. A seizure may occur on one side on one occasion and the opposite side in the next attack. The impairment of consciousness and autonomic changes are not as severe in unilateral seizures as in generalized seizures. Unilateral seizures primarily affect infants and young children. The reason they are restricted to this age group is not known.

Partial Seizures

Partial seizures are caused by discharges from one anatomical and/or functional system of neurons. The neurons may be quite widely distributed in the cerebral cortex and subcortical structures, but do not involve an entire hemisphere. Partial seizures may be classified into attacks with simple symptomatology and those with complex symptomatology.

Seizures with simple symptomatology start and end abruptly and usually last less than one minute. Consciousness is not usually significantly impaired. Manifestations may be primarily motor or sensory or autonomic depending on the group of neurons involved. Motor seizures are characterized by convulsive movements in localized parts of the body. Areas of the body such as the thumb, fingers, lips, and great toe, which are represented by a large cortical area in the precentral gyrus, are often involved. In some motor seizures (jacksonian seizures), the muscle spasms characteristically pass progressively from one part of the body to another. Sensory seizures may involve any sensory modality and produce such manifestations as tingling or numbness of a part of the body; seeing bright moving spots of light; hearing buzzing, hissing, or ringing noises; or smelling disagreeable odors. Autonomic seizures most commonly affect the gastrointestinal tract; other autonomic functions are rarely affected. Any part of the alimentary tract can be involved. Colicky abdominal pain is characteristic of intestinal involvement (abdominal epilepsy).

Figure 9-5. *The EEG pattern during a generalized tonic-clonic seizure. (From Gastaut H, Broughton R: Epileptic Seizures: Clinical and Electrographic Features, Diagnosis and Treatment, 1972. Courtesy of Charles C Thomas, Publisher, Springfield, Ill.)*

Partial seizures with complex symptomatology usually start and end in a progressive manner and last two minutes or more. Clouding of consciousness usually occurs. The symptoms are mainly psychic, such as illusions, hallucinations, behavioral automatisms, affective disturbances, or intellectual disturbances.

Status Epilepticus

Status epilepticus is a state of prolonged continuous seizure activity or a series of attacks in such rapid succession that consciousness is not regained or no recovery occurs between seizures. Status epilepticus can occur with partial, unilateral, or generalized seizures. An uncontrolled status epilepticus involving a partial seizure usually does not cause major impairment of general health. Grand mal status epilepticus, on the other hand, can be fatal after 48 to 72 hours.

The mechanism by which seizures are normally terminated is not known. One early theory is that with gradually increasing hypoxia and decreasing glucose the brain cells run out of energy. This theory, however, does not explain the abrupt manner in which seizures end. It is now believed that a mechanism of active inhibition is responsible for seizure termination. Status epilepticus represents a failure of the seizure-terminating mechanism. Suddenly discontinuing anticonvulsive medication (particularly phenobarbital) can contribute to such a failure.

Causes of Epileptic Seizures

Although the exact nature and extent of the genetic component in epilepsy is not know, most authorities agree that an inherited predisposition is important in determining whether a person will have an epileptic seizure, regardless of the particular environmental precipitating factor(s). Some people have a very low epileptic threshold (i.e., a greater hereditary risk) and may have seizures in the absence of any obvious environmental precipitating factor. In other cases the epileptic threshold is high and severe environmental distur-

bances are necessary to evoke a seizure (i.e., a lower hereditary risk).

According to the etiology, epileptic seizures can be divided into two causal groups: organic and nonorganic (functional). The cause is considered to be organic when pathological structural changes are present in the brain. When no obvious organic cerebral damage can be demonstrated, the cause is said to be functional. Functional epileptic seizures result from a genetic disorder or acquired metabolic disturbance. Isolated seizures are caused either by metabolic factors that suddenly increase neuronal excitability (i.e., lower the epileptic threshold) or organic lesions that cause local irritation and excitation of cerebral neurons. Chronic epilepsy either has a genetic cause or is due to an organic lesion. Seizures due to metabolic or organic factors are sometimes called *symptomatic* epilepsy, as opposed to *genetic* or familial epilepsy. This distinction is rather arbitrary, however, because strong evidence exists that genetic factors influence the probability that epileptic seizures will occur in a person with an acquired metabolic or organic disorder. (Many people have metabolic disturbances or organic brain damage without having seizures.) On the other hand, the seizures of genetic epilepsy are probably symptomatic of a biochemical defect that in some way alters brain metabolism, neuronal membrane stability, or nerve-impulse transmission, but the nature of the defect is not yet known.

Epileptic seizures are much more common in childhood than adulthood. The neurons of the brain are very excitable during the first two years of life. The infant brain also has fewer inhibitory mechanisms. Therefore, some factors that will cause seizures in infants and young children (e.g., hypocalcemia, fever) will not produce seizures in older children and adults.

Genetic (Idiopathic) Epilepsy

As just mentioned, in some cases the functional defect causing epileptic seizures is not known, but the person has a strong inherited predisposition to epileptic seizures. Some children have such a low epileptic threshold that seizures apparently occur spontaneously, in the absence of any obvious precipitating factor. With increasing age the likelihood of such spontaneous seizures diminishes. In other children, sudden noise or bright light may precipitate a seizure. Others have a higher epileptic threshold and a more obvious triggering factor (e.g., fever, fatigue) is necessary to evoke an epileptic seizure.

Metabolic Factors

Many metabolic disturbances evoke epileptic seizures; the seizures produced are usually generalized (except in very young infants). Pyridoxine (vitamin B_6) deficiency is sometimes the cause of severe seizures in neonates and infants. Disorders of amino acid and protein metabolism, such as PKU and other inborn errors of metabolism (see Chapter 6), are frequently associated with epileptic seizures. Fluid and electrolyte imbalances, such as hypernatremia and water intoxication (see Chapter 12), may also cause seizures. Hypocalcemia (see Chapter 16) is often the cause of unilateral or partial seizures in the first few weeks of life, but does not cause seizures in older children or adults. Hypoglycemia, poisoning by exogenous toxins such as pesticides, endogenously produced toxic states due to hepatic or renal insufficiency and toxemia of pregnancy, and withdrawal of sedative drugs such as alcohol and short-acting barbiturates are all factors that can precipitate epileptic seizures.

Hyperthermia is a frequent cause of epileptic seizures (febrile convulsions) in children between the ages of 6 months and 3 years. Occasionally febrile convulsions occur in children up to age 5. The fever that precipitates the convulsive seizure is often due to a trivial infection of the upper respiratory tract.

Organic Lesions

Organic lesions usually cause partial seizures, which may or may not become secondarily generalized. Acquired pathological cerebral changes are due to many factors: infection (e.g., encephalitis and meningitis); toxic substances (e.g., lead, alcohol); anoxia; vascular changes (e.g., arteriosclerosis, thrombosis); abscesses; tumors; and traumatic head injuries. Brain damage acquired prenatally or at birth may give rise to epileptic seizures that are not manifested until later in childhood or occasionally even in adulthood.

Trauma, brain tumors, and chronic alcoholism are the most common causes of epileptic seizures in adults. Seizures occurring immediately (within seconds) following a head injury are attributed to mechanical irritation of cerebral structures. Cerebral edema is responsible for seizures that develop 24 to 48 hours after trauma. Posttraumatic seizures having their onset several months after a head injury are due to scarring.

SUGGESTED ADDITIONAL READING

DiBlasi M, Washburn CJ: Using analgesics effectively. Am J Nurs 79 (1): 74–78, 1979.

Dodd MJ: Assessing mental status. Am J Nurs 78(9): 1500–1503, 1978.

Jouvet M: The states of sleep. Sci Am 216(2): 62–72, 1967.

Melzack R: The perception of pain. Sci Am 204(2): 41–49, 1961.

Muehl JN: Seizure disorders in children: prevention and care. MCN 4(3): 154–160, 1979.

Silman J: Reference guide to analgesics. Am J Nurs 79(1): 74–78, 1979.

Trockman G: Caring for the confused or delirious patient. Am J Nurs 78(9): 1495–1499, 1978.

Wilkinson O: Out of touch with reality. Am J Nurs 78(9): 1492–1494, 1978.

UNIT FOUR

DISTURBANCES
OF HOMEOSTASIS

10

Oxygen Imbalance

Oxygen is vital for normal cellular metabolism. The amount of oxygen delivered to the cells is determined by the oxygen content of inspired air, ventilation of the lungs, diffusion of oxygen across the pulmonary membrane, oxygen-carrying ca-pacity of the blood, amount of blood flow to the tissues, and transfer of oxygen from the blood to the cells. Alterations in any of these factors may lead to a disturbance of homeostasis. In addition, anything that interferes with the use of oxygen by

161

the cells may cause serious disturbances of body function.

The body cannot store oxygen the way it can store other substances, such as glucose (as glycogen) and fat. Therefore, oxygen must be constantly supplied to the body tissues. The small amount of oxygen that is dissolved in the body fluids or bound to hemoglobin is quickly used up if the oxygen supply is interrupted. Cardiac and skeletal muscles have a small emergency supply of oxygen bound to myoglobin, but this supply is limited.

The absence of oxygen in the tissues is *anoxia*. The occurrence of anoxia is unlikely except when blood flow stops. A more common situation is *hypoxia*, a reduced oxygen content in the tissues or decreased availability of oxygen to the cells. A deficiency of oxygen in the blood is *hypoxemia*. *Hyperoxia* is an increase or excess of oxygen in the system.

FUNCTIONS OF OXYGEN

Molecular oxygen (i.e., O_2; free oxygen) is used in many oxidation-reduction reactions in the cells of the body. Chemically, *oxidation* is defined as the loss of electrons from an atom or molecule and *reduction* as a gain of electrons. Oxidation and reduction always go together; when one substance is oxidized another must be reduced. Substances that give up electrons (i.e., electron donors) are called reducing agents. Electron acceptors are called oxidizing agents. Oxygen is an important oxidizing agent but many other substances, such as some coenzymes, can also act as oxidizing agents. Food molecules that are used as fuel, such as glucose, are reducing agents. In biological systems, oxidation is often accompanied by the loss of the proton in hydrogen. In other words, oxidation involves the loss of a hydrogen atom, since a hydrogen atom consists of one proton and one electron. Usually two hydrogen atoms (i.e., a pair of electrons) are lost (transferred) in each reaction.

Oxygen serves an essential metabolic function as the final electron acceptor in the process of cellular respiration, whereby energy is derived from the oxidation of food molecules. This energy is used to form adenosine triphosphate (ATP) from adenosine diphosphate (ADP) and inorganic phosphate. Energy is subsequently released when ATP is hydrolyzed to ADP and inorganic phosphate. By coupling the hydrolysis of ATP with cellular reactions that require energy, ATP is used to do cell work (Fig. 10-1).

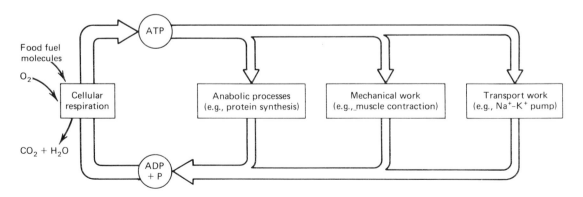

Figure 10-1. *Energy transfer in the cells. Energy released during cellular respiration is used to form ATP. Energy released when ATP is hydrolyzed to ADP and inorganic phosphate (P) is then used to do cell work. (Adapted from Lehninger AL: Bioenergetics, ed 2, © 1971 by W. A. Benjamin, Inc. Reprinted by permission of the Benjamin/Cummings Publishing Co., Inc.)*

Oxygen is also used in several other biochemical oxidation reactions that are not involved in energy production. For example, it is required in the biosynthesis of steroids and fatty acids. Oxygen also functions in the degradation of heme to biliverdin and in detoxification of several substances by oxidative transformation (see Chapter 25). These nonenergy-producing functions of oxygen require a special iron-containing enzyme that is in cells of the liver, kidneys, and intestine. Some cells, such as macrophages, use molecular oxygen in the production of hydrogen peroxide, which may be important in killing microorganisms that are ingested by the phagocytic cell.

Cellular Respiration

The release of energy from food molecules occurs in a stepwise manner involving a series of reactions, as summarized in Figure 10-2. Two important oxidizing agents in these reactions are the coenzymes nicotinamide adenine dinucleotide (NAD) and flavin adenine dinucleotide (FAD). The nicotinamide portion of NAD is derived from niacin, one of the B vitamins. Riboflavin (vitamin B_2) is a necessary precursor in the formation of FAD.

The first phase in the breakdown of glucose is the process of glycolysis, which yields pyruvic acid. During glycolysis, which occurs in the cytoplasm of the cell, two NAD molecules are reduced to $NADH_2$ and four ATP molecules are formed per molecule of glucose. Two molecules of ATP are required to start the reaction, however, so that the net yield is two ATP molecules per molecule of glucose. The supply of NAD is limited; therefore, for glycolysis to continue, the $NADH_2$ must be reoxidized so that it can be used again. When oxygen is available (*aerobic respiration*), electrons from $NADH_2$ are passed to the cytochromes of the respiratory chain and are ultimately accepted by oxygen. When oxygen is not available (*anaerobic glycolysis*), pyruvate is reduced to lactic acid and the $NADH_2$ is reoxidized to NAD in the process.

When oxygen is available, pyruvic acid is converted to acetate. Thiamine (vitamin B_1) is re-

quired in this process. The acetate is not in the free form but is bound with coenzyme A (CoA) to form acetyl CoA ("active" acetate). Pantothenic acid, another B vitamin, forms part of the structure of coenzyme A. Acetyl CoA is formed from the oxidation of fatty acids and some amino acids, as well as from the oxidation of glucose.

The next phase in the oxidation of food molecules is the operation of the tricarboxylic acid (TCA) cycle (also called Krebs cycle or the citric acid cycle), which occurs in the mitochondria. The acetate portion of acetyl CoA is transferred to oxaloacetic acid to form citric acid. Citric acid undergoes a series of reactions and oxaloacetic acid is regenerated. During this process only one ATP molecule is formed per molecule of acetate entering the cycle, but several coenzyme molecules are reduced. The reduced coenzymes are reoxidized when they pass their electrons to the enzymes of the respiratory chain.

The transfer of electrons along the respiratory chain constitutes the third phase of cellular energy production. The enzymes of the respiratory chain, which are located on the inner membranes of the mitochondria, are iron-containing proteins called cytochromes. As electrons are transferred along the respiratory chain the iron in the cytochromes is alternately oxidized and reduced. This process provides the energy for the formation of ATP from ADP and inorganic phosphate. For every molecule of $NADH_2$ that is reoxidized by the respiratory chain, three molecules of ATP are produced; two ATP molecules are produced per molecule of $FADH_2$ that is reoxidized. Ultimately the electrons are passed from the last cytochrome in the chain to oxygen. The oxygen then combines with hydrogen ions to form water. The process of ATP formation in the respiratory chain is called *oxidative phosphorylation*. It is the major source of ATP for the cell and can only proceed when oxygen is available. Under some circumstances, the energy generated during the transfer of electrons along the respiratory chain is not utilized for the formation of ATP, but is lost as heat instead. This situation is referred to as *uncoupling of oxidative phosphorylation*. Under aerobic conditions (i.e., in the

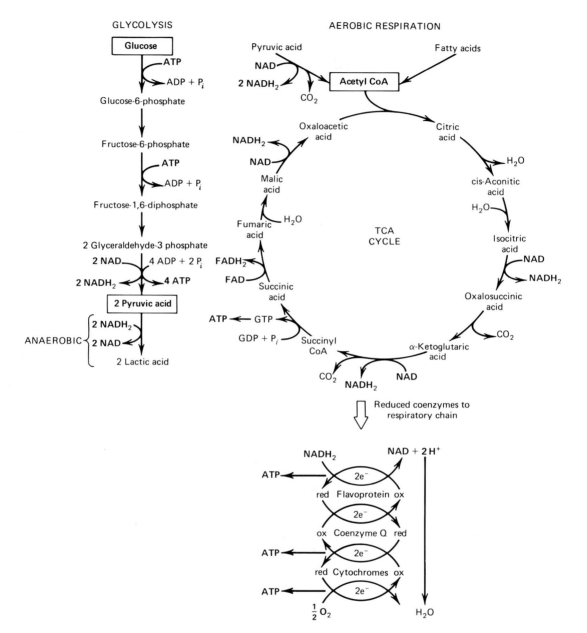

Figure 10-2. *Summary of the reactions involved in the release of energy from food molecules. See text for explanation. Several intermediate reactions have been omitted. FADH₂ passes its electrons directly to coenzyme Q. Four cytochromes are involved in the respiratory chain after coenzyme Q. Pᵢ represents inorganic phosphate; ox, oxidized; red, reduced.*

presence of oxygen) 36 ATP molecules are formed per molecule of glucose, in contrast to 2 ATP molecules formed by anaerobic glycolysis. Oxidation of fatty acids yields more ATP per molecule than oxidation of glucose.

CONSEQUENCES OF HYPOXIA

Consequences at the Cellular Level

Little is known about the effects of hypoxia on the nonenergy-producing functions of oxygen in the cell. Presumably synthetic and detoxification reactions requiring oxygen will be impaired by a deficiency of oxygen.

The major disruption of cellular functions by hypoxia results from impairment of aerobic respiration, with subsequent depletion of the cellular ATP supply. As a result, all the energy-requiring processes of the cell are impaired. If hypoxia is not too severe or does not last too long, cells may be temporarily nonfunctional or functioning at a submaximal level, but the damage is reversible. Severe hypoxia, however, can result in cell death. Lack of ATP to operate the sodium pump results in an influx of sodium into the cell. (Normally the intracellular concentration of sodium is low and the extracellular concentration is high. This concentration gradient is maintained by the activity of the sodium pump, which actively transports sodium out of the cell.) When sodium enters the cell, water follows by osmosis and the result is cellular swelling. Membrane-bound intracellular structures such as mitochondria and the endoplasmic reticulum also swell. Activation of anaerobic glycolysis, with production of lactic acid, lowers the pH inside the cell. The decreased pH interferes with the functioning of many enzymes and alters membrane permeability; increased membrane permeability allows calcium to diffuse into the cell. Calcium uncouples oxidative phosphorylation and therefore decreases the production of ATP even further. Further swelling of

the endoplasmic reticulum occurs and ribosomes are shed from its surface. Thus protein synthesis is disrupted, not only because of a lack of energy but also because the necessary machinery is damaged. The mitochondria swell further, become distorted, and may rupture. Thus the machinery necessary for energy production is ruined. Swelling may lead to rupture of the cell or cell death may result from leakage of enzymes from the lysosomes due to increased membrane permeability. The powerful digestive enzymes from the lysosomes are activated by the decreased pH in the cell and consequently bring about the disintegration of the cell.

When cell-membrane permeability is increased or when cells rupture, intracellular enzymes enter the extracellular fluid. Clinically, the serum levels of several enzymes are monitored to estimate the amount of hypoxic tissue damage that has occurred. For example, myocardial cells contain the enzymes glutamic-oxaloacetic transaminase (GOT), lactic dehydrogenase (LDH), and creatine phosphokinase (CPK), as well as other enzymes. Following myocardial infarction the serum levels of these enzymes rise. GOT and LDH are also abundant in the lungs, liver, pancreas, and kidneys. Therefore, hypoxic damage to these tissues also results in increased concentrations of GOT and LDH in the serum. Only the heart, brain, and skeletal muscles contain CPK.

Systemic Manifestations of Hypoxia

Clinical manifestations of hypoxia are a reflection of abnormal organ functioning due to impairment of oxygen-dependent cellular reactions and of adaptive mechanisms by which the body attempts to maintain homeostasis.

Nervous System Manifestations
As stated in Chapter 9, a constant supply of oxygen is essential to maintain normal brain metabolism. Oxidative phosphorylation is necessary to provide enough ATP (i.e., energy) for two important functions: operation of the sodium-potassium pump to maintain the necessary con-

centration gradients of these ions for nerve-impulse transmission; and synthesis of chemicals necessary for synaptic transmission. Hypoxia, therefore, causes impairment of normal nerve-impulse transmission, which is manifested by lassitude, decreased mental activity, impaired judgment, and signs of faulty neuromuscular coordination such as clumsiness and a slowed reaction time. Sometimes drowsiness occurs, sometimes euphoria. As a result of acute hypoxia a person usually becomes very restless. Convulsive seizures may occur in some people.

With severe hypoxia or anoxia, loss of consciousness occurs quickly. When the oxygen supply is interrupted, for example, during cardiac arrest, the amount of residual oxygen in the capillaries of the brain is used up in 10 to 15 seconds. Brain metabolism is disrupted and coma ensues. Irreversible damage to brain parenchyma can quickly occur if the supply of oxygen is not resumed. Another consequence of severe hypoxia is increased permeability of brain capillaries with resultant cerebral edema.

Other nervous tissue, such as the retina, also has high oxygen requirements. Visual disturbances may therefore accompany hypoxia.

Muscular Manifestations

ATP is required for muscle contraction. When the oxygen supply, and therefore the supply of ATP, is limited the result is muscular weakness and fatigue. Skeletal muscles have a greater capacity for anaerobic glycolysis than most other tissues and therefore are less susceptible to damage by hypoxia. They also have a limited supply of stored energy in the form of creatine phosphate. Creatine phosphate is only formed when the concentration of ATP in the cell is high, however, and therefore once the stored supply is used it cannot be regenerated if hypoxia is prolonged.

Respiratory Manifestations

Hypoxia is frequently accompanied by shortness of breath or difficult, labored breathing (*dyspnea*). Hypoxia stimulates ventilation, therefore, an ab-

normal increase in the rate and depth of respiration (*hyperpnea*) may occur. (Hyperpnea cannot occur, of course, if the hypoxia is due to a neuromuscular disorder of ventilation.)

Normally, slight increases in arterial PCO_2 provide the major stimulus for breathing, but when the arterial PO_2 drops below about 60 mm Hg (normally it is 95 to 100 mm Hg), hypoxia also stimulates ventilation. When increased arterial PCO_2 (hypercapnia) accompanies a low arterial PO_2, the effect of the low oxygen tension in stimulating breathing is enhanced. In some people with chronic retention of carbon dioxide (e.g., those with chronic obstructive pulmonary disease), the medullary chemoreceptors no longer respond to a high level of CO_2 and hypoxemia becomes the major stimulus to breathing.

Hypoxia is usually accompanied by acidosis (see Chapter 15). Acidosis also stimulates respiration and may be a contributing factor in producing hyperpnea.

The total oxygen content of the blood is determined by the amount of oxygen combined with hemoglobin plus the amount of oxygen dissolved in the plasma. Oxygen tension (PO_2) of the blood is determined by the amount of dissolved oxygen. The chemoreceptors in the carotid and aortic bodies respond to oxygen tension, not to the total oxygen content of the blood. Therefore, anemia does not stimulate ventilation because the arterial PO_2 is normal (unless the anemia is accompanied by some other condition), but the total oxygen content of the blood is reduced due to a lack of hemoglobin.

Hypoxia that is severe enough to cause unconsciousness may depress the respiratory center. Consequently breathing may become slow and irregular and finally stop.

Cardiovascular Manifestations

In response to hypoxia the heart rate increases (tachycardia), cardiac output increases, and peripheral vasodilation occurs. These responses are adaptive mechanisms that increase blood flow in an attempt to increase tissue oxygenation. With chronic hypoxia the number and size of capillaries increase, thus delivering more blood to the hypoxic tissues.

Hypoxia causes constriction of pulmonary blood vessels. All the alveoli are not always ventilated to the same extent. Blood flowing through poorly ventilated alveoli is not able to pick up much oxygen and the resulting hypoxia causes local vasoconstriction. Consequently, less blood flows through the capillaries in poorly ventilated alveoli and instead is shunted to well-ventilated alveoli. This mechanism normally serves a useful purpose in that it helps to adjust blood flow to air flow and thereby maximize oxygenation of the blood. Unfortunately, hypoxia of all or most of the alveoli, such as may occur in some types of lung disease, can cause generalized pulmonary vasoconstriction. As a result, pulmonary vascular resistance is increased and pulmonary arterial pressure is elevated. With chronic hypoxia this situation can lead to right ventricular hypertrophy because the right ventricle has to work harder to pump blood into the pulmonary circulation against the increased resistance. Eventually right ventricular failure may occur.

Hematological Manifestations

Hypoxia causes an increase in the number of circulating red blood cells. This increase is an adaptive mechanism that increases the oxygen-carrying capacity of the blood. In response to acute hypoxia, immature red blood cells (reticulocytes) are released into the blood. If the hypoxia persists, more red blood cells are formed and the number of mature circulating red blood cells is increased.

All the factors regulating the formation and release of mature erythrocytes are not known, but at least one plasma substance, called *erythropoietin*, is known to stimulate maturation and release of erythrocytes. The exact site of formation of erythropoietin in the body is not known. It is possibly secreted by the kidneys but may also be produced by the liver and/or spleen. It is possible that the kidneys do not produce erythropoietin, but rather an enzyme (renal erythropoietic factor or erythrogenin) that converts a plasma substance produced by the liver into active erythropoietin.

Hypoxia stimulates production of erythropoietin, which in turn stimulates formation, maturation, and release of red blood cells from the marrow. If the hypoxia is due to an abnormal decrease in the number of circulating red blood cells (e.g., due to hemorrhage), this mechanism restores the normal number of erythrocytes. If hypoxia is due to inadequate oxygenation of the blood in the presence of a normal number of erythrocytes (e.g., low oxygen content of inspired air such as occurs at high altitudes), this mechanism produces an increase above the normal number of red blood cells (*polycythemia*). As a result, the hematocrit may be elevated. Plasma volume often increases also when hypoxia is prolonged; therefore, the hematocrit may be normal.

An increase in the hematocrit increases the viscosity of the blood and therefore increases peripheral resistance. An increase in resistance due to polycythemia may be a contributing factor in the development of pulmonary hypertension and subsequently right ventricular hypertrophy in people with chronic hypoxic lung disease.

Cyanosis

Cyanosis is a bluish discoloration of the skin and mucous membranes due to an excessive concentration of deoxygenated (reduced) hemoglobin in the capillaries. Cyanosis often accompanies hypoxia, but hypoxia can occur without cyanosis. Cyanosis depends on the concentration of reduced hemoglobin, irrespective of the amount of oxygenated hemoglobin. Definite cyanosis is usually visible when the concentration of deoxygenated hemoglobin in the blood exceeds 5 g/100 ml. Sometimes mild cyanosis can be detected when only 3 to 4 grams of deoxygenated hemoglobin are present per 100 ml of blood. When the amount of hemoglobin in the blood is increased, a greater amount of reduced hemoglobin will be present at a given oxygen saturation and therefore a greater degree of cyanosis will occur. Thus, people with polycythemia develop cyanosis very readily. On the other hand, people with anemia rarely become cyanosed because they do not have a sufficient amount of hemoglobin.

Cyanosis can be classified as central or peripheral. When it is caused by decreased saturation of systemic arterial blood with oxygen (e.g., with a disturbance of pulmonary function), it is said to be *central*. Cyanosis produced as a result of increased extraction of oxygen from the blood at the capillary level is said to be *peripheral*. Peripheral cyanosis may occur as a result of slow blood flow in the extremities due to vasoconstriction.

Cyanosis is most easily seen where the layer of tissue over the capillaries is thinnest and most transparent. Central cyanosis is best detected in the mucous membrane of the undersurface of the tongue and in the conjunctivae. Cyanosis of the lips, nailbeds, earlobes, and tip of the nose may be either central or peripheral.

CAUSES OF HYPOXIA

As stated at the beginning of this chapter, several factors and processes determine the amount of oxygen reaching the tissues. Disturbances of any of these factors or processes may cause hypoxia.

When tissue oxygenation is inadequate because the systemic arterial oxygen tension is decreased and the hemoglobin is only partially saturated, the condition is called *hypoxic hypoxia*. Hypoxic hypoxia may result from a decreased oxygen content of inspired air, inadequate ventilation of the lungs, impaired pulmonary diffusion, altered perfusion of the lungs, or any combination of these.

When the systemic arterial oxygen tension is normal and the hemoglobin is almost completely saturated, but the oxygen content of the blood is decreased due to a lack of hemoglobin, the term *anemic hypoxia* is used.

Circulatory hypoxia describes the condition in which tissue oxygenation is decreased because of inadequate blood flow. The oxygen content of the blood may be normal, but the amount of blood, and therefore the amount of oxygen, reaching the tissues is decreased.

In some situations, despite normal blood flow and adequate oxygenation of the blood, the amount of oxygen actually taken up by the cells or the capacity of the cells to use oxygen may be decreased. The effects on the cells are the same as if inadequate oxygen were available. The term *histotoxic hypoxia* is used when the cells are unable to use oxygen that is delivered to them.

Decreased Uptake and Utilization of Oxygen by Cells

Movement of oxygen from the capillary blood to sites of utilization inside the cells is by the process of diffusion. The rate of diffusion will depend on the diffusion gradient (i.e., the difference between the PO_2 of the capillary blood and the PO_2 inside the mitochondria), the surface area available for diffusion, and the diffusion distance. Under normal conditions, the PO_2 of capillary blood is high enough to provide an adequate diffusion gradient. The surface area for diffusion is mainly determined by the number of perfused capillaries per unit mass of tissue. As previously mentioned, during prolonged hypoxia the number of capillaries may increase and thereby provide an increased surface area for diffusion. Any condition that increases the diffusion distance, for example tissue edema, will decrease the rate of oxygen transfer to the cells. In this situation the rate of delivery may not be sufficient to keep up with cellular demand.

A number of toxins interfere with the use of oxygen by the mitochondria. Cyanide is a potent inhibitor of one of the enzymes of the respiratory chain and prevents transfer of electrons to molecular oxygen. As a result, oxidative phosphorylation stops. Arsenic also inhibits oxidative phosphorylation, but the block is not as complete as with cyanide. Barbiturates inhibit electron transfer from $NADH_2$ to the respiratory chain.

Thyroid hormone is an important regulator of oxygen consumption by the cells. The exact mechanism of action of this hormone is not known, but it is possibly involved with coupling the production of ATP to the operation of the respiratory chain. When inadequate amounts of thyroid hormone are available, cellular energy production by oxidative phosphorylation is decreased. Deficiency of niacin will result in a decreased amount of NAD and therefore may impair cellular energy production and oxygen use.

Decreased Blood Flow

Adequate delivery of oxygen to the tissues depends on sufficient blood flow. A generalized circulatory deficiency, for example, due to cardiac insufficiency or shock, will result in ischemia, and therefore hypoxia, in most or all the tissues of the body. Shock is discussed in Chapter 14.

Localized impairment of blood flow may result from occlusion or abnormal constriction of one blood vessel. In this case only the tissue served by that blood vessel will be affected by ischemia and hypoxia. The effect on the total person will depend on which tissue is ischemic. Occlusion of a blood vessel may be caused by a thrombus or an embolus, as already discussed in Chapter 7. Atherosclerosis is often responsible for severe narrowing of the lumen of arteries, with resultant ischemia.

In *Raynaud's phenomenon* (or disease), painful paroxysmal vasospasms occur, particularly in the fingers, but also occasionally in the toes, the ears, or the tip ot the nose. Intense spasm of small arteries and arterioles in the affected part occurs in response to cold or emotional stress and produces extreme blanching. Cyanosis then occurs due to the extremely slow blood flow in the capillaries. After a few minutes blood flow resumes; the part becomes hyperemic and may appear very red. The pain becomes more severe at this stage.

Normally, severe tissue ischemia does not occur even with very strong sympathetic stimulation because local regulatory mechanisms cause opposing vasodilation as the PO_2 declines and metabolic products accumulate in the tissue. The balance that is achieved prevents damage due to ischemia.

Raynaud's phenomenon represents an extreme sensitivity to sympathetic stimulation, with the result that an imbalance occurs between sympathetic vasoconstriction and local vasodilation, and tissue blood flow is almost completely stopped. Usually hypoxic tissue damage is mild, but in severe cases of Raynaud's disease the skin of the affected part may become ulcerated. The condition may become progressively worse over the years, until the vessels are continuously constricted. This situation may lead to gangrene.

Decreased Oxygen-Carrying Capacity of the Blood

Oxygen is transported in physical solution in the water of the blood and in reversible chemical combination with hemoglobin in the red blood cells. Most of the oxygen is carried in combination with hemoglobin because oxygen is not very soluble in water. Each hemoglobin molecule can combine with four molecules of oxygen. Hemoglobin is said to be *fully saturated* when it is completely oxygenated (i.e., carrying as much oxygen as it possibly can); when not completely oxygenated, it is said to be *partially saturated*. The degree of saturation is expressed as percentage saturation.

Several factors determine the degree of saturation of the hemoglobin; the most important is the PO_2 of the blood. A graph of hemoglobin saturation plotted against PO_2 gives an S-shaped curve called an *oxygen-hemoglobin dissociation curve* (Fig. 10-3). The shape of the curve and the affinity of hemoglobin for oxygen are largely determined by the structural and chemical properties of the hemoglobin molecule and are of considerable physiological significance. As can be seen from the curve, at a low PO_2 (such as exists in the tissues) hemoglobin does not combine to a very great extent with oxygen. Therefore oxygen is readily released to the tissues. As the PO_2 increases from 10 to 60 mm Hg, the degree of saturation increases rapidly, and at a PO_2 of 60 mm Hg hemoglobin is about 90% saturated with oxygen. Any further increase in PO_2 will bring about only a slight in-

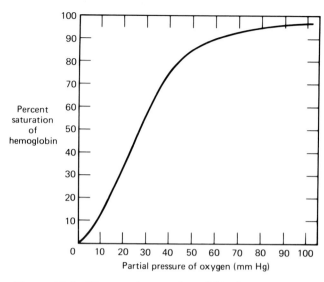

Figure 10-3. *The normal oxygen-hemoglobin dissociation curve.*

crease in oxygen uptake. Thus, under usual conditions, as the blood flows through the lungs hemoglobin is easily saturated with oxygen at the normal alveolar PO_2 (104 mm Hg). Even if the alveolar or arterial PO_2 is decreased due to pulmonary disease or other factors, hemoglobin saturation will not be seriously affected until the PO_2 drops below 60 mm Hg.

The affinity of hemoglobin for oxygen is influenced by temperature and pH. Increased temperature or decreased pH (i.e., increased acidity) decreases the affinity of hemoglobin for oxygen and causes the dissociation curve to be shifted to the right. In other words, at any given PO_2 the degree of saturation is less. Therefore, dissociation of oxygen from hemoglobin is facilitated in actively metabolizing tissues, which have a higher temperature and lower pH than tissues at rest. Decreased temperature and increased pH cause the curve to be shifted to the left; that is, they increase the affinity of hemoglobin for oxygen so that even at a low PO_2 the percent saturation of hemoglobin is high. Although this situation enhances oxygenation of the blood in the lungs, it decreases tissue

oxygenation because oxygen is not released from the hemoglobin as easily.

Another factor that influences hemoglobin saturation is a substance called 2,3-diphosphoglycerate (DPG), which is produced during glycolysis. Most cells contain very small amounts of DPG, but erythrocytes contain much larger quantities. DPG combines reversibly with hemoglobin and facilitates the release of oxygen. Therefore, an increase in the amount of DPG shifts the oxygen-hemoglobin dissociation curve to the right and favors the release of oxygen in the tissues. The amount of DPG in the red blood cells increases in response to hypoxia or an increased need for oxygen.

Any condition that reduces the affinity of hemoglobin for oxygen or decreases the amount of hemoglobin in the blood will diminish the oxygen-carrying capacity of the blood and may cause hypoxia. A reduction in the concentration of hemoglobin below the normal value is called *anemia*. Some disorders increase the affinity of hemoglobin for oxygen so that release of oxygen to the tissues is impaired and tissue hypoxia results.

Altered Affinity of Hemoglobin for Oxygen

The affinity of hemoglobin for oxygen can be altered by various poisons or by structural abnormalities of the hemoglobin molecule. Hemoglobin has a much greater affinity for carbon monoxide than it does for oxygen. Therefore, in *carbon monoxide poisoning* the hemoglobin combines with carbon monoxide instead of with oxygen. Since there are four combining sites per hemoglobin molecule, the hemoglobin may combine with both carbon monoxide and oxygen at the same time. When this situation occurs, hemoglobin binds the oxygen more tightly. Consequently, tissue hypoxia results not only because the amount of oxygen in the blood is decreased, but also because the oxygen that is being carried by the hemoglobin is not readily released to the tissues. Hemoglobin combined with carbon monoxide has a bright red color, therefore people with carbon monoxide poisoning may appear very pink, not cyanosed, although they are hypoxic.

The iron in hemoglobin is normally in the ferrous state (Fe^{2+}). When it is oxidized to the ferric state (Fe^{3+}) it cannot bind oxygen. Hemoglobin containing ferric iron is called *methemoglobin*. Many chemicals and drugs, including amyl nitrite, aniline, nitrobenzene, acetanilid, phenacetin, and salicylates, can oxidize the iron in hemoglobin. If a substantial proportion of the hemoglobin is in the form of methemoglobin, hypoxia may result. Cyanosis appears when the methemoglobin concentration is 1.5 g/100 ml of blood.

Several inherited structural defects of hemoglobin cause the iron in hemoglobin to be stabilized in the ferric state. These disorders are collectively called *hemoglobin M disease*, but they are not all the same. With some types of hemoglobin M, oxygen affinity is decreased; with other types, oxygen affinity is normal. Only about 30% to 40% of the hemoglobin is in the abnormal form and only two of the four oxygen-combining sites are affected. Therefore the oxygen-carrying capacity of the blood is only decreased by 15% to 20%. Affected people are always cyanosed but otherwise usually do not show any symptoms.

Anemia

The normal erythrocyte count and hemoglobin concentration depend on age, sex, and altitude. Near sea level, the normal number of erythrocytes ranges from 4.6 to 6.2 million/mm³ for adult males; 4.2 to 5.4 million/mm³ for adult females; and 3.8 to 5.2 million/mm³ for children of both sexes from 3 months to 13 years. The normal hemoglobin concentration ranges from 14 to 17 g/100 ml for adult males; 12 to 15 g/100 ml for adult females; and 10 to 14.5 g/100 ml for children.

Anemia may result from excessive loss or destruction of red blood cells or from impaired production of hemoglobin or red blood cells. Red blood cell production can increase up to six to eight times the normal rate to compensate for an increased loss. Therefore a person can tolerate considerable loss of erythrocytes before anemia will occur and a slow, steady loss of red blood cells will not necessarily produce anemia.

The manifestations of anemia depend on its severity (i.e., the degree of reduction in the amount of hemoglobin), its rate of development, the ability of adaptive mechanisms to compensate for the reduction in oxygen-carrying capacity, and the person's degree of activity (i.e., oxygen requirements). Physiological compensatory mechanisms include increased heart rate and increased cardiac output. A reduction in the number of erythrocytes reduces the viscosity of the blood and tissue hypoxia causes vasodilation, so that peripheral resistance is decreased and blood velocity is increased. All these factors increase blood flow through the tissues to help maintain adequate oxygenation. In addition, the concentration of DPG in the erythrocytes increases so that more oxygen is released to the tissues.

Usually the only signs of mild anemia are pallor and a slightly increased heart rate. When the hemoglobin concentration falls to about 7.5 g/100 ml a person quickly experiences shortness of breath on exertion. Marked weakness occurs when the hemoglobin falls below 6 g/100 ml. At about 3 g/100 ml shortness of breath occurs at rest and below this value cardiac failure occurs. (If a person already has an underlying cardiac or pulmonary disorder cardiac failure can occur much sooner.) A hemoglobin concentration of less than 2 g/100 ml is not usually compatible with life. Headache, dizziness, and low-grade fever are other manifestations that may occur with anemia.

In addition to classifying anemia according to cause, anemia may be classified according to the appearance of the erythrocytes. The size of the red blood cells is designated as *normocytic* (normal), *microcytic* (small), or *macrocytic* (large). The color of the cell depends on the hemoglobin concentration within the cell. If the concentration is normal, cells are *normochromic*. When the concentration of hemoglobin in the cells is less than normal, the cells appear pale and are designated *hypochromic*.

Anemia due to impaired erythropoiesis. Many factors can interfere with normal red blood cell production. *Iron deficiency* is one of the most common causes of anemia. Iron is an essential part of hemoglobin; when it is lacking, the developing red blood cells are not able to produce the normal amount of hemoglobin and the result is a hypochromic-microcytic anemia.

Deficiency of vitamin B_{12} or folic acid impairs production and maturation of blood cells. When vitamin B_{12} deficiency is due to a lack of intrinsic factor the resulting condition is called *pernicious anemia*. Intrinsic factor is necessary for absorption of vitamin B_{12}; it is normally secreted by parietal cells in the fundus of the stomach.

Vitamin B_{12} metabolism and folic acid metabolism are interrelated; both vitamins are required for DNA synthesis. A deficiency of either vitamin impairs DNA synthesis and thus interferes with cell division. Red blood cell precursors are unable to divide at the normal rate and consequently grow larger than normal. Hemoglobin synthesis is not affected, however, and the red blood cells contain a normal concentration of hemoglobin. Many of the abnormal erythrocyte precursors are destroyed by phagocytosis within the marrow and so fewer

red blood cells than normal are released into the circulation. Those entering the blood are large and oval in shape. Some small cells also occur, possibly from fragmentation of the large cells. The abnormal cells are fragile and have a reduced life span. A macrocytic-normochromic anemia therefore develops as a consequence of both impaired production and decreased survival time of red blood cells. In addition to the usual manifestations of anemia already mentioned, the serum bilirubin level may be increased and excretion of urobilinogen in the feces and urine increased due to excessive destruction of immature red blood cell precursors.

Hypoplastic (or *aplastic*) anemia results from a reduction in blood cell production due to a lack of hematopoietic stem cells in the bone marrow. The condition may be congenital or acquired. In most cases of marrow hypoplasia not only erythrocyte production but also production of granulocytes and thrombocytes is decreased (pancytopenia). Affected people are therefore prone to infections and have a bleeding tendency as well as anemia.

Congenital marrow hypoplasia appears to be hereditary, but the exact nature of the genetic defect is not known. The marrow hypoplasia is often accompanied by other congenital anomalies (Fanconi's syndrome) and is associated with a high incidence of chromosome abnormalities. Acquired hypoplastic anemia can be caused by a variety of physical and chemical agents. Some agents consistently produce marrow hypoplasia provided that the dose is adequate. These agents include ionizing radiation (see Chapter 23); many drugs, such as alkylating agents (e.g., nitrogen mustard), antimetabolites (e.g., methotrexate and cytosine arabinoside), and mitotic inhibitors (e.g., urethane and colchicine derivatives); and chemicals such as benzene and related compounds. Other drugs and chemicals produce marrow hypoplasia in sensitive people but not in everyone receiving the drug. A well-known example is the antibiotic chloramphenicol, but many other drugs have also been implicated. The exact mechanism(s) by which this second group of toxins produces hypoplastic anemia in some susceptible people is not known. Some cases of acquired marrow hypoplasia may be caused by viral infections or autoimmune disorders. Often the cause is not known.

Marrow hypoplasia that affects only the erythrocytic stem cells is much less common. In most cases the cause is unknown, although some cases are associated with tumors of the thymus. It has been postulated that the thymic tumor produces antibodies against the red blood cell precursors.

Erythropoiesis may be impaired as a result of neoplastic processes. In some types of leukemia (e.g., granulocytic leukemia) primitive marrow stem cells that normally provide the precursors for several types of blood cells may be diverted into producing only one type of cell to the exclusion of the others. In other cases, such as lymphocytic leukemia and metastatic tumors of the marrow, normal marrow cells may be displaced (i.e., "crowded out") by abnormal cells. Even in the absence of metastasis to the red bone marrow, most malignant neoplasias are associated with anemia due to depression of marrow function. The mechanism by which marrow depression is produced is not known.

A mild to moderate, normochromic-normocytic type of anemia occurs secondary to many conditions, such as chronic infection, rheumatoid arthritis, renal insufficiency, and chronic liver disease. The anemia in these cases appears to be due to a depression of bone marrow function, but the exact mechanisms are not known. Anemia is also usually associated with alcoholism. This anemia is usually secondary to nutritional deficiencies or associated liver disease, but alcohol may also depress erythropoiesis directly.

The *thalassemias* are a group of hereditary disorders of hemoglobin synthesis that result in chronic hypochromic anemia. The globin (protein) portion of hemoglobin contains four polypeptide chains. In the normal adult most of the hemoglobin contains two alpha (α) chains and two beta (β) chains (Hb A), as shown in Figure 10-4. In addition, small amounts of fetal hemoglobin (Hb

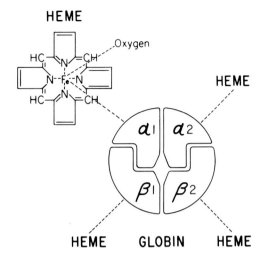

Figure 10-4. *Schematic representation of hemoglobin A. (From Linman JW:* Hematology: Physiologic, Pathophysiologic, and Clinical Principles. *New York, Macmillan Publishing Co., Inc. Copyright © 1975, James W. Linman.)*

F) and another hemoglobin (Hb A_2) are present. Hb F contains two α chains and two gamma (γ) chains; Hb A_2 consists of two α chains and two delta (δ) chains. In thalassemia the rate of production of one of the globin chains is decreased, but the unaffected chains are synthesized at normal rates.

Several types of thalassemia occur, depending on which polypeptide chain is affected; most often it is the β chain. As a result of the decreased production of an α-, β-, and/or δ-globin chain the amount of hemoglobin in each red blood cell is decreased, causing a hypochromic anemia. The unaffected chains accumulate in the cell and precipitate on the erythrocyte membrane. They also interfere with erythrocyte metabolism. Consequently the cells are deformed and have a decreased survival time. The anemia is therefore due to increased hemolysis as well as to impaired production of hemoglobin. When the defect occurs in β-chain synthesis, an increased amount of Hb F is present in the person's blood. This persistence of Hb F appears to be a compensatory mechanism.

The usual manifestations of anemia and chronic hemolysis (see below) dominate the clinical picture of thalassemia. The heterozygous genetic condition results in a mild anemia (thalassemia minor). In the homozygous condition the disease is severe (thalassemia major) and usually results in early death.

Anemia due to excessive loss or destruction of blood cells. Excessive loss of red blood cells occurs with hemorrhage. After acute hemorrhage the normal blood volume is usually replaced within 20 to 60 hours after bleeding stops. The immediate restoration of blood volume is due to the formation of new plasma; formation of new blood cells takes longer. Therefore, the already decreased number of red blood cells is diluted, and the hematocrit and erythrocyte count gradually decrease over a period of one to three days post hemorrhage. Each red blood cell contains the normal amount of hemoglobin, but the hemoglobin concentration of the blood is decreased due to the decreased number of cells. The result is a normochromic-normocytic anemia. If erythropoiesis is not impaired by some other disorder and hemorrhage does not recur, the red blood cell count, hematocrit, and hemoglobin content of the blood return to normal in three to six weeks.

Chronic bleeding does not result in a normochromic-normocytic anemia. With a slow rate of blood loss the marrow is able to increase production of red blood cells enough to compensate. Eventually, however, the iron stores of the body may be depleted and a hypochromic-microcytic anemia may develop as a result of iron deficiency.

Anemia resulting from excessive destruction of red blood cells is called *hemolytic anemia*. Many abnormal conditions can shorten the life span of the erythrocytes. Anemia will only occur, however, if the rate of destruction is greater than the maximum production capacity. When increased production balances the rate of destruction so that the blood count remains normal, the hemolytic condition is said to be compensated. In some cases the increased marrow activity may cause bone pain and may produce widening of the medullary cavities of the bones.

Enlargement of the spleen (splenomegaly) almost always accompanies chronic hemolytic conditions. The splenomegaly is usually caused by the need to remove an excessive number of abnormal or damaged red blood cells. In some cases it may reflect the need for extramedullary erythropoiesis. (The spleen is a normal site of erythrocyte production in the fetus but loses this activity just before birth. In times of need, however, the spleen can revert to its erythropoietic function and supplement the erythropoietic activity of the red bone marrow.) In other cases splenomegaly may be a basic facet of some underlying disease and may cause the excessive red blood cell destruction (e.g., Gaucher's disease).

Hemolytic anemia may occur as a result of hereditary disorders of red blood cell structure or function. The defect may be in hemoglobin structure, such as in sickle cell anemia (see Chapter 6), or may be due to deficiency of an erythrocyte enzyme. In some disorders, for example, hereditary spherocytosis, the exact nature of the genetic defect is not known. The abnormal cells are primarily destroyed during passage through the spleen.

Acquired hemolytic disorders may be due to isoimmune reactions, for example, transfusion reactions and erythroblastosis fetalis; or due to autoimmune disorders (see Chapter 30). Acquired hemolysis can also be caused by chemical and physical factors. A number of chemicals can interfere with erythrocyte metabolism (e.g., phenylhydrazine and copper) or alter the erythrocyte membrane (e.g., lead and some snake venoms) and cause hemolysis. Heat can damage red blood cells; therefore, acute hemolysis may occur in people who have been badly burned. Acute hemolysis occurs if large amounts of water enter the blood, presumably due to osmotic swelling and rupture of the cells. This type of hemolysis may occur in people who survive fresh-water drowning and may occur as a complication of transurethral resections. Hemolysis is associated with some infections, particularly those in which the microorganisms directly parasitize red blood cells (e.g., malaria). Hemolytic anemia may also accompany cholera, typhoid fever, and gas gangrene.

Chronic uncompensated hemolysis is manifested by nonspecific signs and symptoms of anemia. Acute hemolysis, however, may cause chills, fever, prostration, and pain in the back, abdomen, or extremities. The reason for these manifestations is not known. The rapid decrease in the number of erythrocytes may cause hypovolemia, with resultant shock. Other manifestations of hemolysis are due to the excessive amounts of hemoglobin being catabolized. The plasma level of unconjugated bilirubin rises and therefore the affected person may be jaundiced (see Chapter 26). The liver is able to conjugate and excrete two to three times the normal amount of bilirubin, however, so that jaundice may not occur if liver function is adequate. In addition to the elevated bilirubin level, the amount of urobilinogen excreted in the feces and the urine is increased.

In some cases of hemolytic anemia hemoglobin may appear in the urine. Hemoglobin that is released directly into the plasma immediately binds with a plasma protein called haptoglobin. The hemoglobin-haptoglobin' complex is too large to enter the glomerular filtrate and so is not excreted through the kidneys but is removed from the blood by liver and reticuloendothelial cells. When all the circulating haptoglobin is bound with hemoglobin, excess free hemoglobin enters the glomerular filtrate. Subsequently the hemoglobin is reabsorbed by epithelial cells in the proximal renal tubules. When the concentration of free hemoglobin in the plasma is greater than 25 mg/100 ml, the renal threshold is exceeded and hemoglobin is lost in the urine. The hemoglobin that is reabsorbed is catabolized in the tubular epithelial cells and the iron is deposited as ferritin or hemosiderin. Some iron may be transported to other sites and reused, but some is lost in the urine when epithelial cells are shed, causing hemosiderinuria. Hemosiderinuria occurs with chronic hemolysis, whereas hemoglobinuria is a manifestation of acute hemolysis.

Decreased Oxygenation of the Blood

Adequate oxygenation of the blood requires adequate ventilation of the lungs, adequate diffusion across the respiratory membrane, and adequate blood flow through the lungs. Disturbances of any of these functions may lead to hypoxemia, but pulmonary disease may be present without causing hypoxemia if compensatory mechanisms are adequate. Although the mechanisms by which disturbances of these functions produce hypoxemia can be considered separately, in many clinical situations more than one mechanism is involved.

Pulmonary Diffusing Capacity

Oxygen from the alveolar air must diffuse through a thin layer of surfactant and fluid lining the alveolus, across the alveolar epithelium, through a thin interstitial space, and then across the capillary basement membrane and endothelium to enter the blood. These barriers are collectively called the *respiratory membrane*. Then the oxygen has to diffuse through the plasma and across the erythrocyte membrane to combine with hemoglobin. The rate of diffusion of oxygen across the respiratory membrane will be influenced by the surface area of the membrane, the thickness of the membrane (i.e., the diffusion distance), and the diffusion gradient. The diffusion gradient is the difference between the PO_2 in the alveolar air and the PO_2 of the capillary blood. The volume of a gas (in this case oxygen) diffusing through the respiratory membrane per minute per mm Hg pressure difference is called the *pulmonary diffusing capacity*.

Any condition that decreases the pulmonary diffusing capacity may cause hypoxemia. Pulmonary diffusing capacity can be decreased as a result of decreased surface area of the respiratory membrane. Such a decrease occurs if part or all of a lung is consolidated. *Consolidation* is a condition in which the normally soft spongy tissue has become firm or solid because the alveoli are filled with tissue or fluid. Consolidation may be caused by cancer, but it is usually due to inflammation. Inflammation of the lung parenchyma is called *pneumonia* or *pneumonitis*. Pneumonia is usually due to viral or bacterial infection. The surface area for diffusion will also be decreased by destruction of lung tissue by disease processes such as emphysema, cancer, or tuberculosis.

Collapse of part or all of the lung (*atelectasis*) will decrease the surface area for diffusion. Entry of air into the pleural space (*pneumothorax*) will increase the intrapleural pressure and cause the lung to collapse. Atelectasis can also be caused by complete obstruction of an air passage. The gases in the alveoli distal to the obstruction will gradually be absorbed into the blood and since entry of air is blocked the alveoli collapse. The alveoli may reexpand if the obstruction is removed. Atelectasis may also be caused by a deficiency of surfactant, a lipoprotein substance secreted by the lungs that lowers the surface tension inside the alveoli. Thus when surfactant is lacking the surface tension in the alveoli is increased, making the lungs less distensible during inspiration and prone to collapse during expiration. Atelectasis due to surfactant deficiency is a prominent feature of *hyaline membrane disease* (respiratory distress syndrome of the newborn). In addition to the atelectasis in this condition a transparent, glassy lining (hyaline membrane) forms in the alveoli, alveolar ducts, and bronchioles. The hyaline material is believed to be derived from blood proteins.

The respiratory membrane is thickened by pulmonary edema and by interstitial fibrosis. *Interstitial fibrosis* (alveolocapillary block) is a condition in which fibrous tissue is deposited in the interstitial space between the alveolar epithelium and the capillary membrane, usually due to an inflammatory or allergic process. It may occur following inhalation of noxious fumes, irritating inorganic dusts such as silicates or asbestos, or allergenic organic dusts. It was once thought that thickening of the respiratory membrane decreases the diffusing capacity and causes hypoxemia because it increases the diffusion distance and therefore increases the time for diffusion to occur. In recent years this concept has been challenged. Diffusion of oxygen through the respiratory membrane occurs so rapidly that an incredibly thick membrane would be required to seriously impair oxygenation of the blood. Pulmonary edema and interstitial fibrosis can cause hypoxemia, but by a different mechanism. In these conditions alveolar expansion is restricted, resulting in hypoventilation. Hypoxemia may then result from an altered ventilation-perfusion ratio (see below) and/or decreased surface area for diffusion.

Shunting of Blood

Blood is said to be shunted when it passes from the right to the left side of the heart without picking up oxygen. A small amount of venous blood (about 2% of the cardiac output) normally does not flow through the pulmonary capillaries and therefore does not pick up any oxygen. This blood, which is called the *venous admixture*, is shunted through the heart and enters the left side of the heart by way of the thebesian veins or is shunted through parts of the lungs and enters the pulmonary veins by way of the bronchial veins. Therefore, although the blood leaving the pulmonary capillaries normally has a P_{O_2} of about 104 mm Hg, the systemic arterial P_{O_2} is about 95 to 100 mm Hg.

Conditions that cause excessive shunting of blood and increase the venous admixture can cause hypoxemia. Venous admixture is increased in some congenital heart diseases, such as tetralogy of Fallot, or if the foramen ovale fails to close after birth so that blood is shunted from the right to the left side of the heart without going through the pulmonary circulation. In pulmonary arteriovenous aneurysm, blood is shunted from the pulmonary artery to the pulmonary veins, with resultant hypoxemia.

Ventilation-Perfusion Ratio

Blood flow through the lungs is not uniformly distributed, nor are the alveoli uniformly ventilated.

The ratio of alveolar ventilation to pulmonary capillary blood flow is called the *ventilation-perfusion ratio*. If little or no blood flows through the capillaries in well-ventilated alveoli (a high ventilation-perfusion ratio), the air delivered to those alveoli is wasted (alveolar dead space); that is, it contributes little to the oxygenation of the blood, yet takes ventilation away from other alveoli. On the other hand, if poorly ventilated alveoli receive a good blood supply (a low ventilation-perfusion ratio), the blood flowing through the capillaries in those alveoli will not pick up much oxygen and the physiological effect will be shunting of blood. These two situations are illustrated in Figure 10-5. Oxygenation of the blood will be most effective if most of the blood flows through the capillaries in well-ventilated alveoli and very little blood flows through the capillaries in poorly ventilated alveoli (i.e., the ideal situation is a ventilation-perfusion ratio of one). As stated previously, a low alveolar PO_2 causes vasoconstriction of adjacent blood vessels so that blood is redistributed from poorly ventilated alveoli to better ventilated alveoli. A low pH enhances this effect.

Even in healthy people the ventilation-perfusion ratio is not the same in all parts of the lung, but the differences are not large enough to seriously affect oxygenation of the blood. As discussed in Chapter 22, distribution of blood flow through the lungs is influenced by position. In the upright position very little blood flows through the upper part of the lung; blood flow is greater at the bottom. Alveolar ventilation is also less at the apex of the lung than at the base, but the change in ventilation does not match the change in blood flow, so that alveoli in the apex are overventilated in relation to blood flow and alveoli in the base are underventilated in relation to their perfusion. In the middle portion of the lungs ventilation and perfusion are well matched. In the supine position more blood flows through the posterior parts of the lungs than through the anterior parts, but the regional differences are not as great as in the upright position.

Disturbances of pulmonary blood flow that de-crease blood flow to well-ventilated alveoli will increase the alveolar dead space and increase the ventilation-perfusion ratio. Pulmonary blood flow may be altered, for example, by thrombosis or embolism. Localized disturbances will not cause hypoxemia if ventilation and perfusion of other parts of the lungs are adequate. Total ventilation will have to increase, however, to compensate for the large amount of wasted ventilation. Therefore hyperpnea may occur and the person may feel short of breath.

Abnormal conditions that result in poor ventilation of many alveoli while pulmonary blood flow remains relatively normal (i.e., conditions that produce a low ventilation-perfusion ratio) will cause the blood to be shunted through the lungs without picking up much oxygen and produce systemic arterial hypoxemia. For example, conditions that cause hypoventilation (see below) can produce a low ventilation-perfusion ratio.

Disturbances that cause nonuniform ventilation-perfusion ratios throughout the lungs will cause hypoxemia regardless of whether total pulmonary ventilation and total pulmonary blood flow are normal. Ventilation-perfusion ratios may be abnormally high in some parts of the lung, and simultaneously abnormally low in other parts of the lung in people with pulmonary disease.

Altered ventilation-perfusion ratios have a greater effect on arterial oxygen saturation than they do on arterial carbon dioxide levels because of the differences in the transport of these two gases. As already described, most of the oxygen in the blood is carried in combination with hemoglobin; very little is dissolved in the plasma. Although the overventilated alveoli will have a higher than normal PO_2, hemoglobin saturation will not be increased very much because hemoglobin is already almost completely saturated at the normal alveolar PO_2. In the underventilated alveoli the PO_2 will drop below normal as will the hemoglobin saturation. Therefore when blood coming from capillaries in underventilated alveoli is mixed with blood from overventilated alveoli, the hemoglobin saturation and PO_2 will be less than normal.

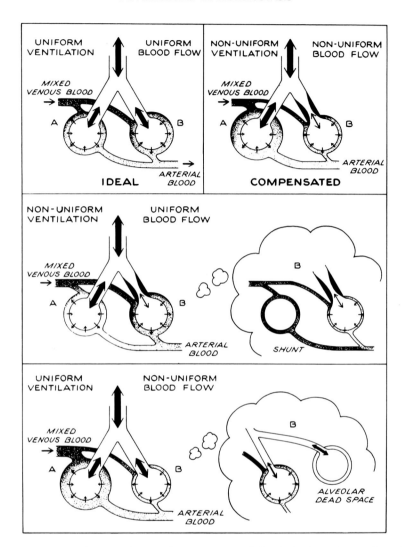

Figure 10-5. *Ventilation-perfusion relationships.* Top left, *ideal relationship, with uniform ventilation and perfusion to both alveoli. Top right, uneven ventilation and uneven perfusion but properly matched. Center, nonuniform ventilation. Alveolus A has too much ventilation for its blood flow. Alveolus B, with inadequate ventilation to match its blood flow, is divided on the right into two "pretend" alveoli: one with enough blood flow to match its ventilation and the other with the remaining blood flow and no ventilation. Bottom, nonuniform perfusion. Alveolus A has too much blood flow for its ventilation. Alveolus B, with inadequate blood flow to match its ventilation is divided on the right into two "pretend" alveoli: one with just enough ventilation to match its blood flow and the other with the remaining ventilation and no blood flow. (Reproduced with permission from Comroe JH, Jr: Physiology of Respiration, An Introductory Text, ed 2. Copyright © 1974 by Year Book Medical Publishers, Inc., Chicago.)*

With carbon dioxide the situation is different. Carbon dioxide is 20 times more soluble than oxygen; therefore, a larger proportion of carbon dioxide is dissolved in the plasma. The dissolved carbon dioxide reacts with water to form carbonic acid, which then dissociates into bicarbonate plus free hydrogen ions. This reaction is freely reversible and the concentrations of carbon dioxide and bicarbonate in the blood are in equilibrium. Most of the carbon dioxide in the blood is in the form of bicarbonate; about one-third is carried in combination with hemoglobin. Overventilated alveoli will have a lower than normal PCO_2 and so the blood leaving the capillaries in these alveoli will have a lower than normal PCO_2. Underventilated alveoli will have a higher than normal PCO_2, as will the blood flowing past these alveoli. When blood coming from overventilated alveoli mixes with blood coming from underventilated alveoli the result will be near normal. In other words, sufficient hyperventilation of well-perfused alveoli can compensate for poorly ventilated alveoli in the elimination of carbon dioxide, but cannot significantly increase oxygen saturation.

In the early stages of pulmonary disease, therefore, hypoxemia may be present but the PCO_2 may be normal. As a result of compensatory hypernea, the PCO_2 may even be lower than normal. In later stages, however, resistance to breathing increases and the person may not be able to increase ventilation enough to compensate. Then carbon dioxide retention occurs, and the person has a high arterial PCO_2 as well as a low arterial PO_2.

Chronic Obstructive Pulmonary Disease

The term *chronic obstructive pulmonary disease* (COPD) encompasses those conditions characterized by chronic or recurrent obstruction to airflow within the lungs. Other terms that may be used are chronic obstructive lung disease (COLD) and chronic airways obstruction (CAO). The conditions that are commonly included under this title are chronic bronchitis, emphysema, and asthma. These conditions can occur separately but often may occur in combination.

Chronic bronchitis is characterized by chronic or recurrent excess bronchial mucus production, usually associated with coughing. To be considered chronic it must occur on most days for at least three months per year for at least two years in succession. Chronic bronchitis is associated with enlargement of the mucus glands in the trachea and bronchi. Small airways are narrowed and become plugged with mucus. All airways are not equally affected, so that ventilation-perfusion ratios are seriously disturbed. Airway narrowing is more severe during expiration than inspiration. Consequently expiration is prolonged due to increased resistance to outflow of air and the residual volume and functional residual capacity are increased. When the amount of residual air in the lungs is increased, then the amount of fresh tidal air mixing with the residual air in the alveoli represents a smaller fraction than normal. Consequently the alveolar PO_2 decreases and the alveolar PCO_2 increases.

All the factors involved in the development of chronic bronchitis are not understood, but irritation of the tracheobronchial tree is an important factor. Affected people commonly have a long history of heavy smoking.

Emphysema is characterized by a permanent, abnormal increase in the size of air spaces distal to the terminal bronchioles, accompanied by destruction of septal tissue. The part of the lung that is involved is the *acinus*, the respiratory unit where gas exchange occurs. An acinus is made up of the respiratory bronchioles, alveolar ducts, and alveolar sacs (Fig. 10-6).

Two major patterns of emphysema have been described. *Centriacinar (centrilobular) emphysema* primarily involves the proximal portion of the acinus. The respiratory bronchioles are enlarged and become confluent as the walls between them are destroyed. This type of emphysema mainly affects the upper parts of the lungs, occurs primarily in people who smoke, is more common in men than women, and is frequently associated with chronic bronchitis.

Panacinar (panlobular) emphysema involves the

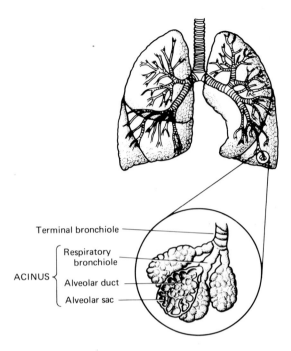

Terminal bronchiole

ACINUS { Respiratory bronchiole

Alveolar duct

Alveolar sac

Figure 10-6. *The structure of the lung, showing an acinus, the respiratory unit where gas exchange occurs.*

entire acinus. Enlargement of air spaces and destruction of septa occur more or less uniformly throughout the acinus. This type of emphysema is more predominant in the lower parts of the lungs but can occur throughout. It affects women almost as often as men. Panacinar emphysema usually develops at an earlier age than centriacinar emphysema and is not necessarily associated with cigarette smoking, although it occurs earlier in smokers than nonsmokers. It is not commonly associated with bronchitis. Panacinar emphysema is often associated with a heriditary deficiency of a plasma protein called alpha antitrypsin.

The lungs contain large numbers of leukocytes and leukocytes contain protein-digesting enzymes (proteases) that are capable of digesting lung tissue. It is hypothesized that α-antitrypsin normally inhibits the proteases released by leukocytes. When insufficient amounts of α-antitrypsin are available, release of proteases from the leukocytes

may then cause destruction of lung tissue and produce emphysema.

The tissue destruction in emphysema causes a loss of elastic recoil of the lungs. As a result, the intrapleural pressure increases more than normal during expiration and compresses the bronchioles and bronchi. Destruction of supporting tissue contributes to the airway collapse. As a result, resistance to airflow is high during expiration and air is trapped in the lungs. Therefore the residual volume and functional residual capacity are increased. Another consequence of the loss of elastic recoil is that the lungs become overdistended.

Not all parts of the lung are equally affected; therefore, ventilation-perfusion ratios are very uneven in different parts of the lung. Destruction of alveolar septa decreases the surface area for gas exchange; in addition, destruction of pulmonary capillaries occurs. Together these factors cause a decrease in pulmonary diffusing capacity.

Asthma is characterized by recurrent attacks of widespread narrowing of the airways due to bronchospasm. Asthma is often, but not always, associated with allergy. Allergy is most often associated with asthma that develops during childhood. Childhood-onset asthma affects boys more often than girls; about 30% of affected children continue to have symptoms in later life. Adult-onset asthma is less commonly associated with allergy, but is more likely to progress to COPD; it affects women more often than men.

One feature of asthma is hyperreactivity of bronchial smooth muscle. Bronchospasm is not the only cause of airway obstruction, however. People with asthma produce thick tenacious mucus, which blocks the airways. Areas of atelectasis may occur due to obstruction of small airways with plugs of mucus. Airway obstruction is not uniform throughout the lungs so that ventilation-perfusion ratios are abnormal. Again, the airways are narrower during expiration than inspiration, resulting in an increase in residual volume and functional residual capacity and overinflation of the lungs.

COPD is often manifested as either of two extreme clinical syndromes. Cyanosis and edema are characteristic of one syndrome (*"blue bloaters"*). People who manifest this syndrome tend to have a fairly heavy body build. Arterial PO_2 is decreased and the PCO_2 is increased. Respiratory acidosis that occurs as a result of the carbon dioxide retention is usually compensated (see Chapter 15). Polycythemia may occur and the hematocrit may be elevated. Usually the right atrial pressure is increased and there is right ventricular hypertrophy. Edema is believed to be usually due to right ventricular failure (see Chapter 12), but there may be other contributing factors. Edema may be due to a direct effect of hypercapnia, but the mechanism is not known. It has been noted, however, that the amount of water retention is correlated with the arterial PCO_2 level.

The other COPD syndrome is characterized by severe breathlessness with the absence of cyanosis (*"pink puffers"*). The arterial PCO_2 is normal. The arterial PO_2 may be slightly below normal at rest and decreases further on exertion. Right ventricular hypertrophy may be present but heart failure usually does not occur until the terminal stages. People with the "pink puffer" syndrome tend to have a thin body build.

The "blue bloater" syndrome is often attributed to chronic bronchitis and the "pink puffer" syndrome to emphysema, but this designation is not necessarily always correct. Many people with chronic bronchitis are "pink puffers," while many "blue bloaters" have both chronic bronchitis and emphysema. It has been suggested that the disease processes may be similar but that individual differences in ventilatory response to the altered blood-gas levels may be responsible for the two different syndromes. It may be that "blue bloaters" fail to respond normally to an elevated arterial PCO_2, whereas "pink puffers" respond normally or have an increased response. Another possibility is that the hypoxic drive to breathing is depressed in "blue bloaters" but normal in "pink puffers."

Hypoventilation

Minute ventilation is equal to the tidal volume times the respiratory rate. Not all the tidal volume reaches the alveoli, however, because of the ana-tomical dead space. The amount of fresh air entering the alveoli (*alveolar ventilation*) is equal to the tidal volume minus the dead-space volume. Therefore a decrease in the depth of breathing can significantly decrease alveolar ventilation. For example, if a person has a respiratory rate of 30 breaths per minute and a tidal volume of 200 ml (i.e., rapid, shallow breathing), the minute ventilation is 6,000 ml/minute. With an anatomical dead space of 150 ml, however, the alveolar ventilation is only 1,500 ml/minute. In contrast, if the person has a respiratory rate of 10 breaths per minute and a tidal volume of 600 ml, the minute ventilation is still 6,000 ml/minute but the alveolar ventilation is 4,500 ml/minute. In other words, the depth of breathing is more important than the rate of breathing in determining alveolar ventilation.

When the amount of air entering the alveoli is reduced (*hypoventilation*), the fraction of fresh tidal air mixing with the residual air in the alveoli is decreased. As a result, the alveolar PO_2 is lowered and less oxygen diffuses into the blood. As discussed previously, saturation of hemoglobin with oxygen will not be seriously impaired until the PO_2 drops below 60 mm Hg. Hypoventilation can have various causes: abnormalities of respiratory control; paralysis of respiratory muscles; airway obstruction; and decreased compliance of the lungs and chest wall.

Depression of the respiratory center. Depression of the respiratory center will decrease the rate and depth of breathing and breathing may become irregular. The result may be hypoxia. Inactivation of the respiratory center will cause breathing to stop (*apnea*).

Many drugs, if given in excess, can decrease the sensitivity of the respiratory center and cause hypoventilation. Examples are opiates, narcotics, barbiturates, tranquilizers, and anesthetics. Also, as previously mentioned, the respiratory center may lose its sensitivity to stimulation by carbon dioxide in people with chronic hypercapnia.

Increased intracranial pressure due to brain edema, a tumor, or any other condition can depress or inactivate the respiratory center. The respiratory center may be damaged directly by pressure, or damage may be due to ischemia as a result of compression of blood vessels. Head injuries may directly damage the respiratory center or may cause increased intracranial pressure.

Infections of the CNS may cause respiratory depression through the production of toxins or through increased intracranial pressure.

Paralysis of respiratory muscles. Impaired functioning of the respiratory muscles may lead to uneven expansion of different areas of the lungs with resultant abnormalities of the ventilation-perfusion ratio, or it may lead to severe underventilation of the alveoli with resultant hypoxia and carbon dioxide retention.

Unequal ventilation of the lungs with resultant ventilation-perfusion disturbances occurs when the thoracic muscles contract unequally. This situation may exist in dermatomyositis, myasthenia gravis, or muscular dystrophy when the intercostal muscles are not equally involved and have varying strengths.

Severe alveolar hypoventilation may occur as a result of paralysis of the respiratory muscles due to poliomyelitis, polyneuritis, spinal cord injuries, or administration of muscle relaxants. Artificial respiration is necessary to prevent severe hypoxia and carbon dioxide retention in these cases.

The diaphragm is the principal muscle of respiration. It will be paralyzed if the phrenic nerves are cut or damaged. The phrenic nerves may be affected by diseases, such as meningitis, that affect the anterior horn cells of the spinal cord; or by conditions, such as diphtheria, lead poisoning, or beriberi, that directly damage the nerves.

Decreased compliance of lungs and chest wall. The distensibility of the lungs and chest wall is called *compliance,* and is expressed as the change in volume of the lungs per unit change in intraalveolar pressure. Normally the total compliance of the lungs and chest wall is 0.13 liter/cm of water pressure. Whenever the compliance is decreased, the respiratory muscles must work harder and expend

more energy to expand the lungs. In some cases hypoventilation may occur in spite of increased respiratory effort.

Oxygen is required by the respiratory muscles; when they work harder they require more oxygen. If the increase in oxygen consumption by the respiratory muscles equals or exceeds the amount of oxygen gained by the increased ventilatory effort, compensation will no longer be possible. In some respiratory diseases, therefore, the increased work of breathing may contribute to hypoxia.

Pulmonary fibrosis restricts expansion of the lungs and decreases compliance. Excessive deposition of fibrous connective tissue in the lungs may follow any condition that causes inflammation or necrosis of lung tissue, such as irradiation, or inhalation of irritating substances.

Alveoli may become filled with fluid due to pulmonary edema or due to inflammatory exudate resulting from pneumonia. The presence of fluid in the alveoli increases the resistance to expansion and therefore decreases compliance. In addition, the fluid displaces air from the alveoli and decreases the lung capacity.

Thoracic skeletal abnormalities may increase resistance to movement of the ribs and restrict expansion of the lungs. In addition to acute conditions such as traumatic injuries to the chest and spine, chronic conditions suich as kyphoscoliosis, rheumatoid spondylitis, and tuberculous osteomyelitis of the spine can cause distortion of the thoracic cage. Kyphoscoliosis is often caused by weakening of the spinal muscles due to poliomyelitis.

Scoliosis is an abnormal lateral curvature of the spine. Severe scoliosis of the thoracic spine causes distortion of the rib cage, with the ribs being widely separated on the convex side and crowded together on the concave side of the spine. Kyphosis is an abnormal increase in the posteriorly directed convex curvature of the thoracic spine; it crowds the ribs anteriorly and causes the chest and sternum to bulge forward. Minor degrees of scoliosis or kyphosis do not significantly impair pulmonary function. In *kyphoscoliosis,* however, these two conditions occur together and the effects appear to be additive. With severe kyphoscoliosis, crowding of the ribs on one side compresses the underlying lung, while on the opposite side the ribs are spread apart and the lung is overdistended (Fig. 10-7).

Kyphoscoliosis increases the resistance to expansion of the lungs and chest wall, resulting in an increase in the work of breathing. Breathing tends to be rapid and shallow and the vital capacity and total lung capacity are decreased. Hypoxemia and hypercapnia may therefore develop as a result of alveolar hypoventilation. Hypoxemia also results from mismatching of ventilation and perfusion. In addition to moderate impairment in the distribution of inspired air, compression of pulmonary blood vessels causes uneven blood flow.

Deficient Oxygen Content of Inspired Air

At sea level the partial pressure of oxygen in atmospheric air is about 159 mm Hg (this value varies slightly depending on humidity); in alveolar air it is about 104 mm Hg. When the PO_2 in the atmospheric air is decreased, alveolar PO_2 and subsequently arterial oxygen saturation will decrease.

The oxygen content of the air will decrease in poorly ventilated enclosed spaces if oxygen is being consumed. The PO_2 also decreases with increasing altitude: for example, at an altitude of 20,000 feet the PO_2 of atmospheric air is 73 mm Hg and the alveolar PO_2 is only 40 mm Hg. At this pressure, arterial blood is only 70% saturated with oxygen. At 30,000 feet, atmospheric PO_2 is 47 mm Hg, alveolar PO_2 is 21 mm Hg, and arterial oxygen saturation falls to 20%. By breathing pure oxygen instead of air at this altitude, however, arterial oxygen saturation may be maintained at 99%. Obviously, mountain climbers and people flying in unpressurized aircraft will be subject to hypoxia.

At 8,000 feet the arterial oxygen saturation is about 93% and pulmonary ventilation increases. Above about 12,000 feet other signs of hypoxia are manifested: fatigue, drowsiness, muscular incoordination, and sometimes headache and nausea. As a result of hyperventilation a person blows off more carbon dioxide and respiratory alkalosis occurs (see Chapter 15). A person remaining at high altitude for more than a few days adapts to the low PO_2, and it has fewer adverse effects on the body. Pulmonary ventilation and the diffusing capacity for oxygen increase. In addition, red blood cell production and plasma volume gradually increase, as previously described. When a person remains at a high altitude for months or years, the number of capillaries also increases, as mentioned previously.

HYPEROXIA

Although oxygen is essential for life, too much oxygen can be toxic. Oxygen toxicity can result from prolonged use of high concentrations of oxygen for therapy or from increased pressures of oxygen encountered in unusual environments such as in deep-sea diving. Oxygen toxicity takes time to develop; therefore a high PO_2 can be tolerated for a short time. The higher the PO_2, however, the shorter the duration of safe exposure. Oxygen toxicity can be delayed by periodic brief interruptions of oxygen administration.

As mentioned previously, hemoglobin is almost completely saturated at the normal PO_2, and very little oxygen is dissolved in the plasma. A high PO_2 cannot increase the amount of oxygen carried by hemoglobin, but it can significantly increase

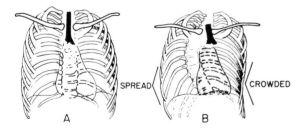

Figure 10-7. (A) Normal chest contour. (B) Kyphoscoliosis. (From Cherniack RM, et al: Respiration in Health and Disease, ed 2. © 1972 by the W.B. Saunders Company, Philadelphia.)

the amount of oxygen dissolved in the plasma. For a newborn (especially a premature infant), even a slight increase in the PO_2 may represent a state of relative hyperoxia, because in utero the fetus exists in a state of relative hypoxia.

Hyperoxia produces both physical and chemical effects, which are manifested by pulmonary changes, central nervous system toxicity, and damage to the eyes.

Mechanisms of Damage

Physical Effects
Air is composed of about 79% nitrogen; at sea level the partial pressure of nitrogen in atmospheric air is about 600 mm Hg. Nitrogen is not readily absorbed into the body because it is not very soluble in body fluids; in contrast, oxygen is absorbed rapidly. The volume of gas-containing spaces in the body (e.g., alveoli, paranasal sinuses, and middle ear) is therefore maintained primarily by nitrogen.

Inhalation of pure oxygen will result in a washing out of nitrogen from the air spaces of the body; the spaces will contain only oxygen, carbon dioxide, and water vapor. If communication of these spaces with the external environment is blocked (e.g., by secretions, edema, or spasm) the gases in them are rapidly absorbed. The result will be collapse of part of a lung or pain, hemorrhage, and exudation due to reduced pressure in spaces, such as the sinuses and middle ear, that have rigid walls.

Chemical Toxicity
Excessive oxygen interferes with cell metabolism. Many enzymes are oxidized by a high PO_2, including several enzymes required for operation of the TCA cycle. Consequently the enzymes are inactivated and several metabolic processes are impaired. In addition, a high PO_2 in the tissues may cause oxidation of some lipids. As a result, structures that have a high lipid content, such as cell membranes, may be altered. Altered membrane permeability may be a consequence of this structural change.

Effects of Hyperoxia

Pulmonary Effects
Inhalation of 80% oxygen for more than 12 hours may cause irritation of the respiratory passages, as manifested by coughing, sore throat, and nasal congestion. Bronchopneumonia (inflammation of the lungs that begins in the terminal bronchioles) or pleural effusion (an abnormal amount of fluid in the pleural space) may result after breathing 100% oxygen for more than 24 hours. Longer exposures may impair gas exchange. As already mentioned, atelectasis may occur if airway obstruction develops.

In experiments with animals, severe oxygen toxicity has resulted in pulmonary structural changes, loss of surfactant, pulmonary edema, and atelectasis. Eventually death of the animals resulted from carbon dioxide retention, acidosis, and hypoxia.

Central Nervous System Effects
At pressures greater than two atmospheres (i.e., greater than 1,520 mm Hg), oxygen has a toxic effect on the central nervous system. Such high pressures may be encountered in hyperbaric oxygen therapy or in the use of oxygen in diving.

Oxygen toxicity to the CNS is manifested as generalized convulsive seizures with loss of consciousness. A variety of signs and symptoms, such as twitching of the lips, eyelids, or small muscles of the hands; tingling of the hands; nausea; and dizziness may precede the generalized seizures. The person is alert until the onset of the convulsive seizure. (With hypoxia, mental impairment and drowsiness precede the onset of a convulsive seizure.)

Effects on the Eyes
A high PO_2 causes reversible vasoconstriction in the eyes of adults. Prolonged exposure to very high

oxygen pressure causes contraction of the visual fields, with loss of peripheral vision.

The eyes of premature infants are much more seriously affected by hyperoxia. Prolonged exposure to high concentrations of oxygen leads to the development of *retrolental fibroplasia,* which can cause blindness.

A high concentration of oxygen causes constriction of the retinal blood vessels. The immature vessels then become obliterated, resulting in retinal hypoxia. Hypoxia acts as a stimulus to the growth of new capillaries; therefore, when the infants are later placed in a normal atmosphere, wild, disorganized regrowth of the blood vessels occurs. The blood vessels extend beyond the retinal surface into the vitreous body (normally the blood vessels do not leave the retina). In most cases the proliferative process subsides and the retina spontaneously reverts to normal. In some cases, however, retinal hemorrhages occur and fibrous scar tissue forms, causing retinal detachment and blindness.

SUGGESTED ADDITIONAL READING

Perutz MF: Hemoglobin structure and respiratory transport. *Sci Am* **239**(6): 92–125, 1978.

Waldron MW: Oxygen transport. *Am J Nurs* **79**(2): 272–275, 1979.

Windle WF: Brain damage by asphyxia at birth. *Sci Am* **221**(4) 76–84, 1969.

11

The Body Fluids and Fluid Shifts

Water is vital in the functioning of the human body. It is the solvent for many body chemicals; since these chemicals must be in solution for biochemical reactions to occur, water is essential to metabolism. Water is also necessary for body temperature regulation (see Chapter 24). By providing tissue turgor, water contributes to the structure and form of the body. Alterations in the distribution of body water or changes in body fluid volume can lead to disturbances of homeostasis.

BODY FLUID COMPARTMENTS

The total body water (TBW) is functionally divided into two compartments: the water (fluid) inside the cells, or *intracellular fluid* (ICF); and the water outside the cells, or *extracellular fluid* (ECF). Anatomically, the separation of ICF into discrete cells surrounded by membranes provides the basis for specialization of cellular function. The ECF, however, is like a continuous phase that bathes

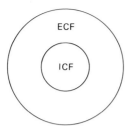

Figure 11-1. *The extracellular fluid (ECF) surrounds the cells, which contain intracellular fluid (ICF).*

the cells. It forms the "internal environment" that surrounds the cells (Fig. 11-1). The fluid outside the cells is constantly in motion, which is important in maintaining homeostasis.

Volume and Distribution of Body Fluid

The normal water content of the body varies with age, sex, and amount of fat in the body. The body water content in children and adults of various ages is summarized in Tables 11-1 and 11-2. The values given in these tables are only approximate, and it is important to realize that considerable individual variation exists.

Children have a higher proportion of body water than adults (Fig. 11-2). In a normal newborn, water represents approximately 79% of the body weight. A premature infant has an even higher proportion of body water. A large portion of this water is in the extracellular compartment.

Table 11-1. Approximate Body Water Content of Children as Percent of Body Weight[a]

Age	TBW	ECF	ICF
Newborn	79	45	34
2–30 days	74	40	34
1–12 mo	63	30	33
1–2 yr	59	24	35
2–8 yr	62	25	37

[a]Data derived from various sources listed in bibliography.

Table 11-2. Approximate Body Water Content of Adolescents and Adults as Percent of Body Weight[a]

Age	TBW	ECF	ICF
Males:			
10–16 yr	59	26	33
20–35 yr	60	28	32
35–50 yr	55	25	30
70+ yr	51	25	26
Females:			
10–15 yr	56	25	31
20–35 yr	50	25	25
35–50 yr	48	23	25
60+ yr	43	21	22

[a]Data derived from various sources listed in bibliography.

In the first 12 months a rapid decrease in TBW occurs, mainly due to a decrease in the amount of ECF in relation to body weight. A gradual decrease in the proportion of body water continues throughout life. In old age the decrease is mainly due to a decrease in ICF.

A slight difference in body water content exists between the sexes from birth throughout childhood, with boys having a higher proportion of body water than girls. In adults the sexual difference in body water content is very marked; this difference is attributed to differences in body fat content. Adipose (fat) tissue has a very low water content, and women usually have a higher proportion of body fat than men. It follows, also, that

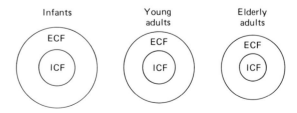

Figure 11-2. *The proportion of body water progressively decreases with age.*

Table 11-3. Effect of Body Fat on Body Water Content in Young Adult Females[a]

	Average Ht (meters)	Average Wt (kg)	Water Content as Percent Body Weight		
			TBW	ECF	ICF
Thin subjects	1.67	42.2	64	35	29
Average Subjects	1.67	65.7	50	25	25
Obese Subjects	1.67	109.8	38	29	17

[a]Data derived from Ljunggren H et al: *Acta Endocrinol* **25**: 187–223, 1957.

an obese person of any age (male or female) will have a lower proportion of body water than a thin person of the same age. For this reason, some physiologists prefer to speak of body water content in terms of "lean body mass." For adults (male or female) water represents approximately 70% of the lean body mass. As an example of the effect of body fat content on body water content, the body water content of lean, average, and obese young women is shown in Table 11-3.

Total body water can be measured fairly accurately, but it is much more difficult to determine how much water is in the intracellular compartment and how much is in the extracellular compartment. ICF volume cannot be determined directly; it is estimated by measuring TBW and ECF volume and then taking the difference. ECF volume is determined by the dilution principle (Fig. 11-3). A known amount of a test substance is administered. After allowing adequate time for

the substance to become distributed throughout the fluid compartment being measured, a sample of the body fluid is taken and the concentration of the substance is determined. The final concentration will depend on the size of the fluid compartment; the greater the volume of fluid, the lower the concentration of the test substance will be.

Although the dilution principle is simple, it is difficult to find a substance that is uniformly distributed throughout the ECF within a reasonable length of time and that does not enter the cells. Therefore, the values obtained for ECF volume are critically dependent on the substance used. A variety of test substances have been used to measure the ECF volume, including inulin, sucrose, mannitol, thiosulfate, radioactive sodium, radioactive chloride, radioactive bromide, and thiocyanate. The values obtained range from 16% to 28% of the body weight for a 70-kg (154-lb) adult male, depending on the substance used. Since none of these substances measures the ECF volume exactly, physiologists usually refer to the inulin space, the bromide space, the thiocyanate space, and so forth. (In spite of this difficulty, it is possible to measure *changes* in ECF volume using a particular test substance and in the clinical situation such measurements can be useful.)

Since the volume of ICF cannot be determined directly, the value obtained depends on what value is chosen for the ECF volume. As a result of the factors just mentioned, values of ICF and ECF volume are only estimates, and the values given in Tables 11-1 and 11-2 may differ from values given in some other textbooks. The values for ECF vol-

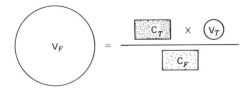

Figure 11-3. *The dilution principle.* V_F *represents the volume of the fluid compartment being measured;* C_T, *the concentration of the test substance administered;* V_T, *the volume of the test substance administered;* C_F, *the concentration of the test substance in the body fluid compartment.*

ume given in these tables represent the bromide space. Unfortunately, data based on measurements using the same test substance are not available for all age groups. The trend of decreasing body water with increasing age, however, can be seen from the measurements that are available. The values for ECF volume in Table 11-3 represent the chloride space.

Extracellular Fluid

Not only is total body water divided into the intracellular compartment and the extracellular compartment but the extracellular compartment is further subdivided into several components. The major components are the plasma and the interstitial-lymph fluid, but the extracellular compartment also includes the fluid of dense connective tissue and bone, as well as specialized transcellular fluids.

Plasma

Plasma is the liquid portion of the blood, which is contained in the *intravascular compartment*. Total blood volume is made up of blood cell volume in addition to plasma volume; the blood cell volume is primarily due to erythrocytes. The relationship between plasma volume and red blood cell volume is given by the *hematocrit*, which is the percentage of blood volume that is red blood cells. For example, if the hematocrit is 40% it means that 40% of the blood volume is red blood cell volume; the remaining 60% is plasma volume.

Plasma volume averages about 45 to 50 ml/kg (i.e., 4.5% to 5.0% of the body weight) throughout childhood and about 45 ml/kg for adults. Blood volume in children is approximately 75 ml/kg of body weight, but considerable individual variation is found. A slight increase occurs around puberty, especially in males, due to an increase in the hematocrit.

For the average adult whose weight is close to ideal for height, blood volume is approximately 70 ml/kg of body weight. Adipose tissue has a smaller blood content than other tissues, so that the blood volume per kilogram of body weight is less for an

obese person and more for a thin person. The blood volume is normally slightly greater in men than women beause men usually have a higher hematocrit and smaller proportion of body fat than women. For an average young adult male the total blood volume is about 5 liters, of which 3 liters is plasma.

Interstitial-Lymph Fluid

Interstitial fluid occupies the spaces between the cells. Only a small portion of it is actually in the form of free-flowing fluid. Most of the water is bound with the protein (primarily collagen) and mucopolysaccharide (primarily hyaluronic acid) of the interstitial space to form a gel.

Lymph is the fluid within the lymphatic vessels. It is derived from interstitial fluid and returned to the blood.

Interstitial-lymph fluid volume is estimated to be about 12% of the body weight (i.e., 120 ml/kg) for a young adult male; for an infant it may be as much as 25% of the body weight (i.e., 250 ml/kg).

Dense Connective Tissue and Bone Fluid

Anatomically, bone and dense connective tissue contain relatively few cells and a large amount of intercellular material. A significant amount of water is bound to this intercellular material. The water in these spaces is exchangeable with the interstitial fluid (i.e., water molecules move back and forth between the two compartments). Some of the test substances used to measure ECF volume (e.g., inulin and sucrose) enter the dense connective tissue very slowly and do not penetrate into the bone fluid space, however, so that some measurements of ECF do not include the fluids in these spaces. The values given in Tables 11-1 and 11-2 do include dense connective tissue and bone fluid. An estimate of the amount of dense connective tissue and bone fluid for a healthy young adult male is 9% of the body weight (i.e., 90 ml/kg).

Transcellular Fluids

Transcellular fluids are specialized extracellular fluids that have been formed by the transport activity of cells. This component includes mucus, digestive juices, serous fluid, synovial fluid, secretions of the genitourinary tract, cerebrospinal fluid, and the ocular fluids. An estimated total value for transcellular fluid volume is 15 ml/kg of body weight for an average adult.

The fluid in the lumen of the gastrointestinal tract comprises the largest proportion of transcellular fluid. Accurate measurements of this fluid volume are difficult and the quantity varies according to food intake, but an approximate value is 7.4 ml/kg of body weight when a person is fasting. This value represents the amount of fluid in the gastrointestinal tract at a given time. Since gastrointestinal fluid is constantly being secreted and reabsorbed, however, it is more useful to know the daily production of digestive juices when considering fluid balance. In adults, approximately 6 to 8 liters/day of digestive juices are secreted into the gastrointestinal tract, but most of the water is normally reabsorbed. The rate of secretion of gastrointestinal fluids relative to TBW or ECF volume appears to be higher in children than in adults.

Composition of Body Fluids

Many minerals and small organic molecules are dissolved in the body fluids. In addition, some body fluids contain protein. Most of these dissolved substances are ionized.

An *ion* is an atom or group of atoms that carries an electrical charge. Ions with negative charges are called *anions*; those with positive charges are called *cations*. *Valence* is the combining power of an atom (or group of atoms, e.g., HCO_3^-, that react chemically as a unit) and is determined by the number of electrons the atom shares or contributes in chemical union. An ion with a valence of one is said to be *monovalent*, for example, sodium (Na^+), potassium (K^+), bicarbonate (HCO_3^-), and chloride (Cl^-). A *divalent* (or bivalent) ion has a valence of two, for example, calcium (Ca^{2+}), magnesium (Mg^{2+}), and sulfate (SO_4^{2-}).

A solution that contains ions is capable of conducting an electric current; therefore it is called an electrolytic solution. Acids, bases, and salts that dissociate into ions when dissolved in water are called *electrolytes*. Thus, body fluids are electrolytic solutions and have electrolytes dissolved in them.

Units of Measure

Atomic weights are the relative weights of the atoms of the elements on an arbitrary scale in which carbon is assigned the value of 12. *Molecular weight* is the sum of the atomic weights of the elements that make up a molecule of a substance. For example, a water molecule is made up of two hydrogen atoms and one oxygen atom. The atomic weight of hydrogen is 1 and the atomic weight of oxygen is 16; therefore the molecular weight of water is 18. A mole is the amount of a substance that contains the molecular weight in grams. For example, one mole of water is 18 g. A millimole is 1/1,000 of a mole, or the weight of the substance in milligrams. The *molarity* (M) of a solution is the number of moles of solute per liter of solution. Molarity varies slightly with temperature because liquids expand with increasing temperature. The *molality* (m) of a solution is the number of moles of solute per kilogram (1,000 g) of solvent; it does not change with temperature.

The *equivalent weight* of a substance is its combining weight. Atoms or groups of atoms entering into chemical combination always do so in quantities proportional to their equivalent weights. The equivalent weight of an element forming a simple ion is equal to its atomic weight divided by the valence. For example, the atomic weight of sodium is 23 and the equivalent weight of Na^+ is 23; the atomic weight of calcium is 40 and the equivalent weight of Ca^{2+} is 20. The equivalent weight of a complex ion is equal to its formula weight divided by the valence. For example, the formula weight of sulfate is 96 and the equivalent weight of SO_4^{2-} is 48.

An *equivalent* (Eq) of a substance is the equivalent weight expressed in grams. It is the amount of the substance that can combine with or replace one gram of hydrogen. (Hydrogen has an atomic weight of one and the hydrogen ion is a monovalent cation, i.e., H^+.) A *milliequivalent* (mEq) is

1/1,000 of an equivalent, or the equivalent weight expressed in milligrams. For example, one milliequivalent of Na^+ is 23 mg.

One milliequivalent of a substance will react with or combine with exactly one milliequivalent of another substance. For example, 1 mEq Ca^{2+} (20 mg) will combine exactly with 1 mEq Cl^- (35.5 mg). For this reason it is convenient to express electrolytes in terms of milliequivalents per liter. When expressed as milliequivalents, total cations equal total anions. This numerical equality does not exist when substances are expressed in terms of milligrams per 100 ml or milligrams per liter.

When the osmotic activity of a solution is under consideration the most useful unit of measure is the *osmole* (Osm) or *milliosmole* (mOsm). (One milliosmole is 1/1,000 of an osmole.) The osmotic pressure exerted by a solute depends on the number of *particles* (i.e., molecules or ions) in a solution and an osmole is a unit used to express the number of solute particles. One osmole equals the number of particles in one mole of undissociated solute. (One mole of any substance contains the same number of molecules, irrespective of its weight.) For example, the molecular weight of glucose is 180 and 1 mole of glucose equals 180 g. Glucose does not dissociate in solution (i.e., does not form ions), therefore 1 mole (180 g) of glucose equals 1 Osm. If a solute dissociates, the number of osmoles is determined by the number of particles (ions) formed upon dissolution. For example, 1 mole (58.5 g) of sodium chloride (NaCl) equals 2 Osm because NaCl dissociates into Na^+ and Cl^- ions. One mole (111 g) of calcium chloride ($CaCl_2$) equals 3 Osm because $CaCl_2$ dissociates to give one Ca^{2+} ion and two Cl^- ions (i.e., three particles) for each molecule. The *osmolarity* of a solution is the number of osmoles of solute per liter of solution; it varies slightly with temperature. The *osmolality* of a solution is the number of osmoles of solute per kilogram of solvent; it does not vary with temperature.

Electrolytes of the Body Fluids

Table 11-4 shows the approximate compositions of ICF and the plasma and interstitial portions of the ECF. The composition of ICF is difficult to determine precisely and varies from tissue to tissue; however it has been shown that the compositions of ECF and ICF differ considerably (Fig. 11-4).

The major cations of ICF are potassium (K^+)

Table 11-4. Approximate Composition of Body Fluids

	Plasma (mEq/liter)	Interstitital Fluid (mEq/liter)	Intracellular Fluid (mEq/liter)
Total Cations:	153	156	200
Sodium	142	145	12
Potassium	4	4	150
Calcium	5	5	4
Magnesium	2	2	34
Total Anions:	153	156	200
Chloride	104	117	4
Bicarbonate	26	29	12
Phosphate	2	2	95
Sulfate	1	1	20
Protein	14	1	55
Other	6	6	14

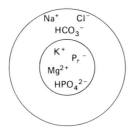

Figure 11-4. *The compositions of the extracellular fluid and intracellular fluid are different. Pr⁻ represents proteinate.*

and magnesium (Mg^{2+}). Very little sodium is present in ICF. The cations are balanced mainly by the anions phosphate (varying proportions of $H_2PO_4^-$, HPO_4^{2-}, and PO_4^{3-}), sulfate (SO_4^{2-}), and proteinate (ionized protein). In contrast, the important cation of the ECF is sodium (Na^+); the ECF has very little potassium. The major anions of ECF are chloride (Cl^-) and bicarbonate (HCO_3^-). A variety of organic acids are also present in the ECF; they are derived from metabolic reactions in the cells. The major one is lactic acid; other common ones are pyruvic acid, acetoacetic acid, and citric acid.

Plasma contains proteins, but the concentration of plasma proteins is about one-fourth that in the ICF. Interstitial fluid differs from plasma in that it contains little or no protein. Small molecules and ions diffuse easily between the plasma and the interstitial fluid, but the capillary membrane is impermeable to the large protein molecules. Proteins carry a net negative charge at the pH of body fluids (i.e., they are anions), and anions must equal cations to maintain electrical neutrality. Since the plasma contains proteinate and the interstitial fluid does not, it follows that the concentrations of the other electrolytes must differ slightly between the plasma and the interstitial fluid in order to maintain electrical neutrality (the Gibbs-Donnan effect). This situation is the case, as can be seen from Table 11-4.

Movement of Fluids Between Compartments

The body water is not static; water molecules are constantly moving back and forth between the various fluid compartments. In a state of health, the movement of water molecules in one direction is balanced by movement of molecules in the other direction. Movement of water between compartments is mainly due to osmotic pressure and hydrostatic pressure. In physiology these pressures are usually measured as millimeters of mercury (mm Hg), although other units of measure can be used.

Hydrostatic pressure is the pressure exerted by a fluid. As more molecules are packed into a given volume of fluid, the pressure becomes greater. In a column of fluid, the hydrostatic pressure will be proportional to the depth of the fluid because of the weight of the fluid above the point of measurement.

Osmosis is the net movement of water (solvent) from a more dilute solution (i.e., a solution of lower osmolarity) to a more concentrated solution (i.e., a solution of higher osmolarity) when the movement of solute is restricted by a membrane. As water moves into the compartment containing the more concentrated solution, the volume of the solution increases until the inward flow is balanced by an outward flow due to hydrostatic pressure. *Osmotic pressure* is the pressure that develops in a solution as a result of osmosis into that solution. Osmotic pressure develops in the solution that originally contains the higher concentration of the solute that does not diffuse freely through the membrane. As stated previously, osmotic pressure is determined by the number of solute particles in a given amount of solution. *Potential osmotic pressure* is the maximum osmotic pressure that could develop in a solution if it were separated from pure water by a semipermeable membrane.

Movement of Water Between ECF and ICF
Water moves into and out of cells by the process of osmosis. The cell membrane is highly permeable

to water but restricts the movement of some solute molecules.

Within the cell are many protein anions that cannot cross the cell membrane. Therefore, a potential osmotic pressure exists within the cell. If this pressure were not balanced by an equal pressure in the ECF, water would move into the cell and the cell would swell and eventually rupture. To solve this problem, positive sodium ions are actively transported out of the cell. Consequently, the inside of the cell becomes electrically negative (due to the negatively charged protein ions) relative to the outside. This negative charge inside the cell repels the chloride anions, so that they do not move into the cell, but stay in the ECF. In addition, potassium cations are attracted by the negative charge inside the cell and so inward movement of potassium ions is enhanced. Sodium ions also diffuse into the cell, but they are pumped out as fast as they can enter. Therefore, the ICF has a high concentration of potassium ions and the ECF has a high concentration of sodium ions, as mentioned previously. The high concentrations of sodium and chloride ions create a potential osmotic pressure in the ECF to balance the potential osmotic pressure within the cell. Therefore the movement of water molecules into the cell is normally balanced by an equal movement of water molecules out of the cell (i.e., net movement of water is zero) and the ICF volume does not change.

Two solutions that have the same potential osmotic pressure are said to be *isoosmotic*, or *isotonic*. Clinically, a solution is considered to be isotonic when it has the same potential osmotic pressure (i.e., the same osmolarity) as the body fluids in health. For a healthy person, the osmolarity of the body fluids is 285 to 290 mOsm/liter (except for some transcellular fluids, interstitial fluid of the renal medulla, and the final urine).

When two solutions have unequal potential osmotic pressures, the one with the higher pressure (i.e., the greater osmolarity) is said to be *hypertonic*, or *hyperosmotic*. The one with the lower pressure (i.e., the lower osmolarity) is said to be *hypotonic*, or *hypoosmotic*. Water will move from a hypotonic solution to a hypertonic solution. If a cell is placed in a hypotonic solution (i.e., a solution with a lower osmolarity than the ICF), water will move into the cell and the cell will swell. If a cell is placed in a hypertonic solution (i.e., a solution with a higher osmolarity than the ICF), water will leave the cell and the cell will shrink. Thus, if the ECF becomes hypertonic relative to the ICF, water will move out of the cells into the ECF. Conversely, if the ECF becomes hypotonic relative to the ICF, water will move into the cells (Fig. 11-5).

Transcapillary Fluid Exchange

Distribution of fluid between the plasma and interstitial fluid compartments of the ECF depends on the balance of forces governing exchange of fluid across capillary membranes. Capillary membranes are very permeable to water and most of the plasma solutes, except the plasma proteins and substances bound to them. The major force causing the movement of fluid from the plasma to the interstitial fluid is a hydrostatic pressure gradient due to the capillary blood pressure. The primary force responsible for the movement of water from the interstitial fluid to the plasma is an osmotic pressure gradient created by the plasma proteins.

The total osmotic pressure of the ECF is due to all the solute particles: electrolytes, small mole-

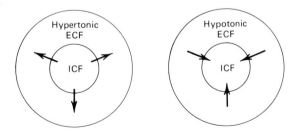

Figure 11-5. *Movement of water between the ECF and ICF. Arrows indicate the direction of net movement of water.*

cules, and proteins. The electrolytes and small molecules are freely diffusible between the plasma and interstitial fluid, so that they exert the same osmotic force on both sides of the capillary membrane. Since the capillary membrane restricts the movement of plasma proteins and the interstitial fluid contains very little protein, however, the plasma has a greater potential osmotic pressure than the interstitial fluid. This osmotic pressure gradient tends to draw water from the interstitial fluid into the plasma. The osmotic pressure created by the proteins is called the *colloid osmotic pressure,* or *oncotic pressure.*

The normal concentration of plasma proteins is approximately 7 g/100 ml and the plasma oncotic pressure is about 28 mm Hg. Capillary permeability and therefore the protein concentration of the interstitial fluid varies slightly from one tissue to another. On the average, however, the colloid osmotic pressure of the interstitial fluid is about 4.5 mm Hg, opposing the plasma oncotic pressure. Therefore, the net colloid osmotic pressure (i.e., the *effective oncotic pressure*) drawing water into the capillaries is approximately 23.5 mm Hg.

The movement of fluid from the interstitial spaces into the capillaries due to the plasma oncotic pressure is opposed by the hydrostatic pressure of the blood (i.e., blood pressure), which tends to force fluid out of the capillaries. Capillary hydrostatic pressure varies depending on the arterial blood pressure and the degree of constriction of the precapillary sphincter, but is thought to normally average about 25 mm Hg at the arterial end of the capillary. The hydrostatic pressure in the interstitial space is thought to be about −7 mm Hg (i.e., 7 mm Hg less than atmospheric pressure), although this value is still controversial. Therefore a hydrostatic pressure gradient (*effective hydrostatic pressure*) of approximately 32 mm Hg favors the movement of fluid out of the capillaries. Since the effective hydrostatic pressure at the arterial end is greater than the effective plasma oncotic pressure by about 8.5 mm Hg, there is a net movement of fluid out of the capillaries into the interstitial space.

Capillary hydrostatic pressure decreases from the arterial to the venous end of a capillary. At the venous end, capillary hydrostatic pressure is thought to be about 10 mm Hg, while the hydrostatic pressure of the interstitial fluid stays about the same. Therefore, at the venous end the effective hydrostatic pressure is about 17 mm Hg, which is 6.5 mm Hg less than the effective oncotic pressure. Consequently, at the venous end there is a net movement of fluid from the interstitial space into the capillaries. The forces governing transcapillary fluid exchange are summarized in Figure 11-6. The net pressure gradient forcing fluid out of the capillaries is a little greater than the net pressure gradient drawing fluid into the capillaries. Consequently, slightly more fluid leaves the capillaries than reenters. This excess fluid and any proteins that leak out of the capillaries are returned to the blood by way of the lymphatic vessels.

Fluid exchange across the capillary membranes of the pulmonary circulation is governed by the same forces that determine transcapillary fluid exchange in the systemic circulation, but the magnitude of the forces is different. The plasma oncotic pressure is the same, but capillary hydrostatic pressure is lower in the pulmonary circulation. The mean pulmonary capillary hydrostatic pressure is about 7 to 10 mm Hg, while the interstitial hydrostatic pressure is thought to be about −3 mm Hg. Therefore, the effective hydrostatic pressure is approximately 10 to 13 mm Hg, which is less than the plasma oncotic pressure. This apparent imbalance in favor of retention of fluid in the capillaries led to the concept that the lung is a "dry" organ. Results of research in recent years, however, have led to a reassessment of this concept. It is now known that a thin layer of moisture covers the alveolar surfaces. More importantly, it is known that a constant flow of lymph drains from the lungs. Therefore fluid must be entering the interstitial space. Based on the protein content of lymph

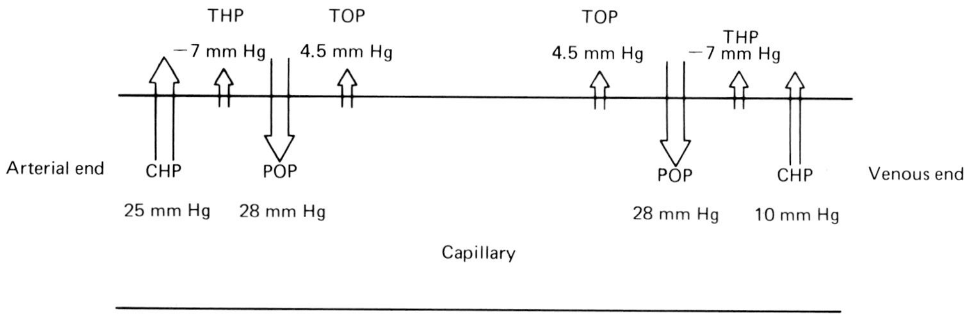

Effective hydrostatic pressure = 25 − (−7) = 32.0 mm Hg

Effective oncotic pressure = 28 − 4.5 = 23.5 mm Hg

Net force outward = 8.5 mm Hg

Effective hydrostatic pressure = 10 − (−7) = 17.0 mm Hg

Effective oncotic pressure = 28 − 4.5 = 23.5 mm Hg

Net force inward = 6.5 mm Hg

Figure 11-6. *Summary of the forces governing transcapillary fluid exchange. CHP, capillary hydrostatic pressure; THP, tissue hydrostatic pressure; POP, plasma oncotic pressure; TOP, tissue oncotic pressure. Arrows indicate direction of force.*

flowing from the lungs, it is estimated that the colloid osmotic pressure of the interstitial space is about 19 mm Hg. (Presumably protein is leaking out of the pulmonary capillaries into the interstitial space.) Therefore, the effective oncotic pressure is only about 9 mm Hg, which is less than the effective hydrostatic pressure. Consequently more fluid leaves the capillaries than reenters and the excess is drained by way of the lymphatics.

ABNORMAL DISTRIBUTION OF ECF

The forces governing transcapillary fluid exchange and therefore determining the distribution of fluid between the plasma and interstitial fluid compartments have just been described. Any factor that disrupts the normal balance of these forces will lead to an abnormal shift of fluid from the plasma to the interstitial space or from the interstitial space to the plasma. Edema is produced when fluid shifts from the plasma to the interstitial space.

Edema

Edema is the accumulation of an abnormally large amount of fluid in the interstitial space. Edema may be localized, such as occurs with a local inflammatory reaction; or it may be generalized, such as occurs with congestive heart failure or the nephrotic syndrome. Massive generalized edema is also called *anasarca.* In some cases of generalized edema (e.g., due to extensive burns or the nephrotic syndrome) the intravascular volume is decreased. In other words, the edema represents a shift of fluid from the plasma to the interstitial compartment; the total ECF volume may be normal or abnormal. In other cases of generalized edema (e.g., due to congestive heart failure), the intravascular volume is normal or increased and the total ECF volume is increased. (See Chapter 12 under Fluid Volume Excess.)

As stated previously, most of the interstitial fluid is bound to proteins and mucopolysaccharides of the tissue spaces to form a gel. Only a small portion of it is in the form of free fluid, which moves in tiny rivulets between the gel and the cells. The gel structure is important, because it holds the interstitial fluid in place. When edema develops, a small amount of the excess fluid is probably bound with the gel, but as the amount of edema fluid increases the fluid moves freely throughout the tissues. Gravity causes the fluid to move to the lowermost, or dependent, portions of the body. This condition is called *dependent edema.*

If a finger is pressed on the skin over an edematous area, the edema fluid moves away from the area beneath the pressure point. If the finger is then suddenly removed, a small depression, or pit, is evident at the place where the finger had been pressing. This phenomenon is called *pitting edema* (Fig. 11-7). Gradually the fluid flows back into the area and the pit disappears.

Pulmonary Edema

Pulmonary edema is an abnormal accumulation of extravascular liquid in the lungs. The excess liquid first collects in the interstitial spaces of the interalveolar septa. If the amount of liquid increases, some of it enters the alveoli, giving rise to the signs of moist rales and frothy sputum. Pulmonary edema can only occur when the rate of formation of interstitial liquid is greater than the capacity of the lymphatics to remove the excess liquid. The rate of lymph flow from the lungs can probably increase up to about 10 times the usual rate, thus providing a safety factor against the development of pulmonary edema. The usual cause of pulmonary edema is increased capillary hydrostatic pressure, for example due to congestive heart failure. Pulmonary edema can also result from increased capillary permeability, for example due to inflammation.

Plasma-to-Interstitial-Fluid Shift

When an excessive amount of fluid leaves the capillaries, a compensatory increase in the flow of lymph occurs (unless the lymphatics are blocked) to return the excess fluid to the circulation. The degree to which lymph flow can increase is lim-

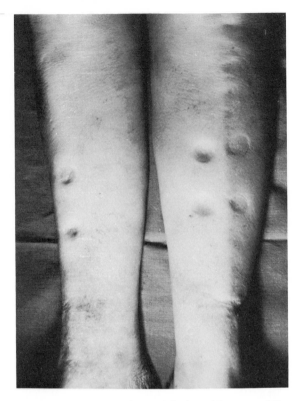

Figure 11-7. *Pitting edema of the legs. (Courtesy of Dr. J. Burton, Vancouver General Hospital, Vancouver, B.C., Canada.)*

ited, however, so that eventually the excess fluid that leaves the intravascular compartment accumulates in the interstitial space, producing edema.

Localized shifts of fluid to the interstitial space (i.e., localized edema) are accompanied by a slight transient reduction in plasma volume. The plasma volume is quickly restored to normal by compensatory retention of salt and water by the kidneys, brought about by increased secretion of antidiuretic hormone (ADH) and aldosterone (see Chapter 12). When the fluid shift is generalized and when large amounts of fluid shift to the interstitial space, however, hypovolemia results. *Hypovolemia* is an abnormally decreased volume of circulating blood. Since fluid leaves the intravascular compartment but blood cells do not, the hematocrit and the hemoglobin concentration may be elevated.

As a consequence of hypovolemia, stroke volume falls, cardiac output decreases, and tissue perfusion is reduced. Heart rate increases as a compensatory mechanism to maintain cardiac output. Symptoms of hypovolemia are related to decreased blood flow to the tissues. With mild degrees of hypovolemia a person may experience lassitude, easy fatigability, thirst, and dizziness or syncope on standing. When the hypovolemia is more severe or when the shift occurs acutely (e.g., due to trauma or burns), shock can result (see Chapter 14).

The four basic causes of a plasma-to-interstitial-fluid shift are increased capillary hydrostatic pressure, decreased plasma protein concentration, increased capillary permeability, and lymphatic obstruction. In some circumstances more than one of these factors can be operating to produce a shift of fluid to the interstitial space.

Increased Capillary Hydrostatic Pressure

Increased capillary hydrostatic pressure can result from arteriolar dilatation or increased venous pressure. The most common cause of arteriolar dilatation is inflammation; the release of histamine in allergic reactions is another cause. This mechanism results in localized edema.

Increased venous pressure occurs in the legs and feet due to prolonged standing (see Chapter 22). Venous obstruction (e.g., due to thrombosis) causes increased venous pressure behind the obstruction and can cause localized edema. Cardiac failure is a common cause of increased venous pressure, leading to generalized edema. (Congestive heart failure is discussed in Chapter 12; see under Isotonic ECF Volume Excess. Increased venous pressure is not the only factor involved in the excessive accumulation of interstitial fluid in this condition.)

As fluid shifts from the plasma to the interstitial space, the interstitial hydrostatic pressure rises until it is high enough to balance the excessive capillary hydrostatic pressure. When this level is achieved a new equilibrium is established across the capillary membrane and the amount of fluid that accumulates in the interstitial space is limited.

Decreased Plasma Protein Concentration

As stated previously, the plasma proteins exert an osmotic pressure that is responsible for holding fluid in the vascular compartment. Whenever the plasma protein concentration is decreased, the plasma oncotic pressure decreases and the balance of forces governing transcapillary fluid exchange is shifted in favor of movement of fluid out of the capillaries. A decreased plasma protein concentration (*hypoproteinemia*) can result from decreased formation of plasma proteins by the liver, as occurs in cirrhosis (see Chapter 8) and malnutrition (see Chapter 17); or excessive loss of protein, either through the gastrointestinal tract or the kidneys. Hypoproteinemia also occurs as a result of fluid losses through burned areas and is partly responsible for the plasma-to-interstitial-fluid shift that occurs with extensive burns (see Chapter 24).

Plasma proteins constantly leak into the secretions of the gastrointestinal tract. Normally most of these proteins are broken down in the intestinal tract and the amino acids that are released are reabsorbed and reutilized. In a wide variety of gastrointestinal disorders, however, this leakage of protein is increased and a considerable loss of plasma proteins may occur (*protein-losing gastroenteropathy*).

The nephrotic syndrome. The nephrotic syndrome is characterized by severe proteinuria (protein in the urine), hypoproteinemia, generalized edema, and an elevated serum lipid level (hyperlipidemia). It is not a single disease entity but results from a wide variety of conditions: renal diseases such as chronic glomerulonephritis or lipoid nephrosis; systemic diseases such as diabetes mellitus, amyloidosis, or lupus erythematosus; circulatory disturbances, such as renal vein thrombosis; toxins, such as bismuth, gold, and mercury; and infections, such as syphilis and malaria. The common factor, regardless of the cause, is glomerular damage, which allows the escape of large amounts of protein (mainly albumin) into the urine. More than 3.5 grams of protein are lost per day; the result is hypoproteinemia and a considerable decrease in the plasma oncotic pressure. Consequently fluid shifts into the interstitial space, causing generalized edema and a reduction in the plasma volume. As a result of the decreased plasma volume, renal blood flow is reduced and the renin-angiotensin mechanism is activated. Angiotensin stimulates aldosterone production, leading to sodium retention by the kidneys. ADH release is also stimulated, leading to water retention. The retention of sodium and water cannot correct the plasma volume deficit, however, because the primary defect (hypoproteinemia) persists and the fluid retained by the kidneys simply moves into the interstitial space, increasing the edema. Therefore the kidneys continue to conserve sodium and water, and the amount of edema fluid increases. Eventually the rise in interstitial hydrostatic pressure limits the amount of edema. The cause of the hyperlipidemia associated with the nephrotic syndrome is not known.

Increased Capillary Permeability

Capillary permeability can be increased due to inflammation, allergic reactions, trauma, or burns. As a result, protein leaks from the plasma into the interstitial space and the plasma oncotic pressure decreases while the colloid osmotic pressure of the interstitial fluid increases. Therefore the effective oncotic pressure is greatly reduced and fluid cannot be held in the intravascular compartment.

Lymphatic Obstruction

As stated previously, the amount of fluid leaving the capillaries is normally slightly greater than the amount that reenters. This excess fluid is returned to the circulation by way of the lymphatics, as is the small amount of protein that normally escapes from the capillaries. Obviously, if the lymphatic channels are blocked, this fluid and protein will accumulate in the interstitial space. The accumulation of protein increases the colloid osmotic pressure of the interstitial fluid. Since this pressure opposes the plasma colloid osmotic pressure, the effective oncotic pressure will be decreased and less fluid will be held in the capillaries. Edema due to lymphatic obstruction is localized.

An infection called filiariasis, which is caused by a nematode (roundworm), is a common cause of lymphatic obstruction. Another cause of lymphatic obstruction is the surgical removal of lymph nodes. In some types of surgery for the removal of cancerous tissue, the lymph nodes draining the area are also removed to prevent possible spread of the cancer. Consequently lymph flow from the surrounding area will be blocked. For example, following a radical mastectomy (removal of a cancerous breast and associated structures, and axillary lymph nodes), the arm on the affected side may become severely edematous due to obstruction of lymph flow. New lymph channels develop, however, and the swelling usually subsides after about two to three months.

Interstitial-Fluid-to-Plasma Shift

The basic causes of a shift of fluid from the interstitial space to the plasma are decreased capillary hydrostatic pressure and increased plasma osmotic pressure.

Decreased capillary hydrostatic pressure can result from decreased arterial blood pressure. The resultant shift of fluid from the interstitial space to the intravascular compartment increases blood volume and thereby helps to raise the arterial pressure. Therefore, in this situation the fluid shift acts as a compensatory mechanism to help maintain normal arterial pressure. (See also Chapter 13 under Physical Mechanisms.)

Infusion of substances such as serum albumin or dextran, which remain in the plasma and do not enter the interstitial fluid, will result in an increase in the plasma colloid osmotic pressure. Consequently fluid is drawn from the interstitial space into the plasma. These substances are used therapeutically as volume expanders in the treatment of hypovolemia. If excessive amounts are infused, however, cirulatory overload may occur. The signs of circulatory overload are an elevated blood pressure, bounding pulse, and venous engorgement. Pulmonary edema may occur due to increased pulmonary capillary hydrostatic pressure.

Another cause of interstitial-fluid-to-plasma shift is the "remobilization of edema fluid" that occurs about the third to fifth day post burn or post trauma. In the first 48 hours following a burn or massive injury, fluid shifts from the plasma to the interstitial space. Later when capillary tone and permeability return to normal and the tissue pressure rises to equal the capillary pressure, fluid shifts back into the intravascular compartment. Circulatory overload can occur as a result of this shift.

SUGGESTED ADDITIONAL READING

Isacson LM, Schulz K: Treating pulmonary edema. *Nursing 78* 8(2): 42–46, 1978.

Precious A: Nephrotic syndrome in a child: when nursing vigilance counts. *Nurs Mirror* 147(17): 30–33, 1978.

Seybert PL, Gardón KM, Jackson BS: The LeVeen shunt: new hope for ascites patients. *Nursing 79* 9(1): 24–31, 1979.

12

Disturbances of Fluid Volume and Osmolarity

Water intake and water loss must be balanced in order to keep the volume of the body fluids constant and thus to maintain homeostasis. A major source of body water is the oral ingestion of free fluids and water in foods. Another source is the water formed within the body from the oxidation of carbohydrate, protein, and fat. For a person in hospital, administration of parenteral fluids may be an important source of water.

Water is lost from the body in several ways. A

considerable amount is lost by diffusion and evaporation from the skin and lungs. This process is called *insensible water loss* because the person is not aware of it. Infants and children have a larger surface area in relation to body mass and therefore have a proportionately greater amount of insensible water loss than adults. Hyperpnea, intubation, tracheostomy, and assisted ventilation will cause an increased loss of water from the lungs. Insensible water loss from the lungs is decreased if the inspired air is humidified. In addition to insensible water loss, varying amounts of water are lost through the skin by sensible perspiration. The amount of perspiration is governed by the need to control body temperature (see Chapter 24) and not by the need to maintain water balance. Water losses through the skin (both sensible and insensible) increase during fever and also when the temperature of the external environment is increased.

A small amount of water is normally lost in the feces. This amount can be drastically increased if a person has diarrhea.

Urine is an important means of water loss. A certain amount of urine must be excreted each day in order to eliminate waste substances. This amount is called *obligatory water excretion*. It varies according to the solute load (i.e., the amount of wastes to be excreted) and the ability of the kidneys to concentrate urine, but averages approximately 700 ml/day for an adult. In addition, a variable amount of water is lost in the urine depending on the body's need to conserve or excrete water. This additional amount is called *facultative water excretion*. The kidneys are the major regulators of body water balance. Conditions that interfere with normal kidney function may lead to excessive water loss or abnormal fluid retention.

Regulation of water balance appears to operate primarily to maintain the osmolarity of the body fluids within a narrow range. Although the volume of each fluid compartment is determined by its water content, the solute concentration determines the amount of water that is held in the compartment.

Isotonicity must be maintained between the intracellular fluid (ICF) and extracellular fluid (ECF); alterations of ECF osmolarity influence the distribution of water between the ECF and ICF, as described in Chapter 11. Therefore the osmolarity of the ECF must be monitored and controlled. The major solutes of the ECF (i.e., the major determinants of ECF osmolarity) are sodium salts, therefore sodium metabolism is closely related to the regulation of fluid volume. Two hormones, aldosterone and antidiuretic hormone (ADH), are essential for the regulation of sodium and water balance.

Even when a person is excreting maximally concentrated urine, some free water must be ingested to replace insensible water losses and obligatory urine losses. The signal for the need to ingest water is thirst; the thirst mechanism is very important in the regulation of body fluid volume and osmolarity.

REGULATION OF VOLUME AND OSMOLARITY OF BODY FLUIDS

Renal Mechanisms

The functional unit of the kidney is the *nephron*; it is a tubular structure with an associated blood supply (Fig. 12-1). The glomerulus, Bowman's capsule, and proximal and distal convoluted tubules of a nephron are located close to each other in the kidney cortex. The loop of Henle, however, dips into the renal medulla. The collecting ducts lie parallel to the loops of Henle and extend from the cortex to the tips of the renal papillae.

The glomerulus and glomerular capsule of most nephrons lie in the outer part of the cortex. These *cortical nephrons* have a short loop of Henle, which dips only into the outer region of the medulla. About 15% of the kidney nephrons have their glomerulus and glomerular capsule in the inner part of the cortex, next to the medulla. These *juxtamedullary nephrons* have a long loop of Henle, which dips deep into the medulla. The ability of

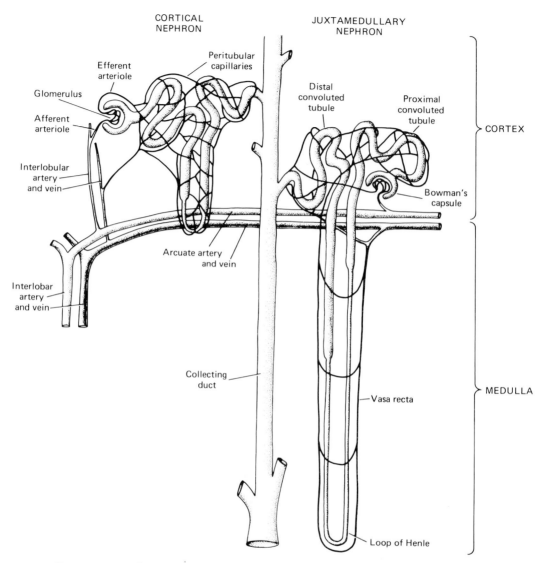

Figure 12-1. *Schematic representation of two nephrons, showing a cortical nephron and a juxtamedullary nephron.*

the kidneys to concentrate urine depends primarily on the functioning of the juxtamedullary nephrons.

The Urine Concentrating and Diluting Mechanism

The initial step in the formation of urine involves the filtration of water and solutes from the glomer-

ulus into the lumen of Bowman's capsule. This glomerular filtrate has essentially the same composition as plasma except that it contains very little protein. As the filtrate passes through the proximal convoluted tubule, any protein that is present is actively reabsorbed. Active reabsorption of many other solutes also occurs in the proximal convoluted tubule. This active transport of solutes establishes an osmotic gradient so that water is drawn out of the tubule and reabsorbed. Therefore, the fluid within the proximal tubule and the interstitial fluid of the kidney cortex are isoosmotic with the plasma, and the volume of fluid entering the loop of Henle is about 20% to 25% of the original filtrate.

As a result of activities in the loop of Henle, the volume of the filtrate is reduced by about a further 5% and the fluid entering the distal convoluted tubule is hypotonic relative to the plasma and to the cortical interstitial fluid. A varying amount of water may pass from the distal tubular fluid to the surrounding interstitial fluid by osmosis and be reabsorbed. Therefore the fluid leaving the distal tubule and entering the collecting duct may be hypotonic or isotonic with the plasma.

The interstitial fluid in the renal medulla is hypertonic relative to the plasma and interstitial fluid in other parts of the body. Not only is the medullary fluid hypertonic but the concentration of solutes also progressively increases in going from the outer medulla to the tips of the papillae. As previously mentioned, the collecting ducts pass through the renal medulla. Therefore, as urine flows through the collecting duct, water can move by osmosis from the lumen of the duct into the interstitial fluid (and subsequently be carried away by the blood, i.e., be reabsorbed) until the concentration of the urine in the collecting duct equals the concentration in the surrounding medullary interstitial fluid. Thus the kidneys can form urine that is hypertonic to the fluids in other parts of the body.

The concentration gradient in the medullary interstitial fluid is essential to the formation of hypertonic (i.e., concentrated) urine. This concentration gradient is established by the operation of a *countercurrent mechanism* in the loops of Henle of the juxtamedullary nephrons. Fluid moves through the loop of Henle in such a way that the flow (i.e., current) in the ascending limb is in the opposite direction (i.e., counter) to the flow in the descending limb. The descending limb of the loop of Henle is freely permeable to water and solutes, but the ascending limb is impermeable to water

and actively transports sodium chloride from the tubular lumen into the interstitial fluid.

Although in reality fluid is constantly flowing through the loop of Henle, the operation of the countercurrent mechanism is easier to understand if the flow is considered to be intermittent, with the gradient of osmolarity being established while the flow is stopped (Fig. 12-2). In the first step, suppose the loop of Henle is filled with fluid from the proximal convoluted tubule and then flow stops. Initially the fluid throughout the loop of Henle has a concentration of about 300 mOsm/liter (i.e., it is isotonic with the plasma). In step two, sodium chloride is actively transported out of the ascending limb into the interstitial fluid, making the fluid in the ascending limb less concentrated and the interstitial fluid more concentrated. While this process is occurring, sodium chloride passively diffuses into the descending limb and water moves from the descending limb into the interstitial fluid (i.e., is drawn out by osmosis) until the osmolarity of the interstitial fluid and fluid in the descending limb are equal. The ascending limb is able to actively transport sodium chloride into the interstitial fluid until a concentration gradient of about 200 mOsm/liter is established. Therefore, the final concentration of the fluid in the ascending limb is about 200 mOsm/liter and the concentration of the fluid in the descending limb and of the interstitial fluid is about 400 mOsm/liter.

In step three, flow occurs again. Some of the dilute fluid leaves the ascending limb and enters the distal tubule, concentrated fluid from the descending limb enters the ascending limb, and new fluid enters the descending limb from the proximal tubule. In step four, movement of sodium chloride and water occurs once more until a gradient of 200 mOsm/liter between the ascending limb and interstitial fluid is reestablished at each level. As can be seen from Figure 12-2, through the repetition of these steps a considerable longitudinal gradient of osmolarity can be established in the medullary interstitial fluid, while at any given level the gradient between the interstitial fluid and the fluid of the ascending limb does not exceed 200 mOsm/

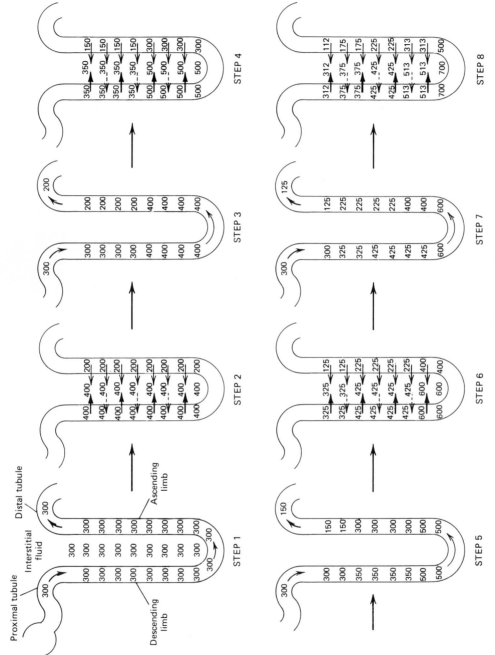

Figure 12-2. *Stepwise operation of the countercurrent system in the loop of Henle. See text for explanation. Numbers refer to osmolarity of fluid;* ⟶ *passive diffusion of water;* ⟶ *active transport of NaCl;* ⟶ , *passive diffusion of NaCl.*

liter. The longer the loop of Henle, the greater the longitudinal concentration gradient will be.

If blood were to flow in one direction through the renal medulla, the concentration gradient in the interstitial fluid would be dissipated. The peritubular capillaries associated with the loops of Henle of the juxtamedullary nephrons, however, form hairpin loops called the vasa recta, which are parallel to the loops of Henle. The vasa recta act as a second countercurrent system to maintain the medullary concentration gradient. As blood flows down into the medulla, water moves out of the vasa recta into the interstitial fluid by osmosis, and sodium chloride diffuses into the blood (i.e., the blood becomes concentrated). As blood flows back up toward the cortex, however, sodium chloride diffuses out of the vasa recta and water enters by osmosis. The net result is that the sodium chloride is left behind in the medullary interstitial fluid but water is carried away by the blood. Blood flow through the vasa recta is normally very slow; if the rate of flow is increased, the magnitude of the longitudinal concentration gradient in the medullary interstitial fluid will be decreased. Similarly, if the glomerular filtration rate (and therefore the rate of flow of fluid through the loop of Henle) is increased, the magnitude of the longitudinal concentration gradient will be decreased because there will be less time available for equilibrium to be established between the tubular fluid and the interstitial fluid. The magnitude of the longitudinal concentration gradient in the medullary interstitial fluid determines the degree to which the urine can be concentrated.

The urine concentrating mechanism is summarized in Figure 12-3. Isotonic fluid from the proximal tubule enters the descending limb of the loop of Henle. As the fluid passes down the descending limb it becomes more concentrated. As it moves up the ascending limb, however, the fluid becomes more dilute because sodium chloride is transported out and water cannot enter. This dilute fluid (hypotonic relative to plasma) flows into the distal convoluted tubule.

When water needs to be conserved, ADH is released from the neurohypophysis (see below) and increases the permeability of the distal tubule and collecting duct to water. Therefore, as the dilute fluid flows through the distal tubule, water moves from the tubule lumen into the cortical interstitial fluid by osmosis and the fluid leaving the distal tubule is isotonic. As the fluid passes down the collecting duct, more water moves from the lumen of the duct into the interstitial fluid by osmosis because of the concentration gradient in the medullary interstitial fluid. In other words, water is reabsorbed (retained) and a small volume of concentrated (i.e., hypertonic) urine is excreted.

When water needs to be excreted, ADH release is suppressed and the distal tubule and collecting duct are relatively impermeable to water. Therefore, very little water is reabsorbed as the fluid flows through the distal tubule and collecting duct and a large amount of dilute (i.e., hypotonic) urine is excreted.

Sodium Excretion

The amount of sodium excreted in the urine depends on the glomerular filtration rate (GFR; i.e., the amount of sodium filtered) and on the amount of sodium reabsorbed as the filtrate flows through the renal tubules. Sodium excretion will be increased if the GFR increases or if tubular reabsorption of sodium decreases. When both of these events occur simultaneously, sodium excretion is greatly enhanced. Conversely, if the GFR decreases and/or if tubular reabsorption increases, the amount of sodium excreted will decrease.

GFR is determined by the hydrostatic pressure in the glomerular capillaries, the hydrostatic pressure in Bowman's capsule, and the plasma oncotic pressure. The hydrostatic pressure in the glomerular capillaries forces fluid from the capillaries into Bowman's capsule; this force is opposed by the plasma oncotic pressure and the hydrostatic pressure in Bowman's capsule. Normally the glomerular capillary hydrostatic pressure exceeds the other two pressures and glomerular filtration occurs. Glomerular capillary hydrostatic pressure is the major factor involved in the control of GFR.

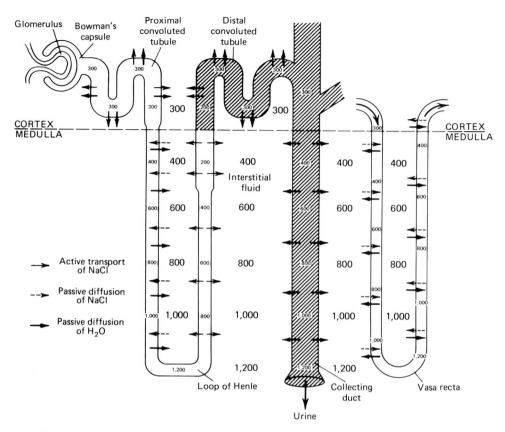

Figure 12-3. *Summary of the urine concentrating mechanism. Numbers refer to osmolarity of fluid in milliosmoles. Under the influence of ADH, cells in shaded area are permeable to water. Therefore, water is drawn out of collecting duct by osmosis (i.e., reabsorbed) due to the gradient of osmolarity established in the medullary interstitial fluid by the countercurrent mechanism in the loop of Henle, and a concentrated urine is formed. The vasa recta act as a second countercurrent system so that water is carried away by the blood but solutes are left behind in the medullary interstitial fluid.*

Decreased arterial blood pressure and/or constriction of the afferent arterioles will decrease glomerular capillary hydrostatic pressure and therefore cause a decline in the rate of glomerular filtration. Conversely, an elevated arterial blood pressure, dilation of the afferent arterioles, and/or constriction of the efferent arterioles will increase glomerular capillary hydrostatic pressure and therefore cause an increase in the GFR.

Reabsorption of sodium is an active process; that is, energy is required to transport sodium from the renal tubular fluid into the interstitial fluid. Active transport of positive sodium ions creates an electrical gradient, so that negative chloride or bicarbonate ions follow along by passive diffusion. (In contrast to the situation in the proximal and distal tubules, recent evidence suggests that sodium chloride movement from the ascending limb of the loop of Henle may occur by active transport of chloride followed by passive diffusion of sodium. Although the mechanism is different, the result is the same.) Reabsorption of sodium chloride creates an osmotic pull that is responsible for the passive reabsorption of water.

About two-thirds of the renal sodium reabsorption occurs in the proximal convoluted tubules. Here reabsorption of sodium salts and water occur in isoosmotic proportions. In the distal tubule and collecting ducts, water reabsorption is influenced by ADH, as already mentioned. ADH does not influence sodium reabsorption, however, so that sodium may be reabsorbed while excess water is excreted. Reabsorption of sodium from the distal tubules is influenced by adrenal mineralocorticoid hormones, primarily aldosterone (see below).

In the distal tubules sodium appears to be reabsorbed in exchange for the secretion of potassium or hydrogen ions. This exchange is not a directly coupled transport process, however. When the positive sodium ions are reabsorbed the tubular fluid becomes relatively negative. The electrical gradient thus established tends to pull positive potassium ions from the tubular cells into the tubular lumen by passive diffusion. (Recall that the ICF has a high concentration of potassium.) The cellular potassium concentration is restored by active transport of potassium ions from the interstitial fluid into the tubular cells. (Secretion of hydrogen ions into the urine is discussed in Chapter 15.)

Diuresis

Diuresis is an increase in the volume of urine formed. The increased volume of urine can result from decreased reabsorption of water, which leads to increased loss of solute-free water, or water diuresis. Another cause of increased urine volume is decreased reabsorption of solutes, which limits the osmotic gradient between the tubular fluid and interstitial fluid and leads to an increased loss of solutes and water, or osmotic diuresis. Increasing the GFR can also cause diuresis.

The usual cause of water diuresis is excessive fluid intake. Excessive intake of water or hypotonic fluids will dilute the ECF and suppress the release of ADH. Consequently, even though an osmotic gradient exists between the tubular fluid

and the medullary interstitial fluid, very little water is reabsorbed because the distal tubules and collecting ducts are impermeable to water when ADH is absent. The result is a large volume of dilute (hypotonic) urine. Other factors that decrease the amount of circulating ADH also cause a water diuresis (see below).

As stated previously, reabsorption of solutes from the glomerular filtrate creates an osmotic pull that is responsible for the reabsorption of water. Therefore, decreased reabsorption of sodium will cause an osmotic diuresis. (A number of drugs used as diuretic agents exert their effects by decreasing sodium reabsorption.) In addition, if the filtrate contains a large amount of solute that is poorly reabsorbed, the solute creates an osmotic pressure in the tubular fluid that prevents the reabsorption of water (i.e., it causes obligatory water loss). For example, in diabetes mellitus the presence of a large amount of glucose in the tubular fluid causes an osmotic diuresis. (The term diabetes refers to the excessive urine excretion. Diabetes mellitus is discussed in Chapter 18.)

Hormonal Mechanisms

Antidiuretic Hormone

As previously mentioned, antidiuretic hormone (ADH; vasopressin) acts on the distal tubules and collecting ducts of the kidneys and increases renal reabsorption of water. A certain amount of ADH is always circulating in the blood. When water needs to be conserved the amount of ADH increases; when water needs to be excreted, the amount decreases.

ADH is secreted by cells in a region of the hypothalamus, travels down the nerve fibers in the hypophyseal stalk, and is stored in the neurohypophysis (posterior pituitary). It is released from the neurohypophysis in response to nervous stimulation from the hypothalamus.

ADH release is influenced by the osmolarity and volume of the ECF, and by several other factors. Certain cells of the hypothalamus act as *osmoreceptors*, which respond to changes in the osmolarity of the ECF. When the osmolarity increases (i.e., the ECF becomes hyperosmotic), the osmoreceptors stimulate the release of ADH. Therefore water is conserved by the kidneys, and if the person drinks enough water, the ECF is diluted until the osmolar concentration returns to normal. Decreased osmolarity of the ECF (i.e., hypoosmotic ECF) inhibits the release of ADH. Therefore excess water is excreted by the kidneys until the osmolarity of the ECF returns to normal.

Baroreceptors are located in the carotid sinuses and aortic arch (high-pressure receptors), and also in the left atrium and the pulmonary veins (low-pressure receptors). These receptors respond to stretch or tension in the wall of the receptor organ, therefore they can act as pressure receptors or volume receptors. (See also Chapter 13 under The Baroreceptor Reflex.) In addition to sending impulses to the cardiovascular control center in the medulla, these receptors send impulses to the area of the hypothalamus that influences ADH secretion. The baroreceptors in the low-pressure system especially are very sensitive to small changes in blood volume.

A decrease in the rate of impulse transmission from the baroreceptors increases the secretion of ADH and leads to water retention. Decreased arterial blood pressure secondary to decreased blood volume (hypovolemia) and/or a decreased cardiac output, and decreased tension in the walls of the left atrium and pulmonary veins secondary to decreased intrathoracic blood volume stimulate ADH release by this mechanism. Reduced intrathoracic blood volume can be due to hemorrhage, the upright position (see Chapter 22), or positive-pressure breathing.

An increased number of impulses from the baroreceptors decreases ADH secretion and leads to water loss. Increased arterial blood pressure secondary to ECF volume expansion and an increased cardiac output, and increased tension in the walls of the left atrium and pulmonary veins secondary to increased intrathoracic blood volume inhibit ADH release by this mechanism. Intrathoracic

blood volume is increased in the recumbent position (see Chapter 22), as a result of negative-pressure breathing, and due to acute exposure to cold, which causes peripheral vasoconstriction and shifts the blood centrally. Hypervolemia also causes an increased intrathoracic blood volume.

Several other factors influence ADH release. Emotional stress usually stimulates ADH release, although occasionally it acts as an inhibitor. Pain, increased temperature of the blood flowing through the hypothalamus, and drugs such as cholinergic agents, β-adrenergic agents, morphine, barbiturates, and nicotine stimulate the release of ADH and therefore can lead to water retention. Decreased temperature of the blood flowing through the hypothalamus and drugs such as alcohol, diphenylhydantoin, and α-adrenergic agents inhibit the release of ADH and therefore can lead to water diuresis.

Diabetes insipidus is a condition caused by a failure in the production or release of a sufficient quantity of ADH to maintain normal renal conservation of water. It is characterized by water diuresis. An affected person drinks an excessive amount of water to compensate for the excessive renal water loss. Often the cause of diabetes insipidus is not known, and it may be due to a congenital or familial disorder. Diabetes insipidus can be caused by injury to the hypothalamus or neurohypophysis or by tumors associated with these structures.

Nephrogenic diabetes insipidus is a rare congenital or familial disorder in which the person secretes large amounts of ADH but the kidneys do not respond to ADH. The result is the same as if no ADH were prsent; that is, excessive renal water loss and compensatory excessive water intake.

Aldosterone

Aldosterone is a steroid hormone produced by the adrenal cortex. It is the most potent mineralocorticoid. Aldosterone increases reabsorption of sodium by the distal renal tubules and enhances excretion of potassium and hydrogen ions. Another effect of aldosterone is increased absorption of sodium from the gastrointestinal tract and increased fecal excretion of potassium. In addition, aldosterone causes a decreased sodium concentration and increased potassium concentration in saliva and in sweat. Thus, the overall effect of aldosterone is to conserve body sodium and enhance potassium excretion.

Aldosterone secretion is influenced by angiotensin II, by the levels of sodium and potassium in the ECF, and by adrenocorticotropic hormone (ACTH). Release of renin by the kidneys leads to the production of angiotensin II. (See Chapter 13 for a discussion of the renin-angiotensin system.) Angiotensin II acts on the adrenal cortex to stimulate aldosterone secretion. Renin release (and therefore the circulating level of angiotensin II) is increased by decreased renal arterial pressure, β-adrenergic stimulation by sympathetic nerves or circulating catecholamines, and a low concentration of sodium in the distal renal tubules. The resulting increased secretion of aldosterone enhances sodium reabsorption, which can lead to increased osmotic reabsorption of water and increased blood volume. The increased blood volume contributes to raising the renal arterial pressure, which subsequently suppresses renin release.

Aldosterone secretion is also stimulated by a low sodium concentration and/or high potassium concentration in the ECF. This stimulation appears to be due to a direct effect on the adrenal cortex. A decreased sodium level and elevated potassium level occurring at the same time have an additive stimulatory effect on aldosterone production. Conversely, an increased sodium level and decreased potassium level occurring together have an additive inhibitory effect on aldosterone production. If the levels of both sodium and potassium are decreased, aldosterone secretion is inhibited. Thus it appears that the effect of potassium concentration predominates over the effect of sodium concentration in determining the rate of aldosterone secretion.

ACTH primarily controls the secretion of glucocorticoids by the adrenal cortex, but it also has a slight stimulatory effect on aldosterone se-

cretion. Normally, however, ACTH plays a minor role in determining the rate of aldosterone secretion.

The Thirst Mechanism

The mechanisms governing fluid intake and fluid output must be coordinated in order to regulate the volume and osmolarity of the body fluids. Not surprisingly, therefore, conditions that lead to fluid retention by the kidneys also stimulate the desire to drink.

Thirst is a conscious sensation of the need for water, which leads to the motivated behavior of drinking. Not all fluid ingestion occurs in response to thirst, however. Drinking is often a habit associated with eating and other activities, so that water intake is usually adequate under normal conditions.

The various stimuli that influence water ingestion are integrated in the "thirst center" in the hypothalamus. The thirst center is located very close to the area that controls ADH secretion and the two areas overlap slightly. Stimulatory and inhibitory impulses are sent from the thirst center to the cerebral cortex, giving rise to the conscious sensation of thirst or absence of thirst.

The conditions that evoke thirst are cellular dehydration and hypovolemia. An increase in the osmolarity of the ECF results in a shift of water out of the cells (cellular dehydration) and stimulates thirst. Even if the volume of total body water is increased, hyperosmotic ECF will cause cellular dehydration and produce thirst. As little as a 1% to 2% reduction in ICF volume can stiumulate thirst; severe degrees of cellular dehydration produce extreme thirst. Cellular dehydration results in the shrinkage of cells throughout the body, including thirst osmoreceptors in the hypothalamus. Shrinkage of the osmoreceptors stimulates thirst. When enough water has been ingested to restore the osmolarity of the body fluids to normal, the thirst will be satisfied.

Decreased ECF volume due to isoosmotic fluid loss, and decreased blood volume, whether due to an actual loss of fluid or to a shift of fluid that results in decreased central blood volume, stimulate thirst. The thirst occurring in response to these situations is possibly mediated by the baroreceptors in the left atrium and pulmonary veins. Thirst also occurs in response to a low cardiac output and to hypotension (low blood pressure). It has recently been found that angiotensin II acts directly on the brain to stimulate thirst. This effect may be the means by which thirst due to hypovolemia, low cardiac output, and/or hypotension is stimulated. These conditions lead to decreased renal arterial pressure, which stimulates renin release and subsequent formation of angiotensin II. Ingestion of water or hypotonic fluids in response to thirst in these situations will produce a hypotonic ECF and a shift of water into the cells. Consequently thirst will be inhibited before the volume deficit is restored. On the other hand, if isotonic solutions (or water plus solids) are ingested, thirst will be satisfied only when the extracellular or intravascular fluid volume is restored.

VOLUME DEFICIT

A decreased volume or water content of a body fluid compartment (e.g., the ECF or ICF) is called *hypovolia*. *Hypovolemia* refers specifically to an abnormal decrease in the volume of circulating blood. A loss of body fluid is often referred to as dehydration, but this term has been used in several ways, which sometimes leads to confusion. Therefore it will not be used here, except to define it. Strictly speaking, *dehydration* means the removal of water from a substance; it is the condition resulting from an excessive loss of body water. When the water loss is accompanied by a loss of electrolytes, so that the net loss of fluid and electrolytes is isotonic, the condition is sometimes called isotonic dehydration; it is the same as what is called isotonic ECF volume deficit in this book. When the net loss of electrolytes is propor-

tionately greater than the net loss of water (i.e., the net fluid loss is hypertonic), the remaining ECF will be hypotonic. This condition may be called hypotonic dehydration; it is the same as what is called sodium deficit in this book. When the net loss of electrolytes is proportionately less than the net loss of water (i.e., the net fluid loss is hypotonic), the remaining ECF will be hypertonic. This condition may be called hypertonic dehydration; it is sometimes referred to as "pure" dehydration and corresponds to what is called water deficit in this book.

Volume deficits can result from a lack of oral intake in the presence of a normal output, but usually they result from abnormal losses (e.g., due to vomiting or diarrhea) in the presence of an intake that is inadequate to compensate for the losses. Severe volume deficits produce hypovolemic shock, which is discussed in Chapter 14.

Water Deficit

In water deficit the *net* fluid loss is hypotonic. The fluid that is lost from the body is not necessarily hypotonic, but the sum of losses from all routes minus total intake produces a net loss of water in excess of electrolytes (i.e., in hypotonic proportions). As water is lost from the body, the ECF becomes hyperosmotic and draws water out of the cells. Therefore the water content of all body fluid compartments is diminished.

Causes
Water deficit can result from decreased intake or increased output of water. *Decreased water intake* may be due to difficulty in swallowing, impairment of the thirst mechanism (e.g., due to brain injury), stupor or coma, extreme debility, or unavailability of water. Increased water output in hypotonic proportions is usually due to excessive losses through the skin, lungs, or kidneys.

Evaporation of water increases when the temperature is increased, therefore insensible water loss through both the skin and the lungs is increased during fever. Hyperpnea increases insensible water loss through the lungs, because it increases the amount of air moving out of the lungs in a given period of time, and the expired air contains water vapor. Therefore, a considerable loss of water can occur through the lungs when a person has a pulmonary disease (e.g., tracheobronchitis) that is accompanied by rapid breathing and fever. Perspiration is a hypotonic secretion, therefore profuse diaphoresis can cause water deficit.

Increased urinary water loss occurs when the ability of the kidneys to concentrate urine is impaired due to kidney disease. Impaired urine-concentrating ability occurs in the diuretic phase of acute renal failure (see Chapter 14 under Effects of Shock on the Kidneys), and may occur in the early stages of chronic pyelonephritis. Increased urinary water loss also occurs when the solute load is increased, for example due to glucose in the urine of people with diabetes mellitus. Water deficit can also occur in unconscious people who are given tube feedings that contain a high concentration of protein and other solutes, with an inadequate amount of water. A high protein intake increases the amount of urea formed (i.e., increases the solute load) and therefore increases the obligatory urinary water loss. Another cause of excessive urinary water loss is diabetes insipidus, which has already been mentioned. Water deficit does not usually occur in this condition unless water intake is restricted.

Adaptive Responses

ADH release is stimulated by the hyperosmolarity of the ECF and by the decreased blood volume that results from the loss of body water. Therefore, water is retained by the kidneys, unless the concentrating ability of the kidneys is impaired due to renal disease.

Hyperosmolarity of the ECF and decreased blood volume also stimulate thirst. Therefore, if possible, a person with water deficit will drink water until the normal body fluid volume is restored.

Effects

As a result of water deficit, the serum sodium concentration is elevated (hypernatremia), reflecting the hyperosmolarity of the ECF. The hematocrit and hemoglobin concentration are elevated as hemoconcentration occurs. Blood volume is decreased; therefore the blood pressure may be low and the pulse rate increased. Renal blood flow and glomerular filtration are decreased due to the diminished blood volume. In addition, ADH release is stimulated and promotes renal retention of water, as just mentioned. Therefore, unless the primary cause of the water deficit is excessive urinary water loss, the volume of urine is small and the urine is concentrated, as reflected by a high specific gravity.

Decreased fluid in the skin results in a loss of skin turgor; thus when the skin is pinched, it tends to remain in folds. This sign is particularly noticeable in infants, who will also have sunken fontanels. Eyeball tension is decreased as a result of decreased ocular fluid, therefore the eyeballs are soft and sunken. The amount of saliva is diminished and the mucous membranes and tongue are dry. Water is necessary for body temperature regulation; therefore fever may be present. Loss of water from brain cells produces lethargy, which progresses to coma when the water deficit is severe. Increased irritability may occur, especially in children.

Water is responsible for a large portion of the body weight; therefore water deficit is accompanied by weight loss. Weight losses occurring over a short period of time are useful in assessing the degree of water deficit.

Isotonic ECF Volume Deficit

Isotonic ECF volume deficit usually results from abnormal losses. The net fluid loss is isotonic. The fluid that is lost in excessive amounts is not necessarily isotonic, but the sum of losses from all routes minus total intake produces a net loss of water and electrolytes in isotonic proportions.

Total ECF volume, including blood volume, is decreased. ICF volume is not affected because the osmolarity of the ECF is not changed.

Causes
Conditions that can cause isotonic ECF volume deficit are vomiting, diarrhea, hemorrhage, loss of fluid through burned areas, and excessive drainage from wounds.

Adaptive Responses
The decreased blood volume elicits several adaptive responses. It stimulates thirst, so that if possible the person will drink fluids to replace body fluid volume. At the same time, ADH release is stimulated, promoting renal retention of water.

Another consequence of decreased blood volume is diminished renal blood flow, which has two effects. Glomerular filtration is decreased, thus favoring fluid retention, and renin release is stimulated. The renin in turn stimulates aldosterone secretion, so that renal reabsorption of sodium increases. The sodium retention promotes fluid retention and maintains the isotonicity of the ECF.

Effects
The serum sodium concentration will be normal, since the fluid loss is isotonic. Except in the case of hemorrhage, the hematocrit is increased due to decreased plasma volume.

Urine volume is low (oliguria) as a result of the decreased glomerular filtration and adaptive mechanisms just mentioned.

As a result of the decreased blood volume, the blood pressure may be low and the fullness of the neck veins is decreased. The person may experience postural hypotension (a fall in blood pressure on changing from a recumbent to an erect position). The pulse rate may be increased as a result of reflex sympathetic stimulation to maintain cardiac output. The person feels weak due to decreased blood flow to the muscles. As mentioned

previously, when the volume deficit is severe, shock results.

Sodium Deficit

In sodium deficit the *net* fluid loss is hypertonic. The fluid that is lost from the body is not necessarily hypertonic, but the sum of losses from all routes minus total intake produces a net loss of electrolytes (primarily sodium salts) in excess of water (i.e., in hypertonic proportions). As sodium is lost from the body, the ECF becomes hypoosmotic. Therefore water moves into the cells and the ICF volume may be increased although the ECF volume, including blood volume, is usually decreased.

Causes
Decreased sodium intake is an unusual cause of sodium deficit. Sodium deficit usually results from excessive losses or from replacement of sodium and water losses with water only. People on diuretic therapy and a low sodium diet, however, may develop sodium deficit.

Excessive amounts of sodium can be lost in gastrointestinal secretions as a result of vomiting, diarrhea, or gastric suction. Sodium deficit may also result from excessive biliary drainage, since the concentration of sodium in bile is higher than the concentration of sodium in the plasma.

Sweat contains about 30 to 70 mEq sodium per liter, which is considerably less than the concentration in the ECF, but sodium deficit can result from profuse diaphoresis, especially if the fluid loss is replaced with water only. Children with mucoviscidosis (cystic fibrosis) have an abnormally high sodium concentration in the sweat; therefore they can develop sodium deficit quite easily in this way.

Lack of aldosterone due to adrenocortical insufficiency (Addison's disease) can cause excessive renal loss of sodium. Excessive loss of sodium in the urine also occurs in some renal diseases, particularly chronic pyelonephritis, but sodium deficit does not usually occur unless salt intake is restricted.

Adaptive Responses

ADH release will be inhibited due to the decreased osmolarity of the ECF, thus promoting excretion of water to return the osmolarity to normal. If the blood volume is very low, however, this factor will have a stimulatory effect on ADH secretion. The amount of ADH released will depend on the balance of these two factors.

Except in the case of adrenocortical insufficiency, aldosterone secretion is stimulated by the mechanisms described previously. Therefore renal conservation of sodium occurs. The person may also have a craving for salt and eat salty foods if possible. The mechanism controlling salt appetite is not understood.

Effects

With sodium deficit, the serum sodium concentration is decreased (*hyponatremia*). Increased renal sodium reabsorption is associated with increased excretion of potassium and hydrogen, so that serum levels of these electrolytes may decrease. Since the plasma volume is usually decreased, the hematocrit and plasma protein concentration may be elevated.

Urine volume is variable. Inhibition of ADH due to the decreased osmolarity of the ECF tends to cause water diuresis. At the same time, however, renal blood flow may be decreased due to the decreased blood volume, with the result that the GFR may be decreased. Therefore, urine volume may be low, normal, or increased.

Due to decreased blood volume, the pulse rate may be increased and the blood pressure decreased, and postural hypotension may occur.

Other manifestations of sodium deficit are muscle weakness and cramps, apathy, headache, anorexia, and nausea. When the sodium deficit is severe, mental confusion, convulsive seizures, stupor, or coma may develop. The exact mechanisms responsible for these effects are not known, but are probably related to impaired cell functioning due to movement of water into the cells. In addition, neurotransmission may be impaired by the low sodium concentration, since sodium ions are involved in nerve-impulse transmission.

VOLUME EXCESS

An increased volume or water content of a given compartment (e.g., the ICF or ECF) is called *hypervolia*. *Hypervolemia* refers specifically to an abnormal increase in the circulating blood volume. An increased volume of body fluid can be due to water excess, retention of fluid in isotonic proportions, or sodium excess.

Water Excess

In water excess the *net* fluid gain is hypotonic. Total fluid intake minus the sum of losses from all routes produces a net gain of water in excess of electrolytes. As water is retained by the body the ECF is diluted and becomes hypotonic. As a result of the hypotonicity of the ECF, water moves into the cells; therefore both ICF volume and ECF volume are increased. When the water excess is relatively severe, the condition is sometimes called *water intoxication.*

Causes

Water excess can be due to excessive intake, but usually it results from renal retention of water. Excessive water intake can occur as a result of excessive intravenous infusion of 5% dextrose in water, as a result of absorption of the irrigating fluid following transurethral prostatic resection, or as a result of excessive administration of tap-water enemas.

Usually it is difficult for a person to drink large enough quantities of water to produce water excess while the kidneys and ADH mechanism are functioning normally. Glomerular filtration increases as a result of increased renal blood flow, and ADH secretion is suppressed, resulting in a large volume of dilute urine and a rapid elimination of the excess water. Some people with psychotic disturbances (e.g., schizophrenia), however, may develop water intoxication as a result of excessive fluid intake.

Water excess may result from an inability of the kidneys to excrete water normally. This situation occurs when renal blood flow is low, for example due to acute congestive heart failure or acute renal failure.

Excessive or inappropriate ADH secretion is a frequent cause of water excess. The amount of ADH circulating at a given time depends on the sum of all the factors influencing ADH secretion and release (see above under Hormonal Mechanisms). For example, hypoosmotic ECF normally depresses ADH secretion and release, bringing about diuresis. If several nonosmotic factors (e.g., fear, pain, drugs) are stimulating ADH release, however, the amount of circulating ADH may be high and water may be retained by the kidneys, even though the ECF is hypoosmotic. ADH secretion is frequently increased in people who are hospitalized. For example, the ADH level is usually increased postoperatively due to several factors that stimulate ADH release, including fear, stress, anesthesia, pain, and drugs such as morphine and meperidine (Demerol). Consequently, water excretion is impaired postoperatively and water excess can result if fluid intake (intravenous or oral) is not carefully monitored and controlled.

Inappropriate secretion of ADH accompanies a variety of inflammatory or neoplastic conditions, for example pulmonary abscess, pulmonary tuberculosis, and tumors of the lung, pancreas, thymus, and duodenum. Excessive ADH secretion may occur as a result of head injuries or central nervous system diseases. In some cases thirst may also be stimulated inappropriately, resulting in excessive water intake (if the person is able to drink) in the presence of impaired water excretion.

Adaptive Responses

Unless the water excess is due to impairment of the normal ADH mechanism, ADH secretion will be inhibited and the excess water will be excreted

by the kidneys. If kidney function is impaired, it may not be possible for the person to excrete the excess water and outside intervention (e.g., dialysis) may be necessary.

The low sodium concentration of the ECF stimulates aldosterone release so that the kidneys conserve sodium. Thirst is suppressed, unless the water excess is due to an impaired thirst mechanism.

Effects

Dilution of the ECF by the excess water is reflected by a low sodium concentration (*dilutional hyponatremia*), low serum protein concentration, and low serum osmolarity. Blood volume is increased and the hematocrit decreased.

If the water excess is due to impaired renal water excretion, the person will have oliguria. If kidney function and ADH secretion are normal, the person will excrete a large quantity of dilute urine. If the water excess occurs acutely, a sudden weight gain may be noticed. Anorexia, nausea, and vomiting, muscular weakness and twitching, mental disturbances, convulsive seizures, and stupor or coma may develop as a result of the swelling of brain cells and the low sodium concentration.

Isotonic ECF Volume Excess

Isotonic ECF volume excess usually results from renal retention of sodium and water. The *net* fluid gain is isotonic. The fluid that is ingested is not necessarily isotonic, but total intake minus the sum of losses from all routes produces a net gain of water and electrolytes in isotonic proportions. Total ECF volume, including blood volume, is increased. ICF volume is not affected because the osmolarity of the ECF is not changed.

Causes

ECF volume excess may occur as a result of excessive intravenous infusions, but usually it is caused by renal retention of sodium and water, for example due to congestive heart failure or renal failure. In the case of congestive heart failure, the reten tion of fluid represents an adaptive mechanism to maintain the circulation.

Adaptive Responses

The increased volume of fluid will depress ADH release, resulting in increased water loss if renal perfusion and renal function are normal. If the kidneys are normal, renal blood flow will be increased due to the increased blood volume. Consequently renin release will be inhibited, aldosterone secretion will decrease, and the kidneys will excrete more sodium. In addition, the increased renal blood flow will increase the GFR, thus promoting urinary excretion of the excess fluid.

In renal failure the normal homeostatic mechanism for maintaining fluid balance is lost; therefore adaptation is not possible. Outside intervention will be required to restore fluid balance.

Effects

Increased ECF volume produces weight gain and edema. The blood pressure may be elevated. Pulmonary edema may develop due to increased capillary hydrostatic pressure.

Congestive Heart Failure

Heart failure may be defined as an inability of the heart to pump an adequate amount of blood to meet ordinary metabolic demands. It is possible for one side of the heart to fail independently of the other side, although failure of one side produces changes that may eventually result in failure of the other side as well.

Heart failure can result from a variety of causes. Common causes of left ventricular failure are myocardial infarction (see Chapter 7) and hypertension (see Chapter 13). Right ventricular failure may result from mitral stenosis, pulmonary valvular stenosis, or pulmonary hypertension secondary to chronic obstructive lung disease (see Chapter 10) or left ventricular failure.

Cardiac output is usually decreased in heart failure, although in some cases (high output failure) the cardiac output may be normal or increased.

This situation occurs when the metabolic demands of the body are increased and increased blood flow is necessary to meet tissue needs, for example due to severe fevers or thyrotoxicosis. Another cause of high output failure is severe anemia (see Chapter 10).

The factors involved in the development of edema and ECF volume excess in congestive heart failure are not completely understood, but the following mechanism appears to be operating. As a result of the decreased cardiac output, renal blood flow is decreased and fluid is retained by the kidneys. The renal retention of fluid may be brought about partly by a reduced rate of glomerular filtration and partly by activation of the aldosterone and ADH hormonal mechanisms. Decreased renal blood flow stimulates the renin-angiotensin system; angiotensin in turn stimulates aldosterone production. Aldosterone increases renal reabsorption of sodium. This situation leads to water retention because the retention of sodium causes a transient increase in the osmolarity of the ECF and stimulates ADH release. Also, as more sodium is reabsorbed the osmotic gradient between the tubular lumen and the interstitial fluid is increased, thus allowing greater reabsorption of water. In addition, the low cardiac output may stimulate ADH release by way of the arterial baroreceptors.

As fluid is retained by the kidneys a progressive increase in blood volume and total ECF volume occurs. The increased blood volume raises mean systemic blood pressure and increases venous return of blood to the heart. Therefore end-diastolic volume and pressure are increased, and stroke volume can increase due to the Frank-Starling mechanism. (In severe heart failure, however, excessive fluid retention can overstretch the myocardial fibers so that the Frank-Starling mechanism is no longer effective.) A new equilibrium is established, with the ventricular pressure remaining high to permit an adequate stroke volume. As a result of the increased ventricular pressure, atrial pressure also rises, which in turn raises venous pressure. Therefore capillary hydrostatic pressure may increase and contribute to the edema formation.

With left ventricular failure, the right ventricle continues to pump blood into the pulmonary circulation with its usual vigor, but the left ventricle is not able to pump blood adequately out into the systemic circulation. Consequently, a redistribution of blood volume occurs, with blood shifting from the systemic circulation into the pulmonary circulation. As a result, mean systemic blood pressure decreases and mean pulmonary blood pressure increases. To compensate for the decreased stroke volume, heart rate increases in an effort to maintain cardiac output. (Cardiac output equals heart rate times stroke volume.)

As a result of the decreased cardiac output and decreased systemic blood pressure, the person experiences muscular weakness and fatigue. (The cardiac reserve is being used to maintain an adequate cardiac output at rest, therefore exercise capacity is limited. See Chapter 22.) Often the extremities are pale and cold, and peripheral cyanosis may occur. Nocturia (excessive urination at night) occurs, probably because renal blood flow improves when the person lies down and aldosterone and ADH secretion are decreased.

Pulmonary congestion causes a cough and also dyspnea. Breathing is usually rapid and shallow because the congestion causes increased mechanical resistance to breathing. When the person lies down, blood is shifted from the periphery to the lungs (see Chapter 22), increasing the pulmonary congestion. Consequently the person may have difficulty breathing while lying flat (*orthopnea*), and usually sleeps in a semireclining position with the head propped up on pillows. With less severe degrees of pulmonary congestion the person may sleep lying flat. Gradually, however, fluid moves from the interstitial space back into the vascular compartment because the venous pressure in the dependent parts of the body is decreased in the recumbent position (see Chapter 22). Therefore, a gradual increase in pulmonary congestion occurs; when it reaches a critical level the person wakes up feeling short of breath and has to sit up. This situation is called *paroxysmal nocturnal dyspnea*.

With severe heart failure the pulmonary capillary pressure rises so high that pulmonary edema develops. Pulmonary edema causes severe dyspnea and apprehension. Moist rales can be heard with a stethoscope on the back over the base of the lungs. Frothy sputum is produced. Occasionally the sputum is tinged with blood, probably due to small hemorrhages from the congested bronchial mucosa. With severe pulmonary edema the person can literally drown if prompt effective treatment is not instituted.

With right ventricular failure systemic venous congestion develops and venous reservoirs such as the liver, spleen, and splanchnic bed become engorged. Therefore the liver and spleen are enlarged. The superficial veins are distended. Normally the neck veins are collapsed when a person is in an erect position. With right-sided heart failure, however, the jugular veins are distended when the person is in the erect position because of the increased venous pressure. Peripheral cyanosis may be evident due to slow blood flow through the skin.

Peripheral edema develops and is usually noticeable first in the dependent parts of the body, such as the feet and ankles. The edema is probably due to increased capillary pressure and renal retention of fluid, as described previously. (With right-sided failure an inadequate amount of blood is transferred to the left side of the heart. Therefore left ventricular output also decreases and stimulates the renal and hormonal mechanisms.) The edema is accompanied by a gain in weight. Congestion and increased pressure in the portal venous system cause effusion of an excessive amount of fluid into the peritoneal cavity (*ascites*), which produces abdominal distention. These external signs of right ventricular failure are shown in Figure 12-4.

Sodium Excess

In sodium excess total intake minus the sum of losses from all routes produces a net gain of sodium salts in excess of water. As a result, the ECF is hypertonic and draws water out of the cells.

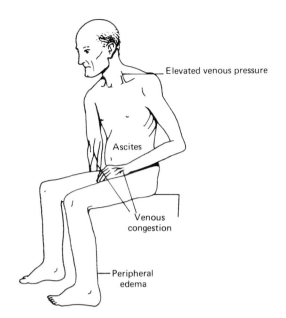

Figure 12-4. *External signs of right ventricular failure.* *(From Rushmer:* Cardiovascular Dynamics, *ed 4.* © *1976 by the W.B. Saunders Company, Philadelphia.)*

Therefore ICF volume is decreased but ECF volume is increased. Total fluid volume increases as adaptive mechanisms restore osmolarity.

Causes

Excessive salt intake due to intravenous therapy or hyperalimentation can cause sodium excess. (Isotonic saline contains 154 mEq sodium per liter, which is greater than the concentration normally found in the ECF.) Excessive renal retention of sodium occurs in primary aldosteronism, a condition caused by an adrenal tumor that secretes aldosterone.

Adaptive Responses

The increased sodium concentration inhibits aldosterone secretion (except in the case of primary aldosteronism) so that more sodium is excreted in the urine. The hyperosmolarity of the ECF stimulates ADH secretion and release, resulting in water retention by the kidneys. Thirst is also stimulated and the person will drink water if possible. As a result of these mechanisms, the ECF sodium concentration is returned to normal, but the ECF volume (including blood volume) is increased.

Effects

The serum sodium concentration is increased only transiently because the adaptive mechanisms quickly restore the normal osmolarity of the ECF. Edema may develop and the blood pressure may be elevated as a result of the increased fluid volume.

SUGGESTED ADDITIONAL READING

Aspinall MJ: A simplified guide to managing patients with hyponatremia. *Nursing 78* 8(12): 32–35, 1978.

Moens J: Coping with diabetes insipidus. *Can Nurse* 75(4): 18–20, 1979.

13

Disturbances
of Blood Pressure

Pressure is a force per unit area. As blood flows through the blood vessels, it exerts a force against the vessel walls. *Blood pressure,* therefore, is the force exerted by the blood on any unit area of a blood vessel wall. Unless specified otherwise, the term blood pressure refers to arterial pressure. Blood pressure is usually measured in millimeters of mercury (mm Hg).

Blood is ejected from the heart into the arteries by contraction of the ventricles during systole; at the same time, blood is flowing out of the arteries into the arterioles. The amount of blood flowing out of the arteries during systole, however, is less than the amount of blood entering the arteries. Therefore during systole the total amount of blood in the arteries increases. As a result, the arteries are distended and the arterial pressure rises. When the ventricles relax during diastole blood no longer enters the arteries but it is still leaving, so that the volume of blood distending the arteries decreases and the blood pressure slowly falls. The elasticity of the arterial walls causes them to passively recoil and close down on the diminishing blood volume. This elastic recoil of the arterial walls maintains the pressure during diastole. The maximum pressure in the systemic arteries occurs as blood is being ejected into the aorta by the contracting ventricle and is called the *systolic pressure.* The lowest pressure in the arteries occurs just before the start of ventricular ejection and is called the *diastolic pressure.* Blood pressure is usually recorded as systolic/diastolic.

The difference between the systolic pressure and diastolic pressure is called the *pulse pressure.* Pulse pressure varies with the stroke volume and with the distensibility of the vessels. In general the pulse pressure increases with an increase in stroke volume. Pulse pressure also increases when the distensibility of the arteries is decreased (i.e., the walls become stiffer), for example due to arteriosclerosis. The arterial walls cannot stretch as much during systole to accommodate the increased volume; therefore a large increase in pressure occurs during systole. In addition elastic recoil is decreased, resulting in a large drop in pressure during diastole.

Mean arterial pressure, or mean blood pressure, is the average pressure during the cardiac cycle. The length of time during systole is usually shorter than the time during diastole; therefore mean pressure is not simply the value halfway between systolic and diastolic pressure. The methods for determining mean arterial pressure are quite complex, but mean pressure can be approximated by adding the diastolic pressure to one-third of the pulse pressure. For example, if the arterial pressure is 120/80 mm Hg, mean arterial pressure is approximately $80 + (1/3 \times 40)$, or 93 mm Hg.

Blood pressure exhibits a wide range of normal values; in addition, it varies with age and sex (Fig. 13-1). Normal blood pressure is lowest in the newborn and slowly but progressively increases with age, probably at least partly due to loss of elasticity of the blood vessels. Until about the age of 40 blood pressure is slightly lower in women than men. Between about 40 and 50 years of age, however, blood pressure rises at a greater rate in

women than men. The reason for the greater rate of change in women at this age is not known, but it is possibly due to the hormonal changes occurring at menopause.

Racial differences in blood pressure have also been observed. For example, Orientals generally have lower blood pressures than Americans and Europeans. It is not known to what extent genetic, environmental, and/or dietary factors are responsible for the differences, but it is suspected that dietary differences play an important role.

For a particular person, blood pressure can vary from moment to moment depending on position and activity (see Chapter 22). For example, blood pressure increases during exercise. Blood pressure shows considerable variation throughout the day; it is highest during activity and usually lowest during sleep. Greater variation occurs in the systolic than in the diastolic pressure.

Emotional factors, pain, and temperature can also influence blood pressure because the cardiovascular control center in the medulla oblongata is influenced by nervous input from the hypothalamus and from the cerebral cortex through connections in the hypothalamus. Anxiety, anger, and excitement usually cause an increase in blood pressure due to enhanced sympathetic nervous activity. Sometimes, however, emotional factors (e.g., fear) cause a precipitous drop in blood pressure, which results in fainting (see Chapter 14 under Neurogenic Shock). Touch may indirectly influence blood pressure as a result of the emotional response elicited by the touch. (For example, consider how a touch by a lover's hand can produce changes of heart rate.)

Pain may cause vasoconstriction, increased heart rate, and increased blood pressure in some cases. Deep pain, such as that caused by distension of abdominal organs or severe trauma to skeletal muscles and joints, however, may cause slowing of the heart and decreased blood pressure, accompanied by weakness, nausea, cold sweat, and fainting. Temperature influences the degree of vasoconstriction in skin blood vessels and therefore can influence blood pressure (see Chapter 24).

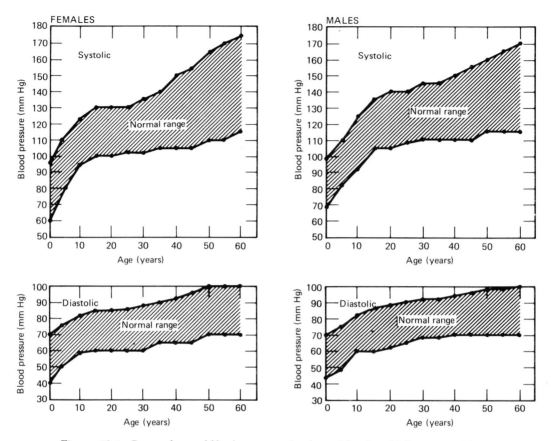

Figure 13-1. *Range of normal blood pressures of males and females of different ages. (Data from various sources listed in Bibliography.)*

Arterial pressure is the driving force for tissue blood flow. Blood flow is determined by the *difference* in pressure, or pressure gradient, between the two ends, not by the absolute pressure in the blood vessel. Blood flows from a region of high pressure to a region of lower pressure; if the pressure at both ends of the vessel were the same, no blood would flow. Blood pressure normally is very close to 0 mm Hg in the vena cavae near the point of entry to the heart. Therefore, the pressure gradient in the systemic circulation is determined by the mean arterial pressure. (Actually the gradient is determined by mean aortic pressure, but the mean pressure in all large arteries is essentially the same as mean aortic pressure.) If the mean arterial pressure falls, tissue blood flow decreases. An ab-

normally low blood pressure is called *hypotension*. Elevation of the mean arterial pressure can increase blood flow, but chronic elevation of blood pressure above the normal range has detrimental effects. A persistently high arterial pressure is called *hypertension*.

REGULATION OF BLOOD PRESSURE

Arterial blood pressure is determined by cardiac output, peripheral resistance, and the volume of blood distending the vessels. Each of these entities is, in turn, influenced by several factors (Fig. 13-2). If one factor is altered, compensatory

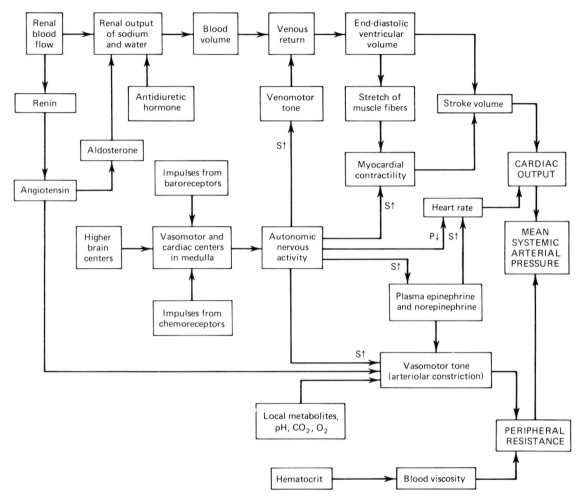

Figure 13-2. *Summary of factors influencing blood pressure. S ↑, Increased by sympathetic stimulation. P ↓, Decreased by parasympathetic stimulation. (See also Chapter 1, Fig. 1-2.)*

changes must occur in some other factor in order to maintain a particular arterial pressure. For example, if peripheral resistance is lowered in one part of the circuit as a result of vasodilation in a particular tissue, then peripheral resistance must be increased by vasoconstriction in other tissues and/or cardiac output must increase in order to maintain mean arterial pressure.

Arterial pressure is regulated by the simultaneous operation of several control systems. Nervous mechanisms and some hormonal mechanisms pro-

vide rapidly acting short-term control of arterial pressure from moment to moment. Other hormonal mechanisms and two intrinsic physical mechanisms provide intermediate-term control. Long-term control of arterial pressure appears to be mediated by a renal–body fluid mechanism.

Nervous Mechanisms

Several nervous reflexes are involved in blood pressure regulation. The most important is the baroreceptor reflex, but other reflexes also influence arterial pressure.

The Baroreceptor Reflex

The walls of large systemic arteries contain baroreceptors (also called pressoreceptors). These receptors are sensitive to stretch and, since pressure within the artery determines the degree of stretch of the wall, these receptors serve as pressure receptors. Baroreceptors are especially abundant in the carotid sinuses, which are located near the bifurcations of the carotid arteries, and in the arch of the aorta; but almost every large artery in the thoracic and neck regions has a few baroreceptors located in its wall.

Changes in pressure alter the rate of nerve-impulse transmission from the baroreceptors. Impulses from the baroreceptors travel to the cardiovascular control center in the medulla and reflexly influence autonomic nervous activity. An increase in arterial pressure causes an increased rate of firing from the baroreceptors. As a result, parasympathetic activity is increased and causes slowing of the heart rate. At the same time, sympathetic activity is inhibited, which contributes to the slowing of the heart rate and may also reduce stroke volume by decreasing myocardial contractility. As a result of these actions, cardiac output decreases. Decreased sympathetic activity also results in vasodilation and thus a decrease in peripheral resistance. Systemic arterial pressure is therefore lowered as a result of decreased cardiac output and decreased peripheral resistance.

A fall in blood pressure produces the opposite result. The baroreceptors fire at a decreased rate and so parasympathetic activity is decreased. Simultaneously, sympathetic activity increases. Consequently, heart rate and possibly stroke volume increase, and vasoconstriction occurs. Therefore arterial pressure is raised because cardiac output and peripheral resistance increase. In addition, sympathetic stimulation causes venoconstriction, which results in decreased venous capacity and increased venous return of blood to the heart. This effect contributes to the increase in cardiac output.

The baroreceptors are sensitive not only to mean arterial pressure, but also to the rate of change of pressure. When the pressure is rising, the baroreceptors respond more than if it is stationary; they respond less to a falling pressure. For example, if the mean arterial pressure is 120 mm Hg and rising, the rate of firing of the baroreceptors is greater than if the mean pressure is stationary at 120 mm Hg.

The baroreceptor reflex is important in counteracting fluctuations in the arterial pressure caused by changes in posture (see Chapter 22) and normal daily activities. This reflex probably only functions for short-term control of blood pressure because of sensory adaptation by the baroreceptors. For example, a large increase in arterial pressure initially causes a great increase in the rate of nerve-impulse transmission by the baroreceptors, but then the rate of firing gradually diminishes even if the blood pressure remains elevated.

In addition to the arterial baroreceptors, cardiopulmonary baroreceptors (also called low-pressure receptors) are located in the atria, ventricles, and pulmonary veins. The precise role of these baroreceptors in blood pressure regulation is not known, but in general they respond to pressure changes in the same way as the arterial baroreceptors. Reflexes initiated by the low-pressure receptors also influence blood volume by their effect on secretion of ADH (see Chapter 12).

The Chemoreceptor Reflex

Chemoreceptors that are sensitive to alterations in the chemical composition of the blood are located in the carotid and aortic bodies. These chemoreceptors are primarily stimulated by decreased arterial oxygen tension, but are also stimulated to a lesser extent by increased arterial carbon dioxide concentration and increased hydrogen-ion concentration (i.e., decreased pH). The chemoreceptors are mainly involved with control of respiration but they also transmit impulses to the cardiovascular control center. Stimulation of the chemoreceptors brings about a reflex increase in arterial pressure by increasing sympathetic nervous activity and decreasing parasympathetic activity.

The CNS Ischemic Response

The CNS ischemic response is not involved in the regulation of normal arterial pressure, but becomes operative at low arterial pressure levels. When blood pressure falls so low that the brain becomes ischemic, potent stimulation of the sympathetic nervous system is brought about by the cardiovascular control center. As a result, arterial pressure is elevated. Thus, the CNS ischemic response acts as an emergency system to restore blood flow to the brain.

Hormonal Mechanisms

The hormones that are known to have a direct effect on blood pressure are epinephrine, norepinephrine, angiotensin, and ADH (vasopressin).

The Norepinephrine-Epinephrine System

Stimulation of the sympathetic nervous system causes the release of epinephrine and norepinephrine (catecholamines) from the adrenal medullae into the blood. Therefore, the effect of sympathetic nervous stimulation on blood pressure is mediated not only by direct nervous action on the heart and blood vessels, but also by these two hormones. Epinephrine and norepinephrine have essentially the same effect on the heart and blood vessels as direct sympathetic nervous stimulation. They circulate in the blood for several minutes before being inactivated, however, so that their effect lasts longer than nervous stimulation alone. In addition, these hormones can reach some parts of the circulatory system, such as the metarterioles, that are not supplied with sympathetic nerves.

Sympathetic nerve endings primarily release norepinephrine, whereas the adrenal medullae mainly release epinephrine and only a small amount of norepinephrine. The actions of these two hormones are similar, but not identical. The differences are believed to be due to the presence of two types of binding sites for these hormones on cell membranes: α-adrenergic receptors and β-adrenergic receptors. It appears that norepinephrine acts only on α-adrenergic receptors, whereas epinephrine acts on both α- and β-adrenergic receptors. Norepinephrine causes vasoconstriction throughout the body, whereas epinephrine causes vasodilation in skeletal muscles under some circumstances. Although norepinephrine increases heart rate, epinephrine has a greater effect on heart rate and also increases the strength of myocardial contraction. As a result of its vasoconstrictive effect, norepinephrine greatly increases peripheral resistance and thereby raises blood pressure. As a result of its vasodilative effect in skeletal muscle, epinephrine may not increase total peripheral resistance and may, in fact, cause total peripheral resistance to decrease. Therefore, epinephrine does not increase blood pressure to as great an extent as norepinephrine does. Epinephrine causes a considerable increase in cardiac output, however, and raises blood pressure by this action. Another difference in the actions of the two hormones is that epinephrine stimulates metabolism to a greater extent than norepinephrine. (Epinephrine is called adrenaline in Britain. In Canada, both names are used. In the United States, Adrenalin is a brand name for a particular preparation of epinephrine. Similarly, in Britain norepinephrine is called noradrenaline.)

The Renin-Angiotensin System

Whereas the nervous mechanisms just described are activated within seconds, the renin-angiotensin system takes about 20 minutes to become fully active. *Renin* is an enzyme produced by the juxtaglomerular cells, which are located in the walls of the afferent arterioles next to the glomeruli in the kidneys. The renin substrate is a plasma globulin called angiotensinogen, which is synthesized by the liver. Renin acts on angiotensinogen to produce *angiotensin I*. Subsequently, angiotensin I is converted to *angiotensin II* by an enzyme (converting enzyme) present in the lungs and also in the plasma. Angiotensin II is rapidly broken down (i.e., within minutes) by several enzymes, collectively called angiotensinase, which are present in the blood and the tissues.

Under normal conditions angiotensinogen and converting enzyme are present in excess and so the amount of angiotensin II that is produced is determined by the amount of circulating renin. Renin is released into the circulation in response to decreased renal arterial pressure (i.e., decreased renal blood flow); β-adrenergic stimulation by sympathetic nerves or circulating catecholamines; and low sodium concentrations in the distal renal tubules, as sensed by the macula densa cells. The plasma renin level also shows diurnal variation, being lowest during sleep and showing a peak at about noon. After release, renin circulates in the blood for about an hour and is removed mainly by the liver.

Angiotensin II is a potent vasoconstrictor and raises blood pressure by increasing peripheral resistance. To a lesser extent it also causes venoconstriction, thereby increasing venous return and cardiac output. These effects are produced directly by an immediate action of angiotensin II on vascular smooth muscle and indirectly by an action on the CNS to stimulate sympathetic nervous activity. In addition, angiotensin II influences body salt and water balance in two

ways: it has a direct effect on the kidneys to promote sodium and water retention and it stimulates secretion of aldosterone by the adrenal cortex. Aldosterone, in turn, promotes reabsorption of sodium by the kidneys, as discussed in Chapter 12. Therefore, the renin-angiotensin system also affects blood pressure through its influence on blood volume. When blood pressure rises as a result of these actions, renal blood flow increases and renin release declines. In addition, angiotensin II exerts a direct inhibitory effect on renin release in a negative feedback manner.

Recent studies suggest that rather than angiotensin II, one of its breakdown products (sometimes called angiotensin III) may be the primary mediator of increased secretion of aldosterone by the adrenal cortex. Angiotensin III, however, does not appear to cause a significant degree of vasoconstriction.

The renin-angiotensin system is summarized in Figure 13-3. This system appears to be especially important for maintenance of blood pressure in conditions of sodium depletion; for people in sodium balance the role of angiotensin is not as crucial. The concentration of sodium in the body fluids appears to influence the response to angiotensin. The vascular smooth muscle seems to be

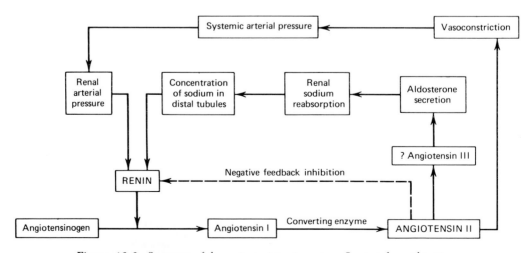

Figure 13-3. *Summary of the renin-angiotensin system. See text for explanation.*

more responsive to angiotensin II when the sodium concentration is elevated.

Antidiuretic Hormone (Vasopressin)

Low arterial pressure causes increased secretion of antidiuretic hormone (ADH; vasopressin) by the hypothalamus and release of this hormone from the neurohypophysis (posterior pituitary). ADH acts directly on the blood vessels, causing vasoconstriction and therefore raising systemic arterial pressure by increasing peripheral resistance. In addition to this immediate direct effect on blood pressure, ADH causes retention of water by the kidneys (see Chapter 12) and therefore is involved in long-term control of arterial pressure by the renal–body fluid mechanism (see below).

Prostaglandins

The prostaglandins are a group of related lipid compounds that are formed in many tissues. They are hormonelike substances that take part in numerous processes within the body. Several classes of prostaglandins are known, including prostaglandin E (PGE), prostaglandin F (PGF), and prostaglandin A (PGA).

Some prostaglandins cause arteriolar dilation and appear to be involved in autoregulation of blood flow in a number of organs, including the kidneys. Although the precise role of the prostaglandins is controversial, they are possibly involved in blood pressure control. PGF tends to raise blood pressure, mainly by causing constriction of the veins, which increases venous return and therefore increases cardiac output. PGE and PGA both cause vasodilation and a decrease in blood pressure, although they differ in their onset and duration of action and in some of their other effects. PGE and PGA compounds also promote excretion of sodium and water. PGA circulates for a longer time than PGE before being degraded and it has been suggested that PGA interacts with the renin-angiotensin system to maintain normal blood pressure (i.e., normal blood pressure may represent a balance between the hypotensive effect of PGA and the hypertensive effect of angioten-

sin). In addition, PGA possibly interacts with angiotensin in the control of aldosterone release.

Physical Mechanisms

Control of arterial pressure is influenced by two intrinsic physical mechanisms: capillary fluid shift and vascular stress-relaxation. These mechanisms usually start acting within a few minutes, but it takes an hour or longer for their full effects to be achieved.

Capillary Fluid Shift

A change in arterial pressure is usually accompanied by a change in capillary pressure. As a result, the balance of forces governing fluid exchange across the capillary membrane is disturbed and the net movement of fluid between the blood and the interstitial fluid compartment is altered (see Chapter 11). For example, a large increase in arterial pressure causes an increase in capillary hydrostatic pressure, so that an increased amount of fluid moves from the capillaries into the interstitial space. Consequently the blood volume decreases and blood pressure is brought back toward normal. Gradually a new state of equilibrium is established, but the initial fluid shift has a beneficial effect in maintaining the blood pressure within the desired range.

Vascular Stress-Relaxation

When blood pressure changes due to a rapid change in blood volume, the blood vessels gradually adjust their size to accommodate the amount of blood that is available and the blood pressure returns almost to its previous level. This adaptation by the blood vessels occurs mainly in the veins and only slightly in the arteries. Changes in arterial pressure due to blood volume changes, however, are usually accompanied by pressure changes in the veins and venous reservoirs.

This adaptive mechanism is due to the ability of smooth muscle to change length without a great change in tension. When a smooth muscle is first stretched the tension increases greatly, but within a few minutes the tension reverts almost to its previous level even though the muscle is now longer. This phenomenon is called *stress-relaxation.* Conversely, when a smooth muscle is no longer stretched it shortens and immediately loses most of its tension, but within one minute or more the tension returns. This situation is called *reverse stress-relaxation.*

Thus, following a rapid increase in blood volume (e.g., due to massive transfusion), the blood vessels are distended and arterial pressure rises. Gradually, however, the smooth muscle of the vein walls adjusts to the new length, the veins are able to accommodate the increased blood volume, and the blood pressure returns to its previous level even though the blood volume may be as much as 30% greater than normal.

On the other hand, following an acute decrease in blood volume by as much as 15% (e.g., due to hemorrhage), blood pressure initially falls. Within 10 minutes to an hour, however, the blood vessels and venous reservoirs contract down around the diminished blood volume due to reverse stress-relaxation. This mechanism assists the nervous and hormonal mechanisms in raising the mean systemic blood pressure back toward normal.

The Renal-Body Fluid Mechanism

When the circulatory system is disturbed, the renal–body fluid mechanism for control of arterial pressure takes several hours to become very effective. During this time the body depends on the rapidly acting and intermediately acting nervous and hormonal mechanisms to maintain normal arterial pressure. The renal–body fluid mechanism, however, appears to be very important in the long-term control of blood pressure.

Basically, the renal–body fluid mechanism operates in the following manner. A change in arterial pressure alters renal output of water and electrolytes. This effect is brought about by an altered rate of glomerular filtration due to the change in renal blood flow, and by changes in aldosterone and ADH secretion, as mentioned previously (see

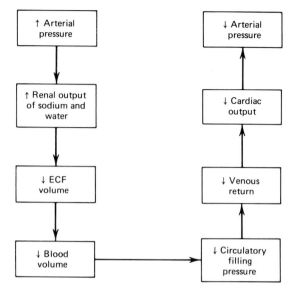

Figure 13-4. *Influence of the renal–body fluid mechanism on blood pressure.* ↑, *Increased.* ↓, *Decreased.*

also Chapter 12). Consequently, extracellular fluid volume (including blood volume) changes. This change influences the circulatory filling pressure (i.e., the degree to which the blood fills the circulatory system), which in turn affects venous return and cardiac output. The change in cardiac output alters the blood pressure (Fig. 13-4).

For example, an increase in blood pressure causes the kidneys to excrete increased amounts of water and electrolytes. This increase in renal output tends to cause the extracellular fluid (ECF) volume to decrease, but whether the ECF volume actually decreases depends on the balance between fluid intake and output. A decrease in ECF volume will result in a corresponding decrease in blood volume since the ECF is distributed between the vascular and interstitial fluid compartments. A decrease in blood volume causes a decrease in circulatory filling pressure, which reduces venous return of blood to the heart. Consequently, cardiac output decreases and arterial pressure is reduced.

Conversely, a reduction in arterial pressure

below normal causes retention of water and electrolytes by the kidneys. Provided that fluid intake is adequate, blood volume, circulatory filling pressure, venous return, and cardiac output all increase; and arterial pressure is restored to normal.

HYPOTENSION

A certain critical level of arterial pressure is necessary to ensure adequate blood flow for normal functioning of vital organs such as the brain, heart, liver, and kidneys. Ordinarily arterial pressure is maintained at a level that is higher than necessary to provide adequate tissue perfusion; thus, a safety margin exists. As stated previously, low blood pressure impairs blood flow to the tissues. There is no absolute numerical value that forms the dividing line between "normal" blood pressure and hypotension, however. The extent and rate of decrease in blood pressure, local condition of the blood vessels, and adequacy of compensating mechanisms all determine the arterial pressure level at which tissue perfusion is critically reduced. The manifestations of hypotension result from impaired blood flow (e.g., dizziness and fainting due to cerebral ischemia) or from activation of compensatory mechanisms (e.g., rapid heart rate and sweating due to sympathetic stimulation brought about by the baroreceptor reflex).

Low arterial pressure by itself is not necessarily a pathological condition; some normal adults have blood pressures as low as 90/60 mm Hg with no known cause and no apparent ill effects. Chronic hypotension that occurs without any associated disease (*idiopathic hypotension*) may in fact be favorable because it decreases the load on the heart. Statistical studies suggest that otherwise healthy people with chronic hypotension may live longer than people with higher blood pressure.

Chronic hypotension may be associated with a variety of conditions such as severe cardiac failure, constrictive pericarditis, adrenocortical insufficiency, and malabsorption syndrome. In these cases hypotension is merely one sign of the primary disorder.

Postural, or *orthostatic, hypotension* is an acute reduction in arterial pressure that occurs when a person stands; blood pressure is adequate when the person is lying down. This condition is discussed in Chapter 22.

Shock is a state of circulatory failure such that tissues are damaged due to inadequate blood flow. Hypotension usually, but not necessarily always, accompanies shock. (See Chapter 14.)

Hypotension can sometimes be caused by external pressure to the carotid sinuses (*carotid sinus syndrome*). In this condition the baroreceptors are excited by strong pressure on the neck over the bifurcations of the carotid arteries. This excitation brings about reflex peripheral vasodilation and slowing of the heart, as though to correct an elevated pressure. As a result of this inappropriate response, the blood pressure falls abruptly and the person may faint. In some abnormal situations the baroreceptors may be so sensitive that even mild external pressure (e.g., a tight collar) may be enough to evoke syncope. In some cases the response of the baroreceptors is so strong that heart actually stops due to excessive parasympathetic activity.

HYPERTENSION

In hypertension either the systolic or diastolic pressure, or both may be elevated. No agreement exists as to what level of blood pressure constitutes hypertension. According to some authorities the line between normal blood pressure and hypertension should be drawn at a systolic pressure of 140 mm Hg and a diastolic pressure of 90 mm Hg; others have suggested values ranging up to 200 mm Hg systolic and 110 mm Hg diastolic as the threshold for hypertension. A relatively mild degree of hypertension is called *benign hypertension.* A severe progressive hypertensive state is referred to as *malignant hypertension.*

Causes of Hypertension

Hypertension can occur secondarily to renal disease, endocrine disorders, neurological disturbances, cardiovascular disorders (e.g., coarctation of the aorta), and toxemia of pregnancy. In most cases, however, the cause is not known and the condition is referred to as *essential,* or *primary, hypertension.* Once hypertension has been initiated by a particular factor, alterations in several other factors might operate together to maintain the elevated blood pressure. Often it is difficult to determine what factor initiated the rise in blood pressure.

Renal Hypertension

Two basic mechanisms appear to be responsible for the development of hypertension in people with kidney disease, although often the full cause of the hypertension is not known. One mechanism is related to decreased renal blood flow, while the other is related to a reduction in functional kidney mass. Both mechanisms are involved to varying degrees in people with renal parenchymal disease, depending on the amount of kidney tissue lost and the adequacy of blood flow through the remaining kidney tissue.

When renal blood flow is reduced, the kidneys secrete large amounts of renin, which causes the formation of angiotensin, as described previously. Hypertension therefore develops due to the excessive amount of angiotensin, which directly raises blood pressure. In addition, the excessive angiotensin leads to production of increased amounts of aldosterone. Therefore sodium and water retention occur; the increased fluid volume contributes to the hypertension. Although the hypertension is initiated by the high level of renin, plasma renin activity may later decline as sodium and water retention occur. The hypertension is maintained by the expanded ECF volume and possibly by other factors. Although the hypertension has detrimental systemic effects (see below), it serves the purpose of increasing renal blood flow to normal levels. Viewed in this way, the hypertension can be seen as an adaptive response to maintain adequate renal blood flow so that the kidney can perform its vital excretory function.

Hypertension secondary to decreased renal blood flow (*renovascular hypertension*) is typified by renal arterial stenosis. The main renal artery or one of its branches may be narrowed; one or both kidneys may be affected. The usual causes of the narrowing are fibromuscular hyperplasia of the arterial wall or atherosclerosis. In fibromuscular hyperplasia the arterial wall is thickened due to an overgrowth of smooth muscle or of the connective tissue of the inner (intimal) lining of the arteries, or of both. Consequently the lumen of the artery is narrowed. This condition occurs most frequently in young women; it rarely occurs in men. Renal arterial stenosis due to atherosclerosis is most common in older men. Stenosis of the renal artery causes a decrease in blood pressure and blood flow distal to the narrowing. As a result, the juxtaglomerular cells are stimulated to secrete excess renin into the blood. Other unknown factors may contribute to the development of the hypertension, since it has been observed that some people with renal arterial stenosis have normal blood pressure.

Hypertension secondary to decreased kidney mass is exemplified by the anephritic state (i.e., both kidneys have been removed). In this case hypertension results primarily from increased fluid volume, although lack of a renal hypotensive agent or agents may be a contributing factor. Following removal of the kidneys, retention of water and electrolytes causes expansion of the ECF volume, resulting in increased blood volume, increased circulatory filling pressure, increased venous return, increased cardiac output, and increased blood pressure, as described earlier. The increased blood pressure is believed to be mainly due to the increased cardiac output initially. If hypervolemia persists, however, vasoconstriction occurs due to local autoregulation. Autoregulation is an adaptive mechanism to maintain normal tissue blood flow. When cardiac output increases, blood flow increases in all the tissues of the body.

When blood flow increases above tissue requirements, vasoconstriction occurs to decrease the flow. As a result, venous return and cardiac output return toward normal, but peripheral resistance is increased; this increase maintains the hypertensive state. Removal of the excess fluid by hemodialysis can restore the blood pressure to normal.

Removal of both kidneys is an extreme situation, but a reduction in kidney mass occurs with some kidney diseases (e.g., chronic pyelonephritis, which causes scarring and atrophy). A loss of kidney mass will not necessarily cause hypertension, however, if the remaining nephrons are functioning normally (e.g., if one kidney is removed and the remaining kidney is functioning normally). Kidney diseases that decrease glomerular filtration (e.g., glomerulonephritis), however, will cause hypertension due to fluid retention. Excess renin may be a contributing factor in some cases. Although the plasma renin level may be low or normal when compared with values obtained from healthy subjects, it is often inappropriately high in relation to the excess body sodium and water.

Endocrine Hypertension

Hypertension can be caused by a rare tumor called a pheochromocytoma, which secretes excessive amounts of epinephrine and norepinephrine. Other forms of endocrine hypertension are related to excessive adrenocorticosteroid hormones.

Pheochromocytomas are tumors of chromaffin cells; they usually occur in the adrenal medulla but may occasionally be found in other parts of the body. Pheochromocytomas are usually benign but are sometimes malignant. They are composed of neuronlike cells that secrete epinephrine and norepinephrine in varying proportions. In some cases the catecholamines are released into the blood continuously, producing sustained hypertension. In other cases the hormones are released intermittently (presumably in response to sympathetic stimulation), causing paroxysmal hypertension. The hypertension is caused by increased peripheral resistance due to vasoconstriction brought about by the catecholamines. In addition, cardiac output may be increased due to increased heart rate and increased myocardial contractility, brought about mainly by epinephrine.

Intermittent catecholamine release is characterized by attacks consisting of a sudden rise in blood pressure, headache, tachycardia (rapid heart rate), sweating, anxiety, nausea, and pain in the epigastric and precordial regions. Some people do not exhibit all these symptoms; the relative amounts of the two hormones will influence the manifestations of the attack. Some affected people may have an elevated fasting blood glucose level because epinephrine causes increased breakdown of liver glycogen and release of glucose into the blood.

Primary aldosteronism (or *hyperaldosteronism*) is a fairly rare condition caused by a small tumor of the adrenal cortex that secretes large amounts of aldosterone. Aldosterone causes increased reabsorption of sodium by the kidneys; the sodium retention is accompanied by water retention, as discussed in Chapter 12. A mild to moderate degree of hypertension therefore occurs as a result of increased ECF volume. Primary aldosteronism also causes hypokalemia (see Chapter 16) and sometimes alkalosis because the kidneys excrete potassium and hydrogen ions in exchange for reabsorption of sodium. In contrast to conditions that cause increased levels of aldosterone secondary to increased renin, plasma renin activity is low in primary aldosteronism.

Hypertension sometimes occurs in *Cushing's syndrome,* a condition resulting from excess cortisol (see Chapter 19). Cortisol is the major glucocorticoid hormone, but it also has some mineralocorticoid activity and therefore can cause fluid retention when it is present in excess. Deoxycorticosterone (DOC; a mineralocorticoid) may be produced in excess if the Cushing's syndrome is caused by excessive adrenocorticotropin (ACTH). ACTH primarily stimulates the adrenal cortex to produce glucocorticoids, but it also stimulates DOC production and to a lesser extent aldosterone production. Therefore mineralocorticoid excess may contribute to the development of hypertension in Cushing's syndrome.

Hypertension also occurs in one form of *congenital adrenal hyperplasia* (see Chapter 19). In this case the hypertension is due to an excessive amount of DOC.

Licorice contains a steroid substance similar to the mineralocorticoids and it can cause salt and water retention. Excess consumption of licorice, therefore, can produce hypertension by increasing ECF volume.

Coarctation of the Aorta

Coarctation of the aorta is a rare congenital condition in which the aorta is severely narrowed or sometimes completely occluded. The constriction usually occurs at the lower end of the aortic arch. The transverse cervical, transverse scapular, intercostal, internal mammary, and superior epigastric arteries are enlarged to provide collateral blood flow around the coarctation. The collateral circulation offers considerable resistance to blood flow from the upper part of the body to the lower part; consequently the blood pressure is elevated in the upper part of the body. Blood presure is normal or low in the lower part of the body.

Toxemia of Pregnancy

Toxemia of pregnancy is a syndrome that consists of hypertension with proteinuria, or edema, or both. It occurs during the third trimester of pregnancy and mainly affects primigravidas, although multiparas are sometimes affected. (Not all cases of hypertension during pregnancy are due to toxemia. A pregnant woman may have essential hypertension or hypertension due to some other cause, but the hypertension may not have been diagnosed before pregnancy.)

The cause of toxemia of pregnancy is not known. It was once believed to be due to some unidentified toxin, hence the name toxemia. Toxemia has two forms: preeclampsia and eclampsia. Hypertension is characteristic of both forms. In addition, generalized seizures or coma occur in eclampsia, but not in preeclampsia.

The exact mechanism by which the hypertension of toxemia is produced is not known. Peripheral resistance is increased and the blood vessels have increased sensitivity to substances such as norepinephrine and angiotensin II, which cause vasoconstriction. Increased peripheral resistance raises the blood pressure, but the cause of the vasopasm that produces the increased peripheral resistance is not known. It does not appear to be due to increased sympathetic nervous activity.

Possibly the hypertension is due to fluid retention. As mentioned earlier, increased ECF volume increases cardiac output, which causes a secondary rise in peripheral resistance due to vasocontriction brought about by local autoregulation. Characteristic changes in the renal glomeruli occur in toxemia. These changes reduce glomerular filtration, which could result in fluid retention. Sodium and water retention do occur in toxemia, but fluid retention also occurs in normal pregnancy without the development of hypertension. Possibly the amount and distribution of retained fluid is different in women who develop toxemia.

In one study that compared normal pregnant women with preeclamptic women, those with hypertension (i.e., those with preeclampsia) had lower concentrations of renin, renin substrate, angiotensin II, aldosterone, and DOC in their plasma. Perhaps the women with hypertension have a greater degree of sodium retention, which would suppress the renin-angiotensin system. As mentioned previously, a high sodium concentration makes the blood vessels more reactive to angiotensin. Therefore, even though the level of angiotensin II is lower in the women with hypertension, it might still have an excessive vasoconstrictive effect on the blood vessels.

Other researchers have suggested that the vasospasm may be due to lack of a vasodilator substance to balance the effects of the vasoconstrictors. Decreased levels of urinary kallikrein have been observed in women with pregnancy-induced hypertension. Kallikrein is an enzyme that catalyzes the formation of kinins from a plasma globulin. The kinins are potent vasodilators. A reduction in the amount of kallikrein would lead to decreased levels of these vaso-dilators.

Essential Hypertension

Essential hypertension is usually manifested as an excessive rise in blood pressure occurring in middle age. It rarely occurs in young people; severe hypertension in a young person is usually secondary to some other condition. In the early stages essential hypertension is usually symptomless; the high blood pressure is usually discovered during a routine examination. Later symptoms reflect the effects of hypertension on the heart and blood vessels (see below).

Essential hypertension shows a familial tendency, but the exact genetic determinant is not known. One group of researchers contends that essential hypertension is a specific disease entity governed by a single dominant gene. According to these people there is a natural dividing line between normal blood pressure and hypertension, and the population falls into two groups: those whose blood pressures increase with age and those whose blood pressures do not.

Other researchers argue that blood pressure is a graded character like height, which is determined by polygenic (multifactorial) inheritance. According to these people, blood pressure follows a normal distribution curve; there is no dividing line between normal and abnormal, and it is not possible to say when the disease begins. Hypertension is seen as a simple quantitative deviation from the average. It represents those people in the upper end of the frequency-distribution curve in whom the genetic and environmental factors contributing to high arterial pressure are most potent.

In the early stage of essential hypertension cardiac output appears to be high. Peripheral resistance may be slightly higher or slightly lower than that observed in people with normal blood pressure. Although the peripheral resistance is within the normal range, it may be abnormally high for the level of cardiac output. (In other words, in a person with normal blood pressure that level of cardiac output would be accompanied by a lower peripheral resistance.) Later the cardiac output decreases to normal levels and peripheral resistance increases. Peripheral resistance is increased even when the blood vessels are maximally dilated, probably because of an increase in the thickness of the wall, which decreases the diameter of the lumen.

Although the cause of essential hypertension is not known, several theories have been proposed. Researchers report conflicting results; therefore, for each theory there is evidence to support it and evidence against it. The conflicting results are probably related to differences in techniques and in the criteria for selection of subjects. It is also possible that essential hypertension is not a single disease entity, and that the etiology is different for different groups of people.

One theory proposes that psychogenic factors are important in the development of hypertension. Emotional factors can raise blood pressure through activation of the "fight-or-flight" response ("defense reaction"), as described in Chapter 2. Frequent elevations of arterial pressure by activation of this response might lead to structural changes of the arterioles. As a result of these changes, the vasoconstrictive effects of even normal levels of circulating substances and normal levels of nervous activity would be amplified. Eventually a state of fixed hypertension would be established.

According to another theory, cardiac output is increased due to an expansion of blood volume. As a result of autoregulation, peripheral resistance increases and subsequently the cardiac output decreases, as described previously. The hypertension is maintained by the increased peripheral resistance. Some people believe that a high salt intake is the precipitating factor in this sequence of events. ECF volume depends on a balance between sodium and water intake and urine output, as discussed in Chapter 12. Urinary output depends partly on the blood pressure level and varies from one person to another depending on the functional capacity of the kidneys to excrete sodium and water loads. Retention of sodium leads to water retention because of an osmotic effect. It has been suggested that the people who develop hypertension have an inherited defect of renal sodium excretion so that the kidneys require a higher than normal blood pressure in order to function adequately. In other words, a high arterial pressure is necessary to maintain sodium balance.

Another possibility is that the compliance of the systemic veins is decreased. In other words, the veins are less distensible, so that for a given blood volume the venous pressure is higher than normal. A decrease in venous compliance causes blood to shift to the central circulation; therefore the filling pressure of the heart and the cardiac output are increased. Another consequence of decreased venous compliance is increased capillary hydrostatic pressure, which results in a shift of fluid from the plasma to the interstitial space.

Many studies have been conducted to determine the role of the renin-angiotensin system in the pathogenesis of hypertension. Most people with essential hypertension have normal plasma renin concentrations, but some have either low or high levels of plasma renin. Some researchers believe that the etiology and prognosis is different for each of these three groups of people. Another suggestion is that the differences in plasma renin level represent different stages in the progression of hypertensive disease. In the early stages renin secretion may be suppressed as a result of the high renal blood flow brought about by the high arterial pressure. In later stages, however, the renin level may rise as arterioles become damaged due to the hypertension (see below, under Effects of Hypertension). As a consequence of arteriolar damage the perfusion pressure may be low in some areas of the kidneys, with resultant stimulation of renin release. The high renin level probably contributes to the elevation of the blood pressure.

Effects of Hypertension

Elevated blood pressure decreases life expectancy. It increases the risk of coronary artery disease and cerebral hemorrhage, and can lead to renal failure. High blood pressure also increases the work load on the heart and can lead to heart failure. Many of the effects of hypertension are consequences of damage to arteries and arterioles. The higher the blood pressure and the longer it remains elevated, the greater will be the severity of the damage to the blood vessels.

Arteriolosclerosis

Moderate degrees of hypertension persisting for months or years lead to the development of *arteriolosclerosis*, a thickening and hardening of the arterioles. The arteriolosclerosis associated with hypertension is due to a process called intimal hyperplasia, in which there is an overgrowth (hyperplasia) of cells of the inner (intimal) lining of the arterioles. As a result, the wall of the arteriole is thickened and the lumen is narrowed, thus limiting blood flow through the arteriole.

Critical narrowing of the afferent arterioles of the kidneys can lead to a gradual loss of nephrons and decreased renal function. This condition is called *benign nephrosclerosis*. It does not occur with mild hypertension but frequently occurs with moderate or moderately severe degrees of hypertension that persist for a long time. It is *not* the same as the nephrosclerosis of malignant hypertension, which is due to fibrinoid necrosis (see below).

Arteriolosclerosis can be detected in the eyes if the optic fundi are viewed with an ophthalmoscope. When the retinal blood vessels are viewed, it is actually the columns of blood within the vessels, not the walls of the vessels, that are seen. When arteriolosclerosis is present the columns of blood appear thinner than normal because the blood vessel walls are thickened and the lumens are narrowed. In addition, where an arteriole crosses a vein, the vein is compressed because the arteriole wall is thicker and stiffer than normal. At such points, an indentation of the venous blood column can be seen; this situation is called arteriovenous (AV) nicking.

Microaneurysms in the Brain

The small cerebral arteries have thinner walls than arteries in other parts of the body. As a person ages these small blood vessels may become weakened and develop minute outpouchings, or *micro-aneurysms*. These microaneurysms occur much more frequently, and at a younger age, in people with hypertension than in those with normal blood pressure. Sustained high blood pressure can lead to rupture of these microaneurysms, causing cerebral hemorrhage. Cerebral hemorrhage is one cause of cerebrovascular accidents (strokes). As mentioned in Chapter 7, however, occlusion of a larger cerebral artery due to thrombosis or embolism is a more common cause of strokes.

Fibrinoid Necrosis

Very severe hypertension (i.e., malignant hypertension) that is sustained for weeks or months is associated with fibrinoid necrosis. Fibrinoid necrosis develops when the diastolic pressure is greater than 130 mm Hg. Necrosis means death of tissue; the term fibrinoid refers to the fact that arteriolar smooth muscle cells are replaced with a material that resembles fibrin.

Fibrinoid necrosis affects arterioles and small arteries. It appears to occur as a result of the strain placed on the blood vessels by sustained extreme elevation of the blood pressure. Fragmentation of smooth muscle fibers occurs in the walls of affected blood vessels. An exudate forms and an inflammatory reaction ensues. The smooth muscle cells degenerate and are replaced with a fibrinous material.

Fibrinoid necrosis narrows the lumen and weakens the wall of the blood vessel. Consequently plasma may leak out, causing edema around the affected artery or arteriole. In some cases red blood cells may also pass through the weakened wall, resulting in small hemorrhages. Another possible complication is thrombosis within the damaged blood vessel, resulting in complete occlusion.

Not all the arterioles in the body are affected by fibrinoid necrosis; the arterioles in some organs are affected more than others. The most serious damage due to fibrinoid necrosis occurs in the kidneys and the brain.

Narrowing of the interlobular arteries and/or afferent arterioles of the kidneys due to fibrinoid necrosis causes diminished glomerular blood flow. Renin secretion may thus be stimulated, initiating a vicious cycle in which the high level of renin causes a further elevation of the blood pressure. The afferent arterioles of the renal glomeruli are especially prone to develop fibrinoid necrosis. When thrombosis occurs subsequent to fibrinoid necrosis in an afferent arteriole, the glomerulus degenerates because it has no other blood supply. Therefore, widespread fibrinoid necrosis in the kidneys results in a loss of renal function, leading to uremia (see Chapter 26).

Fibrinoid necrosis of arterioles in the brain may produce cerebral hemorrhages or cerebral edema due to the leakiness of the damaged blood vessels. Cerebrospinal fluid pressure may be elevated. These complications of severe hypertension produce a syndrome called *acute hypertensive encephalopathy*. The manifestations of this syndrome include severe occipital headaches, transient weakness of a limb, mental dullness, stupor, and possibly convulsive seizures.

Fibrinoid necrosis associated with malignant hypertension also produces characteristic changes in the optic fundi, which can be seen with an ophthalmoscope. Leakage of plasma produces soft, fluffy-looking exudates around arterioles in the retina (*cotton-wool exudates*). Small retinal hemorrhages may occur. The red blood cells accumulate between two nerve fibers so that the hemorrhages have a streaky or linear appearance. Such hemorrhages are called *striate hemorrhages*. Further progression of the hypertension produces *papilledema* (swelling of the optic disc, that is, the point where the optic nerve leaves the eye). The optic disc normally has a sharply defined circular border; when papilledema is present the optic disc appears fuzzy. Partial or complete loss of vision may be the consequence of retinal damage due to fibrinoid necrosis.

Effects on the Heart

Stroke volume is the amount of blood ejected from the ventricle during one beat. It is influenced by the preload and afterload on the heart, as well as by myocardial contractility. *Preload* is the volume of blood in the ventricle just before the start of contraction (i.e., the end-diastolic volume). An increase in the end-diastolic volume will increase stroke volume as a result of the Frank-Starling mechanism. The end-diastolic volume determines the degree of stretch of the cardiac muscle and therefore the length of the muscle fibers. According to the Frank-Starling law of the heart, the length of the muscle fibers determines the amount of mechanical energy released in going from the resting to the contracted state. In other words, the greater the end-diastolic volume the stronger the contraction, up to a point. *Afterload* is the impedance, or resistance, to ejection of blood from the ventricle. It is determined by the arterial pressure, because the pressure in the left ventricle must be higher than that in the aorta before blood can be ejected. The strength of the ventricular contraction is determined by myocardial contractility, which is influenced by several factors in addition to the Frank-Starling mechanism. Changes in myocardial contractility can therefore alter the stroke volume even if the preload and afterload remain constant. An increase in myocardial contractility will cause a greater fraction of the end-diastolic volume to be ejected from the ventricle and therefore increase the stroke volume. Sympathetic nervous activity and circulating catecholamines increase myocardial contractility. Any factor that interferes with myocardial metabolism, such as ischemia, will decrease myocardial contractility.

Hypertension increases the afterload and therefore the left ventricle must work harder to pump blood into the systemic circulation and maintain an adequate stroke volume. As a result of this increased work, the cardiac muscle hypertrophies; that is, the muscle fibers enlarge. Consequently the wall of the ventricle becomes thicker than normal. The hypertrophy increases the strength of contraction so that the heart can do the extra work. The coronary blood supply does not increase to the same extent that the muscle mass increases, however, and a state of relative ischemia of the left ventricle develops. Con-

sequently there is a limit to the ability of the ventricle to maintain a normal stroke volume by this mechanism.

If the blood pressure continues to rise and the ventricle is required to work harder, a second mechanism is used to maintain a normal stroke volume. The ventricle dilates so that it can hold more blood. Therefore the end-diastolic volume is increased and a normal stroke volume is maintained as a result of the Frank-Starling mechanism. Now, however, the stroke volume represents a smaller fraction of the end-diastolic volume and the end-systolic volume increases.

The ability of the left ventricle to maintain a normal stroke volume by means of hypertrophy and dilatation is limited. When the ventricle is overdistended, a point is reached where myocardial contractility is decreased, presumably because the sarcomeres within the muscle fibers are extended so much that the actin and myosin filaments no longer overlap effectively. At this point the Frank-Starling mechanism is no longer effective. Eventually the left ventricle is unable to put out a normal stroke volume and congestive heart failure develops (see Chapter 12).

Hypertension also affects the heart by increasing the risk of coronary artery atherosclerosis. Atherosclerosis is a condition in which cholesterol and other fatty substances are deposited in the intima of large- and medium-sized arteries, forming plaques, or thickenings, called atheromas. The cause of atherosclerosis is not known, but several factors that increase the risk of atherosclerosis are known: one major risk factor is a high concentration of cholesterol or triglycerides in the plasma (see Chapter 18); the other major risk factor is hypertension. It is not known how hypertension increases the susceptibility to atherosclerosis. Possibly the high arterial pressure damages the arteries in some way so that cholesterol and other lipids are deposited in the walls more easily.

Atherosclerosis narrows the arterial lumen, thus reducing blood flow. One consequence of this reduction in blood flow is *angina pectoris*. Blood flow may be adequate at rest, but whenever the demands on the heart are increased (e.g., due to exercise or emotional stress), blood flow is unable to increase enough to meet the increased needs of the myocardium. The result is myocardial hypoxia, which produces chest pain. The pain is also frequently referred to the left shoulder and arm. The pain produced as a result of myocardial ischemia is called angina pectoris.

Atherosclerosis is also a major factor predisposing to coronary thrombosis. The consequence is occlusion of a coronary artery with subsequent myocardial infarction (see Chapter 7 under Effects of Thrombosis).

Effects on the Aorta

The wall of the ascending aorta and aortic arch is structurally different from the descending aorta and other large arteries. The wall of the ascending aorta is composed mainly of elastic tissue, which is very distensible and can stretch easily to accommodate the volume of blood ejected from the left ventricle during systole. The wall of the descending aorta, however, is composed mainly of smooth muscle, which is much less distensible.

High blood pressure causes the aorta to become chronically distended, particularly in the ascending portion. Sustained moderate or severe hypertension stretches the elastic tissues to the breaking point. Consequently fibrous scar tissue forms in the wall, replacing the elastic tissue. This fibrous tissue strengthens the wall, but it also results in the aorta becoming fixed in a distended state. With sustained very severe hypertension the ascending aorta may become so distended that the aortic valve cannot close during diastole, giving rise to an aortic diastolic murmur.

Medial necrosis of the ascending aorta or aortic arch is a serious complication of prolonged severe hypertension. The elastic tissue of the tunica media (middle coat) of the aorta receives its blood supply from arterioles and capillaries that enter from the adventitia (outer coat). Excessive pressure and excessive stretching of the aortic wall may cause compression of these small blood vessels. Consequently, the media becomes ischemic and necrosis occurs. The wall of the aorta is therefore weakened, and if the extreme elevation of the blood pressure persists, the media and intima may be torn apart. Blood enters the media and causes a longitudinal separation of the wall of the aorta. This complication of hypertension is called a *dissecting aneurysm;* it is usually fatal.

SUGGESTED ADDITIONAL READING

Nauright LP: et al: Identifying hypertensive adolescents. *Pediatr Nurs* 5(2): 34–37, 1979.

Sonstegard L: Pregnancy-induced hypertension: prenatal nursing concerns. MCN 4(2):90–95, 1979.

Ward GW, Bandy P, Fink JW: Treating and counseling the hypertensive patient. *Am J Nurs* **78**(5): 824–828, 1978.

14

Shock

Shock is a state of circulatory failure such that tissues are damaged as a result of inadequate blood flow. Basically, three mechanisms can produce shock: decreased circulating blood volume, which causes *hypovolemic* shock; impaired pumping ability of the heart so that it cannot adequately circulate the blood that is available, which gives rise to *cardiogenic* shock; and altered distribution of blood volume, which occurs in *neurogenic* shock and *septic* shock. In the clinical situation more than one of these mechanisms may be operating at the same time to produce shock. For example, following severe trauma shock may result from hypovolemia and from neurogenic factors.

Shock represents a severe disturbance of homeostasis: with inadequate circulation it is impossible to maintain optimum conditions in the internal environment. Negative feedback control mechanisms immediately bring about compensatory adaptive responses in an attempt to restore homeostasis. If the shock is not too severe, these mechanisms prevent further progression of the shock and eventually homeostasis is restored: the person recovers. This condition is called *nonpro-*

gressive, or compensated, shock. If the shock is severe enough, the compensatory mechanisms are inadequate to restore homeostasis and a vicious cycle of positive feedback develops. Inadequate tissue perfusion leads to deterioration of cardiovascular structures so that their functioning is impaired further. Thus the shock itself causes a greater degree of shock. This state is referred to as *progressive*, or *decompensated*, shock. If treatment is inadequate, death eventually results.

HYPOVOLEMIC SHOCK

Normal blood volume is approximately 70 to 80 ml/kg of body weight throughout life for a lean person (less than this amount for an obese person). Individual variation is great, however, so that this value represents only an approximate guideline. For a 60-kg (132-lb) adult the total blood volume is about 4.8 liters (10 pt). Approximately 10% of the normal blood volume can be lost without significant effects. When blood volume is diminished so that it cannot adequately fill the vascular compartment, however, tissue perfusion is impaired and hypovolemic shock results. The degree of shock produced is determined not only by the amount of blood lost, but also by the rate at which it is lost. Rapid loss of 20% of the blood volume may produce more serious shock than a relatively slow loss of up to 40%. When blood loss occurs slowly the body has more time to institute effective compensating mechanisms and is better able to adapt.

Diminished blood volume reduces the mean systemic blood pressure, which causes a decrease in venous return of blood to the heart. As a result, the atrial pressure during diastole decreases, end-diastolic ventricular volume decreases, the force of contraction diminishes, and stroke volume falls. (The end-diastolic ventricular volume determines the degree of stretch of the cardiac muscle and therefore the length of the muscle fibers. According to the Frank-Starling law of the heart, the length of the muscle fibers determines the amount of mechanical energy released in going from the resting to the contracted state. In other words, the greater the end-diastolic volume the stronger the contraction, up to a point. Also, it is obvious that the heart cannot pump out more blood than it contains.) Consequently cardiac output falls, arterial blood pressure declines, and blood flow through the tissues becomes inadequate to meet normal metabolic requirements. As a result of the inadequate supply of oxygen to the cells, anaerobic glycolysis occurs, which produces lactic acid. Metabolic acidosis (see Chapter 15) then develops. (See also Chapter 10 for a discussion of the effects of oxygen lack on cells.)

Causes of Hypovolemic Shock

Hemorrhage is a common cause of hypovolemic shock. Other causes are related to loss of plasma, rather than of whole blood. Large amounts of plasma are lost through burned areas. In addition, a shift of fluid from the vascular compartment to the interstitial space occurs in a person who is severely burned (see Chapter 24). Hypovolemic shock is therefore a hazard for anyone with severe burns. Water deficit (dehydration) can also cause hypovolemic shock due to a reduction in plasma volume; the conditions that lead to water deficit are discussed in Chapter 12. Intestinal obstruction can also result in decreased plasma volume. Intestinal distension, which results from obstruction (see Chapter 21), causes leakage of fluid from the intestinal capillaries into the wall and lumen of the intestine. Thus plasma volume is reduced and hypovolemic shock may result.

Nonprogressive or Compensated Shock

When blood volume is decreased, sympathetic reflexes are activated within seconds. Other mechanisms are also activated to counteract the shock, but they take longer to exert their effects.

Sympathetic Mechanisms

A slight decrease in arterial pressure immediately elicits several compensatory responses (Fig. 14-1). These responses help to maintain the blood pressure despite a continued decrease in cardiac output. Acting by way of the baroreceptors in the carotid sinuses and aortic arch, the lowered blood pressure activates the sympathetic nervous system. Sympathetic stimulation causes constriction of arterioles in most parts of the body, particularly the skin, skeletal muscles, gastrointestinal tract, and kidneys. (Skeletal muscles are supplied with sympathetic nerves that cause vasoconstriction as well as some that cause vasodilation. In the fight-or-flight response described in Chapter 2, vasodilation occurs to increase blood flow to the muscles and prepare them for action. This response is mediated by centers in the cerebral cortex and hypothalamus. In shock, however, vasoconstriction occurs because the object is to maintain arterial blood pressure. This sympathetic response is mediated by the vasomotor center in the medulla.) This vasoconstriction increases the peripheral resistance and thereby helps to maintain systemic arterial pressure. (Recall that systemic arterial pressure is determined by peripheral resistance and cardiac output.)

Sympathetic stimulation also causes venous constriction, which decreases the capacity of the veins so that the diminished amount of blood is better able to fill the circulatory system. Constriction of veins and venous reservoirs (e.g., the spleen) also promotes venous return. In addition, sympathetic stimulation increases the rate and depth of breathing, which assists venous return. Development of metabolic acidosis contributes to the respiratory stimulation (see Chapter 15).

Heart rate and strength of the myocardial contraction are stimulated by sympathetic activity in an effort to maintain cardiac output (i.e., stroke volume times heart rate). Increased heart rate is effective in increasing cardiac output only to a certain point. As the heart rate increases, the time available for ventricular filling between beats decreases. Consequently end-diastolic volume decreases. Stroke volume can be maintained for a time, despite the decreased end-diastolic volume, because the increased myocardial contractility due to sympathetic stimulation causes a larger fraction of the end-diastolic volume to be ejected (i.e., the end-systolic volume is decreased). At very rapid heart rates (greater than about 180 beats/min), however, filling time becomes the limiting factor and stroke volume decreases.

The sympathetic effects are augmented by an increased release of epinephrine and norepinephrine from the adrenal medullae. These mechanisms serve to bring systemic arterial pressure back toward normal and ensure adequate blood flow through the brain and heart, but blood flow through other tissues is decreased because of the peripheral vasoconstriction. In other words, blood is shunted to the brain and heart in order to protect the vital centers, at the expense of other parts of the body.

Other mechanisms contribute to the maintenance of adequate blood flow through the cerebral and coronary circulation. Sympathetic stimulation does not significantly constrict blood vessels in the brain or the heart and in fact may cause vasodilation in the heart. Also, local autoregulation is very effective at maintaining essentially normal blood flow in both these organs, provided that mean arterial pressure does not fall below about 70 mm Hg. When the arterial pressure falls below about 50 mm Hg the CNS ischemic response is activated. Decreased blood flow through the brain results in decreased oxygen and excessive carbon dioxide in the medulla. As a result, the vasomotor center produces even more powerful activation of the sympathetic nervous system, causing vasoconstriction. The vasoconstriction is so intense that blood flow through some peripheral vessels is completely blocked and vasoconstriction in the kidneys is so great that urine production stops.

Other Compensatory Mechanisms

If the blood loss is not too great and the shock is not too severe, compensatory mechanisms eventually restore homeostasis and the person recovers.

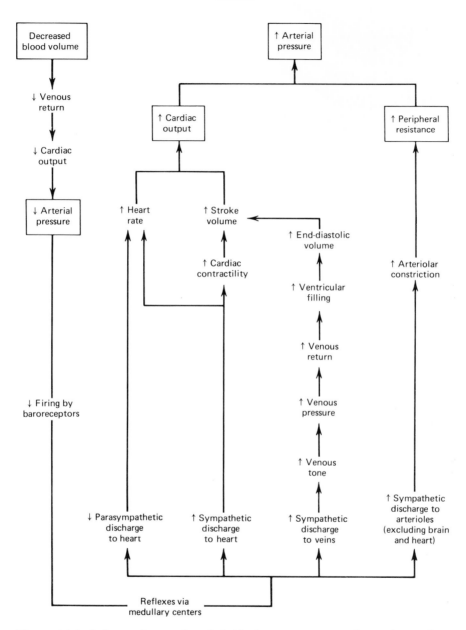

Figure 14-1. *Reflex mechanisms by which blood pressure is returned toward normal in hypovolemia. ↑, Increased. ↓, Decreased. (Adapted from Vander et al.: Human Physiology. Copyright © 1975 by McGraw-Hill, Inc. Used with permission of McGraw-Hill Book Company.)*

Thus a person may recover from mild degrees of shock without treatment, but usually prompt treatment is necessary to correct the underlying cause and prevent progression of the shock. In addition to the sympathetic mechanisms just mentioned, several other mechanisms contribute to the restoration of normal cardiac output, blood pressure, and blood volume.

Fluid is redistributed from the interstitial space to the vascular compartment, thereby increasing plasma volume. This shift occurs because the blood pressure in the capillaries is reduced and the balance of forces governing fluid exchange across the capillary membrane is disturbed (see Chapter 11). Interstitial fluid does not contain protein, however, so that as the fluid shifts to the vascular compartment the plasma is diluted. As a result, the plasma oncotic pressure decreases and further movement of fluid from the interstitial space is hindered. After hemorrhage, however, the liver rapidly synthesizes new protein (primarily albumin) to replace the plasma proteins that have been lost. Consequently the decrease in plasma protein concentration is minimized and more interstitial fluid can shift to the vascular compartment.

Another mechanism that contributes to the restoration of a normal blood pressure is reverse stress-relaxation (see Chapter 13 under Physical Mechanisms). As a result of reverse stress-relaxation, the blood vessels contract down on the remaining blood volume so that the amount of available blood will fill the vascular compartment more adequately.

In response to decreased renal blood flow, the kidneys secrete renin (see Chapter 13). Renin converts a plasma globulin, angiotensinogen, to angiotensin I. Angiotensin I is subsequently converted to angiotensin II, which is a powerful vasoconstrictor; angiotensin II thus causes increased peripheral resistance, which raises systemic arterial pressure. Angiotensin II also causes venous constriction, which promotes venous return. In addition, angiotensin II stimulates secretion by the adrenal cortex of aldosterone, which increases retention of sodium by the kidneys and thus promotes retention of water.

Decreased cardiac output stimulates increased release of antidiuretic hormone (ADH) by the neurohypophysis (posterior pituitary). This effect is mediated by atrial receptors and possibly baroreceptors in the aortic arch and carotid sinuses, as described in Chapter 12. ADH acts on the proximal renal tubules and collecting ducts of the kidneys to increase reabsorption of water; that is, it promotes water retention. ADH also has a vasoconstrictive effect and thus contributes to increasing the arterial pressure. (ADH is also called vasopressin because of this effect.)

Hypovolemia and a low cardiac output also stimulate the thirst center in the hypothalamus (see Chapter 12 under The Thirst Mechanism). As a result, a person in hypovolemic shock experiences extreme thirst and will drink water if she or he is able; thus fluid volume is replaced. Not only water but also electrolytes must be replaced; thus a person recovering from shock usually has a craving for salt. Very little is known about the mechanism involved in controlling salt appetite.

Clinical Manifestations
The primary effects of hypovolemia and the compensatory responses produce the typical signs and symptoms of shock. Systemic arterial pressure and central venous pressure are low as a direct result of reduced blood volume, although in the early stages compensatory mechanisms may maintain systemic arterial pressure near normal levels. Pulmonary wedge pressure is also low.

To obtain pulmonary wedge pressure a catheter is inserted into a branch of the pulmonary artery. Blood flow is occluded either by advancing the catheter to the point that it is wedged in the artery and can go no further or by inflating a balloon surrounding the catheter. The pressure at the tip of the catheter is then recorded. This pressure, which is normally 6 to 12 mm Hg, reflects the pressure downstream within the vascular network and is almost the same as left atrial pressure. Pul-

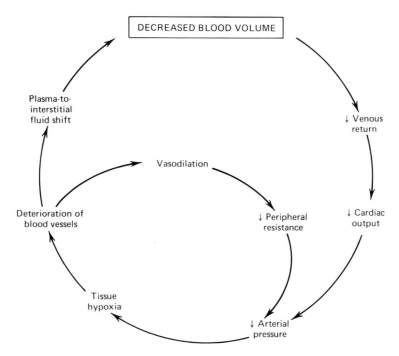

Figure 14-2. *The vicious cycle in decompensated hypovolemic shock.*

monary wedge pressure therefore provides a good assessment of left ventricular end-diastolic pressure and thus an indication of left ventricular functioning.

The pulse is rapid because of sympathetic nervous stimulation. As already mentioned, breathing is rapid and deep. As a result of the rapid deep breathing, large amounts of carbon dioxide are blown off and the arterial PCO_2 may be less than normal. (In other words, the person may have a degree of respiratory alkalosis, which partially compensates for the metabolic acidosis. See Chapter 15.) Arterial blood pH may be less than 7.37, reflecting the metabolic acidosis.

The skin is cold and moist because of decreased blood flow and increased sweating, which is brought about by sympathetic stimulation. Reduced blood flow through the skin causes pallor and perhaps cyanosis because the tissues extract more oxygen from the blood. Decreased blood flow

reduces the amount of oxygen and nutrients available to all of the tissues, so that metabolism is decreased. As a result, less heat is produced and the body temperature may drop. The person also experiences extreme muscular weakness and fatigue as a result of the decreased supply of oxygen and nutrients to the muscles. Urinary output is diminished (oliguria) because of reduced renal blood flow and increased ADH secretion.

Progressive or Decompensated Shock

When shock becomes severe enough, deterioration of circulatory structures causes further progression of the shock and a vicious cycle of positive feedback develops (Fig. 14-2). Several factors contribute to the cardiovascular failure.

As stated previously, systemic arterial pressure is determined by cardiac output and peripheral resistance. In hypovolemic shock the cardiac output is decreased and as a result the blood pressure falls. In compensation, vasoconstriction occurs to increase peripheral resistance and thereby maintain blood pressure. With prolonged severe shock, however, the blood vessels are unable to remain constricted. Vasodilation occurs, peripheral resistance decreases, and arterial pressure declines further. Lack of oxygen and nutrients to the blood vessels themselves can impair smooth muscle function and can lead to vasodilation. Also, with tissue ischemia local concentrations of carbon dioxide and metabolic products such as lactic acid and pyruvic acid are high, causing the pH to decrease (acidosis). The decreased pH is believed to affect arteriolar smooth muscle directly to cause vasodilation. In addition, a variety of intracellular substances, including histamine and lysosomal enzymes, are released into the extracellular fluid as a result of ischemic tissue damage and can bring about vasodilation. These substances, as well as lactic acid, can also cause increased capillary permeability. As a result, fluid shifts from the plasma to the interstitial space, which decreases blood volume and venous return.

Cardiac output continues to fall during progressive shock and contributes to the steady decline of the blood pressure. Decreased venous return is one factor that causes the further decline in cardiac output. As just mentioned, venous return decreases because of increased capillary permeability. In addition, venous dilation occurs as a result of a lack of oxygen and nutrients to the vessels themselves. As a result, blood "pools" in the veins, venous return decreases, and cardiac output diminishes.

Cardiac output also declines because of deterioration of the heart itself. During the first hour or two of shock cardiac deterioration is not significant, but later the myocardium is depressed by toxic substances as well as by inadequate coronary blood flow. As mentioned previously, essentially normal coronary blood flow is maintained by autoregulation as long as the arterial pressure does not fall below about 70 mm Hg; when it does fall below this value, however, coronary blood flow is

diminished and the myocardium is weakened. As the strength of the myocardial contraction decreases, cardiac output decreases further, arterial blood pressure falls lower, coronary blood flow diminishes even more, and the heart is weakened further: a vicious cycle. With a decrease in systemic arterial pressure below about 45 mm Hg, coronary blood flow is so inadequate that the myocardium is damaged. As a result of ischemia, small necrotic lesions develop throughout the heart. Excess lactic acid and toxic substances released by ischemic tissues are carried in the blood to the heart and depress cardiac function. A substance called myocardial toxic factor (MTF) has a direct depressant effect on myocardial contractility. MTF is released into the blood as a result of ischemic damage to the pancreas and/or gastrointestinal tract.

Some researchers believe that endotoxin released by intestinal bacteria contributes to the progression of shock. Bacteria and their products are always entering the blood from the intestines and are carried to the liver by the portal circulation. Normally they are removed or inactivated by reticuloendothelial cells in the liver and do not enter the general circulation. During shock, however, the activity of the reticuloendothelial cells is depressed and endotoxin may enter the general circulation. In addition, absorption of endotoxin from the intestine may be increased during shock. Endotoxin causes vasodilation and also depresses the myocardium. Therefore it contributes to the fall in blood pressure by decreasing both peripheral resistance and cardiac output.

Eventually, in the late stages of shock, a point is reached when systemic arterial pressure is so low that blood flow to the vasomotor center in the medulla is greatly diminished. The vasomotor center is depressed by lack of oxygen and nutrients; it becomes less and less active and finally fails completely. As a result, sympathetic discharges from the vasomotor center decrease and eventually stop. The heart slows and blood vessels dilate. Cardiac output diminishes, peripheral resistance decreases, and the systemic arterial pressure cannot be maintained. The respiratory center may also be depressed as a result of reduced blood flow.

Signs of decompensation, therefore, are further decreased arterial blood pressure and decreased heart rate. Central venous pressure may rise if the failing heart is unable to keep up with the venous return. Gasping or Cheyne-Stokes respiration may occur. A person is usually conscious during the early stages of shock, although mental functioning may be impaired. As shock progresses, however, brain functioning is depressed by lack of blood flow. The person goes into a state of stupor and finally coma. If adequate therapy is not instituted soon enough, shock eventually progresses to death. In some cases death may occur even though therapeutic measures have returned the blood pressure and cardiac output to normal. Presumably a point is reached where tissue damage is so extensive that it is not compatible with life.

CARDIOGENIC SHOCK

Cardiogenic shock results when the pumping ability of the heart is seriously impaired. The cardiac output falls and arterial blood pressure is decreased.

Causes of Cardiogenic Shock

The most comon cause of cardiogenic shock is myocardial infarction (see Chapter 7 under Effects of Thrombosis). Severe cardiac arrhythmias, direct trauma to the heart, and acute cardiac tamponade are other causes. Acute *cardiac tamponade* is compression of the heart caused by rapid accumulation of fluid or blood in the pericardial sac.

With cardiac tamponade, the increased intrapericardial pressure causes compression of the heart and interferes with ventricular filling. Therefore stroke volume decreases, cardiac output falls, and systemic arterial blood pressure declines. The central venous pressure is increased.

Cardiogenic Shock
Due to Myocardial Infarction

As just stated, the most common cause of cardiogenic shock is myocardial infarction. About 10% to 15% of people with acute myocardial infarction develop cardiogenic shock; the mortalilty rate from cardiogenic shock is about 80%. Myocardial infarction usually affects the left ventricle. As mentioned in Chapter 7, the infarcted area of the myocardium is nonfunctional and the surrounding area may be contracting only weakly. Therefore the damaged ventricle is unable to develop sufficient pressure to eject the blood within it and stroke volume falls.

Stroke volume can be increased by increasing the contractility of the myocardium, by increasing end-diastolic volume and pressure, by decreasing the impedance to ejection by the heart (afterload), or by a combination of these actions.

As a result of ineffectual pumping, the left ventricular end-diastolic volume increases. Immediately following myocardial damage, however, venous return is normal because the systemic circulation is not yet altered. If the right ventricle is functioning normally, this amount of blood will be pumped into the pulmonary circulation and enter the left side of the heart (i.e., diastolic inflow will be normal). Thus, left ventricular end-diastolic volume will increase. As a result of the increased volume, end-diastolic pressure will also increase to varying degrees, depending on the compliance (i.e., distensibility) of the left ventricle. Myocardial contractility is therefore enhanced according to the Frank-Starling mechanism. Contractility of the undamaged portion of the myocardium is also increased by reflex sympathetic stimulation. In addition, sympathetic stimulation enhances venous return by causing venoconstriction, as previously described. Therefore diastolic inflow is maintained and the end-diastolic volume remains elevated. Now, however, the stroke volume represents a smaller fraction of the end-diastolic volume and so the end-systolic volume also remains elevated. Thus a new equilibrium may be established; stroke volume and venous return are once again equal, but the end-diastolic and end-systolic volumes remain elevated. These mechanisms may maintain an adequate stroke volume and cardiac output as long as the person remains resting. When myocardial damage is severe, however, stroke volume and cardiac output are seriously diminished in spite of these mechanisms and cardiogenic shock results.

Since the end-diastolic and end-systolic volumes remain elevated, the pressure in the left ventricle increases and left atrial pressure also rises. Consequently, the pressure also rises in the pulmonary circulation due to backpressure. Pulmonary wedge pressure is therefore increased. Central venous pressure (i.e., right atrial pressure) may also increase. If venous return decreases because of the decline in cardiac output, however, central venous pressure may be unchanged.

An elevation in the pulmonary blood pressure can cause pulmonary edema (see below under Effects on the Lungs). Therapy is therefore usually aimed at maintaining the pulmonary wedge pressure between 15 and 19 mm Hg. Pressures in this range maximize the effect of the Frank-Starling mechanism on stroke volume but are not usually high enough to cause pulmonary edema.

In some cases, secondary factors may precipitate a state of shock in a person with myocardial infarction. For example, if the person's fluid intake has been inadequate or output has been excessive due to diuretic therapy, hypovolemia may precipitate shock. If the shock is secondary to hypovolemia, pulmonary wedge pressure will not be increased.

Response to Cardiogenic Shock

Cardiogenic shock elicits the same compensatory responses that are activated in hypovolemic shock. That is, hormonal factors and increased sympathetic nervous activity bring about increased heart rate, increased myocardial contractility, and peripheral vasoconstriction. With the exception that central venous pressure and pulmonary wedge pressure are usually increased in cardiogenic shock, but are decreased in hypovolemic shock,

signs and symptoms are essentially the same: weak rapid pulse, low arterial pressure, rapid breathing, pallor, cold clammy skin, weakness, and oliguria. In cardiogenic shock, the pulse is often irregular. Mental function is often impaired.

Decompensation occurs much more readily in cardiogenic shock than in hypovolemic shock. The already damaged heart can undergo serious deterioration with even a slight decrease in arterial pressure. The increased heart rate and increased contractility brought about by sympathetic stimulation (or drug therapy) result in increased myocardial metabolism (i.e., increased oxygen demand). If coronary blood flow is not increased, the extent of myocardial damage may increase. In the case of myocardial infarction, reduction of arterial pressure to 80 to 90 mm Hg can set off a vicious cycle of cardiac deterioration due to diminished coronary blood flow, whereas in a normal heart serious deterioration does not usually occur until the arterial pressure falls below about 45 mm Hg. In hypovolemic shock, treatment aimed at correcting the cause of the shock (e.g., stopping hemorrhage; replacing blood volume) can often prevent progression of the shock. In cardiogenic shock, however, damage to the heart cannot be reversed (although cardiac arrhythmias can be corrected). The vicious cycle in cardiogenic shock is outlined in Figure 14-3.

NEUROGENIC SHOCK

Neurogenic shock is caused by a loss of vasomotor tone. As a result, peripheral resistance is decreased, causing a fall in systemic arterial pressure. In addition, the dilated blood vessels (especially the veins) are capable of holding a larger volume of blood (i.e., vascular capacity increases), so that the normal amount of blood cannot adequately fill the circulatory system. Mean systemic pressure falls and venous return to the heart is decreased. In other words, blood collects in the greatly expanded peripheral blood vessels and there is in-

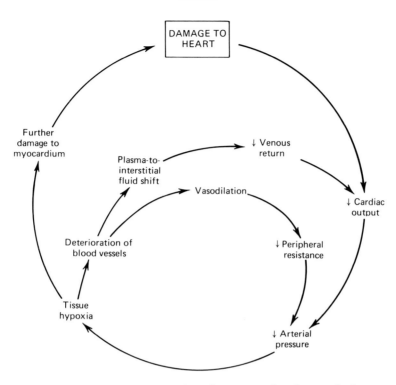

Figure 14-3. *The vicious cycle in decompensated cardiogenic shock.*

adequate return of blood to the heart. This situation is sometimes called *venous pooling,* or *peripheral pooling,* of blood. As a result of the decreased venous return, the cardiac output declines, which contributes to the decrease in arterial pressure.

Anything that causes a sudden decrease in sympathetic outflow can cause loss of vasomotor tone and lead to neurogenic shock. The vasomotor center in the medulla may be sufficiently depressed by deep general anesthesia that neurogenic shock can result. Spinal anesthesia can also cause neurogenic shock by blocking outflow of sympathetic impulses from the CNS. Neurogenic shock can also occur as a result of injury to the spinal cord.

Pain can cause shock. The exact mechanism is not well understood, but apparently pain can sometimes inhibit the vasomotor center. As a result, fewer sympathetic impulses are sent out from the vasomotor center and vasomotor tone is decreased.

Brain damage, especially to the brainstem, can impair functioning of the vasomotor center and cause severe neurogenic shock. Neurogenic shock can also develop after medullary ischemia. Initially ischemia causes intense stimulation of vasomotor sympathetic activity (the CNS-ischemic response described previously) in what might be called a "last-ditch" attempt to restore blood flow to the brain. If the ischemia lasts more than a few minutes, however, vasomotor activity is depressed and neurogenic shock results.

Fainting (syncope) is not neurogenic shock, but rather a transient loss of consciousness due to cerebral ischemia. Fainting may be caused by mild forms of neurogenic shock, however, when it is due to loss of vasomotor tone. Fainting caused by an emotional disturbance (vasovagal syncope) is not caused by loss of sympathetic vasomotor tone. Therefore some authorities do not consider it a form of neurogenic shock, although others do refer to vasovagal syncope as neurogenic shock. Strong emotional disturbances can stimulate the parasympathetic nerves to the heart and sympathetic vasodilator fibers to the skeletal muscles. As a result, the heart rate is slowed, which reduces cardiac output, and blood vessels in skeletal muscles become dilated, which lowers peripheral resistance. Therefore blood pressure falls and fainting results from the decreased blood flow to the brain.

If a person is in an upright position, sudden loss of vasomotor tone results in extensive peripheral pooling of blood and severe shock can occur. When a person is in a horizontal position, however, the effects of gravity in causing pooling of blood are eliminated (see Chapter 22). Therefore cardiac output is not as greatly reduced and only a mild-to-moderate degree of shock results.

Since neurogenic shock is caused by a lack of vasomotor tone, the sympathetic compensatory mechanism is impaired. A person maintained in an upright position could quickly go into the progressive stage of shock and die.

SEPTIC SHOCK

Septic shock is caused by overwhelming infection in which microorganisms and/or their products are present in the bloodstream. The exact mechanisms by which shock is produced are not known. Water deficit often accompanies severe infection and fever. In addition, increased capillary permeability due to the infection may lead to a loss of fluid from the vascular compartment to the interstitial space. Therefore hypovolemia may be a contributing factor in some cases of septic shock. The clinical picture in the early stages is variable, depending on the type of infection and the nature of the underlying condition. The late stage, however, is essentially the same as the decompensated stage of hypovolemic shock.

Causes of Septic Shock

The organisms most commonly causing septic shock are *Escherichia*, *Klebsiella*, *Proteus*, and *Pseudomonas* species of aerobic gram-negative bacilli. These bacteria release an endotoxin that is believed to be responsible for causing shock. Endotoxin is a lipopolysaccharide found in the cell walls of gram-negative bacteria. Less frequently septic shock is caused by gram-positive cocci such as *Staphylococcus aureus.* Not only bacteria, but also occasionally herpesviruses, yeasts such as *Candida albicans,* fungi such as phycomycetes and aspergilli, and protozoa such as *Toxoplasma gondii* and *Pneumocystis carinii* cause septic shock.

The primary source of the blood-borne infection is frequently a urinary tract infection. Peritonitis often leads to septic shock also. The peritonitis usually results by spread of infection from the uterus and fallopian tubes following an instrumental abortion or from rupture of the bowel caused either by intestinal disease or traumatic injury. Generalized infection leading to shock may also arise from spread of a skin infection or burn infection. Intravenous catheters are another source of septicemia, usually due to *Candida*.

Characteristics of Septic Shock

Septic shock is usually characterized by high fever, especially in the early stages. Later, however, the body temperature may be subnormal. (Body temperature may be subnormal in people with burns who develop septic shock.) As a consequence of the fever, metabolism and thus the demand for oxygen are increased. To compensate for this increased oxygen requirement, heart rate is increased and breathing is rapid and deep. The rapid deep breathing may cause respiratory alkalosis (see Chapter 15) in the early stages of septic shock. In later stages, however, metabolic acidosis occurs because of an inadequate supply of oxygen to the tissues or because the cells are unable to utilize oxygen. Some researchers believe that the infection somehow impairs uptake and/or utilization of oxygen by cells, so that tissue damage occurs even though adequate oxygen may be reaching the cells.

In some cases of septic shock vasodilation occurs. Consequently the person appears flushed and feels warm to touch. The skin is dry. The exact reason for the vasodilation is not known, but it is possibly due to release of histamine and kinins. The vasodilation causes decreased peripheral resistance, which lowers systemic arterial blood pressure. Central venous pressure may be high or low. To compensate for the decreased blood pressure sympathetic stimulation occurs. Heart rate and strength of myocardial contraction are increased, which may result in an increased cardiac output. Later, in the decompensated phase, however, cardiac output decreases.

In other cases of septic shock the mechanism is different. Venous pooling of blood occurs (the reasons for this pooling are not well understood) and as a result venous return is reduced. Cardiac output then declines and systemic arterial pressure falls. Central venous pressure is low. Peripheral resistance may be normal, or it may be increased due to compensatory vasoconstriction. Heart rate is rapid. The extremities are usually cold and moist and may be cyanotic. Urinary output is diminished.

Some researchers believe that endotoxin initiates intravascular clotting, which results in disseminated intravascular coagulation (DIC; see Chapter 7). According to these people, DIC is a major factor in the progression of shock. Tissue perfusion is seriously impaired as capillaries become plugged with clots. Focal tissue necrosis occurs as cells adjacent to the blocked capillaries die because of a lack of oxygen and nutrients. As a result, the functioning of many organs is seriously impaired.

As mentioned previously, when decompensation occurs the events are essentially the same as those that occur in hypovolemic shock and the clinical picture is similar: decreased heart rate, low blood pressure, oliguria, pallor and possibly cyanosis, and impaired consciousness. In a few cases the extremities may feel warm, but most often they are cold.

GENERAL EFFECTS OF SHOCK

The basic effect of shock is inadequate blood flow through the tissues. Although peripheral vasoconstriction helps to maintain systemic arterial blood pressure and therefore protects the blood supply to the brain and heart, blood flow through the other organs is reduced by vasoconstriction. The various organs of the body are therefore damaged as a result of ischemia. The degree of damage will depend on the severity of the shock and the length of time a person is in shock. When shock reaches the progressive stage extensive tissue damage can occur. In hypovolemic shock due to loss of plasma only, hemoconcentration occurs, which increases blood viscosity and further slows blood flow.

With ischemia the supply of oxygen to the cells is inadequate and so oxidative phosphorylation is impaired. Eventually the cells must resort to anaerobic glycolysis to produce energy in the form of adenosine triphosphate (ATP). Very little ATP is produced by anaerobic glycolysis, however, as compared with aerobic respiration. Therefore cellular functions are unable to proceed normally because of lack of energy. Anabolic processes and membrane transport functions are impaired. The sodium-potassium pump is unable to operate maximally because of the energy lack, and so potassium ions leak out of the cells and sodium ions enter. Acid metabolic end products accumulate in the tissue fluid because blood flow is too slow to carry them away as quickly as they are formed. The resultant lowered pH alters membrane permeability and enzymes may leak out of the cells. After prolonged lack of oxygen, the lysosomes of the cells rupture, releasing their potent enzymes. These enzymes digest cellular components, and so the cells are completely destroyed.

The acid metabolic and degradation products from the cells cause agglutination (clumping) of blood cells in the capillaries and other small blood vessels. This agglutination of blood cells within the microvasculature is called *sludging* of blood. It occurs particularly in hypovolemic shock (especially when the hypovolemia is due to loss of plasma only) and septic shock. In septic shock bacterial products probably contribute to the blood-cell agglutination. In some cases thrombosis may also occur. As a result of sludging it is even more difficult for the blood to flow through the small vessels and in many cases blood vessels may actually be plugged. Thus, sludging of blood is a further contributing factor to tissue damage.

Every tissue in the body is affected by shock, but in severe shock, damage to the kidneys, liver, and lungs is particularly serious. As already mentioned, when shock is prolonged and becomes progressive, the heart is also seriously damaged.

Effects on the Kidneys

As stated previously, urine output decreases in shock. When blood flow is diminished, pressure falls below the value necessary for glomerular filtration. Tubular necrosis, however, is a more serious complication that may occur as a result of ischemia. The kidneys normally have a very high metabolic rate and therefore are very vulnerable to ischemia and lack of oxygen. Death of tubular epithelial cells occurs, particularly at the terminal parts of the proximal and distal convoluted tubules. The necrotic epithelium sloughs off and may block the tubules. As a result, renal functioning is severely impaired and complete renal shutdown may occur. Water, electrolytes, and nitrogenous substances are retained, producing uremia (see Chapter 26). A person may survive the initial shock state only to die a week or so later because of kidney failure. Fortunately, renal tubular epithelium can regenerate and with modern therapy (e.g., dialysis) many people can be maintained until renal recovery occurs. The condition is still very serious, however.

The pattern of blood flow in the kidneys is altered during shock, with more blood flowing through the medulla than the cortex. As a result of markedly decreased glomerular filtration while blood flow through the renal medulla continues, the gradient of osmolality that normally exists in the extracellular fluid of the renal medulla is lost.

This gradient of osmolality is necessary in the process of concentrating urine (see Chapter 12). Therefore, when normal blood flow resumes, and while the tubular epithelium is regenerating, large volumes of dilute urine are excreted because the urine concentrating mechanism is disrupted. Consequently, water deficit may occur. In addition, until regeneration is complete, the tubular epithelium is unable to reabsorb filtered electrolytes normally and potassium deficit may occur. Gradually the medullary gradient of osmolality is restored and progressive improvement in renal function occurs.

Effects on the Liver

The liver also normally has a high rate of metabolism and is vulnerable to ischemia. Most of the tissue damage occurs in the central portion of each liver lobule. As blood passes through the liver sinusoids it reaches the central portion of the lobule last, therefore the cells in the center of each lobule receive less oxygen than other parts.

A number of metabolic derangements occur because of liver ischemia. The liver is unable to clear toxic substances from the blood at the normal rate because of disrupted cellular functioning. In addition, the ability to deaminate amino acids and to form urea is impaired. Consequently the concentration of amino acids in the blood rises. In the early stages of shock liver glycogen is converted to glucose and hyperglycemia may occur because glucose is being mobilized, but the ischemic tissues are unable to use it. When shock is prolonged, however, hypoglycemia may occur because glycogen stores are depleted and gluconeogensis is impaired in the ischemic liver.

Effects on the Lungs

The changes in respiratory rate during shock have already been mentioned. In addition, lung function is altered as a result of changes of the pulmonary circulation during shock. Later, a few people develop respiratory distress (shock-lung syndrome) anytime up to three or four days after the period of shock.

Effects of Changes
in Pulmonary Circulation

Blood pressure in the pulmonary circulation is normally low because resistance is low. Blood flow through the capillaries is determined by the presssures in the arterial and venous ends of the capillaries and by alveolar air pressure. Pulmonary blood pressure and the distribution of blood flow are influenced by gravity and therefore also by position (see Chapter 22).

In parts of the lung where the pressure in the pulmonary arteries is less than atmospheric pressure throughout most of the cardiac cycle, little or no blood flows through the capillaries and consequently no gas exchange can occur. The volume of air distributed to the alveoli served by these capillaries is called *alveolar dead space.* Alveolar dead space normally exists in the upper part of the lung when a person is in an upright position.

Where pulmonary arterial pressure is greater than atmospheric pressure, blood is forced through the capillaries. The amount of blood flow is determined by the relationship between the alveolar pressure and the pressure at the venous end of the capillary (pressure at the venous end is less than at the arterial end because of capillary resistance). When alveolar pressure is greater than capillary presssure, the capillary is compressed and less blood flows through. When pressure at the venous end of the capillary is greater than alveolar pressure, more blood flows through. The latter situation exists in the base of the lung when a person is in an upright position.

In hypovolemic shock pulmonary blood flow decreases as a result of decreased cardiac output. Pulmonary arterial pressure therefore decreases and the amount of alveolar dead space increases. As a result of the increased alveolar dead space, gas exchange is less efficient and the partial pressure of oxygen (PO_2) in the systemic arterial blood may decrease. In the presence of hyperpnea, however, arterial PO_2 usually remains normal unless some pulmonary pathology is present (see Chapter 10 under Ventilation-Perfusion Ratio). The partial pressure of carbon dioxide (PCO_2) in the systemic arterial blood does not usually increase and if ventilation is increased, the PCO_2 may be decreased, as already mentioned. Also, as previously mentioned, during shock blood is shunted away from nonvital areas to maintain blood flow to the brain and the heart. That is, the amount of blood flow through nonvital areas is reduced. Since the volume of tissue being perfused with blood is reduced, the load of CO_2 being delivered to the lungs is reduced. Therefore the lungs are able to eliminate the CO_2 delivered to them, even though alveolar dead space is increased.

In cardiogenic shock, the inability of the left side of the heart to pump blood effectively causes the left atrial pressure to rise. As a result, pulmonary venous pressure increases, which in turn causes an increase in capillary pressure. If the capillary pressure (or pulmonary wedge pressure) rises too high, more fluid passes out of the pulmonary capillaries into the interstitial space than is returned and edema develops in the alveolar wall. Later, as the fluid accumulates, it may enter the alveolar space (intraalveolar edema).

The actual value of the pulmonary wedge pressure at which pulmonary edema develops depends on the colloid osmotic pressure. Colloid osmotic pressure holds fluid in the capillaries and opposes the effects of the capillary blood pressure in forcing fluid out. People who develop pulmonary edema after acute myocardial infarction may have a decreased colloid osmotic pressure as well as an increased pulmonary wedge pressure. In this circumstance even a slight increase in pulmonary wedge pressure may be sufficient to cause pulmonary edema. (See Chapter 11 for a discussion of the factors influencing fluid exchange across the capillary membrane.) Pulmonary edema also occurs in septic shock, but in this case the mechanism is different. In septic shock capillary permeability is increased, which causes interstitial edema and intraalveolar edema.

Interstitial edema makes the alveolar walls less

pliable and thus lung compliance is decreased. The edema also narrows the terminal airways and therefore increases airway resistance. Consequently, breathing is more difficult. Interstitial and intraalveolar edema interfere with gas exchange (see Chapter 10 under Decreased Oxygenation of the Blood). In addition, the presence of fluid in the alveoli decreases the amount of air they can hold. Consequently systemic arterial PO_2 is decreased, although arterial PCO_2 may not be increased until the terminal stages.

Shock-Lung Syndrome

Shock-lung syndrome is a serious complication that occasionally develops after severe trauma and shock. The initial pulmonary changes are as already described. The person may then enter a stable phase when circulatory and respiratory function appear normal. In the next few days, however, acute respiratory distress may develop. Respirations are rapid and labored, arterial PO_2 decreases sharply, and the person becomes restless. Roentgenograms may reveal diffuse opacities of the lungs. If effective treatment is not instituted, respiratory distress increases, hypoxia is severe, arterial PCO_2 increases, severe metabolic acidosis develops, and consciousness is impaired. Death occurs from the severe hypoxia.

Pathological changes within the lungs include vascular congestion and hemorrhages around arterioles, followed a few hours later by interstitial and intraalveolar edema and hemorrhages into the alveoli. Occasionally microthrombi may be present but these are usually quickly removed by the fibrinolytic system. A translucent substance is deposited in the alveolar septa, forming a *hyaline membrane.* The origin of the hyaline material is not known, but it is possibly derived from blood proteins. The fluid in the alveoli provides a fertile medium for bacterial growth and bronchopneumonia is usually a final complication in shock-lung syndrome.

The cause of shock-lung syndrome is not known, although probably many factors contribute to its development. Many researchers consider sepsis a major component. As mentioned previously, endotoxin enters the blood from the gastrointestinal tract during shock and is not removed because liver function is depressed. Oxygen toxicity (see Chapter 10 under Hyperoxia) and circulatory overload as a result of therapeutic measures during the initial shock stage may be contributing factors. In some cases trauma to the lungs may occur at the time of the original injury without immediately producing respiratory symptoms. In such cases shock-lung may represent a delayed response to trauma.

SUGGESTED ADDITIONAL READING

Fay FC: Pulling a patient through acute renal failure. *RN* **41**(11): 61–64, 1978.

Molyneux-Luick M, Knecht J: Hypovolemic shock. *Nursing 77* **7**(11): 33–37, 1977.

Stroud SD: What you need to know to save a shock-lung victim. *RN* **40**(8): 47, 1977.

15

Acid-Base Imbalance

Homeostasis requires that the hydrogen-ion concentration of the extracellular fluids be kept within a fairly narrow range. Deviations from this range can seriously disrupt cell metabolism.

ACIDS, BASES, AND BUFFERS

Definition of Acid and Base

The acidity of a solution is determined by the number of hydrogen ions (H^+) in the solution. (Since a hydrogen atom consists of one proton and one electron, the loss of an electron to form a hydrogen ion leaves only a proton. Therefore the term proton is often used interchangeably with the term hydrogen ion.)

An *acid* may be defined as a substance that dissociates to release hydrogen ions when dissolved in water, and a *base* may be defined as a substance that dissociates in aqueous solution to yield hydroxide ions (OH^-). These definitions are perhaps the most familiar, but they are not the only definitions of acid and base. According to the *Brønsted-Lowry definition*, an *acid* is a substance that can donate protons (i.e., hydrogen ions), and a *base* is any substance that can accept protons. When a Brønsted-Lowry acid gives up a proton it becomes the *conjugate base*. Conversely, when a Brønsted-Lowry base accepts a proton it becomes the *conjugate acid*. For example, carbonic acid (H_2CO_3) dissociates to release hydrogen ions and bicarbonate ions (HCO_3^-); bicarbonate is the conjugate base of carbonic acid:

$$H_2CO_3 \rightleftharpoons H^+ + HCO_3^-$$
$$\text{acid} \qquad\qquad \text{base}$$

The Brønsted-Lowry definition is the most useful one for understanding physiological acid-base regulation, and it will be used in this book.

The term *alkali*, in the strictest sense, refers to strong mineral bases containing the alkali metals (e.g., sodium hydroxide). In general usage, however, the term alkali is used synonymously with the term base. In this book the terms *alkali* and *base* will be used interchangeably.

Water can dissociate into hydrogen ions and hydroxide ions:

$$H_2O \rightleftharpoons H^+ + OH^-$$

Since the hydrogen ion is hydrated to form a *hydronium ion* (H_3O^+), the reaction is more correctly written as

$$H_2O + H_2O \rightleftharpoons H_3O^+ + OH^-$$

but for simplicity the first equation is most often used. From this reaction it can be seen that water can act as both an acid and a base. Normally water is only slightly dissociated.

When an acid releases hydrogen ions in solution it is essentially donating its hydrogen ions to water to form hydronium ions. In other words, water has a greater affinity for hydrogen ions than the acid does. A base has a greater affinity for hydrogen ions than water molecules do, and so accepts hydrogen ions from water.

A *strong acid* is an acid that dissociates almost completely and releases many hydrogen ions in solution. For example hydrochloric acid (HCl) and sulfuric acid (H_2SO_4) are strong acids. When hydrochloric acid is added to water, only H^+ and Cl^- ions exist in the solution; no intact HCl molecules are present. An acid that is only slightly ionized (dissociated) and releases few hydrogen ions in solution is called a *weak acid*. For example, acetic acid ($HC_2H_3O_2$) is a weak acid. When acetic acid is added to water, most of the molecules remain intact; only a small fraction of them dissociate to form hydrogen ions and acetate ions. Lactic acid and carbonic acid are other examples of weak acids. There is no clear-cut division between strong and weak acids. Acids exhibit a range of strengths; some may be moderately dissociated in solution. (Do not confuse the terms strong and weak with the terms dilute and concentrated, which express acid concentration. For example, 5 M acetic acid is a concentrated solution of a weak acid; 0.005 M hydrochloric acid is a dilute solution of a strong acid.)

A *strong base* readily accepts hydrogen ions and combines with them; a *weak base* combines only slightly with hydrogen ions (i.e., it is a weak proton acceptor). The conjugate base of a strong acid will be a weak base, whereas the conjugate base of a weak acid will be a strong base. The hydroxide ion (OH^-) combines readily with hydrogen ions to form water; therefore hydroxide is a strong base. On the other hand, chloride ion (Cl^-), the conjugate base of the strong acid HCl, is a very weak base. (Although chloride is a base by the Brønsted-Lowry definition, in physiological systems it does not function as a base and is not usually regarded as such.)

A *salt* consists of the positive ion of a base and the negative ion of an acid. It is formed when an acid and base interact chemically in solution to neutralize each other. If hydroxide ions are present they combine with the hydrogen ions to form water. For example:

$$H^+Cl^- + Na^+OH^- \rightarrow Na^+Cl^- + H_2O$$
$$\text{acid} \qquad \text{base} \qquad \text{salt} \qquad \text{water}$$

Expressing Hydrogen-Ion Concentration

A common way of expressing the hydrogen-ion concentration of a solution is to use the pH scale, in which *pH* is defined as the negative logarithm of hydrogen-ion concentration:

$$pH = -\log [H^+]$$

The square brackets around H^+ in this equation (or any chemical equation) indicate concentration in moles per liter unless otherwise specified. The hydrogen-ion concentration of pure water under ordinary conditions is 0.0000001 (or 10^{-7}) mole/liter. The negative logarithm of 10^{-7} is 7, therefore water has a pH of 7. Since hydrogen ions and hydroxide ions are in equal concentration in pure water, it is neutral in reaction. When the pH is less than 7 the solution is acidic; when the pH is greater than 7 the solution is basic, or alkaline.

It is important to realize that pH varies inversely with the hydrogen-ion concentration. In other words, as the hydrogen-ion concentration increases and the solution becomes more acidic, the pH value decreases. Conversely, as the hydrogen-ion concentration decreases and the solution becomes less acidic (i.e., more alkaline), the pH value increases. Another point that is important to realize is that a small change in pH represents a relatively large change in hydrogen-ion concentration because pH is a logarithmic scale.

Although many people use the pH scale, others prefer to express hydrogen-ion concentration in molar terms. Since the concentration of hydrogen ions in the body fluids is so small (about one-millionth the concentration of other electrolytes, such as sodium, potassium, chloride, and bicarbonate), the hydrogen-ion concentration of the body fluids is expressed as nanomoles per liter or nanoequivalents per liter. A nanomole (nmol) is 10^{-9} mole (one-millionth of a millimole). Since the valence of the hydrogen ion is one, 1 nmol equals 1 nanoequivalent (nEq) for hydrogen ions. (See Chapter 11 under Composition of Body Fluids for a discussion of moles and equivalents.) The relationship between pH and hydrogen-ion concentration is shown in Table 15-1. The normal pH of the body fluids is about 7.4, which corresponds to a hydrogen-ion concentration of 40 nmol/liter. The range that is compatible with life is about pH 6.8 to pH 7.8, or a hydrogen-ion concentration of 160 to 16 nmol/liter, but the extremes of this range are associated with severe disturbances of homeostasis.

Buffers

A chemical *buffer* is a substance that prevents rapid or great change in the pH of a solution. A buffer system (or pair) usually consists of a weak acid together with its conjugate base. For example, the bicarbonate buffer system consists of carbonic acid (H_2CO_3) and bicarbonate (HCO_3^-). Since carbonic acid is a weak acid it is only slightly dis-

Table 15-1. Relationship between pH and Hydrogen Ion Concentration

pH	Hydrogen-Ion Concentration	
	moles/liter	nmol/liter
1	0.1	
2	0.01	
3	0.001	
4	0.0001	
5	0.00001	
6	0.000001	1000
6.8	0.000000160	160
6.9	0.000000125	125
7.0	0.000000100	100
7.1	0.000000080	80
7.2	0.000000063	63
7.3	0.000000050	50
7.4	0.000000040	40
7.5	0.000000032	32
7.6	0.000000026	26
7.7	0.000000020	20
7.8	0.000000016	16
8	0.000000010	10
9	0.000000001	1
10	0.0000000001	
11	0.00000000001	
12	0.000000000001	
13	0.0000000000001	
14	0.00000000000001	

sociated and there are very few hydrogen ions in the solution.

As an example of how a buffer works, consider what happens when hydrochloric acid (HCl) is added to a solution containing the bicarbonate buffer system. Since HCl is a strong acid it dissociates almost completely, releasing many hydrogen ions into the solution. If the solution were not buffered, this great increase in the number of hydrogen ions would change the pH drastically. But the hydrogen ions (protons) released by the HCl are immediately accepted by bicarbonate, which is the conjugate base of carbonic acid, and the weak acid H_2CO_3 is formed:

$$H^+ + Cl^- + HCO_3^- \rightarrow H_2CO_3 + Cl^-$$

(A cation such as Na^+ or K^+ would be present to maintain electrical neutrality.) In other words, the strong acid HCl is replaced by the weak acid H_2CO_3, which dissociates only slightly. Therefore, few hydrogen ions are added to the solution. Although the pH may change a little, the change is slight compared to what the change would be if no buffer were present. (It is important to realize that pH is determined only by the concentration of *free hydrogen ions;* hydrogen atoms that are chemically combined in a molecule do not contribute to pH.) If an excessive amount of HCl were added, however, all of the bicarbonate would be used up and there would be nothing to combine with the remaining hydrogen ions. Then the pH would show a large change.

If a strong base were added to the solution containing the bicarbonate buffer system, more carbonic acid would dissociate to release hydrogen ions as they are used in reaction with the base. Therefore any sharp drop in the hydrogen-ion concentration (or rise in pH) would be prevented.

A buffer system works most effectively when the concentration of the weak acid equals the concentration of the conjugate base.

REGULATION OF HYDROGEN-ION CONCENTRATION

The hydrogen-ion concentration of the body fluids must be maintained within narrow limits for normal cellular function. Hydrogen ions have a high reactivity, especially with proteins. When the hydrogen-ion concentration changes, proteins gain or lose hydrogen ions. This gain or loss alters the charge distribution on the protein molecule and can change the shape of the molecule. Consequently protein function is altered. Since all enzymes are proteins, and since cell function depends on the activity of enzymes, changes in hydrogen-ion concentration can alter cell metabolism by altering enzyme activity. Therefore it is essential that the body have some means of regulating the hydrogen-ion concentration.

Three processes are involved in regulating the pH of the body fluids: chemical buffering by the body buffer systems; control of the carbon dioxide concentration in the blood by alterations in pulmonary ventilation; and control of the bicarbonate concentration in the blood by changes in renal excretion of acid or alkali.

Sources of Acid and Base

Physiologically, two classes of acids are important in the body: carbonic acid (H_2CO_3) and fixed (noncarbonic) acids. Carbonic acid is in equilibrium with carbon dioxide and water in the body fluids and also can dissociate into hydrogen ions and bicarbonate ions. This relationship is expressed as follows:

$$CO_2 + H_2O \rightleftharpoons H_2CO_3 \rightleftharpoons H^+ + HCO_3^-$$

Large amounts of carbon dioxide are continuously formed from the metabolism of carbohydrates and fats. If this carbon dioxide were not excreted, a progressive accumulation of acid would occur in the body, because some of the carbon dioxide combines with water to form carbonic acid. Carbon dioxide is continuously eliminated through the lungs, however, and the carbon dioxide concentration of the blood is regulated by changes in the rate of pulmonary ventilation.

Fixed acids consist of all acids in the body other than carbonic acid, for example, sulfuric acid, lactic acid, and acetoacetic acid. The major production of fixed acids in the body comes from catabolism of proteins. Metabolism of sulfur-containing amino acids released by protein catabolism results in the formation of sulfuric acid. Lactic acid is produced as a result of glycolysis during vigorous exercise or under conditions of hypoxia. Usually the production of lactic acid results in only a transient increase in the amount of fixed acids in the body because the lactic acid is metabolized to

carbon dioxide and water after exercise stops or the hypoxic condition is corrected. Acetoacetic acid and β-hydroxybutyric acid (ketone bodies) are produced from fat catabolism during fasting or when carbohydrate cannot be metabolized normally (e.g., in diabetes mellitus). The amounts of fixed acids that are produced each day are much less than the amount of carbon dioxide that is produced. In addition to the fixed acids produced in the body, some may be ingested in the diet. Hydrogen ions produced from the dissociation of fixed acids are excreted by the kidneys.

The major source of alkali production in the body is the catabolism of dietary organic anions such as lactate, citrate, and isocitrate to carbon dioxide and water. These organic anions are usually accompanied by the cations potassium and sodium. They are present in all foods but are particularly abundant in fruits and vegetables. The catabolism of these organic anions involves the consumption of hydrogen ions, which is equivalent to the production of alkali. For example, the net effect of lactate catabolism is given in the following equation:

$$C_3H_5O_3^- + H^+ + 3O_2 \rightarrow 3CO_2 + 3H_3O$$

For people who eat a large amount of protein (e.g., a high meat intake), the production of sulfuric acid and other fixed acids is usually much greater than the amount of alkali produced from the catabolism of dietary organic anions. Therefore these people have a net production of fixed acid. On the other hand, for people whose intake of fruits and vegetables greatly exceeds meat intake (or for people who are vegetarians), the production of alkali due to organic anion catabolism is greater than the production of fixed acid. Therefore these people have a net production of alkali, which must be eliminated by the kidneys.

Body Buffers

The major buffer systems in the body are the bicarbonate system, the phosphate system, the proteins, and hemoglobin. The body buffers minimize changes in the pH of the body fluids until excess hydrogen ions or base can be excreted. Buffering is a *temporary* defense; if the excess acid or base were not excreted, the buffering capacity of the body fluids would be diminished as the buffers are used. The excess acid or base must be eliminated from the body to restore the members of the buffer pairs to their normal concentrations.

The *bicarbonate buffer pair* consists of the weak acid H_2CO_3 and its conjugate base HCO_3^-, as previously mentioned. It is the major buffer of the extracellular fluid (ECF), particularly in the interstitial fluid compartment. Although the bicarbonate system is an important buffer for fixed (noncarbonic) acids and for alkali, it cannot buffer carbonic acid. If the hydrogen ions that are released from carbonic acid combine with bicarbonate, carbonic acid is simply regenerated.

The amount of carbonic acid in the body fluids is very small, but it is in equilibrium with a much larger amount of dissolved carbon dioxide:

$$CO_2 + H_2O \rightleftharpoons H_2CO_3$$

In a chemical equilibrium, the relative proportions of the reactants and products remain constant. (For example, in the general reaction $A + B \rightleftharpoons C + D$, $[C][D]/[A][B]$ = constant.) If the concentration of one substance changes, reaction occurs until the equilibrium proportions are reestablished. In the carbonic acid–carbon dioxide equilibrium, if the carbonic acid concentration decreases or the carbon dioxide concentration increases, more carbon dioxide reacts with water and more carbonic acid is formed (i.e., the reaction, as written above, shifts to the right). Conversely, if the carbonic acid concentration increases, or the carbon dioxide concentration decreases, the reaction shifts to the left. Therefore, the concentration of carbonic acid plus that of dissolved carbon dioxide forms the total "carbonic acid pool" that is available for buffer action. The concentration of carbonic acid in the body fluids is very small and most of the carbonic acid pool is determined by the amount of dissolved carbon dioxide. (The parameter that is actually measured in clinical determinations is the partial pressure of carbon dioxide, PCO_2. The concentration of dissolved carbon dioxide, in millimoles per liter, equals 0.03 PCO_2.)

Earlier it was stated that maximal buffering occurs when the concentrations of the members of the buffer pair are equal. The bicarbonate concentration in the ECF is approximately 20 times the concentration of the total carbonic acid pool, therefore the bicarbonate buffer system in the body is not working in its optimal range. Despite this fact, the bicarbonate buffer system is very important because the concentrations of the members of the buffer pair can be regulated independently. The carbon dioxide concentration (i.e., the total carbonic acid pool) of the ECF is regulated by changes in pulmonary ventilation, and the bicarbonate concentration is regulated by changes in renal excretion. In addition, a change in the bicarbonate buffer system will be reflected by changes in the other buffer systems. All buffer pairs in a solution are in equilibrium with the same hydrogen-ion concentration. (This fact is called the *isohydric principle.*) A change in the hydrogen-ion concentration affects all of the buffers in the solution, changing the molar ratio of weak acid to conjugate base for each buffer pair. Therefore, if the hydrogen-ion concentration of the ECF is to be kept constant, the ratio of the carbonic acid concentration (i.e., the total carbonic acid pool) to bicarbonate concentration must be kept constant.

The *phosphate buffer system* consists mainly of the dihydrogen phosphate ($H_2PO_4^-$) and monohydrogen phosphate (HPO_4^{2-}) buffer pair. Dihydrogen phosphate is a weak acid and monohydrogen phosphate is its conjugate base:

$$H_2PO_4^- \rightleftharpoons H^+ + HPO_4^{2-}$$

In addition to this inorganic phosphate buffer pair, several organic phosphate compounds can function as buffers in the body. The concentration of phosphates in the ECF is low, therefore the phosphate buffer system is not an important extracellular buffer. The concentration of phosphates within the cells is high, however, and phosphate is a major intracellular buffer.

The *proteins* actually consist of a series of buffer pairs because the side chains of some of the amino acids that make up protein molecules can accept or release hydrogen ions and act as buffers. The proteins are powerful buffers over a wide range of pH. The concentration of protein inside the cells is high and so the proteins are important intracellular buffers. In addition, the plasma proteins contribute to the buffering of the blood.

A protein molecule is a polyanion; that is, it carries many negative charges. When an acid is being buffered, certain amino acid side chains accept hydrogen ions and the protein becomes less anionic (i.e., it has fewer negative charges). When alkali is being buffered, hydrogen ions are released from some of the amino acid side chains and the protein becomes more polyanionic (e.g., it has more negative charges). Although the protein buffer system is very complicated, it is usually symbolized as a simple buffer pair, with HPr representing the weak acid and Pr^- (proteinate) representing the conjugate base. The equilibrium is written as

$$HPr \rightleftharpoons H^+ + Pr^-$$

Hemoglobin of the red blood cells is a protein buffer that is very important in buffering carbonic acid in the blood. It is discussed later, under Buffering of Carbonic Acid.

In addition to the intracellular and extracellular buffers just mentioned, the *carbonate in bone* can function as a buffer. When acid is being buffered, carbonate (CO_3^{2-}) is released from bone into the ECF. The release of carbonate is accompanied by the release of calcium or sodium ions from bone or by the uptake of phosphate by bone. When alkali is being buffered (e.g., excess bicarbonate), more carbonate is deposited in bone. These processes may be summarized as follows:

$$Bone{-}Ca{-}O{-}CO_2{-}Na+ H^+ + Cl^-$$
$$\rightleftharpoons Bone{-}Ca{-}Cl+ Na^+ + HCO_3^-$$

Buffering of Fixed Acids

Fixed acids are produced within the cells, therefore the hydrogen ions released from these acids are initially buffered by the intracellular protein and phosphate buffer systems. The acids are released from the cells and enter the ECF, where they are primarily buffered by the bicarbonate buffer system. For example, sulfuric acid (H_2SO_4) produced from the metabolism of sulfur-containing amino acids is buffered as follows:

$$H_2SO_4 + 2HCO_3^- \rightarrow SO_4^{2-} + 2H_2CO_3$$

Although this buffering minimizes the increase in the hydrogen-ion concentration of the ECF, renal excretion of hydrogen ions must be adjusted to match acid production, otherwise the bicarbonate concentration will be progressively depleted.

Buffering of Carbonic Acid

The metabolic processes involved in energy production in the body result in the formation of large amounts of carbon dioxide each day. As stated earlier, some of this carbon dioxide combines with water to form carbonic acid. Normally the amount of carbon dioxide eliminated through the lungs balances the amount of carbon dioxide produced. Until it is eliminated, however, the carbon dioxide being transported in the blood must be buffered to prevent large changes in the pH.

The processes occurring as carbon dioxide enters the systemic capillaries are shown in Figure 15-1. As arterial blood enters the systemic capillaries, carbon dioxide from the tissues enters the blood. Simultaneously, oxygen is released from hemoglobin and diffuses from the blood into the tissues. The carbon dioxide entering the blood diffuses first into the plasma, where a small amount of carbon dioxide combines with water to form carbonic acid. The carbonic acid dissociates to give bicarbonate and hydrogen ions; the hydrogen ions are buffered by the plasma proteins. The for-

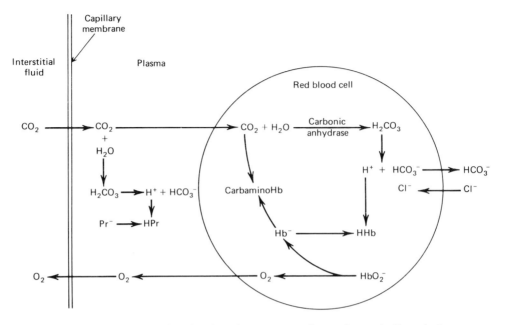

Figure 15-1. *Uptake of carbon dioxide in the systemic capillaries, showing buffering by hemoglobin. Negative charges would be balanced by positive sodium ions (in plasma) or potassium ions (in red blood cells).*

mation of carbonic acid in the plasma occurs slowly, however, and most of the carbon dioxide diffuses into the red blood cells.

Some of the carbon dioxide entering the erythrocytes reacts with an amino group of hemoglobin (Hb) to form carbaminohemoglobin and some of it reacts with water to form carbonic acid. The red blood cells contain an enzyme called *carbonic anhydrase*, which catalyzes the formation of carbonic acid from carbon dioxide and water. Therefore this reaction occurs much more quickly in the red blood cells than in the plasma. The carbonic acid dissociates to give hydrogen ions and bicarbonate ions. Much of the bicarbonate diffuses out of the erythrocytes into the plasma. Since bicarbonate ions are negatively charged, chloride anions diffuse from the plasma into the red blood cells to maintain electrical balance. This movement of chloride in exchange for bicarbonate is called the *chloride shift.*

The hydrogen ions that are released from carbonic acid in the red blood cells are buffered by hemoglobin. Deoxygenated (reduced) hemoglobin is a weaker acid than carbonic acid, otherwise this buffering could not occur. (In other words, the conjugate base form of hemoglobin has greater affinity for hydrogen ions than bicarbonate does.) This reaction can be symbolized as follows:

$$Hb^- + H^+ \rightleftharpoons HHb$$

As a result of this buffering, the pH of venous blood is only slightly lower than the pH of arterial blood.

In the pulmonary capillaries these reactions are reversed (Fig. 15-2). Oxygen diffuses from the alveoli into the blood and combines with hemoglobin in the red blood cells. The properties of hemoglobin are altered when oxygen combines with it. Oxyhemoglobin is a stronger acid than

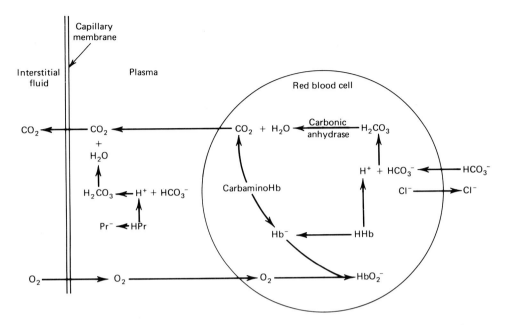

Figure 15-2. *Release of carbon dioxide in the pulmonary capillaries, showing buffering by hemoglobin.*

both reduced hemoglobin and carbonic acid. Therefore, as oxygen is taken up, hydrogen ions are released from the hemoglobin. These hydrogen ions are accepted by bicarbonate to form carbonic acid. The carbonic acid is converted to carbon dioxide and water; this reaction is catalyzed by carbonic anhydrase in the red blood cells. The carbon dioxide then diffuses into the alveoli.

Pulmonary Control of Hydrogen-Ion Concentration

Changes in the carbon dioxide concentration in the body fluids influence the hydrogen-ion concentration because of the equilibrium between carbon dioxide, carbonic acid, and bicarbonate:

$$CO_2 + H_2O \rightleftharpoons H_2CO_3 \rightleftharpoons H^+ + HCO_3^-$$

Changes in pulmonary ventilation alter the rate of excretion of carbon dioxide and therefore influence the hydrogen-ion concentration of the body fluids. If ventilation increases, more carbon dioxide is eliminated and the amount of carbon dioxide dissolved in the body fluids decreases. Consequently the reaction is pulled to the left and the hydrogen-ion concentration of the body fluids is reduced:

$$\downarrow CO_2 + H_2O \leftarrow H_2CO_3 \leftarrow H^+ + HCO_3^-$$

Conversely, if ventilation decreases, less carbon dioxide is eliminated and it accumulates in the body fluids. Consequently the reaction is pushed to the right and the hydrogen-ion concentration increases:

$$\uparrow CO_2 + H_2O \rightarrow H_2CO_3 \rightarrow H^+ + HCO_3^-$$

Normally, pulmonary ventilation is adjusted so that carbon dioxide is eliminated from the body as fast as it is produced and the carbon dioxide concentration of the arterial blood is kept constant. The negative feedback control mechanism by which the arterial PCO_2 is regulated is described in Chapter 1.

Two sets of receptors are involved in the control of ventilation. Peripheral receptors of secondary importance are located in the carotid and aortic bodies. These receptors respond mainly to a decrease in the arterial PO_2 (partial pressure of oxygen) and to a lesser extent to an increase in the PCO_2 and an increase in the hydrogen-ion concentration (i.e., a decrease in the pH). Under usual conditions, however, impulses from these receptors have only a minor influence on ventilation.

The primary receptors are central chemoreceptors located in the brain. A high arterial PCO_2 stimulates these receptors and brings about an increase in ventilation. Conversely, when the PCO_2 is low, ventilation is decreased. The central chemoreceptors are influenced more by the PCO_2 of the cerebrospinal fluid (CSF) than by the PCO_2 of the blood. Carbon dioxide diffuses freely across the blood-brain and blood-CSF barriers, so that a change in the arterial PCO_2 is reflected by a similar change in the PCO_2 of the CSF. Unlike blood, the CSF lacks nonbicarbonate buffers. Therefore a change in the PCO_2 causes a greater change in the hydrogen-ion concentration of the CSF than of the blood. It appears that the response of the central chemoreceptors to changes in the PCO_2 is mediated by this change in the hydrogen-ion concentration of the CSF.

An increase in the hydrogen-ion concentration due to an increase in the amount of fixed acids also stimulates ventilation, even if the arterial PCO_2 is normal. Consequently more carbon dioxide is eliminated, the arterial PCO_2 decreases, the reaction described previously shifts to the left, and the hydrogen-ion concentration is brought back toward normal. Conversely, a decreased hydrogen-ion concentration usually reduces ventilation. Consequently, carbon dioxide accumulates in the body, the carbonic acid level of the body fluids increases, and the hydrogen-ion concentration is brought back toward normal.

Renal Control of Hydrogen-Ion Concentration

The pH of the urine can vary from 4.4 to 8.0, depending on the need to conserve or excrete hydrogen ions. For people who eat meat (i.e., the usual Western diet), there is a net production of acid in the body. This acid is excreted in the urine, resulting in a urine with a pH of about 6. Vegetarians have a net production of alkali in the body, resulting in excretion of bicarbonate and an alkaline urine.

Production of an Acid Urine

When excess acid is present in the body, the kidneys excrete more hydrogen ions in the urine. For each hydrogen ion excreted, a bicarbonate ion is reabsorbed. Thus, acid is excreted and base is conserved in order to maintain the optimum hydrogen-ion concentration in the ECF.

Acidification of the urine depends on active secretion of hydrogen ions in the proximal and distal convoluted tubules and collecting ducts. The gradient of hydrogen-ion concentration that can be established between the peritubular fluid (i.e., ECF) and the fluid of the tubular lumen is limited; the kidneys are unable to produce a urine more acid than pH 4.4. Therefore, the presence of urinary buffers that combine with the secreted hydrogen ions and prevent a sharp drop in the urinary pH increases the amount of acid that can be excreted. The most important buffers in the urine are phosphate and ammonia.

The mechanism of hydrogen-ion secretion and bicarbonate reabsorption is shown in Figure 15-3. Within the renal tubular epithelial cells, carbon dioxide combines with water to form carbonic acid. This reaction is catalyzed by the enzyme carbonic anhydrase. The carbonic acid dissociates to give hydrogen ions and bicarbonate ions. The hydrogen ions are secreted from the cells into the tubular fluid. For each hydrogen ion secreted a sodium ion is taken up from the tubular fluid and reabsorbed. This exchange of sodium for hydrogen

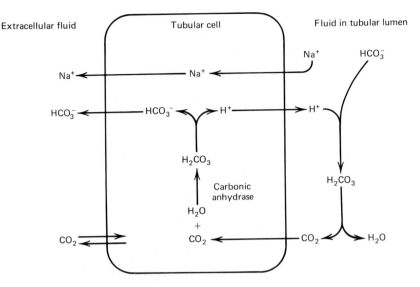

Figure 15-3. *Mechanism of hydrogen-ion secretion and bicarbonate reabsorption by the renal tubules. Note that the net concentration of free hydrogen ions in the tubular fluid does not change because the secreted hydrogen ions combine with bicarbonate in the tubular fluid.*

appears to be a loosely coupled process that occurs to maintain electrical balance. The secreted hydrogen ions combine with bicarbonate in the tubular fluid to form carbonic acid. This carbonic acid is converted to carbon dioxide and water. (In the proximal tubules, this reaction is catalyzed by carbonic anhydrase that is present on the luminal surface of the tubular cells. Carbonic anhydrase is not present in the distal tubular lumen, although it is present inside the cells.) Most of the carbon dioxide diffuses back into the tubular cells. The bicarbonate that is generated within the cells diffuses into the ECF surrounding the tubule; it is accompanied by the sodium that is reabsorbed from the tubular fluid. The *net effect of this process is that bicarbonate is reabsorbed,* although the bicarbonate ions that are in the tubular fluid are not the ones that enter the ECF.

About 85% to 90% of the bicarbonate that enters the glomerular filtrate is reabsorbed in the proximal tubule by this mechanism. No net change in the hydrogen-ion concentration of the tubular fluid occurs at this point. In the distal tubules and collecting ducts this process continues until all of the filtered bicarbonate is reabsorbed. Any excess hydrogen ions that are secreted react with other substances in the tubular fluid and the urine is acidified. These hydrogen ions also come from the dissociation of carbonic acid within the tubular cells, so that for every secreted hydrogen ion that combines with some substance other than bicarbonate in the tubular fluid, a new bicarbonate is added to the plasma (i.e., the kidneys generate bicarbonate).

Some of the excess hydrogen ions combine with phosphate or accompany other anions (e.g., sulfate) in the tubular fluid and are excreted as *titratable acid.* (Combination of hydrogen ions with sulfate produces sulfuric acid, which is a strong acid. Therefore the sulfate and hydrogen ions remain dissociated; the free hydrogen ions lower the pH of the urine.)

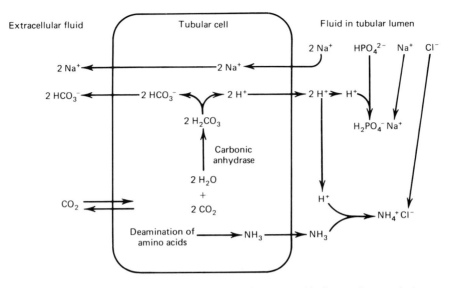

Figure 15-4. *Generation of bicarbonate by the renal tubules and buffering of urinary hydrogen ion by phosphate and ammonia.*

Some of the hydrogen ions combine with ammonia (NH_3) to form ammonium ions (NH_4^+). The ammonia is generated within the tubular cells from the deamination of amino acids, particularly glutamine. The ammonia formed within the cells diffuses into the tubular fluid, where it combines with hydrogen ions to form ammonium ions. The ammonium ions are accompanied by chloride or other anions in the tubular fluid, so that neutral ammonium salts are excreted. This mechanism is very important because it allows acid to be excreted without lowering the pH of the urine. Therefore more hydrogen ions can be secreted into the tubular fluid. If the hydrogen-ion concentration of the ECF is increased for more than one or two days, formation of ammonia by the tubular cells increases, so that more acid can be excreted. The mechanism of this adaptation is not known.

Figure 15-4 illustrates the buffering of the urine by phosphate and ammonia. Note that for each hydrogen ion secreted a bicarbonate ion is added to the ECF. Therefore, the *net effect of these reactions is to increase the ECF bicarbonate concentration.*

Factors Influencing Hydrogen-Ion Secretion

Among the factors that influence the rate of hydrogen-ion secretion by the renal tubular cells are the concentrations of carbon dioxide and potassium in the ECF, the amount of aldosterone available, and some drugs. Whatever increases hydrogen-ion secretion will also increase bicarbonate reabsorption because these processes are linked, as just described. Conversely, whatever decreases hydrogen-ion secretion will decrease bicarbonate reabsorption.

Since the hydrogen ions secreted by the tubular epithelial cells come from the dissociation of carbonic acid, the amount of carbon dioxide available to form carbonic acid will influence hydrogen-ion secretion. When the carbon dioxide concentration of the ECF is elevated, carbonic acid is formed at a faster rate and more hydrogen ions are secreted. Conversely, when the ECF carbon dioxide concentration is decreased, formation of carbonic acid proceeds more slowly and fewer hydrogen ions are secreted.

In the distal tubules and collecting ducts,

potassium ions as well as hydrogen ions are secreted in exchange for sodium-ion reabsorption (see Chapter 16 under Potassium Intake and Excretion). When the level of potassium in the body fluids is increased, more potassium is secreted and fewer hydrogen ions are secreted. Conversely, a low level of potassium results in decreased potassium secretion and enhanced hydrogen-ion secretion.

Aldosterone increases reabsorption of sodium by the distal renal tubules (see Chapter 12). Since hydrogen-ion secretion is coupled with sodium reabsorption, increased reabsorption of sodium enhances hydrogen-ion secretion. Therefore, any factor that increases aldosterone secretion (e.g., a low circulating blood volume) will result in increased hydrogen-ion secretion. Conversely, decreased aldosterone secretion leads to diminished sodium reabsorption and decreased renal tubular secretion of hydrogen ions.

Many diuretic drugs, particularly the carbonic anhydrase inhibitors, decrease hydrogen-ion secretion and bicarbonate reabsorption.

Production of an Alkaline Urine

An increase in the amount of alkali in the body results in an elevated plasma bicarbonate concentration. This situation alters the carbon dioxide–carbonic acid–bicarbonate equilibrium and results in an increase in the ratio of bicarbonate to dissolved carbon dioxide. Consequently the amount of bicarbonate entering the glomerular filtrate is greater than the quantity of hydrogen ions secreted into the tubular fluid, and not all the filtered bicarbonate can be reabsorbed. (Bicarbonate reabsorption depends on hydrogen-ion secretion, as previously described.) The excess bicarbonate is excreted in the urine, making the urine alkaline.

Complementary Functions of Pulmonary and Renal Control Mechanisms

In the discussion of the bicarbonate buffer system earlier, it was stated that the *ratio* of the total carbonic acid pool (i.e., the concentration of dissolved CO_2) to the bicarbonate concentration must be kept constant to maintain a constant pH in the ECF. If the ECF hydrogen-ion concentration is increased (i.e., the pH is decreased), it can be returned toward normal by decreasing the carbon dioxide concentration and/or by increasing the bicarbonate concentration. Conversely, if the ECF hydrogen-ion concentration is decreased (i.e., the pH is increased), it can be brought back toward normal by raising the carbon dioxide concentration and/or decreasing the bicarbonate concentration. The carbon dioxide concentration (i.e., the total carbonic acid pool) is controlled by the pulmonary mechanism, whereas the kidneys control the bicarbonate concentration.

When excess acid enters the ECF it reacts with bicarbonate to form carbonic acid, thus lowering the bicarbonate concentration. In response to this situation, pulmonary ventilation increases and more carbon dioxide is eliminated. Thus the desired ratio of carbonic acid to bicarbonate is maintained, but the concentrations of both carbon dioxide and bicarbonate are decreased. In the kidneys, the quantity of hydrogen ions secreted exceeds the amount of bicarbonate filtered, so that not only is all the filtered bicarbonate reabsorbed but bicarbonate also is generated by the kidneys and added to the ECF. This mechanism restores the plasma bicarbonate concentration to its usual level.

Conversely, when excess alkali is present in the ECF, the bicarbonate concentration is elevated. The pulmonary response is decreased ventilation, so that carbon dioxide is retained in the body and the level of the carbonic acid pool rises. Thus, the carbonic acid/bicarbonate ratio is returned toward normal. The kidneys excrete the excess bicarbonate and the bicarbonate concentration of the ECF is restored to its usual level.

The pulmonary mechanism responds immediately to changes in the ECF hydrogen-ion concentration. It is not completely effective at restoring the hydrogen-ion concentration to the desired level, however, because as the hydrogen-ion concentration returns toward normal, the stimulus for increased or decreased ventilation is diminished. The renal mechanism, on the other hand, takes longer to achieve its effects (one to several days) but is capable of restoring the ECF hydrogen-ion concentration to normal if the excess of acid or alkali is not too great. There is a limit to the amount of acid or base the kidneys can handle; if this limit is exceeded, severe disturbances of acid-base balance can occur.

ACID-BASE IMBALANCE

The important parameters determining a person's acid-base status are the pH (or hydrogen-ion concentration), PCO_2, and bicarbonate concentration of the ECF. The normal range of values for these parameters in arterial blood are: pH 7.37 to 7.43; hydrogen-ion concentration 37 to 43 nEq/liter; PCO_2 36 to 44 mm Hg; and bicarbonate concentration 22 to 26 mEq/liter. For venous blood the normal ranges are: pH 7.32 to 7.38; hydrogen-ion concentration 42 to 48 nEq/liter; PCO_2 42 to 50 mm Hg; and bicarbonate 23 to 27 mEq/liter. These "normal" ranges are based on populations eating the usual Western diet, which contains meat. These people have a net production of acid in the body, as mentioned previously. For vegetarians the normal pH and bicarbonate concentration may be slightly higher, due to a net production of alkali in the body.

The bicarbonate concentration of the blood is not measured directly; most laboratories measure the total carbon dioxide content. Total carbon dioxide equals the concentration of bicarbonate plus the concentration of dissolved carbon dioxide (i.e., 0.03 PCO_2) plus the concentration of carbonic acid. Since the carbonic acid concentration is very small, it is usually ignored. The bicarbonate concentration then equals total CO_2 minus 0.03 PCO_2. (The bicarbonate concentration can also be calculated from the Henderson-Hasselbalch equation when the pH and PCO_2 are known, but a dis-

cussion of this equation is beyond the scope of this book.)

Disturbances of acid-base balance can be considered in terms of changes in the PCO_2 and changes in the bicarbonate concentration of the ECF. As discussed previously, the ratio of the PCO_2 (i.e., total carbonic acid pool) to the bicarbonate concentration reflects the hydrogen-ion concentration. Also, the body regulates the ECF hydrogen-ion concentration through pulmonary elimination or retention of carbon dioxide and renal excretion or generation of bicarbonate.

Acid-base imbalances in which the primary change is in the PCO_2 are designated respiratory disturbances. When the primary change is in the bicarbonate concentration the acid-base disturbance is designated metabolic. Whenever a change in the PCO_2 or bicarbonate concentration occurs, the body responds with adaptive mechanisms to counteract the change, as already described. These adaptive responses tend to offset any change in pH (or hydrogen-ion concentration) that would be caused by the primary disturbance. Therefore it is possible to have an acid-base disturbance with a normal blood pH or hydrogen-ion concentration. The actual pH will depend on the magnitude of the primary disturbance and the extent to which the adaptive response to that initial disturbance is able to counteract the change; usually the adaptive response is not able to return the pH completely to normal. When the adaptive mechanisms have returned the pH toward normal, the acid-base disturbance is said to be *compensated.*

Acidosis is an abnormal condition that tends to produce an increase in the hydrogen-ion concentration (or decrease in pH) of the ECF. In *metabolic acidosis* the primary disturbance is a decrease in the bicarbonate concentration due to a loss of bicarbonate from the ECF or a gain of fixed acids by the ECF. In *respiratory acidosis* the primary disturbance is an increase in the PCO_2 (i.e., the total carbonic acid pool) due to impaired elimination of carbon dioxide.

Alkalosis is an abnormal condition that tends to

Table 15-2. Characteristics of Acid-Base Imbalances

	Metabolic Acidosis	Respiratory Acidosis	Metabolic Alkalosis	Respiratory Alkalosis
Primary disturbance	Decreased $[HCO_3^-]$	Increased PCO_2	Increased $[HCO_3^-]$	Decreased PCO_2
Adaptive response	Decreased PCO_2	Increased $[HCO_3^-]$	Increased PCO_2	Decreased $[HCO_3^-]$
pH	Decreased	Decreased	Increased	Increased
Hydrogen-ion concentration	Increased	Increased	Decreased	Decreased

produce a decrease in the hydrogen-ion concentration (or increase in pH) of the ECF. In *metabolic alkalosis* the primary disturbance is an increase in the bicarbonate concentration due to a gain of bicarbonate by the ECF or a loss of fixed acid from the ECF. In *respiratory alkalosis* the primary disturbance is a decrease in the PCO_2 due to excessive elimination of carbon dioxide.

A *single*, or *simple*, acid-base disturbance is caused by one primary factor. Characteristics of the four single acid-base disturbances are summarized in Table 15-2. When two primary factors are responsible for an acid-base imbalance, the disturbance is designated as *mixed*. For example, a person with uncontrolled diabetes mellitus may have a simple metabolic acidosis due to the accumulation of ketone bodies in the ECF. If this person also has respiratory insufficiency due to chronic lung disease, she or he may have a mixed metabolic and respiratory acidosis.

An actual decrease in the pH of the arterial blood is called *acidemia;* an increase in the arterial pH is *alkalemia*. *Hypercapnia* refers to an excess of carbon dioxide in the blood (i.e., an increased arterial PCO_2). *Hypocapnia* refers to a low arterial PCO_2.

Acid-base disturbances are described in terms of changes in the ECF, but many of the effects of these disturbances are due to changes in intracellular pH, which alter cell function. The intracellular pH is lower than the pH of the ECF.

Also, the pH within the cell is not uniform, because the cell is subdivided into discrete organelles with different functions (e.g., mitochondria, endoplasmic reticulum, nucleus). Clinically, it is the pH of the ECF (i.e., blood) that is measured, because measurement of the intracellular pH is difficult. Changes in the pH of the ECF, however, usually reflect parallel changes in the intracellular pH. When the pH of the ECF is decreased (i.e., the hydrogen-ion concentration is increased), some of the excess hydrogen ions enter the cells, causing a decrease in intracellular pH as well. When hydrogen ions enter the cells, potassium ions leave the cells to maintain electrical balance, and so the ECF potassium concentration may be elevated. (Sodium ions also move out of the cells, but the intracellular sodium concentration is normally so low compared to the concentration in the ECF that this efflux of sodium ions is insignificant.) When the extracellular pH is increased (i.e., the hydrogen-ion concentration is decreased), hydrogen ions move out of the cells, causing a parallel increase in the intracellular pH. Potassium and sodium ions enter the cells to maintain electrical balance.

Metabolic Acidosis

In metabolic acidosis, the pH tends to be low (i.e., the hydrogen-ion concentration is increased). The primary disturbance is a decrease in the bicarbonate concentration. The adaptive response is to increase ventilation; therefore the PCO_2 is also decreased.

Metabolic acidosis can be classified according to the *anion gap*. As stated in Chapter 11, when electrolyte concentrations are given in milliequivalents per liter, total anions equal total cations. Routine electrolyte determinations, however, do not include all of the electrolytes in the plasma. Usually only sodium, potassium, chloride, and total CO_2 (i.e., bicarbonate) are measured. The anion gap represents the anions that are present in the plasma but are not usually measured (e.g., phosphate, sulfate, proteinate, and creatinine). The actual gap equals the sum of sodium and potassium (i.e., cations) minus the sum of chloride and bicarbonate (i.e., measured anions). In everyday practice, however, potassium is usually deleted from the calculation; that is, the sum of chloride and bicarbonate is subtracted from sodium. Using this latter calculation, the normal anion gap is about 12 mEq/liter.

In some cases of metabolic acidosis, the chloride concentration increases to compensate for the decrease in bicarbonate. In this situation, the anion gap is normal. In other cases the bicarbonate concentration is decreased, the chloride is normal, and the anion gap is increased. The increased anion gap may be due to an increased concentration of an anion that is normally present in small amounts (e.g., lactate from the dissociation of lactic acid; acetoacetate and β-hydroxybutyrate from the dissociation of ketone bodies) or due to the presence of an unusual (abnormal) anion as a result of exogenous poisoning (e.g., salicylates; formate from the metabolism of methanol).

Causes

Metabolic acidosis can be caused by excessive loss of bicarbonate, excessive production of fixed acids in the body, accumulation of exogenous acids (or exogenous toxins that produce acid when metabolized), or decreased excretion of hydrogen ions.

Excessive loss of bicarbonate. Bicarbonate can be lost from the gastrointestinal tract or through the kidneys.

Digestive secretions such as bile, pancreatic juice, and secretions of the small intestine contain high concentrations of bicarbonate (higher than the concentration in plasma). Therefore, losses of these secretions as a result of diarrhea, tube drainage, or fistulas can lead to bicarbonate depletion.

Decreased reabsorption of bicarbonate in the proximal renal tubules produces a condition called *proximal renal tubular acidosis* (proximal RTA). As stated earlier, normally about 85% to 90% of the filtered bicarbonate is reabsorbed in the proximal tubules in exchange for secretion of hydrogen ions. This process can also occur in the distal tubules, but the capacity of the distal tubules to reabsorb bicarbonate is low compared to the capacity of the proximal tubules. When the proximal tubules fail to reabsorb most of the bicarbonate, the amount of filtered bicarbonate reaching the distal tubules exceeds their capacity to reabsorb it. Consequently bicarbonate is lost in the urine and the urine is alkaline, but the bicarbonate concentration of the ECF drops and acidosis develops. When the plasma bicarbonate concentration falls to 15-20 mEq/liter, the amount of filtered bicarbonate no longer exceeds the reabsorptive capacity of the renal tubules, a new steady state is established, and the kidneys are able to produce an acid urine.

Proximal RTA is seen most commonly in children. It can occur secondarily to a wide variety of metabolic disorders. In some cases it is an inherited defect; often the cause is not known. Proximal reabsorption of a variety of other substances, such as phosphate, amino acids, and glucose, may also be impaired.

Excessive production of fixed acids. Fixed acids are buffered by the bicarbonate buffer system. When production of fixed acids increases, the bicarbonate in the ECF is consumed. Therefore acidosis will develop if the kidneys are unable to excrete the excess hydrogen ions and generate bicarbonate at a rate fast enough to match acid production. Development of metabolic acidosis by this mechanism is usually due to overproduction of either the ketoacids (ketone bodies) β-hydroxybutyric acid and acetoaecetic acid, or lactic acid.

Production of ketoacids results from incomplete oxidation of fatty acids. The metabolic acidosis that occurs is called *ketosis,* or ketoacidosis. The most common cause of ketosis is diabetes mellitus (see Chapter 18). Starvation is another cause (see Chapter 17). Mild ketosis may develop during a short-term fast. Occasionally ketoacidosis occurs as a result of alcohol (ethanol) ingestion combined with poor dietary intake. Ethanol inhibits gluconeogenesis (formation of glucose from noncarbohydrate sources) by the liver and enhances fat catabolism. These factors, together with decreased dietary intake of carbohydrate, favor the oxidation of fat rather than glucose for energy and result in increased production of ketoacids.

Lactic acid is the end product of anaerobic glycolysis (see Chapter 10 under Cellular Respiration). Some lactic acid is always being produced in the body. The lactic acid dissociates into hydrogen ions, which are buffered by bicarbonate, and lactate. The lactate is carried to the liver, where some of it is metabolized to carbon dioxide and water, and some of it is converted back to glucose. Both reactions produce bicarbonate and thus restore the bicarbonate that was used in buffering the acid. The capacity of the liver to metabolize lactate may be exceeded, however, if lactic acid production is increased. The result will be *lactic acidosis.*

Lactic acidosis can occur when delivery of oxygen to the tissues is impaired. The most common cause is shock (see Chapter 14). Excess lactic acid may also be produced in diabetes mellitus, acute pancreatitis, and leukemia. Toxic doses of phenformin (an oral hypoglycemic agent) can also increase lactic acid production. Occasionally lactic acidosis occurs in the absence of any obvious underlying disorder (*idiopathic lactic acidosis*).

Accumulation of exogenous acids. Excessive amounts of acid may accumulate in the body as a result of overdoses of certain drugs, ingestion of certain poisons, or administration of certain hyperalimentation fluids.

Aspirin (acetylsalicylic acid) is converted to salicylic acid within the body. Excessive amounts of salicylic acid not only have a direct effect on the pH of the ECF but also cause organic acids to accumulate by interfering with carbohydrate metabolism. In addition, salicylates stimulate the respiratory center, causing hyperventilation and a decreased PCO_2. Therefore, salicylate intoxication may produce metabolic acidosis or respiratory alkalosis, or a mixed acid-base disturbance. The effects of salicylate poisoning on acid-base balance are influenced by the age and the previous condition of the person and by the severity of the poisoning.

Overdosage of ammonium chloride can cause metabolic acidosis because hydrogen ions are released as the ammonium ions are metabolized to urea in the liver. Metabolism of paraldehyde produces organic acids. Therefore overdosage with this drug can also produce metabolic acidosis.

Methanol (wood alcohol) is converted to formaldehyde and formic acid in the body. Ingestion of this toxin leads to metabolic acidosis due to accumulation of formic acid. Ethylene glycol (the major component of antifreeze) is another poison that is metabolized to acidic products and produces metabolic acidosis.

Some parenteral hyperalimentation fluids containing synthetic amino acids have more cationic amino acids (e.g., arginine, lysine, and histidine) than anionic amino acids or other organic anions. (The extra cations are balanced by inorganic anions such as sulfate and chloride.) Metabolism of the cationic amino acids releases hydrogen ions, whereas metabolism of organic anions consumes hydrogen ions. Therefore, a net excess of hydrogen ions is produced due to metabolism of the extra cationic amino acids, and acidosis may result.

Decreased excretion of hydrogen ions. Urinary excretion of hydrogen ions is impaired in renal failure, in distal renal tubular acidosis, and in hypoaldosteronism.

Chronic progressive renal disease from any cause usually produces some degree of metabolic acidosis as the glomerular filtration rate is decreased. The major cause for the decreased ability of the kidneys to excrete acid appears to be decreased production of ammonia to buffer the secreted hydrogen ions. In some people, impaired reabsorption of bicarbonate in the proximal tubules may be a contributing factor. Kidney diseases that primarily affect tubular function (e.g., chronic pyelonephritis) usually cause a greater impairment of hydrogen-ion excretion than diseases that primarily affect glomerular function (e.g., chronic glomerulonephritis).

In *distal renal tubular acidosis* (distal RTA), the basic defect is an inability to develop the usual hydrogen-ion concentration gradient between the peritubular fluid (i.e., ECF) and the tubular lumen. Consequently the amount of acid excreted cannot keep up with the production of fixed acids in the body and metabolic acidosis develops. As with proximal RTA, distal RTA can be a genetic defect or can occur secondarily to a wide variety of metabolic disorders. Sometimes the cause is not known.

Hypoaldosteronism is a deficiency of aldosterone in the body. It occurs with Addison's disease, in which secretion of all adrenocortical hormones is diminished (see Chapter 19). Impaired secretion of renin, which may occur in some cases of kidney failure, can cause secondary hypoaldosteronism because the renin-angiotensin system stimulates aldosterone secretion (see Chapter 12). Administration of drugs that act as aldosterone antagonists (e.g., spironolactone) has the same effect as lack of aldosterone. Since aldosterone stimulates sodium reabsorption and enhances hydrogen-ion secretion, a deficiency of aldosterone results in decreased excretion of hydrogen ions.

Adaptive Response

Excess hydrogen ions stimulate the respiratory center by their effects on both the peripheral and central chemoreceptors. Therefore ventilation is increased. The depth of breathing is increased to a greater degree than the rate of breathing, producing characteristic deep, sighing respirations (*Küssmaul respirations*). This respiratory stimulation is more pronounced with acute metabolic acidosis than with chronic acidosis. The result is that more carbon dioxide is eliminated, the carbonic acid/bicarbonate ratio is returned toward normal, and consequently the pH is returned toward normal.

Unless the acidosis is due to renal dysfunction, the kidneys respond by increasing hydrogen-ion secretion and ammonia production, as described previously. This mechanism results in the addition of bicarbonate to the plasma to return the bicarbonate concentration toward normal, and production of a very acid urine. If the acidosis is due to renal dysfunction, however, the urine may be inappropriately alkaline.

When the renal tubules reabsorb sodium, an anion must accompany it into the ECF (or a cation must be excreted) to maintain electrical balance. Chloride and bicarbonate are the major anions of the ECF and the glomerular filtrate. When the bicarbonate concentration is decreased, as it is in metabolic acidosis, more chloride must be reabsorbed along with sodium, unless some other reabsorbable anion is present in the filtrate. Therefore, in some cases of metabolic acidosis, the plasma chloride level is increased (*hyperchloremia*). When hyperchloremia accompanies acidosis the anion gap is normal, as mentioned previously.

Effects

Signs and symptoms of acidosis are produced by the adaptive mechanisms, as just described, and by the effects of the decreased pH on metabolism. The major effect of acidosis is depression of the CNS. Lethargy, disorientation, stupor, or coma occurs, depending on the degree of acidosis. Very severe acidosis depresses the respiratory center.

Cardiac arrhythmias may occur, presumably due to the shift of potassium ions out of the cells as hydrogen ions enter. (See Chapter 16 for a discussion of potassium imbalance.) The increased hydrogen-ion concentration causes peripheral vasodilation. Therefore the skin may be warm and flushed, and hypotension may occur. The heart rate may be increased in order to increase the cardiac output and offset the reduction in blood pressure caused by the peripheral vasodilation.

Bone disorders often develop with chronic acidosis, possibly related to the buffering of excess hydrogen ions by the carbonate in bone. Chronic acidosis in children retards growth.

Other signs and symptoms may be present, depending on the nature of the disorder that caused the acidosis.

Respiratory Acidosis

The primary disturbance in respiratory acidosis is retention of carbon dioxide, which produces an increased arterial PCO_2. The adaptive response is to increase the excretion of hydrogen ions and the generation of bicarbonate by the kidneys, therefore the plasma bicarbonate concentration is also increased. The pH tends to be decreased (i.e., the hydrogen-ion concentration is increased).

Causes

Respiratory acidosis occurs when the rate of production of carbon dioxide in the body is greater than its rate of elimination by the lungs. This situation can be caused by depression of the respiratory center, primary lung disease or airways obstruction, or disorders of the respiratory muscles and chest wall. (See Chapter 10 for a discussion of how these factors affect respiratory function.)

Depression of the respiratory center can be caused by drugs, head injuries, or organic brain diseases. As a result, the rate and depth of respiration decrease, producing alveolar hypoventilation.

Pulmonary diseases can interfere with gas exchange in several ways, by causing alveolar hypoventilation, by disturbing the ventilation-perfusion ratio, or by decreasing the surface area for gas exchange. As explained in Chapter 10, these disturbances affect oxygenation of the blood to a greater extent than elimination of carbon dioxide, but alveolar hypoventilation leads to carbon dioxide retention. Pulmonary edema also impairs gas exchange and can lead to respiratory acidosis.

Disorders of the respiratory muscles and chest wall restrict expansion of the lungs, producing alveolar hypoventilation. Again, the result is carbon dioxide retention.

Adaptive Response

Since the cause of the acidosis is impaired respiratory function, the only adaptive response that can be made is to increase renal excretion of acid. As more hydrogen ions are excreted in the urine as titratable acid and ammonium, bicarbonate is added to the plasma. Therefore the plasma bicarbonate concentration rises, which returns the carbonic acid/bicarbonate ratio, and thus the pH, toward normal. This mechanism takes about 6 to 12 hours to have any noticeable effect, however, and several days to achieve its full potential. Therefore, acute respiratory acidosis can be very severe, but with chronic respiratory acidosis the pH may return to normal, or almost to normal (i.e., the respiratory acidosis is compensated).

Correction of the respiratory acidosis can usually only be achieved when the underlying respiratory disorder is corrected. In some cases ventilation can be assisted by mechanical means. Often, however, the respiratory condition is chronic, and the acid-base disturbance cannot be corrected.

Effects

Neurological effects of respiratory acidosis are usually more severe than those caused by metabolic acidosis. This difference appears to be due to the fact that carbon dioxide readily crosses the blood-CSF barrier, whereas bicarbonate crosses very slowly. Therefore, with respiratory acidosis the pH of the CSF changes as rapidly as the pH of the blood, whereas with metabolic acidosis the change in pH of the CSF lags behind the change in pH of the blood.

Severe acute respiratory acidosis produces a syndrome called carbon dioxide narcosis. Early symptoms are weakness, fatigue, headache, and sometimes blurred vision. Irritability, lethargy, and confusion follow. Eventually mental derangements, tremors, asterixis (a peculiar flapping tremor), and delirium or somnolence may occur. The EEG is abnormal. The pressure of the CSF may be elevated and papilledema may be seen, possibly because hypercapnia increases cerebral blood flow.

As with metabolic acidosis, cardiac arrhythmias and peripheral vasodilation may occur, with resultant hypotension.

Metabolic Alkalosis

In metabolic alkalosis the primary disturbance is an increase in the bicarbonate concentration in the ECF, due to retention of bicarbonate or loss of hydrogen ions. Therefore the pH tends to be elevated and the hydrogen-ion concentration decreased. The adaptive response is to retain carbon dioxide, therefore the P_{CO_2} is increased.

Causes

Excessive loss of hydrogen ions can occur from the gastrointestinal tract or through the kidneys. Bicarbonate accumulates because of renal retention of bicarbonate or occasionally excessive administration of alkali. In most clinical situations metabolic alkalosis is produced by a combination of hydrogen-ion loss and failure to excrete bicarbonate.

Renal retention of bicarbonate. A major cause of metabolic alkalosis is failure to excrete bicarbonate due to chloride depletion (*hypochloremia*). When the kidneys reabsorb sodium, either an anion (Cl^- or HCO_3^-) must accompany it or a cation (K^+ or H^+) must be excreted to maintain electrical balance. When the ECF chloride concentration is decreased, the amount of chloride entering the glomerular filtrate is also decreased. Therefore fewer chloride ions are available for reabsorption with sodium ions. Consequently all the bicarbonate in the filtrate is reabsorbed, and more potassium and hydrogen ions are secreted in exchange for sodium reabsorption. Secretion of hydrogen ions after all the bicarbonate has been reabsorbed results in the generation of bicarbonate and therefore an increase in the plasma bicarbonate concentration, as previously described.

When the chloride deficit is accompanied by ECF volume deficit, the kidneys avidly reabsorb sodium, thus causing secretion of more potassium and hydrogen ions. In this situation, maintenance of ECF volume takes precedence over maintenance of acid-base balance.

Diuretic therapy is a common cause of chloride depletion and metabolic alkalosis. Furosemide and ethacrynic acid, in particular, cause large losses of chloride and can produce severe metabolic alkalosis. Thiazide diuretics inhibit chloride reabsorption only slightly but can produce a mild metabolic alkalosis, especially if salt intake is restricted.

The concentration of chloride in gastric juice (120–160 mEq/liter) is greater than the plasma chloride concentration. Therefore ECF chloride deficit can result from loss of gastric juice due to vomiting or suction.

Another cause of chloride deficit is a rare congenital condition called *chloridorrhea*. This condition is characterized by diarrhea, with the stools having a high concentration of chloride and a low pH, apparently due to defective reabsorption of chloride and faulty secretion of bicarbonate in the intestinal tract. As a result, metabolic alkalosis develops.

Excessive alkali administration. Ingestion of excessive amounts of absorbable alkali or intravenous administration of alkali causes alkalosis only when the rate of intake exceeds the rate at which the kidneys are able to excrete bicarbonate. Alkalosis is rarely produced by this mechanism unless renal function is impaired.

Occasionally ingestion of antacids containing calcium carbonate causes hypercalcemia and metabolic alkalosis (*milk-alkali syndrome*). Decreased renal function appears to be important in the development of this condition.

Loss of hydrogen ions. Aldosterone and other mineralocorticoid hormones enhance sodium reabsorption and increase the secretion of hydrogen ions and potassium ions by the distal renal tubules. Excesses of mineralocorticoid hormones result in increased renal secretion of hydrogen ions and can produce metabolic alkalosis. In *primary hyperaldosteronism*, excessive secretion of aldosterone is usually attributable to an adrenal tumor. This condition is characterized by hypertension (due to salt and water retention; see Chapter 13), hypokalemia, and metabolic alkalosis. Occasionally aldosterone excess is caused by hypersecretion of renin by the kidneys. Renin release leads to the formation of angiotensin, which stimulates aldosterone secretion. With one type of *congenital adrenal hyperplasia* there is excessive secretion of the mineralocorticoid deoxycorticosterone (see Chapter 19), and metabolic alkalosis may occur.

Licorice contains a steroid that exerts the same action as mineralocorticoid hormones. Chronic excessive ingestion of licorice can produce hypertension, hypokalemia, and metabolic alkalosis, mimicking primary hyperaldosteronism.

Cortisol is the major glucocorticoid produced by the adrenal cortex, but it also has slight mineralocorticoid activity. With cortisol excess (Cushing's syndrome) this mineralocorticoid activity may become significant and produce metabolic alkalosis.

Potassium depletion can also cause loss of hydrogen ions from the ECF and lead to metabolic alkalosis, if a stimulus for increased sodium reabsorption occurs at the same time (e.g., ECF volume deficit). A certain number of cations (Na^+, K^+, or H^+) must be excreted in the urine to balance anions in the glomerular filtrate that are poorly reabsorbed (e.g., phosphate, sulfate, and some organic anions). When sodium is being avidly reabsorbed due to ECF volume deficit or some other cause, this cation is not available for excretion. If potassium deficit occurs at the same time, then the requirement for cation excretion is met by increased secretion of hydrogen ions. When hydrogen ions are secreted by the renal tubules, bicarbonate is added to the ECF, as described earlier. The result is metabolic alkalosis. When the potassium deficit is not too severe, administration of saline to correct the volume deficit will allow the kidneys to excrete bicarbonate and restore acid-base balance. With severe potassium deficits, however, acid-base balance cannot be restored until the potassium deficit is at least partially corrected.

Gastric suction or vomiting of gastric contents only (e.g., due to pyloric stenosis) results in a loss of hydrogen ions and an increase in the bicarbonate concentration of the ECF. (In some cases, vomiting results in loss of fluid from the small intestine as well as from the stomach. In this situation bicarbonate is also lost and alkalosis does not occur.) Gastric juice contains a high concentration of hydrochloric acid and also contains sodium chloride and potassium chloride. For each hydrogen ion secreted into the gastric juice, a bicarbonate is added to the ECF. Ordinarily this secretory mechanism produces only a transient increase in the plasma bicarbonate concentration. When the acid gastric contents move into the duodenum, pancreatic secretion of bicarbonate is stimulated. Therefore, under usual conditions, no net change in acid-base balance occurs due to the secretion of acid by the stomach. When gastric juice is lost due to vomiting or suction, however, the stimulus for secretion of bicarbonate by the pancreas is lacking. The result is a net loss of hydrogen ions and gain of bicarbonate by the body. Metabolic alkalosis will not occur if the kidneys are able to excrete the excess bicarbonate. Loss of gastric fluid, however, can also result in chloride deficit, potassium deficit, and ECF volume deficit, caused not only

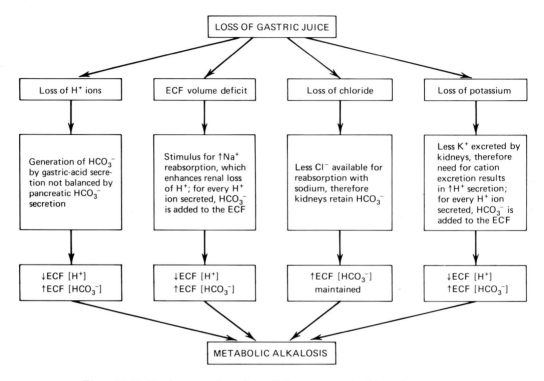

Figure 15-5. *Development of metabolic alkalosis as a result of loss of gastric juice.*

by losses but also by lack of intake while losses by other routes continue. Under these conditions the kidneys retain bicarbonate and metabolic alkalosis occurs (Fig. 15-5).

Adaptive Response

The adaptive response to metabolic alkalosis is decreased ventilation (hypoventilation), which causes the PCO_2 to rise. It is mainly the depth of respiration that is decreased; the rate of respiration is altered only slightly. This adaptive response is limited in its ability to return the carbonic acid/bicarbonate ratio and the pH toward normal because hypoventilation causes hypoxia, which acts as a stimulus to respiration. Therefore in metabolic alkalosis the PCO_2 rarely rises above 60 mm Hg.

Effects

Alkalosis causes increased irritability of the central and peripheral nervous systems. This effect is

much less pronounced with metabolic alkalosis than with respiratory alkalosis, however, presumably because bicarbonate crosses the blood-brain and blood-CSF barriers much more slowly than carbon dioxide, as mentioned previously. This neurological effect of alkalosis may be manifested by numbness and tingling of the fingers, toes, and circumoral region, and possibly by cramps in the arms and legs.

In addition to symptoms of alkalosis, often the predominant symptoms in affected people are those of associated hypokalemia and/or ECF volume deficit (e.g., muscle weakness and postural dizziness).

Respiratory Alkalosis

In respiratory alkalosis the primary disturbance is a low PCO_2 (hypocapnia) due to hyperventilation. The bicarbonate concentration is decreased as an adaptive response. The pH tends to be elevated and the hydrogen-ion concentration decreased.

Causes

Respiratory alkalosis occurs when the rate of elimination of carbon dioxide is greater than the rate of production of carbon dioxide in the body. Alveolar ventilation in excess of the body's need for carbon dioxide elimination is called *hyperventilation*. (An increase in ventilation that meets a physiological need exactly is not considered hyperventilation; the general term for increased ventilation is hyperpnea.) Hyperventilation causes a decrease in the P_{CO_2} and consequently the carbon dioxide–carbonic acid–bicarbonate equilibrium is shifted to the left:

$$\downarrow CO_2 + H_2O \leftarrow H_2CO_3 \leftarrow H^+ + HCO_3^-$$

As bicarbonate ions combine with hydrogen ions to form carbonic acid, the hydrogen-ion concentration and bicarbonate concentration fall. The ECF hydrogen-ion concentration is much less than the ECF-bicarbonate concentration; therefore the proportionate decrease in hydrogen-ion concentration is greater than the proportionate decrease in bicarbonate concentration. As the hydrogen ions are used in this reaction, hydrogen ions are released from intracellular buffers to combine with bicarbonate. The decrease in hydrogen-ion concentration causes an increase in the pH. The rise in pH begins 10 to 20 seconds after the onset of hyperventilation and reaches its maximal value in 10 to 15 minutes.

Hyperventilation can be caused by primary stimulation of the respiratory center in the brain due to psychogenic factors, organic brain disorders (e.g., encephalitis, subarachnoid hemorrhage), or drugs (e.g., salicylates). The respiratory center is also stimulated by progesterone; therefore mild respiratory alkalosis occurs in normal pregnancy.

Another cause of hyperventilation is reflex stimulation of the respiratory center by the peripheral chemoreceptors as a result of arterial hypoxemia. When hypoxemia is attributable to alveolar hypoventilation it is associated with hypercapnia, but when it is attributable to living at high altitude, interstitial lung disease, pulmonary embolism, congestive heart failure, or congenital heart defects with shunting of blood, hyperventilation and respiratory alkalosis may occur. (See also Chapter 10 under Decreased Oxygenation of the Blood.) In some cases of localized pulmonary disease irritation of intrathoracic stretch receptors may contribute to the increase in ventilation.

Hyperventilation can occur when a person is receiving ventilatory assistance by mechanical means, particularly when the rate and depth of breathing are set by the ventilator.

Hyperventilation can also occur in states of increased metabolism, such as fever or thyrotoxicosis, in which the demand for oxygen is increased. Sepsis due to gram-negative bacteria is another cause of respiratory alkalosis. In this case the mechanism responsible for hyperventilation is not understood. Respiratory alkalosis often accompanies cirrhosis of the liver for unknown reasons.

Adaptive Response

As a result of the decreased P_{CO_2} fewer hydrogen ions are secreted by the renal tubules and less bicarbonate is reabsorbed. Thus the kidneys conserve hydrogen ions and excrete bicarbonate, producing an alkaline urine. This response lowers the ECF bicarbonate concentration further and brings the pH back toward normal, but it occurs relatively slowly. Therefore the renal adaptive response becomes significant only if the respiratory alkalosis lasts several days or longer. With chronic respiratory alkalosis (e.g., due to pregnancy or living at high altitude) the renal mechanism is often able to restore the pH to normal (i.e., the respiratory alkalosis is compensated).

Effects

Respiratory alkalosis causes increased irritability of the central and peripheral nervous systems. This increased irritability is manifested by sensory symptoms such as numbness and tingling of the extremities and circumoral area and by motor symptoms such as muscle cramps and carpopedal spasm. These manifestations are indistinguishable from the tetany caused by hypocalcemia (see Chapter 16). Feelings of light-headedness may also be experienced. The occurrence of these symptoms appears to be proportional to the increase in pH; therefore they are manifested more often with acute respiratory alkalosis than with the chronic form. In addition, hyperventilation can provoke epileptic seizures in susceptible people.

People who hyperventilate for psychogenic reasons may experience headache, shortness of breath, and chest pain. These symptoms are believed to be emotional in origin, rather than being caused by the alkalosis.

Acute respiratory alkalosis is accompanied by an increased concentration of lactate in the blood caused by increased production of lactic acid. The mechanism responsible for this increased lactic acid production is not known, but several mechanisms are likely responsible, including a direct effect of the low PCO_2 and decreased delivery of oxygen to the cells. The decreased oxygen delivery could be caused by vasoconstriction and by decreased release of oxygen from hemoglobin. When the pH is increased, hemoglobin has a stronger affinity for oxygen (see Chapter 10 under Decreased Oxygen-Carrying Capacity of the Blood). The hydrogen ions released from the lactic acid help to offset the pH change caused by the respiratory alkalosis.

Often a decrease in the plasma phosphate concentration occurs with respiratory alkalosis. This decrease appears to be caused by a shift of phosphate into the cells.

Mixed Acid-Base Disturbances

Mixed acid-base disturbances occur when two primary factors are operating simultaneously.

With mixed metabolic acidosis and respiratory acidosis the bicarbonate concentration is decreased because of one etiology and simultaneously the PCO_2 is increased due to an independent disturbance of ventilation. Both of these primary factors increase the hydrogen-ion concentration and decrease the pH; therefore the pH is usually extremely low. This situation may occur, for example, in a person with diabetic ketoacidosis who has respiratory insufficiency due to pulmonary disease.

With mixed metabolic alkalosis and respiratory alkalosis the bicarbonate concentration is increased and the PCO_2 is decreased. Since both of these factors decrease the hydrogen-ion concentration, the pH may be very high. This situation may occur, for example, when a person with persistent vomiting hyperventilates due to emotional factors.

With mixed metabolic acidosis and respiratory alkalosis the bicarbonate concentration is decreased and the PCO_2 is increased. In this situation the effects of the two primary disturbances on the pH oppose each other. Therefore the pH may be normal, decreased, or increased, depending on the relative magnitude of each of the primary disturbances. Mixed metabolic acidosis and respiratory alkalosis typically occurs in infants with salicylate intoxication.

With mixed metabolic alkalosis and respiratory acidosis the bicarbonate concentration is increased and the PCO_2 is decreased. Again, in this situation the two primary disturbances have opposing effects on the pH and the pH may be normal, decreased, or increased. This mixed acid-base disturbance may occur in people with respiratory failure who are concomitantly receiving therapy with diuretics and/or steroids.

SUGGESTED ADDITIONAL READING

del Bueno DJ: A quick review on using blood-gas determinations. *RN* **41**(3): 68–70, 1978.

16
Mineral/Electrolyte Imbalance

The composition of the body fluids is described in Chapter 11. Electrolyte balance in the extracellular fluid (ECF) depends on the equilibrium between minerals that are bound to body components and those that exist as free ions in the body fluids, as well as on a balance between intake and output. Several hormones influence electrolyte metabolism and balance. Electrolyte imbalances can result from excesses or deficiencies of these hormones or from imbalances between intake and losses of electrolytes. A variety of electrolyte imbalances can result from abnormal losses of body fluids.

Sodium is discussed in Chapter 12, because sodium balance is closely related to water balance. Hydrogen ion, bicarbonate, and chloride are discussed in Chapter 15. This chapter is concerned with imbalances of potassium, calcium, phosphate, and magnesium.

POTASSIUM

Potassium ion (K^+) is primarily an intracellular electrolyte; only about 2% of the total body potassium is present in the ECF. The intracellular potassium concentration is 150–160 mEq/liter, in contrast to an extracellular potassium concentration of 4–5 mEq/liter.

Potassium ion is very important in cell metabolism. It is required for the activity of some intracellular enzymes and also participates in the regulation of protein and glycogen synthesis. Potassium is also a necessary cofactor with insulin for the movement of glucose into cells. In addition, potassium ion is important for normal neuromuscular irritability. In this latter respect what is important is the *ratio* of the intracellular to the extracellular potassium concentration.

Potassium Homeostasis

The plasma potassium concentration is determined by the movement of potassium into and out of the cells and by the balance between intake and excretion (Fig. 16-1). Potassium excretion and its distribution between the ECF and ICF (intracellular fluid) are influenced by several hormones and by sodium balance and acid-base balance.

Movement of Potassium Between ICF and ECF

The high concentration of potassium within the

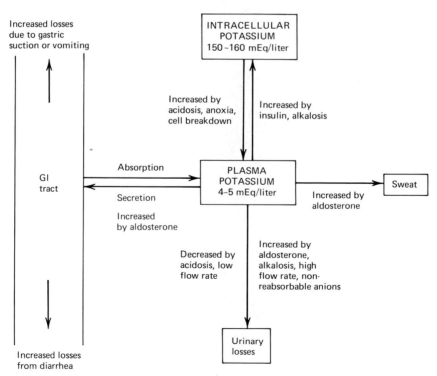

Figure 16-1. *Summary of factors influencing the plasma potassium concentration.*

cells is due to the functioning of the sodium-potassium pump, which extrudes sodium from the cells and moves potassium in by active transport. Conditions impairing the function of the sodium-potassium pump (e.g., anoxia) lead to a loss of potassium from the cells.

Normally the potassium in the ECF is in equilibrium with the potassium inside the cells. Following ingestion of a large amount of potassium, most of the electrolyte rapidly enters the cells. This movement into the cells prevents a large increase in the plasma potassium concentration until the excess potassium can be excreted by the kidneys. Loss of potassium from the ECF is accompanied by movement of potassium out of the cells, thus minimizing the decrease in the plasma potassium concentration. Therefore, under usual circumstances the plasma potassium concentration reflects body stores. In some situations, however, this relationship is disturbed and the plasma potassium concentration is not a good index of total body potassium. Conditions that alter the relationship between total body potassium and the plasma potassium concentration are changes in acid-base balance, hormonal balance, and the rate of cell breakdown. This relationship is also altered in a variety of chronic diseases that are associated with disturbed sodium metabolism.

Influence of acid-base balance.   In acidosis, some of the excess hydrogen ions in the ECF move into the cells and are buffered by intracellular buffers (see Chapter 15). Since hydrogen ions are positively charged, their movement into the cells causes a transient electrochemical imbalance. To restore electrochemical balance, potassium cations move out of the cells into the ECF. In this situation, the intracellular potassium concentration may be below normal and the total body store may be depleted, but the plasma potassium concentration may be normal or slightly elevated.

With alkalosis, hydrogen ions move out of the cells into the ECF and potassium and sodium ions move into the cells to maintain electrochemical balance. Despite this enhanced movement of potassium into the cells, potassium deficit usually occurs because potassium excretion is increased in alkalosis. In this situation the body store is depleted and the plasma potassium concentration is usually low.

Influence of hormones.   Insulin is the major hormone influencing distribution of potassium between the ECF and ICF. Insulin promotes the movement of potassium into liver cells and skeletal muscle cells. Administration of insulin, therefore, causes a lowering of the plasma potassium concentration, even though the body store of potassium is not depleted. Conversely, with insulin deficiency (i.e., in people with diabetes mellitus), entry of potassium into the cells is slow after a large intake of potassium and the plasma potassium concentration rises more than normally. Therefore, with insulin deficiency the intracellular potassium concentration may be low and the body store may be depleted, yet the plasma potassium concentration may be elevated.

Insulin appears to be involved in the regulation of the plasma potassium concentration. An elevated level of plasma potassium increases insulin secretion; the insulin, in turn, promotes entry of potassium into the cells, thus lowering the plasma potassium concentration. Conversely, a low plasma potassium concentration decreases insulin secretion, so that less potassium enters the cells and if intake is adequate the plasma potassium level can rise. These actions constitute a negative feedback control mechanism for maintaining the plasma potassium concentration at the desired level. Another hormone involved in the regulation of the plasma potassium concentration is aldosterone; this hormone influences urinary excretion of potassium (see below).

Movement of potassium into the cells is also enhanced by growth hormone, catecholamines, and androgens.

Rate of cell breakdown.   The integrity of cell membranes is essential for the maintenance of the normal distribution of electrolytes between the ECF and ICF. Whenever the rate of cell breakdown is increased, more potassium is released into the ECF and the plasma potassium concentration rises. The degree to which the plasma potassium level rises depends on the ability of the kidneys to excrete the excess potassium and on the ability of other cells to take up potassium.

Chronic diseases. A variety of chronic diseases such as cirrhosis, heart failure, and malabsorption are associated with potassium depletion, yet the plasma potassium concentration may be normal. Not only is the intracellular potassium concentration low but also the concentration of sodium in the cells may be elevated, possibly due to a defect in the sodium-potassium pump. Conditions such as heart disease and cirrhosis are also associated with altered sodium balance, which influences renal excretion of potassium.

Potassium Intake and Excretion

Potassium is readily available in a variety of foods and is readily absorbed from the small intestine. It is also secreted into the gastrointestinal tract in the digestive juices, but normally this secreted potassium is reabsorbed.

The primary route of excretion of potassium is through the kidneys. About 90% or more is eliminated in the urine; the rest is lost in feces and sweat. Although losses of potassium in the feces and sweat represent only a small fraction of the total, under some conditions these losses may be significant. Sweat contains about 5–10 mEq of potassium per liter; this amount is increased under the influence of aldosterone. Significant potassium losses can occur when sweat production is chronically increased, for example, in people engaged in strenous physical activity in a hot climate. Fecal potassium losses are increased by diarrhea, steatorrhea, or chronic laxative abuse. In addition, abnormal losses of any gastrointestinal secretions, for example, due to vomiting or tube drainage, can also lead to excessive potassium losses.

In the kidneys potassium is freely filtered at the glomerulus. Almost all of it is reabsorbed by an active process in the proximal portions of the nephron; most of the potassium that appears in the urine is secreted distally. Potassium is both reabsorbed and secreted in the distal convoluted tubules and collecting ducts. Changes in the amount of potassium excreted in the urine are mainly due to changes in the distal potassium secretion. Normally, when potassium intake is high renal secretion of potassium increases; when intake is low, secretion decreases to maintain potassium balance.

Renal tubular secretion of potassium. Although movement of potassium from the peritubular interstitial fluid into the tubular cells is an active process, the final step—that is, movement of potassium from the cells into the tubular lumen—appears to occur by passive diffusion. The amount of potassium secreted depends on three factors: the concentration gradient, which is determined by the difference between the concentration of potassium in the cells and the concentration in the tubular fluid; the electrical potential difference across the tubular epithelial membrane; and the permeability of the luminal cell membrane to potassium.

As previously mentioned, the intracellular potassium concentration is high. On the other hand, since most of the potassium in the glomerular filtrate is reabsorbed in the proximal part of the nephron, the fluid reaching the distal tubule has a very low potassium concentration. Therefore a considerable concentration gradient favors movement of potassium from the cells into the tubular fluid (i.e., secretion of potassium). Any factors that increase the concentration gradient, either by increasing the intracellular potassium concentration or decreasing the tubular potassium concentration, promote potassium secretion. Conversely, any factors that decrease the concentration gradient promote potassium retention.

A high intake of potassium causes a transient increase in the plasma potassium level and stimulates uptake of potassium by the cells. Therefore the intracellular potassium concentration rises and more potassium is secreted into the urine. Conversely, with a low potassium intake the plasma potassium level is decreased, less potassium is taken up by the cells, and less potassium is secreted into the urine. (The kidneys are unable to conserve potassium totally, however, and a minimum of 5–15 mEq of potassium is excreted in the urine per day, even when the body store of potassium is depleted.)

Acidosis causes potassium to leave the cells, as previously mentioned, and decreases secretion of potassium into the urine. Conversely, alkalosis causes more potassium to enter the cells and increases urinary potassium excretion.

As already mentioned, the potassium concentration of the fluid reaching the distal tubules is very low. As potassium is secreted into the tubular fluid, however, the potassium concentration of the tubular fluid rises. Therefore the concentration gradient decreases and further secretion is slowed. When the flow of fluid through the distal tubule increases, however, the secreted potassium is washed away, a favorable concentration gradient is maintained, and more potassium is excreted. Conversely, a low rate of flow decreases potassium excretion.

An electrical potential difference normally occurs across the tubular epithelial membrane, the tubular lumen being relatively negative to the peritubular fluid. Potassium as a positively charged ion is influenced by this electrical gradient. The electrical gradient is established by the active reabsorption of sodium ions. Negative chloride ions follow along with the sodium ions, but not all the reabsorbed sodium ions are accompanied by chloride or other anions. Therefore movement of positively charged sodium ions from the tubular fluid into the peritubular interstitial fluid makes the tubular fluid relatively negative. Positively charged potassium ions then move down the electrical gradient into the tubular fluid. The overall effect is that potassium ions are secreted in exchange for reabsorption of sodium ions. Increased distal-tubular sodium reabsorption enhances potas-

sium excretion. In addition, the presence of increased amounts of poorly reabsorbed anions (e.g., sulfate) or nonreabsorbable anions (e.g., some drugs, such as carbenicillin) in the tubular fluid makes the lumen more negative and increases excretion of potassium.

Not only potassium ions but also hydrogen ions are secreted in exchange for reabsorption of sodium (see Chapter 15). The proportions of potassium and hydrogen ions that are secreted depend on the relative concentraions of these ions in the body fluids. In acidosis, more hydrogen ions and fewer potassium ions are secreted into the urine. Conversely, in alkalosis fewer hydrogen ions and more potassium ions are secreted.

Aldosterone increases excretion of potassium in the feces, sweat, and urine. Aldosterone appears to enhance transport of potassium from the peritubular interstitial fluid into the renal tubular cells and to increase luminal membrane permeability to potassium. Aldosterone also promotes sodium reabsorption by the distal renal tubules, which enhances potassium excretion by the exchange process just described.

Aldosterone secretion is influenced by the ECF potassium concentration, as well as by several other factors (see Chapter 12). A high potassium concentration stimulates aldosterone secretion, which in turn promotes potassium excretion and restores the potassium level to normal. Conversely, a low potassium concentration inhibits aldosterone secretion. These actions constitute a negative feedback control mechanism for the maintenance of a normal plasma potassium concentration.

Potassium Imbalance

As stated earlier, the plasma potassium concentration does not always reflect the total body potassium store. Since the plasma potassium concentration is easily measured and the total body potassium is not, however, potassium imbalances are described in terms of hypokalemia and hyperkalemia. *Hypokalemia* is an abnormally low concentration of potassium in the plasma, usually defined as less than 3.5 mEq/liter. *Hyperkalemia* is an abnormally high plasma potassium concentration, exceeding 5.5 mEq/liter. Although potassium deficiency impairs cell metabolism, the clinical manifestations of potassium imbalance are primarily due to altered neuromuscular irritability.

Effects on Neuromuscular Irritability

Nerve and muscle cell membranes are polarized; that is, there is a separation of charge across the cell membrane, the interior of the cell being negative relative to the outside. This electrical gradient across the cell membrane is called the *resting membrane potential*; it is largely determined by the ratio of the intracellular to extracellular potassium concentration.

When a stimulus is applied to a nerve, or when acetylcholine is released at synapses and motor endplates, the membrane permeability to sodium is increased and the positive sodium ions rush into the cell down their concentration gradient. As a result, the membrane potential becomes less negative (i.e., it moves toward zero) and the membrane is depolarized. When the membrane potential reaches a critical value, called the *threshold potential*, the membrane potential is rapidly reversed (i.e., the interior of the cell becomes positive). This transient reversal of polarity is called the *action potential*. At the height of the action potential, the mechanism for increased permeability to sodium is shut off and the permeability to potassium increases. Moving down its concentration gradient and the electrical gradient, potassium passively diffuses out of the cell and the membrane potential returns to its resting level (i.e., the cell is *repolarized*). The sodium-potassium pump then restores the normal intracellular composition by pumping sodium out of the cell and pumping potassium in. Only then is the cell capable of generating another action potential. In neurons the action potential is responsible for the nerve impulse; in muscle cells it initiates contraction.

Neuromuscular irritability (or excitability) is determined by the difference between the resting

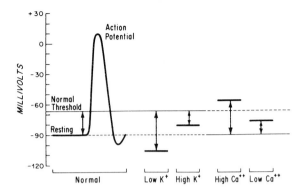

Figure 16-2. *Effects of ECF potassium-ion and calcium-ion concentrations on membrane excitability. The ECF potassium concentration affects the resting potential; the ECF calcium concentration affects the threshold potential. (From Leaf A, Cotran RS: Renal Pathophysiology. New York, Oxford University Press, 1976. By permission.)*

potential and the threshold potential. Hypokalemia makes the resting potential more negative (i.e., the cell membrane is *hyperpolarized*). Therefore the difference between the resting potential and the threshold potential is increased (Fig. 16-2), so that a greater stimulus is required to produce an action potential. In other words, neuromuscular irritability is decreased. Consequently muscle weakness and, in severe cases, flaccid paralysis occur. Conversely, with hyperkalemia the resting membrane potential is less negative, the difference between the resting potential and threshold potential is decreased, and a smaller stimulus will evoke an action potential. In other words, neuromuscular irritability is increased. With severe hyperkalemia, the resting potential may rise to the level of the threshold potential. Consequently the cell cannot repolarize and so is no longer excitable following a single action potential. Therefore, hyperkalemia can also cause paralysis.

The effects of hyperkalemia and hypokalemia depend partly on the speed with which the plasma potassium concentration changes and partly on the levels of other ions. When hypokalemia develops quickly, the decrease in the plasma potassium concentration will cause hyperpolarization of nerve and muscle cell membranes and decreased neuromuscular irritability. With chronic potassium depletion, however, potassium moves out of the cells into the ECF and both the intracellular and extracellular potassium concentrations are decreased. Consequently the ratio of the intracellular to extracellular potassium concentration may be normal and therefore the resting membrane potential will be unchanged. Similarly, chronic hyperkalemia may have fewer adverse effects than acute hyperkalemia because some of the excess potassium moves into the cells.

Neuromuscular irritability is also influenced by the plasma calcium concentration and by the pH of the body fluids. Calcium ions influence the threshold potential. A high plasma calcium concentration decreases neuromuscular irritability and therefore potentiates the effect of hypokalemia but counteracts the effect of hyperkalemia. Generally acidosis decreases neuromuscular irritability and alkalosis increases it. In addition, pH influences the movement of potassium into and out of the cells, as previously mentioned, and therefore influences the plasma potassium concentration.

Effects on the Heart

The altered membrane excitability caused by potassium imbalance also affects cardiac conduction, as reflected by changes in the electrocardiogram (ECG). The normal ECG and the characteristic changes that occur with hypokalemia and hyperkalemia are shown in Figure 16-3.

The electrocardiogram is a record of the electrical activity associated with the cardiac cycle. The P wave represents electrical activity associated with atrial depolarization. The QRS complex represents electrical activity associated with depolarization of the ventricles. Repolarization of the ventricles is represented by the S–T segment and T and U waves. The wave representing atrial repolarization is lost in the QRS complex.

During repolarization, potassium moves out of the cell. Therefore the speed of repolarization depends on the permeability of the membrane to

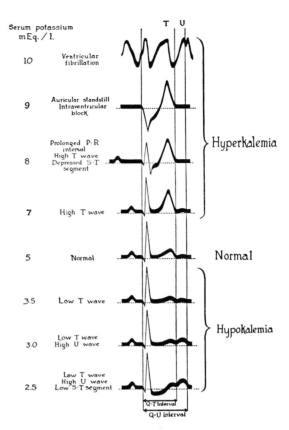

Figure 16-3. *Effects of ECF potassium-ion concentration on the electrocardiogram. (From Burch, GE Winsor T: A Primer of Electrocardiography, ed 6. Philadelphia, Lea & Febiger, 1972.)*

potassium. Membrane permeability appears to be influenced by the plasma potassium concentration. With a low plasma potassium concentration permeability is decreased, movement of potassium out of the cells is retarded, and repolarization is slow. Conversely, when the plasma potassium concentration is high, membrane permeability is increased and repolarization occurs at a faster rate.

Hypokalemia therefore delays ventricular repolarization, producing S–T segment depression, decreased amplitude or inversion of the T wave, increased height of the U wave, and lengthening of the Q–U interval on the ECG. With more severe hypokalemia, the amplitude of the P wave is increased, the P–R interval is prolonged, and the QRS complex is widened. A variety of cardiac arrhythmias, such as premature atrial and ventricular beats and paroxysmal atrial tachycardia, may also occur. Digitalis cardiac glycosides increase the severity of the effects of hypokalemia.

With hyperkalemia the rate of repolarization is increased, producing tall peaked T waves with narrow bases and a decreased Q–T interval on the ECG. As the plasma potassium level increases the S–T segment may become depressed and the P–R interval becomes prolonged. With a further rise in the potassium level, loss of P waves and widening of the QRS complexes occurs. At higher potassium concentrations a biphasic pattern appears, due to fusion of the QRS complex, RS–T segment, and T wave. Finally ventricular fibrillation or cardiac standstill occurs.

As mentioned previously, the effects of potassium imbalance on neuromuscular irritability are influenced by several other factors. Therefore, the plasma potassium concentration at which electrocardiographic changes are seen varies from one person to another. The effects of hyperkalemia are potentiated by low levels of plasma calcium and sodium; by high levels of plasma magnesium; and by acidosis. A high plasma calcium level counteracts the effects of hyperkalemia.

Hypokalemia

Causes. Hypokalemia can result from decreased intake of potassium, increased entry of potassium into the cells, and/or increased losses of potassium from the body.

Dietary intake usually has to be severely restricted before hypokalemia occurs, because most foods contain some potassium and the kidneys can conserve potassium to a certain extent. Renal conservation is not complete, however, so that potassium depletion can occur, for example, if a person is maintained on intravenous fluids without added potassium. In addition, decreased intake

can contribute to hypokalemia caused by excessive losses of potassium.

Persistent hypersecretion of insulin can cause hypokalemia because insulin promotes the movement of potassium into the cells. This situation may occur in people with high intakes of carbohydrate, for example, due to intravenous hyperalimentation. Parenteral administration of insulin or epinephrine lowers the plasma potassium level by the same mechanism.

Hypokalemia can result from treatment of pernicious anemia. As blood cell production increases, potassium is taken up by the newly formed cells. Consequently the plasma potassium concentration falls.

Alkalosis also causes potassium to move into the cells. In addition, urinary excretion increases with alkalosis. Therefore alkalosis and hypokalemia commonly occur together. Not only can alkalosis cause hypokalemia but hypokalemia also can produce alkalosis (see Chapter 15).

Increased loss of potassium can be due to gastrointestinal or urinary losses. The concentration of potassium in the gastric juice is higher than the plasma potassium concentration. Therefore excessive loss of potassium can occur as a result of persistent vomiting (e.g., due to pyloric obstruction) or gastric suction. Also, in this situation intake is impaired.

Chronic laxative abuse results in increased loss of potassium in the feces and can cause hypokalemia. Diarrhea from any cause results in loss of potassium and also bicarbonate or sodium ions. Therefore hypokalemia may occur. Since severe water deficit and acidosis may be present, however, the plasma potassium concentration may be normal (or elevated), although the intracellular potassium store is depleted. As the acidosis is corrected, hypokalemia may become apparent.

Primary aldosteronism (or hyperaldosteronism) and secondary hyperaldosteronism are common causes of excessive urinary losses of potassium. Primary aldosteronism is caused by an adrenal tumor. Secondary hyperaldosteronism commonly occurs with congestive heart failure, cirrhosis, and the nephrotic syndrome. These conditions are associated with low renal blood flow. Consequently, the renin-angiotensin system is activated; angiotensin stimulates production of aldosterone. Excess aldosterone, or other mineralocorticoids, cause increased reabsorption of sodium and secretion of potassium and hydrogen ions by the distal renal tubules. Therefore hypokalemia and metabolic alkalosis usually result.

Most (although not all) diuretic drugs also increase urinary potassium loss. This loss of potassium is partly due to increased flow of fluid through the distal tubules. Also, many diuretics block sodium reabsorption in the proximal portion of the nephron or loop of Henle. Consequently, more sodium is available for reabsorption in the distal tubules; the increased sodium reabsorption here results in increased secretion of potassium and hydrogen ions.

A low plasma magnesium concentration causes increased potassium excretion by an unknown mechanism and can cause hypokalemia.

Effects.   Muscle weakness and fatigue due to decreased neuromuscular irritability are the common symptoms of hypokalemia. The muscle weakness usually occurs first in the legs, particularly in the quadriceps muscles. Occasionally muscle tenderness, cramps, and paresthesias (abnormal sensations) occur. Chronic potassium depletion may actually cause muscle atrophy. With more severe hypokalemia, muscles of the arms and trunk as well as the respiratory muscles are affected. Paralysis may occur, causing respiratory failure.

Decreased neuromuscular irritability also affects the gastrointestinal smooth muscle, causing decreased intestinal motility, abdominal distension, anorexia, nausea, and constipation. Paralytic ileus may occur.

Cardiac arrhythmias and electrocardiographic changes occur, as already described. In addition, weakness of vascular smooth muscle may cause hypotension.

The blood glucose level may be slightly elevated, presumably due to inhibition of insulin secretion by the hypokalemia.

Chronic potassium depletion impairs cell metabolism and organ function. Impaired renal function, including impaired concentrating ability, results in polyuria (excessive urine formation), which in turn stimulates thirst.

Hyperkalemia

Causes.   Hyperkalemia can be caused by increased potassium intake, decreased entry of potassium into the cells or increased movement of potassium out of the cells, and decreased urinary excretion of potassium.

Hyperkalemia is usually caused by decreased urinary excretion of potassium due to renal failure with oliguria. Increased potassium intake usually does not cause hyperkalemia unless urinary excretion or cellular uptake of potassium is impaired. Hyperkalemia can occur, however, if intravenous solutions containing potassium are infused too rapidly. Hyperkalemia may also occur from massive transfusions with stored blood, since potassium is released from the blood cells during storage.

Increased tissue breakdown, causing release of potassium from the cells, can cause hyperkalemia, especially if renal function is impaired. Hyperkalemia commonly occurs after massive trauma such as crushing injuries or burns, in which case acute renal failure may be present along with the tissue breakdown. Hyperkalemia due to increased tissue catabolism can also occur following administration of cytotoxic agents to people with malignant lymphomas.

Insulin deficiency results in decreased entry of potassium into the cells. Therefore people with hyperglycemic nonketotic coma or diabetic ketoacidosis (see Chapter 18) may have hyperkalemia. In the latter case the acidosis contributes to the elevation of the plasma potassium level.

Hyperkalemia and metabolic acidosis often occur together. As mentioned previously, acidosis results in a shift of potassium out of the cells, producing hyperkalemia. In addition, urinary potassium excretion may be decreased, although not necessarily. In some conditions associated with metabolic acidosis, other factors are operating that result in increased potassium excretion. On the other hand, a high level of potassium results in a shift of hydrogen ions out of the cells as potassium moves in. In addition, urinary excretion of hydrogen ions is decreased by hyperkalemia. Therefore metabolic acisosis may result from hyperkalemia.

A few diuretic drugs, such as spironolactone (an inhibitor of aldosterone) and triamterene, are associated with potassium retention, which may lead to hyperkalemia. These drugs inhibit sodium reabsorption and secretion of potassium and hydrogen ions in the distal renal tubules.

Effects. Slight degrees of hyperkalemia cause increased neuromuscular irritability, as already described. This irritability may be manifested by intestinal colic and diarrhea. More severe hyperkalemia produces muscular weakness and paralysis, first affecting the legs, then the trunk and arms. The respiratory muscles are affected last. Hyperkalemia also causes characteristic ECG changes, as previously described. Death may occur due to ventricular fibrillation or cardiac arrest when the plasma potassium level is between 8 and 15 mEq/liter.

CALCIUM, PHOSPHORUS, AND MAGNESIUM

Calcium, phosphorus, and magnesium are considered together because their metabolism is interrelated in some ways.

Normal Metabolism and Control

Plasma levels of calcium, phosphorus, and magnesium depend not only on the balance between gastrointestinal absorption and urinary excretion of these substances but also (particularly in the case of calcium) on their deposition in and release from bone. These processes are influenced by vitamin D, parathyroid hormone, and calcitonin.

Gastrointestinal Absorption

Calcium, phosphorus, and magnesium appear to be absorbed from the small intestine both by carrier-mediated transport and by passive diffusion. Many factors influence the absorption of these minerals and absorption is not complete. Rarely is more than 30% of the dietary intake of calcium absorbed. During periods of growth, or when the body store of calcium is depleted (e.g., as a result of prolonged low dietary intake), the proportion of dietary calcium absorbed is greater than at other times. This adaptation is probably mediated by vitamin D. Calcium absorption decreases with aging, possibly due to altered vitamin D metabolism. Therefore elderly people may have a higher dietary requirement for calcium than young adults. About 65% of the dietary intake of phosphorus is absorbed, and about 35% to 40% of the dietary magnesium.

Calcium must be in the ionized form to be absorbed; therefore, formation of nonionized insoluble complexes with other substances in the lumen of the intestine interferes with calcium absorption. Phytate (a substance found in plants, particularly abundant in grains) and oxalate, if present in large amounts, can decrease calcium absorption in this way. Phytate can also form a complex with magnesium and interfere with its absorption. Malabsorption of fat decreases calcium absorption. Calcium may form complexes with fat, but also vitamin D absorption is impaired by fat malabsorption, and vitamin D is important for absorption of calcium. Some amino acids and some sugars (particularly lactose) enhance calcium absorption.

The form of the phosphorus in the diet influences its availability for absorption. Most phosphorus is absorbed in the form of inorganic phosphate. Some phospholipids may be absorbed in the organic form, but phosphate must be released from proteins and sugars by digestion before it can be absorbed. Nonabsorbable magnesium and aluminum compounds that are used as antacids bind with phosphate in the gastrointestinal tract and interfere with its absorption.

A high phosphate content in the diet may interfere with calcium absorption due to the formation of an insoluble calcium phosphate complex. Normally, however, more phosphate than calcium is absorbed and with the amount of calcium and phosphorus in usual diets, phosphate is unlikely to interfere with calcium absorption. On the other hand, large calcium supplements in the diet may decrease phosphate absorption.

Magnesium is a constituent of most foods except fat, but digestive factors that influence the release of magnesium from food probably affect its availability for absorption. Magnesium absorption is increased by increased protein intake. Magnesium forms an insoluble complex with phosphate; therefore, high concentrations of phosphate in the diet can decrease magnesium absorption. Conversely, high magnesium concentrations can decrease phosphate absorption.

An excessive amount of calcium in the diet appears to inhibit magnesium absorption. Conversely, according to some studies, when the amount of calcium in the diet is low, a high intake of magnesium appears to inhibit calcium absorption. Other studies, however, have shown that when the diet is supplemented with magnesium, calcium absorption increases. Possibly some of the excess magnesium binds with phosphate, phytate, and oxalate in the intestine so that less calcium is bound to these substances and more calcium is available for absorption.

Several hormones influence the absorption of calcium, magnesium, and phosphate. Parathyroid hormone enhances calcium absorption and possibly increases magnesium absorption as well. Calcitonin does not appear to affect intestinal obsorption of calcium, but possibly inhibits magnesium absorption and enhances phosphate absorption. Growth hormone increases the absorption of calcium and magnesium. Aldosterone decreases magnesium absorption. Excessive amounts of glu-

cocorticoids (e.g., as in corticosteroid therapy or Cushing's disease) appear to decrease calcium and phosphate absorption. Vitamin D increases the absorption of calcium and phosphate. It also enhances magnesium absorption, but it is not known whether this effect results from a primary action of vitamin D or whether the action is secondary to increased calcium and phosphate absorption.

Calcium, phosphate, and magnesium are all secreted into the digestive juices. Therefore, if the dietary intake of any of these substances is low, the amount lost in the feces may be greater than the amount ingested.

Bone Formation and Resorption

The structure of bone is briefly described in chapter 8 in the section on healing of fractures. The major bone mineral belongs to a group of calcium phosphate substances called hydroxyapatites, which have the approximate composition $Ca_{10}(PO_4)_6(OH)_2$. Calcium carbonate and minerals such as magnesium and sodium are also present.

Bone is not a static tissue; it is constantly being formed and resorbed. Although longitudinal bone growth stops as a person reaches maturity, the internal remodeling of bone continues, mainly in response to environmental conditions. This remodeling takes place on endosteal surfaces, surfaces of haversian canals, and periosteal surfaces. It is not generalized but occurs at localized sites. For example, new bone may replace old damaged tissue or trabeculae may be resorbed or reinforced in response to changes in stress on the bone. Bone formation takes calcium and phosphate out of the plasma; bone resorption releases calcium and phosphate into the plasma. Therefore the plasma levels of calcium, and to a lesser extent phosphate, are influenced by the relative rates of bone formation and resorption.

The cells involved with bone formation are called *osteoblasts*; those involved with bone resorption are called *osteoclasts*. A third type of bone cells, the *osteocytes*, are necessary for homeostatic regulation of bone metabolism. They seem to be involved with both bone formation and resorption. Osteoblasts secrete large amounts of an enzyme called *alkaline phosphatase* when they are forming bone matrix. When osteoblastic activity is increased the plasma level of this enzyme increases; therefore the serum alkaline phosphatase is a useful measurement in the assessment of metabolic bone disease (see below).

All the factors influencing bone formation and resorption, and the mineralization of bone, are not understood. Mineralization requires a critical concentration of calcium and phosphate in the ECF. Several hormones influence bone metabolism. Parathyroid hormone increases the rate of bone resorption. Calcitonin inhibits bone resorption. The rate of bone formation is increased by growth hormone. Thyroid hormone increases both osteoblastic and osteoclastic activity, presumably due to its general effect of stimulating cell metabolism. Estrogens inhibit bone resorption and therefore promote bone formation. Bone formation is also influenced by androgens.

Urinary Excretion

The amounts of calcium, phosphate, and magnesium excreted in the urine depend on the amounts filtered and on the amounts reabsorbed by the renal tubules. Active secretion of these substances does not appear to take place.

The amount of calcium filtered depends on the plasma calcium concentration and the rate of glomerular filtration. A decreased rate of glomerular filtration or a low level of plasma calcium decreases the amount of calcium in the urine. Conversely, an increased rate of glomerular filtration or a high plasma calcium level increases urinary excretion of calcium. Normally about 98% of the calcium in the filtrate is reabsorbed. Parathyroid hormone increases tubular reabsorption of calcium and therefore decreases urinary losses of calcium.

Calcium excretion appears to be linked with sodium excretion under usual circumstances. Increased urinary excretion of sodium is associated with increased calcium excretion; calcium excretion is decreased with low rates of sodium excretion. Calcitonin increases calcium and sodium excretion, presumably by decreasing tubular reabsorption.

Tubular reabsorption of phosphate is an active process and the amount reabsorbed is variable. Renal tubular reabsorption of phosphate is a major determinant of the plasma phosphate concentration. Parathyroid hormone inhibits the reabsorption of phosphate by the kidneys and therefore increases phosphate excretion.

The amount of magnesium reabsorbed by the renal tubules is variable. The factors influencing magnesium excretion have not been studied as extensively as the factors influencing calcium and phosphate excretion. The amount excreted depends largely on the plasma level of magnesium and therefore reflects magnesium intake. A high calcium intake increases urinary excretion of magnesium, possibly by inhibiting tubular reabsorption in some way. The effect of parathyroid hormone on magnesium excretion is not clear. Calcitonin may increase magnesium excretion. Thyroid hormone appears to inhibit reabsorption and therefore enhance excretion of magnesium.

Vitamin D

Vitamin D exists in several forms, not all of which are active. (Although originally called a vitamin, vitamin D has the characteristics of a hormone and is now regarded as such.) Provitamin D (7-dehydrocholesterol) in (or on) the skin is converted to vitamin D_3 (cholecalciferol) when the skin is irradiated with ultraviolet light. In addition, cholecalciferol (or other forms of vitamin D) may be ingested in the diet. Cholecalciferol is converted to 25-hydroxycholecalciferol (25-$(OH)D_3$) in the cells of the liver. Physiologically, 25-$(OH)D_3$ has very little activity, but it is subsequently converted to 1,25-dihydroxycholecalciferol (1,25-$(OH)_2D_3$) in the kidneys. This latter substance is the active form of the hormone.

Conversion of 25-$(OH)D_3$ to 1,25-$(OH)_2D_3$ appears to be stimulated by parathyroid hormone, a low plasma calcium concentration, and a low plasma phosphate concentration. The 1,25-$(OH)_2D_3$ subsequently enhances gastrointestinal absorption of calcium and phosphate and together with parathyroid hormone stimulates bone resorption, which releases calcium and phosphate into the blood. When the plasma calcium concentration is high, production of $1,25\text{-}(OH)_2D_3$ is inhibited and instead the kidneys form $24,25\text{-}(OH)_2D_3$, which is inactive.

Parathyroid Hormone

Secretion of parathyroid hormone is stimulated by a low plasma calcium concentration and also by a low plasma magnesium concentration. A very low level of magnesium, however, impairs the synthesis of parathyroid hormone, so that the circulating level of parathyroid hormone may be low even if the plasma calcium concentration also drops. High levels of calcium and magnesium inhibit secretion of parathyroid hormone. Adrenergic (i.e., sympathetic) stimulation appears to increase parathyroid hormone secretion, but the exact physiological role of nervous factors in regulating secretion of this hormone is not yet known.

Parathyroid hormone stimulates the release of calcium from bone; increases renal tubular reabsorption of calcium (i.e., decreases urinary excretion of calcium); inhibits renal tubular reabsorption of phosphate (i.e., increases phosphate excretion); and enhances intestinal absorption of calcium. The net effect of parathyroid hormone, therefore, is to raise the concentration of calcium in the extracellular fluids.

Calcitonin

Calcitonin is a hormone secreted by the thyroid gland (not, however, by the same cells that secrete thyroxine). A high plasma calcium concentration stimulates calcitonin secretion. Calcitonin subsequently inhibits bone resorption (i.e., inhibits release of calcium from bone) and inhibits renal tubular reabsorption of calcium (i.e., promotes calcium excretion), thus bringing about a decrease in the plasma calcium concentration. Calcitonin secretion also appears to be influenced by adrenergic stimulation.

Calcium Imbalance

Calcium metabolism is outlined in Figure 16-4. About 99% of the body calcium is in the bones and teeth. The amount of calcium in the soft tissues and ECF represents a small portion of the total body calcium, but this portion is vital.

The total amount of calcium in the plasma is about 9–10.5 mg/100 ml. Approximately half of this calcium is in the ionized form (i.e., about 5 mg/100 ml or 2.5 mEq/liter). About 40% is bound to the plasma proteins and the rest forms complexes with organic anions such as citrate and amino acids. The calcium bound to the plasma proteins cannot leave the vascular compartment. The calcium complexed to various anions is diffusible, as is the free ionized calcium. The ionized calcium (Ca^{2+}) is the functionally important form and the plasma concentration of ionized calcium is carefully regulated. On the other hand, the amount of calcium bound to the plasma proteins depends on the plasma protein concentration. Therefore, the total plasma calcium concentration may increase if the plasma protein concentration increases, but the level of ionized calcium remains normal.

If the plasma calcium level is decreased, secretion of parathyroid hormone is stimulated. This hormone raises the plasma calcium level by mobilizing calcium from bone, by increasing renal tubular reabsorption of calcium, and by enhancing gastrointestinal absorption of calcium, as already described.

If the plasma calcium level is elevated, parathyroid hormone secretion is inhibited and calcitonin secretion is stimulated. Therefore bone resorption is inhibited, renal reabsorption of calcium decreases (i.e., more calcium is excreted), and gastrointestinal absorption decreases. Consequently the plasma calcium concentration falls back toward normal.

Extracellular calcium ion serves many important functions. Calcium is a strong cation, which binds tightly to anions. It is divalent, therefore it can cross-link two separate anions. These properties

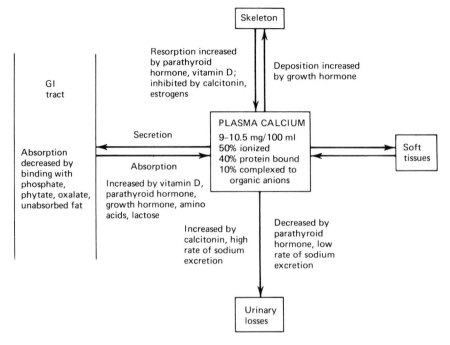

Figure 16-4. *Summary of calcium metabolism.*

make calcium an important "glue" that holds molecules, cell membranes, and cells together. Calcium stabilizes cell membranes and decreases their permeability. When not enough calcium is available, cell membranes become leaky and cells are not as tightly held together. Calcium is also necessary for blood clotting.

Calcium ion is essential for normal neuromuscular function. It influences the movement of sodium across the nerve cell membrane during the conduction of a nerve impulse. The calcium-ion concentration appears to determine the threshold potential of excitable tissues. When the ECF calcium-ion concentration is high, the threshold potential is raised and a stronger stimulus is required to initiate an action potential (nerve impulse). In other words, a high calcium concentration decreases neuromuscular irritability. Conversely, when the ECF calcium-ion concentration is low, the threshold potential is decreased and neuro-

muscular irritability is increased (see Fig. 16-2). Calcium is also necessary for the release of acetylcholine at the synapses.

The calcium concentration of the ECF is higher than the concentration within the cells. The amount of intracellular calcium varies from one type of cell to another. Most of it is bound to some cellular component; very little exists as the free ion. Intracellular calcium is involved in the secretory processes of many glands and is required for muscle contraction. Although calcium is necessary for some intracellular processes, excess calcium ions are very toxic to cells. They inhibit many enzymes, uncouple oxidative phosphorylation (i.e., interfere with ATP production), and bind nucleic acids.

Hypocalcemia

A decrease in the plasma calcium concentration below the normal range is called *hypocalcemia*. A decrease in the plasma protein concentration causes a decrease in total calcium but does not affect the concentration of ionized calcium and does not give rise to clinical signs and symptoms of hypocalcemia. For example, this situation occurs with the nephrotic syndrome and with cirrhosis of the liver.

Causes. The mechanisms commonly responsible for hypocalcemia are inadequate absorption of calcium from the gastrointestinal tract; excessive deposition of calcium in the skeleton as a result of increased bone formation and/or decreased bone resorption; depostition of calcium in soft tissues; insufficient secretion of parathyroid hormone; and failure to respond to parathyroid hormone.

A deficiency of parathyroid hormone is called *hypoparathyroidism.* Often the cause of hypoparathyroidism is not known. In a few cases idiopathic hypoparathyroidism becomes evident in the first year of life and appears to be a sex-linked recessive genetic disorder. Another form of hypoparathyroidism in infants is caused by a congenital absence of the parathyroid glands. In most cases, however, the onset of idiopathic hypoparathyroidism occurs later in life. Hypoparathyroidism sometimes occurs as a complication following thyroid surgery. The parathyroid glands are embedded in the dorsal part of the thyroid gland and their blood supply may be disrupted or they may be inadvertently removed during thyroidectomy. Another cause of parathyroid insufficiency is severe magnesium deficiency, as previously mentioned.

With hypoparathyroidism, gastrointestinal absorption of calcium is decreased, bone resorption is decreased, and urinary excretion of calcium is increased, resulting in hypocalcemia. In addition, renal excretion of phosphate is decreased, causing hyperphosphatemia (an excessive amount of phosphate in the blood).

When the amount of parathyroid hormone in the blood is normal or increased, but the target tissues do not respond to the hormone, the condition is called *pseudohypoparathyroidism.* This disorder, which appears to have a genetic basis, is usually associated with skeletal abnormalities, calcification of soft tissues, and mental retardation, as well as hypocalcemia and hyperphosphatemia.

A high level of phosphate in the ECF enhances bone formation and inhibits bone resorption. Hypocalcemia may therefore occur as a result of hyperphosphatemia. In addition, if the solubility product for calcium and phosphate is exceeded as a result of a high phosphate concentration, calcium phosphate may precipitate in the soft tissues, bringing about a decreased concentration of ionized calcium in the ECF. Hyperphosphatemia frequently accompanies renal failure. Also, vitamin D metabolism may be disturbed when renal disease is present, resulting in decreased intestinal absorption of calcium. Therefore hypocalcemia often occurs with renal failure.

Vitamin D deficiency results in decreased gastrointestinal absorption of calcium and decreased bone resorption. Therefore hypocalcemia can occur because of vitamin D deficiency.

Hypocalcemia frequently occurs in the first 24 to 48 hours after birth (early neonatal hypocalcemia) in premature infants, babies of diabetic mothers, and those with birth asphyxia. The hypocalcemia in premature infants is probably due to immaturity of the parathyroid glands, with subsequent deficiency of parathyroid hormone. Birth asphyxia is accompanied by a high plasma phosphorus concentration, possibly due to breakdown of tissue protein. Usually the hypocalcemia caused by hyperphosphatemia brings about increased secretion of parathyroid hormone, which rapidly raises the plasma calcium level. In newborns, however, the parathyroid glands may not yet be functioning adequately to correct the hypocalcemia. Hypocalcemia may also occur toward the end of the first week (late neonatal hypocalcemia). This hypocalcemia is believed to be due to the high phosphate content of cow's milk formulas.

Some malignant neoplasms of the lungs, breast, and prostate spread to bone and may increase bone formation (osteoblastic metastases). As a result, calcium is deopsited in the skeleton at a rapid rate and hypocalcemia may occur.

Effects. Signs and symptoms of hypocalcemia are primarily due to increased neuromuscular irritability. The plasma calcium concentration at which signs and symptoms develop is variable. A rapid decrease in the plasma calcium level may produce symptoms in some people when the level falls below about 8.5 mg/100 ml, but in some cases of chronic hypocalcemia the plasma calcium concentration may be quite low before signs and symptoms are manifested. The levels of other electrolytes also influence the development of neuromuscular manifestations in hypocalcemia. For example, the effects of hypocalcemia are enhanced by a high potassium concentration, a low magnesium concentration, or increased pH (alkalosis).

The increased neuromuscular irritability associated with hypocalcemia produces a syndrome called *tetany*, which is characterized by paresthesias and spasms of both skeletal and smooth muscles. Sensory symptoms—such as numbness of the fingers, and tingling and burning of the hands, feet, circumoral region, and tongue—usually occur first. Motor symptoms usually begin with skeletal muscle cramps, followed by visible spasms. Carpopedal spasm, which occurs in the hand, is typical (Fig. 16-5). It usually occurs before more generalized spasms of other muscles. Laryngeal muscle spasms may occur, producing hoarseness, breathing difficulty, and possibly death due to asphyxia. Smooth muscle spasms may produce intestinal cramps, biliary colic, or bronchospasm. Convulsive seizures may occur, particularly in infants and children.

Hypocalcemia can cause mental disturbances, such as emotional lability, depression, irritability, memory impairment, confusion, delusions, and hallucinations. These disturbances may occur without signs and symptoms of tetany. In children, chronic hypocalcemia may cause mental retardation.

Chronic hypocalcemia is frequently associated

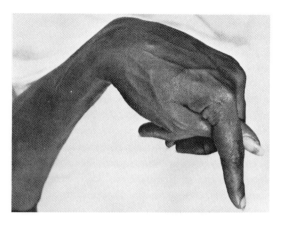

Figure 16-5. *Carpopedal spasm typical of tetany. (From Guyton AC:* Textbook of Medical Physiology, *ed 5. Philadelphia, W.B. Saunders Co., 1976. Courtesy of Dr. Herbert Langford.)*

with abnormalities of the skin, hair, nails, and teeth. In addition, cataracts may develop.

Hypercalcemia
Hypercalcemia is an increase in the plasma calcium concentration above the normal range.

Causes. Three mechanisms are commonly responsible for hypercalcemia: (*1*) excessive absorption of calcium from the gastrointestinal tract, so that the amount absorbed is greater than the amount deposited in the bones and excreted by the kidneys; (*2*) excessive bone resorption, so that calcium is released from the bones at a faster rate than it can be excreted by the kidneys; and (*3*) excessive secretion of parathyroid hormone (*hyperparathyroidism*).

Hyperparathyroidism is classified as primary, secondary, or tertiary. In *primary hyperparathyroidism* excessive secretion of the hormone occurs despite a high plasma calcium concentration, because the normal feedback control is lost. This situation is usually due to a hormone-secreting tumor of one or more of the parathyroid glands. *Secondary hyperparathyroidism* occurs as a compensatory mechanism in response to chronic hypocalcemia (e.g., due to vitamin D deficiency or renal failure). It does not usually produce hypercalcemia because the feedback control mechanism is operating normally. In secondary hyperparathyroidism, hyperplasia of the parathyroid glands occurs. Occasionally the hyperplastic glands develop a tumor or for some other reason fail to respond to the normal feedback control. In this case hypercalcemia develops and the condition is called *tertiary hyperparathyroidism.*

With hyperparathyroidism, the hypercalcemia is a result of increased gastrointestinal absorption and decreased urinary excretion of calcium, and of increased bone resorption. The excessive bone resorption can cause decreased bone density and multiple cysts. Bone pain is common and fractures may occur as a result of trivial injury.

Many malignant neoplastic disorders—particularly carcinoma of the breasts, lung, or kidney; multiple myelomas; lymphomas; and leukemia—are frequently associated with hypercalcemia. In some cases the malignancy may spread to bone and cause bone destruction. Consequently calcium is released from the skeleton at a faster rate than it can be excreted by the kidneys and hypercalcemia occurs. In other cases there is no bone involvement, but the tumor may secrete a substance similar to parathyroid hormone that has the same effect as the hormone.

Hypercalcemia may develop as a result of excessive bone resorption with prolonged immobility (see Chapter 22).

Vitamin D excess can cause hypercalcemia by increasing bone resorption and by increasing gastrointestinal absorption of calcium. The daily dose of vitamin D usually has to exceed 50,000 IU to produce vitamin D toxicity, but in some cases a lower dose can be toxic. Hypercalcemia may occur within two weeks or only after several years of excessive vitamin D administration.

Hypercalcemia sometimes occurs in people with sarcoidosis. Sarcoidosis is a chronic disease of unknown etiology, characterized by multiple granuloma formation. Any tissue may be involved. Bone lesions occur in about 20% of the cases, but hypercalcemia may occur even without bone involvement. The cause of the hypercalcemia is not known, but it is believed to be due to hypersensitivity to vitamin D.

Hypercalcemia due to excessive absorption of calcium is a feature of the *milk-alkali syndrome.* This syndrome can develop in people with peptic ulcers who are treated with large amounts of milk and absorbable antacids, particularly calcium carbonate. The hypercalcemia is accompanied by metabolic alkalosis (see Chapter 15).

Effects. Signs and symptoms of hypercalcemia are mainly caused by decreased neuromuscular irritability, impaired renal function, and deposition of calcium in soft tissues. The plasma calcium concentration at which clinical manifestations develop varies from one person to another. A mild degree of hypercalcemia is often asymptomatic.

Headache and a variety of psychiatric manifestations are common with hypercalcemia. Lethargy, apathy, and depression occur frequently, although some people become agitated and nervous. More severe degrees of hypercalcemia may be associated with disorientation, confusion, delirium, paranoia, and hallucinations. Lethargy and drowsiness may progress to stupor and coma as the plasma calcium level rises.

Decreased neuromuscular irritability results in hypotonicity of the muscles, muscular weakness, and fatigue. Muscular aches and pains may occur. Disturbances of autonomic nervous function and decreased smooth muscle tone cause anorexia, nausea, vomiting, and constipation. Abdominal distension and pain may occur. Hypercalcemia also stimulates the secretion of gastric acid and pepsin, and may be associated with peptic ulcer.

Hypercalcemia also affects heart function. The Q–T interval on the electrocardiogram is shortened, and a variety of cardiac arrhythmias may occur. Hypercalcemia aggravates digitalis toxicity.

Hypercalcemia leads to increased excretion of calcium and excessive calcium in the urine (*hypercalcinuria*). This situation may lead to the development of kidney stones (see Chapter 21).

Hypercalcemia impairs the urine concentrating mechanism and causes polyuria. The high calcium level appears to interfere with sodium chloride transport by the renal tubules, so that the concentration gradient in the renal medulla is decreased. (See Chapter 12 for a discussion of the urine concentrating mechanism.) Together with the anorexia and vomiting, this situation can lead to water deficit. Consequently, thirst is stimulated.

With prolonged hypercalcemia and hypercalcinuria, calcium is deposited in the kidneys. Renal calcification occurs first in the medulla and collecting ducts, where the calcium concentration is highest. Later calcium is deposited in the basement membranes of the proximal tubules and in other regions of the kidneys. The lumens of the tubules and collecting ducts become blocked by calcified cellular debris. The calcium deposits may eventually erode through the tubular epithelium or be surrounded by regenerating epithelium and become interstitial. The interstitial calcium deposits incite an inflammatory reaction, with subsequent fibrosis and scarring. Infection frequently complicates the situation. Renal function is impaired and eventually renal failure, oliguria, and azotemia (an excess of nitrogenous substances in the blood) develop.

Hypertension is a common complication of hypercalcemia. With chronic hypercalcemia the hypertension is mainly due to renal damage and persists after the hypercalcemia is corrected. (See Chapter 13 for a discussion of renal hypertension.) Hypertension can also occur with acute hypercalcemia, however, due to vasoconstriction, which increases peripheral resistance. The vasoconstriction is probably due to catecholamine release, which is enhanced by calcium, but may be partly due to a local action of calcium on the blood vessels. In this case the blood pressure returns to its previous level when the hypercalcemia is corrected.

Calcification of soft tissues (*metastatic calcification*) can occur, especially if the hypercalcemia is accompanied by a normal or elevated plasma phosphate concentration. Calcium salts are de-

posited first in the more alkaline parts of the body, such as the contraluminal side of acid-secreting epithelia (e.g., gastric mucosa, renal tubules, and alveoli of the lungs). Soft tissues around joints are another site of metastatic calcification. Calcium salts are also deposited in the cornea and conjunctiva. Calcium deposits in the cornea form crescent-shaped whitish bands at the lateral margins of the cornea (*band keratopathy*). In the conjunctiva, the deposits have the appearance of glasslike particles and occur in the region of the palpebral fissure. They may cause a gritty sensation in the eyes and produce inflammation. Calcium salts may also be deposited in the skin and cause itching.

Phosphate Imbalance

Phosphorus metabolism is summarized in Figure 16-6. About 85% of the body phosphorus is in the bones and teeth, about 14% is in the cells of the soft tissues, and the remaining 1% is in the ECF.

Phosphorus in the blood is in the form of inorganic phosphate and phosphate bonded to organic molecules (phosphate esters and phospholipids). The term plasma phosphate usually refers to the inorganic form. Inorganic phosphate is present as phosphate (PO_4^{3-}), monohydrogen phosphate (HPO_4^{2-}), and dihydrogen phosphate ($H_2PO_4^-$) and it is difficult to determine the amount of each form precisely. Therefore the total amount of inorganic phosphate is usually expressed as milligrams of phosphorus per 100 ml plasma (or serum). The concentration normally ranges from 3.0 to 4.5 mg/100 ml in adults and is higher in children. Phosphate is mainly an intracellular ion and the plasma phosphate concentration is not controlled as closely as the plasma calcium concentration. Following muscular activity, a recent meal, or administration of insulin and/or glucose, cellular uptake of phosphates is increased as sugar phosphates are formed and consequently the plasma phosphate concentration decreases.

The plasma phosphate concentration is determined by the balance between input due to

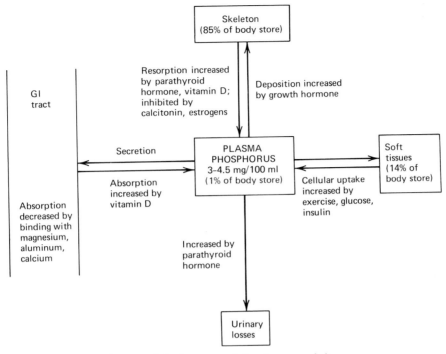

Figure 16-6. *Summary of phosphorus metabolism.*

gastrointestinal absorption, release from bone and soft tissues, and renal tubular reabsorption; and removal due to gastrointestinal secretion, incorporation into bone and soft tissues, and glomerular filtration. Normally the plasma phosphate level is largely determined by the rate of renal tubular reabsorption (i.e., urinary excretion or conservation of phosphate). Renal tubular reabsorption of phosphate is regulated primarily by parathyroid hormone. Secretion of parathyroid hormone is not influenced directly by the plasma phosphate concentration, however, so that the plasma phosphate level appears to be regulated secondarily to plasma calcium.

Phosphate is essential for energy metabolism within the cells and forms part of the ATP molecule (see Chapter 10 under Functions of Oxygen). Phosphate is also essential for the formation of DNA and RNA. Bound to lipids (phospholipids), phosphate is important in the structure of cell membranes. Phosphate is also necessary for bone formation.

Hypophosphatemia

Hypophosphatemia is an abnormally decreased amount of phosphate in the blood.

Causes. The mechanisms most often responsible for hypophosphatemia are malabsorption of phosphate, movement of phosphate into the cells, and decreased renal reabsorption of phosphate.

Phosphorus is widely distributed in foods; therefore dietary lack is an unusual cause of hypophosphatemia. Failure to absorb phosphate, however, can lead to hypophosphatemia. Common causes of phosphate malabsorption are vitamin D deficiency and administration of aluminum and magnesium antacid preparations, which bind with phosphate in the gastrointestinal tract and prevent its absorption. An iatrogenic cause of hypophosphatemia is intravenous hyperalimentation with phosphate-poor solutions. In this case the hypophosphatemia is probably due to movement of phosphate into the cells with glucose. Hypophosphatemia frequently occurs in people with chronic alcoholism; the mechanism is not known, but is possibly related to dietary lack as well as other factors. Decreased renal tubular reabsorption of phosphate (i.e., increased phosphate excretion) occurs with hyperparathyroidism. Decreased renal tubular reabsorption of phosphate can also occur due to a genetic defect and produces familial hypophosphatemic vitamin D–resistant rickets (see below).

Effects. When the plasma phosphate concentration falls, less phosphate is available to the cells and therefore energy metabolism is impaired. The result is profound muscular weakness, malaise, and anorexia. The weakness may be severe enough to cause functional paralysis. Acute respiratory failure may occur, especially if hypophosphatemia is present in a person with pulmonary disease. Cardiac function may be depressed. Neurological abnormalities, such as seizures, may occur.

Hypophosphatemia also affects oxygen transport. The level of diphosphoglycerate in the erythrocytes is decreased. Consequently the affinity of hemoglobin for oxygen is increased (i.e., the oxygen-hemoglobin dissociation curve is shifted to the left) and oxygen is not readily released to the tissues. (See Chapter 10 under Decreased Oxygen-Carrying Capacity of the Blood.) Lack of phosphate also causes alterations in the red blood cell membranes, with resultant hemolysis and anemia. White blood cell function may also be impaired by hypophosphatemia, making an affected person more susceptible to infection. In addition, platelet function may be abnormal, producing a bleeding tendency.

Chronic hypophosphatemia impairs bone metabolism and produces rickets or osteomalacia (see below).

Hyperphosphatemia

Hyperphosphatemia is an abnormally increased amount of phosphate in the blood.

Causes. Hyperphosphatemia occurs mainly as a result of decreased urinary excretion of phosphate. It occurs with hypoparathyroidism and pseudohypoparathyroidism due to increased renal tubular reabsorption of phosphate. With renal failure hyperphosphatemia is caused by decreased glomerular filtration. Hyperphosphatemia also accompanies acromegaly, a condition that results from excessive secretion of growth hormone (see Chapter 19). In this case the hyperphosphatemia is apparently attributable to increased renal tubular reabsorption of phosphate.

Effects. Hyperphosphatemia enhances the deposition of calcium and phosphate in bone and can also cause precipitation of calcium phosphate in the soft tissues. Consequently, hypocalcemia is produced and tetany can occur. Signs and symptoms of hyperphosphatemia are therefore due to hypocalcemia and metastatic calcification, which were described earlier.

Metabolic Bone Disease

The term *metabolic bone disease* refers to bone disorders in which all parts of the skeleton are involved at the molecular level, although clinically, radiographically, and histologically the disease may be evident at only a few sites. The cause of metabolic bone disease is not always known. Known causes include hormonal and nutritional imbalances. Three common types of metabolic bone disease are osteitis fibrosa cystica, osteoporosis, and osteomalacia.

Osteomalacia means softening of bone; it is a condition caused by impaired mineralization of osteoid tissue. When the condition occurs during growth (i.e., childhood), it is called *rickets*. *Osteoporosis* is a condition in which bone mass is decreased, but the composition of the bone remains normal (i.e., the bone is normally mineralized). Osteoporosis and osteomalacia can occur together. *Osteitis fibrosa cystica* occurs in people with advanced hyperparathyroidism and is due to increased bone resorption. Fibrous tissue forms in the areas of bone resorption. Radiographically this condition is characterized by multiple cysts and decreased bone density.

Osteoporosis

Osteoporosis is caused by an imbalance between bone resorption and production. Usually bone resorption is increased and bone production is normal or decreased. The reasons for this imbalance are not known in all cases, and several factors are probably involved. Some researchers believe that calcium deficiency is a cause (i.e., the plasma calcium level is maintained at the expense of bone).

In *primary osteoporosis* no other underlying disease is evident, but bone resorption is increased. Primary osteoporosis occurs almost universally with aging (*senile osteoporosis*). It develops at an earlier age and progresses more quickly in women than in men. In women osteoporosis often becomes evident shortly after menopause (*postmenopausal osteoporosis*), presumably due to diminished estrogen levels (estrogen inhibits bone resorption). Primary osteoporosis occurring in younger people is termed *idiopathic osteoporosis.*

Secondary osteoporosis is associated with a variety of conditions. It frequently occurs in people with Cushing's syndrome and in those receiving corticosteriod therapy. In these cases the osteoporosis appears to be mainly a result of decreased bone formation. Osteoporosis also occurs secondarily to hyperthyroidism. Excessive thyroid hormone has a general effect of increasing cellular metabolism. In the skeleton it causes an increased rate of bone turnover, with bone resorption being slightly more than bone formation. Prolonged immobility is another cause of osteoporosis (see Chapter 22). Osteoporosis also occurs secondarily to malabsorption, vitamin C deficiency, gastrectomy, liver dis-

ease, rheumatoid arthritis, and prolonged heparin administration.

Although osteoporosis affects the entire skeleton, it tends to be most severe in the spine and pelvis. Spontaneous compression fractures of the vertebrae may occur and there is increased susceptibility to fractures of the femur, the ribs, and the lower end of the radius. Kyphosis (an abnormally increased curvature of the thoracic spine) and decreased height may occur due to vertebral compression. Bone pain, especially backache, is a common symptom.

With primary osteoporosis the serum calcium, phosphorus, and alkaline phosphatase levels are within the normal range. With secondary osteoporosis due to Cushing's syndrome, the serum calcium and phosphorus levels may be slightly low, and the alkaline phosphatase level may be slightly increased. With osteoporosis due to hyperthyroidism or immobilization, the serum calcium concentration may be normal or increased.

Osteomalacia and Rickets

The common causes of rickets and osteomalacia are vitamin D deficiency and hypophosphatemia. Vitamin D deficiency may be due to lack of exposure to sunlight, dietary lack, or malabsorption of fat (see Chapter 17). People with chronic renal insufficiency may develop a variety of bony changes, including osteomalacia. In these cases the changes are due to faulty metabolism of vitamin D and other substances. These people may also develop osteitis fibrosa cystica as a result of secondary hyperparathyroidism.

With rickets or osteomalacia due to vitamin D deficiency, the serum calcium and phosphorus levels may be normal or low. Calcium is absent from the urine or is present only in very small amounts. The serum alkaline prosphatase level is characteristically elevated. As mentioned previously, vitamin D enhances intestinal absorption of calcium and phosphate and raises the plasma levels of calcium and phosphorus.

The usual explanation for the development of

rickets and osteomalacia is that the product of calcium and phosphate (Ca × P) of the ECF is below the critical level necessary for the formation of hydroxyapatite crystals in the bone matrix and epiphyseal cartilage. Although this situation occurs with vitamin D deficiency or hypophosphatemia, with renal disease the Ca × P product is usually normal or elevated. Therefore, it is possible that osteomalacia is due to some other mechanism, at least in the case of renal disease. It has been suggested that osteomalacia may be due to an abnormality of osteoid tissue as a result of osteoblastic dysfunction.

Both rickets and osteomalacia are characterized by an excess of poorly mineralized osteoid tissue. (Osteoid is the organic matrix of bone. It is composed of a mucoprotein ground substance in which collagen fibers are embedded.) Uncalcified osteoid resists resorption so that the total amount of bone matrix may be increased.

Normally in an adult most of the bone matrix is calcified, but where new bone is being laid down along the margins of trabeculae and in haversian systems, scattered thin fragments of unmineralized osteoid may occur. These areas are called osteoid borders, or seams. In the early stages of osteomalacia and rickets the number of osteoid borders is increased. Later the osteoid borders become thicker.

Rickets is characterized by defective endochondral bone growth as well as by an increase in osteoid borders. The normal conversion of cartilage to bone fails to occur, resulting in a widening of the epiphyseal plate. The unmineralized osteoid and cartilage are soft and bend easily, producing skeletal deformities (Fig. 16-7).

When rickets develops during infancy the earliest signs are evident in the head and chest. The head has a squared appearance due to an excess of osteoid tissue. The bones of the skull are abnormally soft (craniotabes), so that often the cranium bends under pressure. When the pressure is released it springs back into position. Overgrowth of osteoid tissue at the costochondral junctions causes "beading of the ribs" (rachitic rosary).

Later the ends of long bones become enlarged and thickened; this sign is most evident at the wrists and ankles. Development is slow, the infant stands and walks late, and growth is retarded if the rickets is not treated. When the child begins to walk, the stress placed on the spine, pelvis, and long bones of the legs produces lumbar lordosis and bowing of the legs. When the rickets is prolonged and severe, collapse of the ribs with relative protrusion of the sternum produces pigeon-breast deformity. Dentition may be delayed and abnormal.

Infants with rickets are often irritable, listless, and apathetic. Bone tenderness may be evident and the muscles are hypotonic. Tetany may occur due to hypocalcemia.

Mild degrees of osteomalacia in adults may be asymptomatic. Vague aches and muscular weakness are usually the first symptoms; the muscular weakness is probably due to phosphate deficiency. Later, bone pain becomes the major symptom. It characteristically occurs first in the lumbosacral region and hips, and is aggravated by walking or by attempting to rise from a sitting position. Later the spine and ribs become painful. With severe osteomalacia bone pain is widespread and the person walks with a waddling gait. Skeletal deformities may occur and fractures may result from mild trauma.

Familial hypophosphatemic rickets. Two inherited conditions characterized by hypophosphatemia cause rickets and growth retardation. In *vitamin D–resistant rickets* the basic defect appears to be decreased renal tubular reabsorption of phosphate, which produces hypophosphatemia. The serum calcium level is normal. The child develops a form of rickets that does not respond to physiological amounts of vitamin D, but partial healing occurs when pharmacological doses are administered. This condition is inherited as an X-linked dominant trait.

Vitamin D–dependent rickets is a rare autosomal recessive disorder that is believed to be due to a defect in the enzyme necessary for the conversion of $25\text{-}(OH)D_3$ to $1,25\text{-}(OH)_2D_3$. Both hypophos-

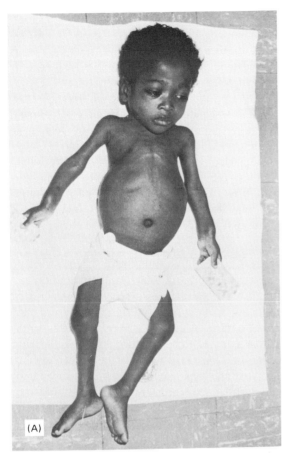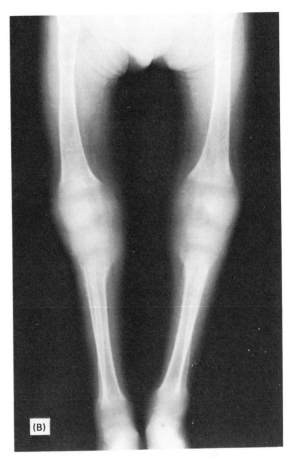

Figure 16-7. A. A 5-year-old boy with vitamin D–dependent rickets. Note small size, bowing of legs, and deformities of forearms. B. X-ray film of legs. Note widened, frayed and cupped ends of long bones. (From Henry D, Elders MJ: Growth retardation syndromes associated with hypophosphatemia. J Ark Med Soc, May 1978.)

phatemia and hypocalcemia occur. This condition resembles vitamin D deficiency but does not respond to physiological amounts of vitamin D. Healing occurs when pharmacological doses of vitamin D are administered.

Magnesium Imbalance

About 57% of the total body magnesium is in the skeleton, about 40% is in the cells of soft tissues, and the rest is in the ECF. The value given for the normal plasma magnesium concentration varies according to the technique used to measure it. A broad range is 1.5–2.5 mEq/liter (1.8–3.0 mg/100 ml), but some researchers consider the normal range to be much narrower, about 1.7–1.9 mEq/liter. Approximately 25% to 35% of the magnesium is bound to plasma proteins; a small amount is complexed to anions such as citrate, phosphate, and sulfate; and the rest is ionized (Mg^{2+}).

As with calcium and phosphate, the plasma

magnesium concentration is determined by the balance between output from glomerular filtration, deposition in bone and soft tissues, and gastrointestinal secretion; and input from gastrointestinal absorption, release from bone and soft tissues, and renal tubular reabsorption. Magnesium is primarily an intracellular electrolyte, and there is apparently no mechanism for mobilizing magnesium from the tissues to maintain the plasma magnesium concentration. In this respect magnesium metabolism is similar to phosphate metabolism. The plasma magnesium concentration is mainly determined by intestinal absorption and urinary excretion.

Within the cells magnesium has an important function as an activator of many enzymes, including some that are involved in energy metabolism. Magnesium is also necessary for the operation of the sodium-potassium pump that is responsible for the movement of potassium into cells. In addition, magnesium is required for nucleic acid and protein synthesis. Magnesium affects neuromuscular irritability in a manner similar to calcium.

Hypomagnesemia

Hypomagnesemia is an abnormally low concentration of magnesium in the plasma.

Causes. The usual mechanisms responsible for hypomagnesemia are malabsorption and increased urinary excretion of magnesium.

Magnesium, like phosphorus, is widely distributed in food and so dietary deficiency is an unusual cause of hypomagnesemia. Prolonged intravenous feeding with magnesium-free solutions, however, can result in hypomagnesemia, especially if the person has abnormal fluid losses, such as gastric suction or diarrhea. Although usual diets contain adequate magnesium any condition that interferes with intestinal absorption can produce hypomagnesemia. Hypomagnesemia often occurs after small-bowel resection.

Increased urinary excretion of magnesium causes hypomagnesemia in association with several conditions. Hypomagnesemia may occur with hyperparathyroidism, possibly because hypercalcemia interferes with renal tubular reabsorption of magnesium. Decreased renal tubular reabsorption of magnesium also occurs with alcoholism. Glycosuria (an abnormal amount of sugar in the urine) is associated with an increase in urinary excretion of magnesium; therefore hypomagnesemia may occur in people with diabetes mellitus, particularly when ketoacidosis is present. After insulin administration more magnesium shifts into the cells and the plasma magnesium level may fall further. Increased urinary loss of magnesium also occurs with diuretic therapy.

Effects. Hypomagnesemia may occur without producing symptoms. The clinical manifestations that do occur are similar to those of hypocalcemia: weakness, tremor, and sometimes tetany and convulsions. Hypomagnesemia may also cause agitation and psychotic personality changes. Lack of magnesium may lead to a loss of potassium from the cells, and hypomagnesemia is sometimes associated with electrocardiographic changes similar to those of hypokalemia. In addition, hypomagnesemia facilitates digitalis toxicity.

Hypermagnesemia

Hypermagnesemia is an abnormally high concentration of magnesium in the plasma.

Causes. Hypermagnesemia is most commonly caused by impaired excretion of magnesium from chronic renal failure; another cause is excessive intake of magnesium-containing compounds (e.g., many antacid preparations). A rare cause of hypermagnesemia is the administration of magnesium sulfate (epsom salts) enemas to infants with congenital megacolon.

Effects. Hypermagnesemia decreases neuromuscular irritability and impairs the release of acetylcholine at neuromuscular junctions. Consequently reflex activity is suppressed. Central nervous system depression occurs, as manifested by drowsiness with moderate elevations of plasma magnesium or coma with severe hypermagnesemia. At very high magnesium levels (greater than 10 mEq/liter), respiratory arrest may occur. Hypermagnesemia can also cause bradycardia (slowing of the heart rate) and produce electrocardiographic changes very similar to those of hyperkalemia. Cardiac arrest can occur when the plasma magnesium concentration reaches 15–20 mEq/liter.

SUGGESTED ADDITIONAL READING

Loomis WF: Rickets. *Sci Am* **223**(6): 76–91, 1970.

Newman JH, Neff TA, Ziporin P: Acute respiratory failure associated with hypophosphatemia. *N Engl J Med* **296**: 1101–1103, 1977.

17

Nutritional Imbalance

Nutrients from the external environment are necessary because they provide not only the materials for growth and maintenance of body tissues but also the energy to carry out metabolic processes. Nutritional balance depends on the availability of nutrients in the diet and on the ability of the body to absorb nutrients and to use nutrients. Nutritional imbalance can result from deficiencies or excesses of nutrients in the diet, failure to absorb dietary nutrients, or inability to use nutrients normally. Inability to use nutrients leads to disturbances of metabolism; these disturbances are discussed in Chapter 18.

NUTRIENTS

The nutrients required by the body are carbohydrates, lipids, amino acids, vitamins, and minerals. The specific amount needed of each nutrient depends on a person's age, activity, and metabolic state. A discussion of specific requirements and food sources of nutrients is beyond the scope of this book.

Carbohydrates

Carbohydrates are organic compounds composed of carbon, hydrogen, and oxygen. Carbohydrate foods are readily available and are the major energy source for the body.

Monosaccharides, or single sugars, are the simplest carbohydrate molecules. Nutritionally, glucose (also called dextrose) is the most important monosaccharide. The structure of this molecule is shown in Figure 17-1. *Disaccharides,* or double sugars, are made up of two monosaccharides linked together. Sucrose (common table sugar), the most common, consists of a glucose molecule linked to a fructose molecule. Lactose, or

milk sugar, is composed of glucose plus galactose. Maltose is made up of two glucose molecules. Monosaccharides and disaccharides are sweet, are soluble in water, and can be crystallized.

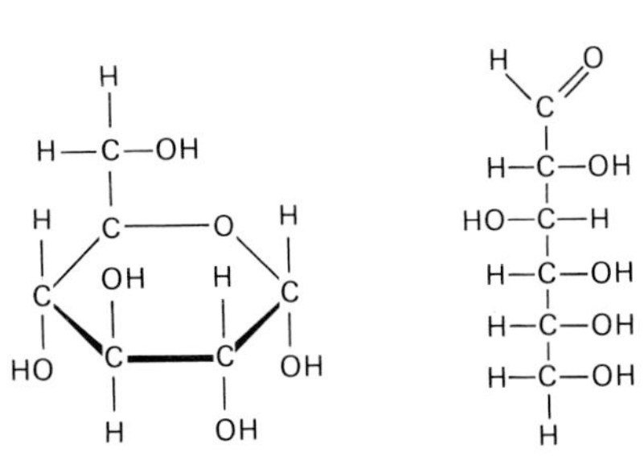

Polysaccharides are complex carbohydrates that consist of many monosaccharide units linked together to form long chains. They are not sweet, are relatively insoluble in water, and cannot be crystallized.

The nutritionally important polysaccharides are starch and glycogen; both are made up of repeating subunits of glucose. Starch is the principal storage carbohydrate of plants. Glycogen is the storage carbohydrate of animals and human beings. In contrast to free monosaccharides, these insoluble polysaccharides cannot diffuse out of the cells and exert no osmotic action within the cells. Starch consists of a mixture of branched chains (amylopectin) and unbranched chains (amylose) that are folded and packed together to form starch grains inside plant cells. Glycogen is similar to amylopectin but is more branched. Glycogen is more soluble than starch and exists as tiny granules in the cytoplasm of animal and human cells.

Cellulose is a polysaccharide used as a structural material in plants. It is also made up of chains of glucose molecules, but the glucose units are linked in a slightly different way than they are linked in starch and glycogen. Cellulose cannot be digested by human beings, but it provides important bulk, which helps to move the food mass along the digestive tract.

Digestion and Absorption

Carbohydrates must be in the form of monosaccharides to be absorbed. Salivary amylase (ptyalin) is an enzyme that catalyzes the hydrolysis of starch to intermediate breakdown products, called dextrins, and to maltose. Food is in the mouth for a very short time and the acid of the stomach inactivates the salivary amylase that is mixed with the food. Therefore, digestion of carbohydrates by this enzyme is limited. Digestion of complex carbohydrates is continued in the small intestine by the

Figure 17-1. *The glucose molecule. Glucose may occur as a ring structure or as a straight-chain aldehyde.*

enzyme pancreatic amylase. This enzyme completes the hydrolysis of starch and glycogen to maltose.

Three enzymes, sucrase, lactase, and maltase (disaccharidases), are located on the luminal side of the membranes of the intestinal mucosal cells. They catalyze the hydrolysis of ingested disaccharides and maltose from starch digestion to their component monosaccharides. Glucose, galactose, and fructose are then absorbed through the intestinal mucosal cells by active transport. They enter the capillaries of the portal venous system and are carried to the liver.

Utilization

In the liver, galactose and fructose are converted to glucose. Some of the glucose is metabolized in the liver and some is released into the general circulation. Glucose from the blood is taken up by all the cells of the body. Insulin is necessary for the transport of glucose into most cells, except those of the liver and central nervous system. As soon as glucose enters a cell, a phosphate group is transferred to it from ATP (adenosine triphosphate) to form glucose-6-phosphate. This process is necessary before glucose can enter the metabolic pathways in the cell. Also, after glucose is phosphorylated it cannot be returned to the blood. Only the liver and kidneys contain the phosphatase enzyme that catalyzes the removal of the phosphate from glucose. Therefore, only these tissues can release free glucose into the blood.

Glucose may be used immediately by the cells or stored as glycogen. The process by which glucose is converted to glycogen is called *glycogenesis*. Glycogenesis occurs in many tissues, most notably the liver and muscles. It usually takes place when the blood sugar level is high or when the glycogen stores of the cells are low.

The hydrolysis of glycogen by the cells is called *glycogenolysis*. In the liver this process yields glucose, which can be released into the blood. In the cells of muscle and other tissues, however, glycogenolysis yields glucose-6-phosphate, which can only be used further within these cells.

The breakdown of glucose for energy is called *glycolysis*. This process, which occurs in all the cells of the body, is described in Chapter 10 (see under Cellular Respiration). Many cells can also oxidize fat and amino acids for energy, but under normal circumstances the brain can only use glucose. Glucose is also the primary energy source for the peripheral nerves, blood cells, and cells of the renal medulla.

Oxidation of glucose yields acetyl CoA (see Chapter 10), which can enter the TCA cycle to produce energy. In the liver and in adipose tissue, acetyl CoA can also be used for the synthesis of fat (*lipogenesis*). Fat synthesis occurs especially when the availability of glucose is high.

Some glucose is used for the production of other compounds needed by the body. For example, the carbon skeletons of some glucose metabolites can be used for the synthesis of certain amino acids. The pentose sugars, ribose and deoxyribose, which are necessary for nucleotide and nucleic acid synthesis (see Chapter 3 under DNA and RNA), can be derived from glucose metabolism. In addition, glucose is used for synthesis of other carbohydrates in the formation of mucopolysaccharides (e.g., heparin) and glycoproteins (e.g., some blood-group substances). Glucose is also used to form glucuronic acid, a substance used in detoxification reactions in the liver (see Chapter 25).

Lipids

Lipids are a structurally heterogeneous group of compounds that are defined on the basis of solubility, as any of a group of organic substances that are soluble in nonpolar solvents. (Water is a polar solvent; see Chapter 25 under General Factors Influencing Absorption.) Lipids are composed mainly of carbon and hydrogen. They also contain oxygen, but in a smaller proportion than in carbohydrates.

Classification

On the basis of chemical composition lipids may be grouped as fatty acids, lipids containing glycerol, lipids not containing glycerol, or lipids combined with other classes of compounds.

Fatty acids. Fatty acids are chains of carbon atoms with hydrogen atoms attached and a carboxyl group (–COOH) at one end. Most fatty acids in edible fat have from 4 to 24 carbons in the chain and most contain an even number of carbon atoms. Those with 4 to 6 carbons are referred to as short-chain fatty acids; those with 8 to 12 carbons as medium-chain fatty acids; and those with more than 12 carbons as long-chain fatty acids.

Fatty acids that have the maximum number of hydrogen atoms attached to each carbon and have no carbon-to-carbon double bonds are said to be *saturated.* In other words, the carbon valence is saturated with hydrogen. Stearic acid and butyric acid are examples of saturated fatty acids. Fatty acids that contain one or more carbon-to-carbon double bonds are said to be *unsaturated* (i.e., the carbon valence is not completely saturated with hydrogen). Fatty acids that contain one carbon-to-carbon double bond are called monounsaturated (e.g., oleic acid); those that contain more than one carbon-to-carbon double bond are called polyunsaturated. Examples of polyunsaturated fatty acids are linoleic acid, which has 18 carbons and 2 double bonds; linolenic acid, which has 18 carbons and 3 double bonds; and arachidonic acid, which has 20 carbons and 4 double bonds. The structures of stearic acid, oleic acid, and linolenic acid are shown in Figure 17-2.

A fatty acid that cannot be synthesized by the body and that is necessary for normal nutrition (i.e., its absence creates a specific deficiency disease) is an *essential fatty acid.* Linoleic acid appears to be the only fatty acid that is essential for human beings. It is used as a precursor for the synthesis of certain other compounds and possibly plays a role in the regulation of cholesterol metabolism.

Lipids containing glycerol. This group includes neutral fats and phospholipids. The major neutral fats are triglycerides, diglycerides, and monoglycerides.

Glycerol is a three-carbon compound with a hydroxyl group (–OH) attached to each carbon atom. A triglyceride is formed by the esterification of three fatty acids with glycerol (Fig. 17-3). The three fatty acids may be the same or different. A diglyceride has two fatty acids attached to glycerol; a monoglyceride has one fatty acid attached to glycerol.

Mixtures of mono-, di-, and triglycerides that are solid at room temperature are usually referred to as fats; those that are liquid at room temperature

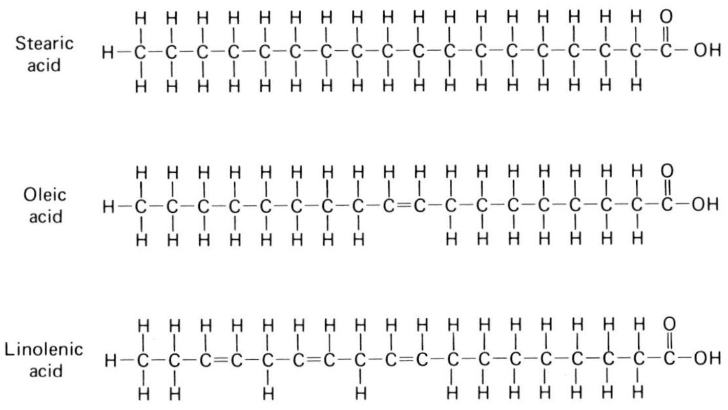

Figure 17-2. *Fatty acids. Stearic acid is saturated, oleic acid is monounsaturated, and linolenic acid is polyunsaturated.*

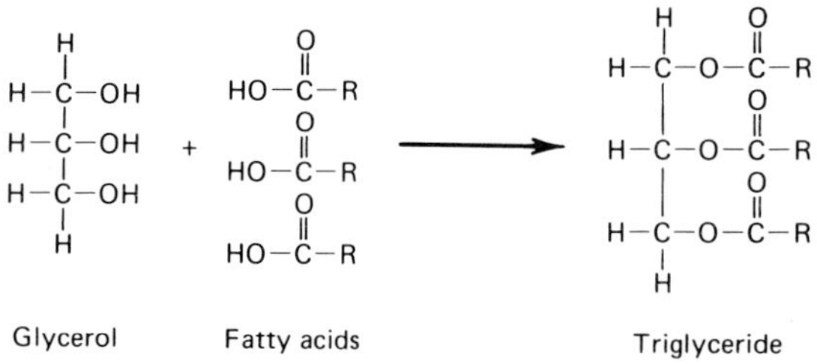

Figure 17-3. *Formation of a triglyceride. R represents the hydrocarbon chains of the fatty acids, which may be the same or different.*

are called oils. The melting point of these substances is influenced by the degree of saturation of their component fatty acids. The greater the degree of saturation, the higher the melting point. Thus, fats contain a high proportion of saturated fatty acids, whereas oils contain a high proportion of unsaturated fatty acids.

Most *phospholipids* consist of glycerol with two fatty acids and one phosphoric acid group attached. Many contain a nitrogenous base. The most widely occurring phospholipids are lecithins, which contain a nitrogenous base called choline (Fig. 17-4).

The structure of phospholipids enables them to associate with water or with nonpolar solvents, because the phosphoric acid part of the molecule is polar (water soluble) and the fatty acid portion is nonpolar (not water soluble). This property is important in the role of phospholipids as structural components of cell membranes and in their involvement in the transport of lipids in the plasma.

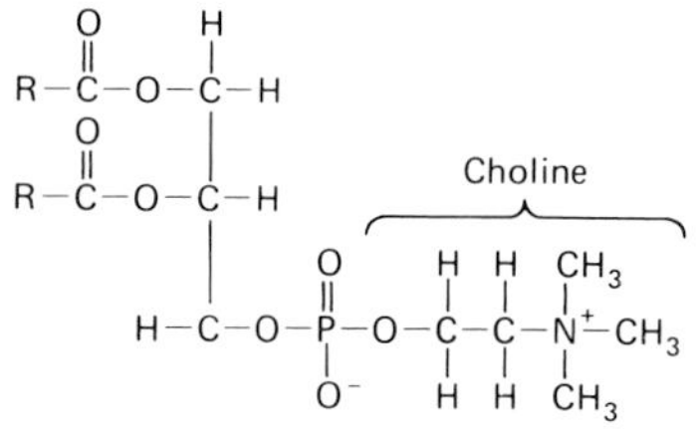

Figure 17-4. *Lecithin. R represents the hydrocarbon chains of the fatty acids.*

Lipids not containing glycerol. This group includes sphingolipids, terpenes, steroids, and waxes. Waxes are not important nutritionally.

Sphingolipids contain the organic base sphingosine or a closely related compound in their structures. Sphingolipids occur in membranes and are found in particularly high concentrations in the brain and nerve tissue, where they form part of the myelin sheath. Sphingomyelins contain phosphoric acid and choline in their structure. Cerebrosides and gangliosides are glycosphingolipids; they have a carbohydrate attached to a sphingolipid.

Terpenes are compounds whose carbon skeletons have a structural relationship to a five-carbon compound called isoprene; many of them contain multiples of five carbon atoms. Examples are carotene and vitamins A, E, and K.

Steroids all have the same basic structure of four fused rings. They differ in the side groups attached to those rings. This group of lipids includes the steroid hormones, bile acids, and sterols. Sterols are steroids with a side chain of 8 to 10 carbon atoms at position 17 and a hydroxyl group (–OH) at position 3, according to the conventional numbering of the carbon atoms. The most important sterol is cholesterol (Fig. 17-5).

Lipids combined with other classes of compounds. Water-soluble proteins conjugated with lipid are called *lipoproteins*. Compounds of lipid conjugated with protein that are insoluble in water but soluble in nonpolar solvents are called *proteolipids*. Lipids conjugated with polysaccharide are called *lipopolysaccharides*.

Digestion and Absorption
Most lipid in the diet is in the form of triglycerides. In addition, small amounts of mono- and diglycerides, phospholipids, and cholesterol are ingested. Triglycerides with long-chain fatty acids are the most common; those with short-chain fatty acids are mainly found in milk fat. Triglycerides with medium-chain fatty acids are uncommon except in certain therapeutic diets. The chain length

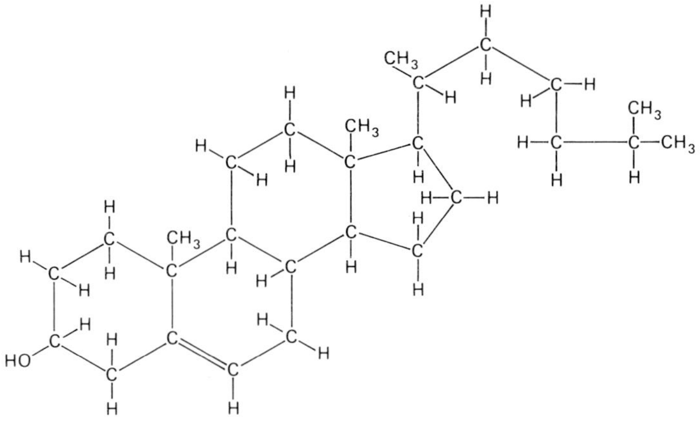

Figure 17-5. *Cholesterol.*

influences the digestion and absorption of triglycerides.

In the stomach, dietary fat is released from protein and carbohydrates by mechanical and chemical actions. An enzyme called gastric lipase, which is secreted in the stomach, can initiate the hydrolysis of triglycerides containing medium-chain or short-chain fatty acids but has little effect on those with long-chain fatty acids.

Chyme (the semifluid mixture of food, saliva, and gastric juice in the stomach) enters the duodenum, where it is mixed with pancreatic juice and bile. Pancreatic juice contains the enzyme pancreatic lipase.

Triglycerides containing short-chain or medium-chain fatty acids are relatively water soluble and are dispersed quite easily in the aqueous contents of the intestine. Triglycerides containing long-chain fatty acids, however, are insoluble and require the detergent action of bile salts to emulsify them. In the small intestine triglycerides and small amounts of diglycerides, monoglycerides, and fatty acids mix with bile salts and phospholipids to form small fat droplets (the oil phase). These droplets are dispersed in the bulk of the intestinal contents (the water phase) to form a stable emulsion. Pancreatic lipase is dissolved in the water phase. Therefore the hydrolysis of triglycerides, which is catalyzed by this enzyme, takes place at the oil-water interface. The finer the emulsion (i.e., the smaller the fat droplets), the greater the surface area available for enzyme action.

The hydrolysis of triglycerides involves the splitting of fatty acids from glycerol. Chemically it is difficult for the middle fatty acid to be split from a triglyceride. Therefore most of the triglycerides are hydrolyzed to monoglycerides and free (or nonesterified) fatty acids. Only a small proportion of the triglycerides is completely hydrolyzed to glycerol and fatty acids.

As the triglycerides are hydrolyzed, the monoglycerides and fatty acids that are released are solubilized by the formation of micelles with bile salts. Micelles are very small aggregates of molecules; they are much smaller than the droplets in an emulsion. The micelles are able to come into close contact with the surfaces of the intestinal mucosal cells, and the monoglycerides and fatty acids enter the mucosal cells. The mechanism of cellular uptake of monoglycerides and fatty acids has not yet been determined. Cholesterol is also solubilized in the micelles and is believed to be absorbed from them. The bile salts pass further along the small intestine and are reabsorbed mainly in the ileum. Bile salts stimulate the digestion and absorption of triglycerides containing

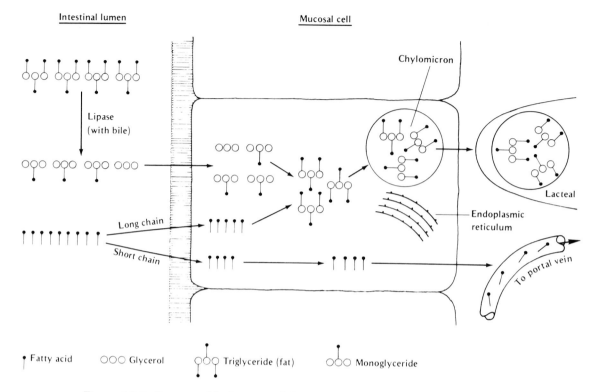

Figure 17-6. *Summary of fat digestion and absorption. (From Landau BR: Essential Human Anatomy and Physiology. Copyright © 1976 by Scott, Foresman and Company. Reprinted by permission.)*

medium-chain or short-chain fatty acids, but because of their water solubility these triglycerides can be digested and absorbed fairly well even when bile salts are lacking.

Inside the mucosal cells the long-chain fatty acids are recombined with monoglycerides and glycerol to form triglycerides. The triglycerides enter the rough endoplasmic reticulum of the cell, where they are wrapped in a protein-phospholipid coat along with a small amount of cholesterol. The resulting lipoprotein particles, which are called *chylomicrons,* are extruded from the mucosal cells and enter the lacteals (lymph capillaries of the intestinal villi). From the lymph the chylomicrons enter the general circulation. The fate of any free glycerol and short-chain and medium-chain fatty acids is different. They pass through the mucosal cells, enter the portal venous capillaries, and are carried to the liver. These processes are summarized in Figure 17-6.

Transport

Lipids are transported in the blood in several forms in association with protein. In the nonfasting state most of the triglycerides in the plasma are contained in the chylomicrons. They are the largest and least dense lipoproteins in the plasma and serve as a transport vehicle for triglycerides and cholesterol from the intestinal mucosa (i.e., exogenous triglycerides) to other tissues of the body. Most triglycerides in the chylomicrons are taken up by adipose tissue, although some are taken up by other tissues. Before the triglycerides can enter the cells, however, they must be hydrolyzed to glycerol and fatty acids. This hydrolysis is catalyzed by the enzyme *lipoprotein lipase*, which is believed to be either bound to the cell membranes or located in the walls of the capillaries.

The *very-low-density lipoproteins* (VLDL, pre-beta-lipoproteins) account for most of the triglyceride in the plasma in the fasting state. The VLDL are mainly assembled in the liver and secreted into the blood. Slight amounts are also formed in the intestine. The function of VLDL is in the transport of endogenous triglycerides; that is, triglycerides derived from body stores or synthesized in the liver. The fate of these triglycerides is similar to that of the triglycerides in the chylomicrons.

The *low-density lipoproteins* (LDL, beta-lipoproteins) carry most of the cholesterol in the plasma. They also contain small amounts of phospholipids, protein, and triglycerides. The LDL originate in the liver; they may result from metabolism of VLDL.

The *high-density lipoproteins* (HDL, alpha-lipoproteins) consist of about 50% protein. The lipid portion is composed mainly of cholesterol and phospholipids. HDL may be involved in the removal of cholesterol from various tissues and its transport to the liver for degradation and excretion.

Free fatty acids (FFA, nonesterified fatty acids) are bound to albumin for transport in the blood.

Utilization

Fat is an important concentrated storage form of energy. A constant turnover of triglycerides occurs in adipose tissue as new fat is stored and stored triglycerides are mobilized for use.

Synthesis and deposition of triglycerides in adipose tissue are favored when the availability of glucose is high. Triglyceride synthesis mainly occurs in the liver, adipose tissue, and intestinal mucosa. Fatty acids must be activated by combining with coenzyme A before they can be esterified with glycerol. Glycerol must be in the active form

of α-glycerophosphate. This compound is an intermediate formed during glycolysis (i.e., the metabolism of glucose) and this pathway is the major source of α-glycerophosphate for triglyceride synthesis. In addition, the liver contains an enzyme that can catalyze the conversion of glycerol to α-glycerophosphate; this enzyme is not present in other tissues.

In addition to the fatty acids derived from the diet, fatty acids can be formed in the body by building the chain two carbons at a time from acetyl CoA. Acetyl CoA for fatty-acid synthesis is mainly derived from glucose metabolism; therefore excess carbohydrates in the diet can be converted to fat for storage. Fatty-acid synthesis requires two B vitamins, biotin and niacin. The niacin forms part of NADPH (the reduced form of nicotinamide adenine dinucleotide phosphate), a coenzyme that is necessary for reduction reactions following each addition of two carbons to the growing fatty-acid chain.

Various fatty acids can also be altered in the body to supply fatty acids that the body needs. An existing fatty acid can be altered by increasing the chain length or by desaturation (i.e., formation of a double bond).

The breakdown of fat (i.e., its mobilization and utilization) is called *lipolysis*. The first step is the hydrolysis of triglycerides to glycerol and fatty acids. This process releases glycerol and fatty acids from adipose tissue into the blood. Glycerol is mainly taken up and metabolized by the liver. It is first converted to α-glycerophosphate, which can either be directly metabolized further through the glycolytic pathway or used to form glucose. α-Glycerophosphate can also be reused in the formation of triglycerides, but under conditions that favor lipolysis this event is unlikely. The fatty acids are rapidly taken up by most tissues of the body and are oxidized for energy. The brain, however, cannot use fatty acids, apparently because they are unable to cross the blood-brain barrier.

The use of fatty acids for energy involves a process called beta-oxidation. This process involves a series of steps; during each step a two-carbon fragment is released as acetyl CoA. The process is continued until the fatty acid is completely broken down. In each step one FAD and one NAD are reduced; reoxidation of these coenzymes results in the formation of five ATP. The acetyl CoA that is formed enters the TCA cycle for further oxidation, which results in the formation of many more ATP molecules.

Two two-carbon units from acetyl CoA may condense to form acetoacetic acid, which subsequently can be converted to acetone or beta-hydroxybutyric acid. These three compounds are referred to as *ketone bodies*. They are normal by-products of fat metabolism that are usually formed in small amounts. In most tissues they can be oxidized further for energy. The liver, however, does not have the necessary enzyme to metabolize ketone bodies. Therefore, ketone bodies produced in the liver diffuse into the blood and are carried to other tissues for oxidation. When oxidation of fatty acids is excessive, as in starvation or in diabetes mellitus, acetyl CoA is formed at a faster rate than it can be fed into the TCA cycle. Consequently a high proportion of acetyl CoA is converted to ketone bodies and they accumulate in the blood. This condition is called *ketosis*.

Cholesterol is metabolized in a variety of ways. In addition to cholesterol from dietary sources, cholesterol is synthesized in the body from acetyl CoA. Probably most tissues can synthesize cholesterol, but the liver is the major site of its production. Cholesterol is a precursor for the synthesis of steroid hormones and vitamin D. In addition, it is converted to bile salts in the liver. Cholesterol is excreted in the bile; some of this cholesterol is reabsorbed, but some is eliminated in the feces.

Amino Acids

Amino acids are organic compounds that contain a carboxyl group ($-COOH$) and an amino group ($-NH_2$) in their structures. They are mainly required for the synthesis of proteins in the body, although they can also be used for energy. In addi-

tion, amino acids provide a source of nitrogen for the synthesis of other nitrogen-containing compounds.

The same 20 amino acids occur in the proteins of all presently existing species of organisms. Several other amino acids also occur in nature; some of them are found in only a few proteins, and others do not occur in protein. Most amino acids found in proteins have the carboxyl and amino group attached to the same carbon atom; that is, they are primary amino acids.

Histidine, arginine, and lysine contain more than one amino group and are *basic* amino acids. Aspartic acid and glutamic acid contain two carboxyl groups and are *acidic* amino acids. Asparagine and glutamine are structurally related to aspartic acid and glutamic acid but contain two amino groups; they are *neutral* amino acids. The rest of the amino acids are also neutral. The aliphatic amino acids are glycine, alanine, valine, leucine, isoleucine, serine, and threonine. Phenylalanine and tyrosine contain an aromatic ring in their structures and tryptophan has two rings in its structure; these three are referred to as *aromatic* amino acids. Methionine and cystine are *sulfur-containing* amino acids. The reduced form of cystine, called cysteine or half-cystine, is counted together with cystine as one amino acid. Proline is slightly different from the other amino acids in that its nitrogen is contained in a ring rather than as a primary amino group.

Two other amino acids, hydroxylysine and hydroxyproline are found in collagen but do not occur in other proteins. They are formed by the hydroxylation of lysine and proline, respectively, after these amino acids have been incorporated into the polypeptide chain.

Amino acids are derived from dietary protein. Histidine, isoleucine, leucine, lysine, methionine, phenylalanine, threonine, tryptophan, and valine are *essential amino acids*. That is, they cannot be synthesized in adequate amounts by the body and must be provided in the diet. In addition to providing essential amino acids, the total amount of protein (or total nitrogen) in the diet must supply enough material for the synthesis of nonessential amino acids and other nitrogen-containing compounds.

Digestion and Absorption

Protein digestion begins in the stomach, although gastric digestion is not essential for the utilization of dietary protein. The stomach secretes an inactive enzyme precursor called pepsinogen, which is activated to the enzyme pepsin by the hydrochloric acid in the stomach. Pepsin catalyzes the breaking of peptide bonds in protein, producing smaller polypeptides called proteoses and peptones.

Protein digestion continues in the small intestine, with enzymes from the pancreas, as well as enzymes secreted by the intestine, being involved. The pancreatic juice contains two inactive enzyme precursors, trypsinogen and chymotrypsinogen. Trypsinogen is activated to trypsin by enterokinase, an enzyme secreted by the duodenum. Trypsin activates chymotrypsinogen to chymotrypsin. Both trypsin and chymotrypsin act on proteins, proteoses, and peptones to produce very small peptides (oligopeptides) and dipeptides.

Carboxypeptidase from the pancreas and aminopeptidase secreted by the intestine act by removing one amino acid at a time from the end of a polypeptide chain. Other peptidase enzymes located on the membranes of the intestinal mucosal cells or in the mucosal cells complete the hydrolysis of oligopeptides and dipeptides to amino acids.

Absorption of amino acids appears to be by carrier-mediated processes. For most of the amino acids the process seems to be energy dependent (i.e., active transport). In addition to free amino acids, some oligopeptides may be taken up by the mucosal cells and hydrolyzed to amino acids within the cells. The amino acids enter the portal capillaries and are carried to the liver.

Utilization

The amino acids in the blood and interstitial fluid are a mixture of amino acids absorbed from the intestine and those released from the cells as a result of breakdown of tissue protein. They form an extracellular amino acid "pool" that is available to all the cells. Amino acids are taken into the cells by active transport. In the cells they are mainly used for the synthesis of protein, although some are used for the synthesis of other compounds. The proteins that are formed are structural and functional components of the tissues. Amino acids are not stored in the body the way fat and carbohydrate are, although tissue proteins can be broken down to provide amino acids for other purposes if necessary.

Metabolism of many amino acids that are not involved in protein synthesis begins with deamination; that is, the removal of the amino group ($-NH_2$). The process of *oxidative deamination* results in the conversion of an amino acid to its corresponding keto acid with the release of ammonia. Ammonia is converted to urea in the liver; the urea is carried in the blood to the kidneys and excreted in the urine. A more important deamination mechanism is *transamination*. In this process the amino group from one amino acid is transferred to a keto acid to form a new amino acid and keto acid (Fig. 17-7). Transamination reactions require pyridoxal phosphate, a form of vitamin B_6, as a coenzyme. Transamination is a means by which nonessential amino acids can be formed in the body. The necessary keto acids can be derived from oxidation of glucose or fatty acids.

Some deamination and transamination reactions yield pyruvic acid or keto acids that are intermediate compounds in the TCA cycle. These substances can either be converted to glucose or fed into the TCA cycle for further oxidation to yield energy.

Many amino acids are involved in other important processes. Some are used for the synthesis of purines and pyrimidines (the bases in nucleic acids). Glycine is used in the formation of porphyrin, an intermediate in the synthesis of heme; it is used in the synthesis of creatine; and it is used in conjugation reactions in the liver (see Chapter 25 under Metabolism of Foreign Chemicals).

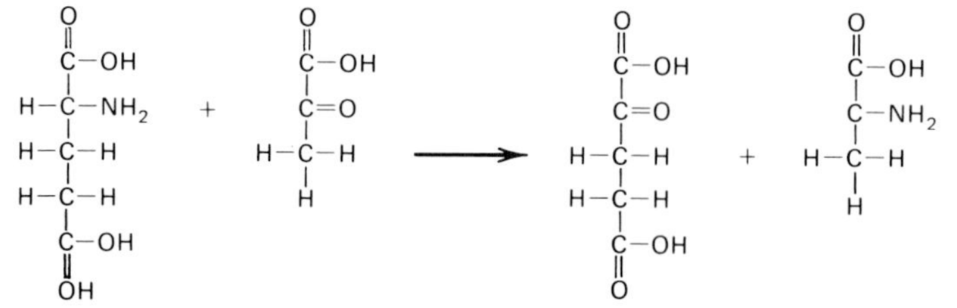

Glutamic acid (amino acid)   Pyruvic acid (keto acid)   α-Ketoglutaric acid (keto acid)   Alanine (amino acid)

Figure 17-7. *Transamination.*

Tyrosine is used in the synthesis of three hormones, epinephrine, norepinephrine, and thyroxine and in the synthesis of dopamine, a neurotransmitter in the brain. It is also a precursor of melanin, the pigment found in skin and hair. Tryptophan can be converted to 5 hydroxytryptamine (serotonin), which may act as a neuroregulator in the brain. Another neuroregulator in the CNS, gamma-aminobutyric acid (GABA), is formed from glutamic acid. Methionine is used in a variety of transmethylation reactions (e.g., in the synthesis of choline) as a donor of methyl groups ($-CH_3$).

Nitrogen Balance

Since dietary protein is the major source of nitrogen in the body, a comparison of nitrogen intake with nitrogen output reflects the metabolism of protein. When the nitrogen intake from protein approximately equals the nitrogen lost in feces and urine, a person is said to be in *nitrogen balance.* This situation is usual for an adult who consumes adequate amounts of the essential amino acids. When nitrogen intake exceeds nitrogen excretion, a person is said to be in *positive nitrogen balance.* This situation occurs when new tissues are being synthesized and the body is retaining nitrogen in the form of new protein, for example, during growth, during pregnancy, and during convalescence from injury or disease when lost tissue is being replaced. When nitrogen loss is greater than nitrogen intake, a person is said to be in *negative nitrogen bal-*

ance. This situation occurs when the rate of tissue breakdown is greater than the rate of new protein synthesis, for example during starvation, during some disease conditions, during the initial period after injury or burns, and for a brief period following surgery.

Vitamins

Vitamin is a general term for a number of unrelated organic substances that are present in small concentrations in foods, that are necessary for normal metabolic functioning, and that cannot be synthesized in the body. They are generally classified as water soluble or fat soluble. The water-soluble vitamins include those of the B complex and vitamin C. The fat-soluble vitamins are A, D, E, and K. Vitamin D is discussed in Chapter 16 and is not considered here.

Absorption and Storage

With the exception of vitamin B_{12}, the water-soluble vitamins appear to be absorbed fairly easily from the small intestine. Storage of these vitamins in the body is limited, although some are stored in the liver. Excess water-soluble vitamins are excreted mainly in the urine.

Vitamin B_{12} is a large molecule that diffuses across the intestinal epithelium to a very limited extent. Its active absorption requires the presence of a mucoprotein called *intrinsic factor,* which is secreted by the stomach. Vitamin B_{12} forms a complex with intrinsic factor in the stomach and the complex is carried to the ileum. Intrinsic factor attaches to the epithelial cells of the ileum and facilitates the uptake of vitamin B_{12}; calcium is also required for this process. The intrinsic factor does not appear to be absorbed.

The fat-soluble vitamins are absorbed in much the same way as dietary fat and seem to require the presence of bile salts. After uptake by intestinal mucosal cells they are incorporated into the chylomicrons and enter the lymph capillaries. Vitamins A, D, and K are stored in the liver; vitamin E is stored in adipose tissue.

Functions

Vitamin A. Several structurally related compounds have vitamin A activity. The most common ones from animal sources are retinol and 3-dehydroretinol (preformed vitamins). Several carotenoid plant pigments (provitamin A) can be converted to vitamin A in the body.

Vitamin A is necessary for the formation of rhodopsin (visual purple) in the rod cells of the retina and therefore is important for vision in dim light. Vitamin A is also required for maintenance of epithelial tissue and maintenance of bone growth, possibly by influencing cellular differentiation and mitosis through an effect on protein synthesis.

Vitamin B complex. The B vitamins function as coenzymes in carbohydrate, fat, and amino acid metabolism. In relation to this function specific vitamins have already been mentioned earlier in this chapter and in Chapter 10.

Thiamine (vitamin B_1) functions as a coenzyme in oxidative decarboxylation reactions; that is, the removal of carbon dioxide from compounds. It is particularly important in carbohydrate metabolism in the conversion of pyruvic acid to acetyl CoA and also in one of the reactions in the TCA cycle.

Riboflavin (vitamin B_2) forms part of the structure of flavin mononucleotide (FMN) and flavin adenine dinucleotide (FAD), two coenzymes involved in oxidation-reduction reactions. FAD is important for electron transport in energy metabolism. FMN is involved in oxidative deamination of amino acids and in other reactions.

Niacin and *niacinamide* are two forms of the same vitamin. They are used to form the coenzymes NAD (nicotinamide adenine dinucleotide) and NADP (nicotinamide adenine dinucleotide phosphate). Both substances act as coenzymes in oxidation-reduction reactions. NAD is involved in oxidative degradation of food molecules for energy, whereas NADP is involved in synthesis reactions (e.g., fatty-acid and steroid synthesis).

Vitamin B_6 is a collective term for three closely related compounds: pyridoxine, pyridoxal, and pyridoxamine. These compounds are used in the body to form pyridoxal phosphate, a coenzyme for transamination reactions and other reactions involved in amino acid metabolism. Pyridoxal phosphate also takes part in the synthesis of porphyrin.

Folic acid acts as a coenzyme in a number of reactions involving the transfer of a single carbon unit. It is necessary for the synthesis of purine nucleotides, which are incorporated into DNA and RNA. Folic acid is also involved in amino acid metabolism.

Cyanocobalamin (vitamin B_{12}) acts as a coenzyme in methylation reactions; that is, the transfer of methyl groups ($-CH_3$). It interacts with folic acid in the synthesis of nucleic acids. Vitamin B_{12} is necessary for CNS functioning, although its exact role is not known.

Pantothenic acid forms part of the structure of coenzyme A. Coenzyme A plays a vital role in many metabolic reactions. Linked to acetate to form acetyl CoA, it is the central compound in energy metabolism and in the synthesis of fatty acids and steroids. Linked to succinate to form succinyl CoA, it takes part in the TCA cycle and in other reactions, including the synthesis of porphyrin.

Vitamin C. Vitamin C (ascorbic acid) has a variety of metabolic functions, which in most cases appear to involve hydroxylation reactions (i.e., the addition of a hydroxyl group (–OH) to a molecule). The exact mechanism by which ascorbic acid participates in these reactions is not understood.

Ascorbic acid is necessaary for the hydroxylation of proline and lysine in the synthesis of collagen, the major protein of connective tissue. In the adrenal medulla ascorbic acid is involved in the conversion of tyrosine to dihydroxyphenylalanine (DOPA). DOPA is subsequently used in the synthesis of epinephrine and norepinephrine. Ascorbic acid is also necessary for the synthesis of steroid hormones of the adrenal cortex. In addition, ascorbic acid appears to be involved in the conversion of cholesterol to bile acids by participating in hydroxylation reactions; it may also be involved in other metabolic processes.

Vitamin E. Several compounds, called tocopherols, have vitamin E activity. Vitamin E acts as an antioxidant that can prevent the oxidation of polyunsaturated fatty acids, vitamin A, and vitamin C. Physiologically vitamin E is believed to function as a lipid antioxidant to prevent the formation of lipid peroxides. Lipids are important structural components of cell membranes, and peroxidation of lipids disrupts membranes. Therefore, vitamin E is important in stabilizing membranes. Selenium, a trace element in the body, acts synergistically with vitamin E in preventing lipid peroxidation.

Vitamin K. This vitamin is necessary for the synthesis of clotting factors II (prothrombin), VII, IX, and X in the liver (see Chapter 7). The exact mechanism of its action is not known.

Minerals

Many minerals occur in varying amounts in the body. Some are important as enzyme activators or form part of an enzyme molecule; others are important structurally. The functions of some minerals in the body are not known. Sodium is discussed in Chapters 11 and 12; chloride is discussed in Chapter 15; and calcium, phosphorus, magnesium, and potassium are discussed in Chapter 16. Iodine is included in the discussion of thyroid function in Chapter 19. Only iron is considered here.

Iron balance is mainly controlled by regulating iron absorption from the gastrointestinal tract. Dietary iron is usually in the ferric form (Fe^{3+}). Gastric acid reduces it to ferrous iron (Fe^{2+}), the form in which it is absorbed. Ascorbic acid enhances iron absorption by reducing ferric iron to ferrous iron. Absorption occurs mainly in the duodenum, where iron is taken into the mucosal cells, probably in combination with amino acids or sugars. Once inside the cells some of the iron is combined with a protein, apoferritin, to form ferritin, which is a storage form of iron. Some of the iron is released into the blood, where it is transported in combination with a plasma protein called transferrin.

The amount of iron absorbed seems to depend on the availability of unsaturated transferrin to carry it from the mucosal cells. Iron remaining in the mucosal cells is lost as the cells are sloughed. Normally only a very small proportion of ingested iron is absorbed, but people with iron deficiency absorb a much higher proportion. The iron that is not absorbed is eliminated in the feces. Trace amounts of iron are lost in urine and sweat. Blood loss due to menstruation, hemorrhage, or blood donations accounts for varying amounts of iron loss from the body.

Bound to transferrin, iron is transported to the body cells for utilization or storage. About 60% to 70% of the iron in the body is incorporated into hemoglobin, about 5% is in myoglobin, about 5% is in cellular enzymes involved in oxidative reactions (e.g., the cytochromes of the respiratory chain), and the rest is stored. The main sites of storage are the liver, spleen, and bone marrow, where iron is stored as ferritin or hemosiderin (a protein-bound ferric oxide). Copper appears to be necessary for the mobilization of stored iron for heme synthesis.

NUTRITIONAL DEFICIENCY

Nutritional deficiency can be due to inadequate dietary intake or failure to absorb ingested nutrients. In addition, a deficiency state can occur if increased utilization or increased loss of specific nutrients is not compensated by increased dietary intake. A description of all the nutritional deficiency diseases is beyond the scope of this book and can be found in any nutrition textbook. Only selected examples of each mechanism are given here.

Inadequate Dietary Intake

In some cases dietary deficiencies are due to unavailability of food. In some cases they are due to lack of knowledge of nutrient requirements and food sources of specific nutrients. In other cases intake may be inadequate due to psychological or physical factors that impair appetite or make eating difficult. Extreme examples of inadequate intake are starvation and protein-energy malnutrition. These conditions not only occur as a result of dietary lack, but can also occur due to failure to absorb nutrients. Therapeutic starvation is occasionally used in the treatment of obesity.

Starvation

Total deprivation of food ultimately results in death, but people can survive starvation for fairly long periods. When food intake is restricted, the nutritional needs of the body are supplied by the body stores. The length of survival depends on the size of the body nutrient stores and the adaptive mechanisms of the body.

The primary need is energy for vital functions. Most tissues can use fat for energy, but the brain requires a continuous supply of glucose. Initially the blood glucose level is maintained by breakdown of liver glycogen, but this supply lasts only a few hours. Then the necessary glucose for the brain must come from gluconeogenesis. Initially gluconeogenesis occurs mainly in the liver and only to a slight extent in the kidneys, but with prolonged fasting most of the gluconeogenesis occurs in the kidneys.

Tissue protein is catabolized, and some of the amino acids that are released are converted to glucose. Most amino acids come from the breakdown of skeletal muscle protein. The amount of alanine released into the blood is more than can be accounted for by the alanine content of the muscle protein, probably because alanine is formed by transamination reactions in the muscle. As stated earlier, muscles cannot release glucose into the blood, but glycogenolysis yields glucose-6-phosphate, which can be metabolized to pyruvic acid. Some of the pyruvic acid is further metabolized for energy in the muscles, but some can be converted to alanine by accepting an amino group from other amino acids derived from breakdown of muscle protein. The alanine is released into the blood and carried to the liver, where it is reconverted to pyruvic acid. The pyruvic acid is then used to form glucose, which is released into the blood (Fig. 17-8). Lactic acid produced by anaerobic glycolysis in the muscles can also be reconverted to glucose in the liver. By these mechanisms a fixed supply of glucose can be recycled. Initially the blood level of alanine is quite high, but as fasting continues the level of alanine falls; the circulating alanine is gradually converted to glucose, which is consumed by the brain.

Simultaneously with the catabolism of muscle protein, fat is mobilized from adipose tissue. The glycerol from lipolysis is converted to glucose in the liver and the fatty acids are used by the tissues that can metabolize them. The increased use of fat results in a buildup of ketone bodies in the blood. When the concentration of ketone bodies reaches a high enough level, possibly within a week, the brain is able to adapt and metabolize them as a source of energy. When this adaptation occurs, less glucose has to be provided from gluconeogenesis. Protein breakdown slows, but it does not stop completely. The ketone bodies in the blood cause ketoacidosis (see Chapter 15 under Metabolic Acidosis).

The initial weight loss during starvation is quite

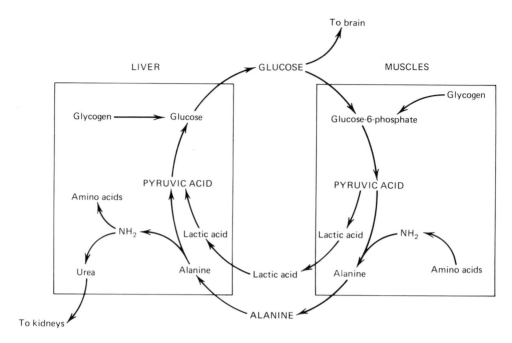

Figure 17-8. *The pyruvic acid–alanine cycle.*

rapid and is mainly due to water loss. Increased protein catabolism results in an increased load of urea to be excreted; also, an increased loss of minerals such as calcium, potassium, and magnesium occurs. Therefore the solute load is increased, causing increased obligatory urinary water loss. As starvation continues weight loss slows and is mainly due to consumption of body fat.

During starvation the caloric requirements of the body are reduced because the basal metabolic rate decreases and metabolically active tissue is lost due to protein breakdown. Starving children stop growing almost immediately. Starving people tend to use available energy more efficiently and engage in less spontaneous activity. The body temperature may be reduced.

Protein-Energy Malnutrition

The term *protein-energy malnutrition* (PEM), or protein-calorie malnutrition, refers to a group of conditions associated with nutritional deprivation in children. According to one classification, *kwashiorkor* is the term used for the condition of children with edema who weigh between 60% and 80% of their expected weight for age. Children without edema who weigh less than 60% of their expected weight for age are considered to have *marasmus*. The term *marasmic kwashiorkor* is used for the condition of children with edema who weigh less than 60% of their expected weight for age. Children who weigh between 60% and 80% of their expected weight for age and who do not have edema are simply classified as underweight.

Marasmus mainly occurs during infancy. Often the child is weaned from the breast early or is never breast-fed and an adequate substitute diet is not available. Poor living conditions are frequently a contributing factor; the home may not have sanitary facilities, running water, or refrigeration. Consequently milk formulas for bottle-feeding become contaminated and produce diarrhea, which further compromises the nutritional status of the child.

Marasmus is caused by a very low intake of protein and calories; it is characterized by extreme wasting of muscles and subcutaneous tissue and stunting of growth. The head usually appears large in proportion to the rest of the body and the eyes are staring. Weakness, motor retardation, and hypothermia (low body temperature) are common. Life-threatening hypoglycemia (an abnormally low blood sugar level) may occur. Infants with marasmus are often apathetic and relatively unresponsive to their environments but have periods of hyperirritability and fretfulness.

Kwashiorkor occurs in older infants and children after they have been weaned from the breast. Due to cultural habits or lack of suitable weaning foods, the child is fed a starchy diet; the diet may be adequate in calories but is deficient in protein. The onset of kwashiorkor is usually precipitated by an acute infection.

Kwashiorkor is characterized by edema, which may mask muscle wasting. Subcutaneous fat may be fairly well preserved. Growth is stunted. The liver is often enlarged and infiltrated with fat. A variety of skin lesions occur. The hair is dry and becomes lighter in color; hair that is normally curly becomes straight. Children with kwashiorkor are usually listless, apathetic, and irritable.

In marasmus the adaptations described earlier for starvation usually occur. Mobilization of protein from muscles maintains the extracellular amino acid pool so that proteins necessary for homeostasis can be preserved. It is believed that kwashiorkor represents a failure of this adaptive mechanism because the high carbohydrate intake inhibits the breakdown of muscle protein. Since dietary protein is inadequate, the level of the extracellular amino-acid pool is low, and the amino acids necessary for the synthesis of essential proteins are not available. In particular, synthesis of albumin by the liver is depressed and the plasma albumin level drops. Consequently the plasma on-

cotic pressure is low, which is partly responsible for the edema in kwashiorkor (see Chapter 11 under Abnormal Distribution of ECF). Retention of sodium and water by the kidneys also contributes, but the mechanism responsible for this fluid retention is not understood.

The liver is a normal site of triglyceride synthesis, but fat is not normally stored in the liver. In kwashiorkor the high carbohydrate intake favors lipogenesis and it is believed that depressed synthesis of the protein necessary for transport of triglycerides out of the liver as VLDL is responsible for the accumulation of fat in the liver.

Marasmic kwashiorkor represents an intermediate form of severe PEM, with clinical features of both marasmus and kwashiorkor. Anorexia (lack of appetite) often accompanies kwashiorkor, and in some cases the child may be too ill to eat as a result of infection. In addition, severe protein deficiency can impair secretion of pancreatic enzymes, which in turn impairs digestion and absorption. Consequently marasmus is superimposed on the kwashiorkor.

Children with PEM often have anemia. Iron deficiency is a factor in some cases, especially in marasmic infants in the first year of life. Other children have adequate stores of iron in the liver but may be unable to utilize the iron for hemoglobin production because they lack copper. In some cases folic acid deficiency is responsible for the anemia. Depression of bone marrow function due to infection is probably a contributing factor. The effects of anemia are discussed in Chapter 10.

PEM reduces resistance to infection. In turn, infection contributes to PEM by depressing appetite, by increasing metabolism, and often by interfering with digestion and absorption of protein. Upper respiratory infections and gastrointestinal infections are common. Diarrhea as a result of the latter leads to ECF volume deficit, acidosis, and electrolyte imbalances (see Chapters 12 and 15). Potassium and magnesium deficits are common.

Vitamin A deficiency may accompany PEM. As a result, the child develops *xerophthalmia*. The first symptom is night blindness. It is due to a decrease in the amount of rhodopsin in the rod cells and an increase in the time required to regenerate rhodopsin after it has been bleached by light. Consequently adaptation to dim light takes longer and vision is impaired in the dark. When vitamin A deficiency is more severe, the conjunctival mucosa becomes keratinized; the normal moist mucosa is replaced with a dry epithelium. Epithelial debris may accumulate as foamy white patches (Bitot's spots) at the edges of the eye. Keratinization of the corneal mucosa follows, producing a dry, opaque cornea and impairing vision. Corneal ulcers may develop and damage may extend to deeper layers, causing softening of the cornea (keratomalacia). Eventually the iris and lens may be damaged. Permanent scarring and blindness result.

Mucous membranes lining the respiratory, gastrointestinal, and genitourinary tracts may also become keratinized due to vitamin A deficiency. Consequently, defense against infection is impaired (see Chapter 28).

Failure to Absorb Nutrients

Failure to absorb nutrients may result from inadequate digestion (*maldigestion*) or from an inability of the products of digestion to cross the intestinal mucosa and enter the lymphatics or portal venous capillaries (*malabsorption*). Maldigestion or malabsorption may be general, affecting all types of foodstuffs, or selective, affecting one particular type of nutrient.

General maldigestion and malabsorption result in weight loss, muscle wasting, and, in children, failure to grow because of inability to absorb sufficient nutrients. Occasionally edema occurs due to inadequate absorption of protein (see discussion of edema in kwashiorkor above). Anemia commonly occurs because of failure to absorb iron, folic acid, and vitamin B_{12}. Insufficient absorption of calcium and vitamin D may lead to osteomalacia and osteoporosis (see Chapter 16).

Vitamin K deficiency leads to bleeding (see Chapter 7). Insufficient absorption of vitamin E occasionally causes hemolysis due to increased fragility of the red blood cell membranes. Vitamin E deficiency is most likely to occur in infants; they may not have a store of vitamin E in the body because it is not easily transported across the placenta and cow's milk contains relatively little of this vitamin. Malabsorption usually has to occur for a relatively long time before vitamin A deficiency is manifested because most people have vitamin A stored in the body. Skin changes may occur due to vitamin A deficiency. Glossitis (inflammation of the tongue), stomatitis (inflammation of the oral mucosa), cheilosis (fissures at the angles of the mouth), and peripheral neuropathy may develop due to deficiencies of B vitamins.

In addition to signs and symptoms resulting from nutritional deficiencies, maldigestion and malabsorption cause diarrhea or steatorrhea. *Diarrhea* is the frequent passage of unformed or liquid stools. Failure to absorb foodstuffs increases the bulk to be eliminated from the intestinal tract. In addition unabsorbed nutrients can interfere with water absorption due to an osmotic effect. Water is mainly absorbed from the large intestine, but when malabsorption occurs in the small bowel the amount of fluid delivered to the colon may exceed its absorptive capacity. *Steatorrhea* is the presence of an excessive amount of fat in the stools. It is characterized by bulky foul-smelling stools; the action of bacteria on fats produces the odor.

General Maldigestion

General maldigestion results from a *deficiency of pancreatic enzymes*, which are necessary for the hydrolysis of proteins, carbohydrates, and fats. Enzyme deficiency can result from a reduction in the number of functional pancreatic cells, for example due to inflammation (pancreatitis), pancreatic cancer, or surgical resection. Obstruction of the pancreatic ducts prevents the flow of pancreatic juice into the duodenum and eventually leads to loss of functional pancreatic cells, as in mucoviscidosis (cystic fibrosis). This condition is discussed in Chapter 21.

Another mechanism responsible for deficiency of pancreatic enzymes is a failure to release cholecystokinin-pancreozymin. Cholecystokinin-pancreozymin is a hormone that is normally released from the duodenal mucosa in response to the presence of fat and products of protein digestion. It is the major stimulus for secretion of pancreatic enzymes and also stimulates the release of bile from the gallbladder. Release of this hormone may be impaired in celiac sprue (see below) or after surgery such as Billroth II gastrojejunostomy.

Lack of bile salts impairs both digestion and absorption of fat. Obstruction of the bile ducts is probably the most common cause of insufficient bile salts. Also, failure to reabsorb bile salts in the ileum may result in loss of bile salts in the stool at a faster rate than the liver can synthesize them and cause a deficiency. Failure to absorb fat results in the loss of an important energy food, but deficiency of the essential fatty acid (linoleic acid) is rarely observed in adults. In infants the skin may become dry and scaly due to linoleic acid deficiency. Deficiencies of the fat-soluble vitamins A, D, E, and K may occur as a result of maldigestion and malabsorption of fat. In addition calcium absorption may be impaired and calcium deficiency may occur because calcium forms complexes with fat in the intestinal tract.

Specific Maldigestion

Specific maldigestion results from a deficiency of a specific enzyme. Isolated enzyme deficiencies are usually congenital and, with the exception of lactase deficiency, are rare.

Deficiency of lactase causes *lactose intolerance.* Lactase is an intestinal enzyme that catalyzes the hydrolysis of lactose, the sugar in milk. A few infants have a congenital deficiency of lactase, but more importantly, most older children and adults are also deficient in lactase. Most infants have a high level of lactase, but after 2 to 4 years of age the amount of lactase produced in the small intestine decreases, possibly as a result of a gene being turned off. About 90% of Caucasians of northern European extraction and 80% of the members of two African tribes continue to secrete lactase and can tolerate lactose, but 70% to 80% of older children and adults of other races and ethnic groups secrete little or no lactase and are lactose intolerant. Following ingestion of milk, undigested lactose moves into the large intestine, where it interferes with water absorption due to an osmotic effect. In addition, intestinal bacteria ferment the sugar, generating organic acids and carbon dioxide. As a result, the person has a bloated feeling, flatulence, abdominal cramps, and explosive diarrhea.

General Malabsorption

General malabsorption may be due to gastrointestinal inflammatory disease or a reduction in the surface area for absorption. Decreased surface area for absorption occurs following intestinal resection and in several intestinal diseases (e.g., celiac sprue) that are characterized by abnormalities of the intestinal mucosa.

Celiac sprue is also called gluten-induced enteropathy, celiac disease, or nontropical sprue. Originally the term celiac disease was applied to a malabsorption syndrome occurring in children. A similar syndrome occurring in adults was called nontropical sprue. It is now recognized that both syndromes are caused by a reaction to gluten, a protein in grains (particularly wheat, rye, barley, and oats). Therefore the syndrome is now usually called celiac sprue or gluten-induced enteropathy.

Gluten and/or breakdown products of gluten are toxic to people with celiac sprue and cause characteristic lesions of the intestinal mucosa. The exact mechanism of the gluten toxicity is not known. The condition appears to be inherited and is possibly due to an enzyme defect or an immune disorder.

After ingestion of gluten by susceptible people,

the villi of the small intestinal mucosa disappear, and the mucosa becomes flat and thickened. Lymphocytes, monocytes, and plasma cells (i.e., inflammatory cells) infiltrate the lamina propria layer of the mucosa. The mucosal epithelium changes from a single layer of columnar cells to several layers of cuboidal cells. The damage is most severe in the proximal portion of the small intestine and is progressively less severe distally. The surface area for absorption is greatly decreased due to the loss of villi. Also, the abnormal epithelial cells are deficient in enzymes and carrier molecules that are necessary for transport of substances across the membranes. Therefore, absorption of monosaccharides, amino acids, and fat is impaired. In addition, water, minerals, electrolytes, and vitamins are not absorbed normally and large amounts of plasma proteins may be lost into the intestinal lumen.

Manifestations of celiac sprue may occur at any age. In children the onset is usually between 6 and 18 months of age, after the introduction of gluten in the diet. Often spontaneous remission occurs in adolescence, but the condition may recur later in adult life. Many adults with celiac sprue give a history of having had the condition in childhood. Signs and symptoms are as previously described for general malabsorption. Steatorrhea, abdominal distension, cramps, anorexia, and weight loss are common manifestations.

Specific Malabsorption

Specific malabsorption is usually due to lack of a carrier molecule that is necessary to transport a specific nutrient across the intestinal mucosa. An example is glucose-galactose malabsorption, which is described in Chapter 6 (see under Inborn Errors Due to Defective Membrane Transport).

Another example of specific malabsorption is failure to absorb vitamin B_{12} due to a lack of intrinsic factor. The resultant vitamin B_{12} deficiency causes pernicious anemia (see Chapter 10 under Decreased Oxygen-Carrying Capacity of the Blood). Lack of intrinsic factor can occur as a rare autosomal recessive inherited condition. Anemia develops at about 2 to 3 years of age, after the supply of vitamin B_{12} stored during fetal development is exhausted. In this condition, gastric acid and pepsin secretion are normal.

Lack of intrinsic factor developing in adulthood is associated with atrophy of the gastric mucosa and deficiency of hydrochloric acid and pepsin. The exact cause of this condition is not known, but it may be due to an autoimmune disorder. (Autoimmunity is discussed in Chapter 30.) Gastrectomy or damage to the parietal cells of the stomach from any cause can also result in a lack of intrinsic factor.

In some cases, production of intrinsic factor may be normal, but the intrinsic factor–vitamin B_{12} complex is unable to bind at receptor sites on the ileal mucosa. Consequently vitamin B_{12} cannot be absorbed.

Manifestations of vitamin B_{12} deficiency are mainly a result of the anemia, which usually has an insidious onset. In addition, lack of vitamin B_{12} can cause neural degeneration. Neurological symptoms such as pain, numbness and tingling of the fingers and toes, stiffness of extremities, loss of vibratory sense, loss of position sense, ataxia, mental impairment, and emotional disturbances may occur.

Increased Utilization of Nutrients

Whenever nutrients are used at a greater than usual rate by the body, nutritional deficiency can occur if intake is not increased. For example, when metabolism is increased, as in fever or thyrotoxicosis, the requirement for calories and B vitamins is increased. If dietary intake is not increased, weight loss, muscle wasting, and vitamin B deficiencies can result.

Utilization of iron, folic acid, and vitamin B_{12} is increased when hematopoiesis is increased, for example in hemolytic anemia (see Chapter 10). If intake is not increased, deficiencies of these nutrients will contribute to the anemia.

Increased Loss of Nutrients

Abnormal losses of nutrients can occur from the gastrointestinal tract or urinary tract or through wound drainage. If the loss is not compensated by increased intake, the result will be nutritional deficiency. For example, chronic blood loss results in a loss of iron from the body and can produce *iron deficiency*. In some cases the blood loss is not obvious, for example when it occurs from gastrointestinal lesions, and iron deficiency anemia may be the first sign that blood loss is occurring.

As iron deficiency develops, iron stores in the liver, spleen, and bone marrow are depleted, and then the plasma iron concentration falls. Synthesis of transferrin is stimulated so that more iron can be absorbed from the gastrointestinal tract. Eventually anemia develops. Decreased activities of iron-containing enzymes also occur, but whether these decreases have pathological significance is not clear. Prolonged iron deficiency causes changes in epithelial tissues. Hair splits and breaks off. The nails become more brittle and the normal curvature may be inverted ("spooning"). Glossitis develops, producing a smooth, sore tongue. Iron deficiency is often associated with atrophic gastritis and lack of gastric acid. It is not known whether this gastritis is a result of iron deficiency because of secondary epithelial changes or whether it is the cause of the deficiency because lack of gastric acid impairs iron absorption. Perhaps both of these events occur. That is, iron deficiency resulting from chronic blood loss (or some other factor) may cause atrophic gastritis, which in turn impairs iron absorption and contributes to the iron deficiency.

NUTRITIONAL EXCESS

When the rate of food intake is greater than the rate of use and loss of nutrients, nutritional excess occurs. Excesses of specific nutrients, such as vitamins (hypervitaminosis) are usually due to ingestion of large doses of dietary supplements. When total caloric (i.e., energy) intake is in excess of energy expenditure, obesity results.

Obesity

Obesity is an excessive accumulation of fat in the body. Not all overweight is due to obesity. Accumulation of fluid in the body or excessive muscular and skeletal development (e.g., in a very athletic person) can also cause overweight. The etiology of obesity involves many factors, not all of which are understood.

Causes

Genetic factors have been identified as determinants of obesity in animals, but the role of genetic factors in human obesity has not been established. Obesity does tend to be familial and probably has a genetic component, but environmental factors are so important (e.g., family eating habits and activity patterns) that it is difficult to determine the genetic influences.

Lack of physical activity is probably a major factor in the development of obesity. Energy is expended for basal metabolism and physical activity. Energy expenditure due to basal metabolism is relatively constant but is influenced by sex, age, and growth. For people of the same sex, age, and body size, physical activity is the major factor responsible for variations in energy expenditure. Not all obese people have a high caloric intake, but physically they may be very inactive so that their caloric requirements are very low.

Endocrine imbalances probably account for overweight in only a small proportion of obese people. Basal metabolism is influenced by several hormones, particularly thyroid hormone. Therefore people with a deficiency of thyroid hormone (hypothyroidism) tend to be overweight (see Chapter 19).

Psychological factors are important in the development of obesity in some, but not all, obese people. Some people overeat in response to stress.

Eating patterns may be another factor in the development of obesity. External environmental stimuli apparently have a greater influence on food intake in obese people than in nonobese people. Obese people appear to respond more to external cues such as the sight, smell, and taste of food than to internal physiological signals of hunger. Nonobese people, on the other hand, tend to respond more to metabolic cues than to external stimuli to eating.

Effects

Some of the effects of obesity are physical consequences of excess body weight. In addition, metabolic changes accompany obesity.

The excessive amount of fat over the chest wall and the pressure on the diaphragm due to accumulation of fat in the abdomen limit the respiratory excursion of the thorax and increase the mechanical work of breathing. As a result, breathing is shallow and hypoventilation may occur. At the same time, oxygen consumption and carbon dioxide production are increased due to the increased body mass. Consequently, hypoxemia and hypercapnia may develop. The hypercapnia produces respiratory acidosis (see Chapter 15). With severe obesity, a person may develop cyanosis, twitching, lethargy, and drowsiness due to hypoxemia and hypercapnia.

Pulmonary vascular resistance is often increased, producing pulmonary hypertension. This effect is presumably due to pulmonary vasoconstriction caused by hypoxemia and hypercapnia. Right ventricular hypertrophy may develop as a consequence of the pulmonary hypertension. Often the systemic blood pressure is also elevated, although the mechanism responsible for the hypertension associated with obesity is not known. Hypertension increases the work of the heart (see Chapter 13). In addition, the load on the heart is increased because of the increased amount of tissue that must be perfused.

With severe obesity, the excessive weight may contribute to orthopedic disorders. For example, osteoarthritis, particularly of the knees and ankles, is aggravated by obesity. Low-back pain may occur. Large calluses may develop over the feet and heels.

Plasma lipid levels are usually moderately elevated in obese people. In addition, the blood glucose level is elevated and glucose tolerance may be impaired. Obese people usually have an elevated plasma insulin level, both in the fasting state and after a glucose load. They seem to require more than the normal amount of insulin to stimulate the use of glucose; both muscle and adipose tissue are resistant to glucose uptake in response to insulin. The precise relationship between the tissue resistance and the elevated insulin level, and the mechanisms responsible for them, are not understood. These abnormalities usually disappear after weight reduction.

SUGGESTED ADDITIONAL READING

Borgen L: Total parenteral nutrition in adults. Am J Nurs **78**(2): 224–228, 1978.

Caly JC: Assessing adult's nutrition. Am J Nurs **77**(10): 1605–1609, 1977.

Dansky KH: Assessing children's nutrition. Am J Nurs **77**(10): 1610–1611, 1977.

Frieden E: The chemical elements of life. Sci Am **227**(1): 52–60, 1972.

Kretchmer N: Lactose and lactase. Sci Am **227**(4): 70–78, 1972.

Young VR, Scrimshaw NS: The physiology of starvation. Sci Am **225**(4): 14–21, 1971.

18

Disturbances
of Metabolism

Metabolism is the sum of all the physical and chemical processes occurring in a living organism. It includes reactions by which energy is made available for cell work and reactions by which substances required for growth and maintenance of the organism are produced. The chemical reac- tions occurring in the body are catalyzed by en- zymes, and metabolic processes are regulated by a number of hormones. Therefore, metabolic distur- bances can result from altered enzyme activity or hormonal imbalances. Many metabolic processes are influenced by diet; substrates for biochemical reactions and energy to carry out metabolic processes come from food. Therefore diet often has an important influence on the development and severity of metabolic disturbances. Any metabolic process can be impaired and disrupt homeostasis; this chapter is concerned with disturbances of lipid and carbohydrate metabolism.

REGULATION OF CARBOHYDRATE AND LIPID METABOLISM

Metabolism of carbohydrates and lipids is briefly reviewed in Chapter 17. Carbohydrate and lipid metabolism are closely interrelated; amino acid metabolism is also influenced by carbohydrate metabolism.

As stated in Chapter 17, carbohydrates and fats are the major sources of energy for the cells. Glucose is essential for the cells of the nervous system, renal tubular epithelium, and red blood cells. Thus, to assure a continuous supply of glucose for the brain, the major factor that is regulated is the concentration of glucose in the arterial blood. When the blood glucose level rises, glucose is converted to glycogen (glycogenesis) and fat (lipogenesis) for storage. When the blood glucose level falls, glycogen is broken down to release glucose (glycogenolysis) and glucose is formed from noncarbohydrate sources (gluconeogenesis). The substances used for gluconeogenesis are amino acids, lactic acid, and glycerol derived from triglycerides. Fatty acids cannot be converted to glucose. Use of fatty acids by the tissues that can metabolize them, however, spares glucose for the tissues that require it. The factors influencing the blood glucose level are summarized in Figure 18-1.

Carbohydrate metabolism is mainly controlled by the hormones insulin and glucagon. Other hormones that influence carbohydrate metabolism are the glucocorticoids, growth hormone, and catecholamines. Thyroid hormone also influences energy metabolism.

The Insulin-Glucagon Ratio

Insulin is secreted by the beta (β) cells and glucagon by the alpha (α) cells of the islets of Langerhans in the pancreas. These two hormones have opposing effects on glucose metabolism and the insulin-glucagon *ratio* appears to be more important in the control of carbohydrate and lipid metabolism than the absolute level of either hormone. Secretion of both hormones is influenced by the concentration of glucose in the blood flowing through the pancreas, as well as by other factors. A high glucose concentration stimulates insulin secretion and inhibits glucagon secretion; a low glucose level inhibits insulin secretion and stimulates glucagon secretion. Insulin secretion is also influenced by potassium. A low level of potassium in the blood limits insulin secretion; a high potassium concentration may stimulate insulin secretion. (See also Chapter 16 under Potassium Homeostasis.)

Insulin enhances the transport of glucose into muscle cells, stimulates oxidative metabolism of glucose, and promotes the conversion of glucose to glycogen. In addition, insulin inhibits the release of amino acids from muscle and favors the incorporation of amino acids into protein. Insulin also increases the transport of glucose into adipose tissue cells and stimulates the conversion of glucose to triglycerides. Insulin stimulates the activity of the lipoprotein-lipase enzyme system and thereby facilitates the uptake of plasma triglycerides by adipose tissue cells.

Unlike its entry into muscle and adipose tissue, glucose can enter the liver cells readily and does not require insulin for transport across the liver cell membranes. Insulin does increase hepatic uptake of glucose, however, by stimulating the rate of glucose phosphorylation and thus increasing the rate of entry of glucose into the metabolic pathways of the liver cells. Insulin stimulates the synthesis of glycogen, triglycerides, and very-low-density lipoproteins (VLDL) in the liver and at the same time suppresses glycogenolysis and gluconeo-

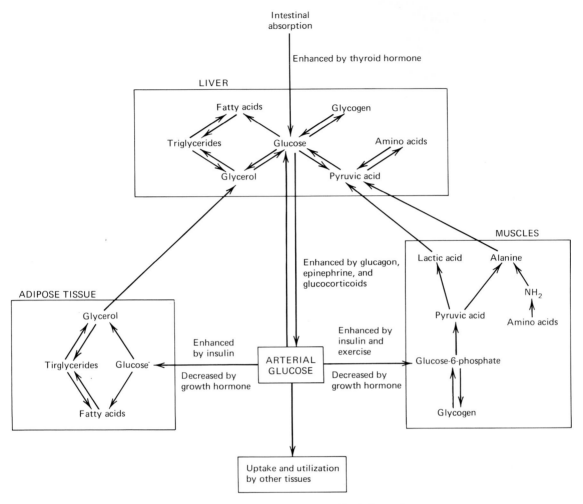

Figure 18-1. *Summary of factors affecting blood glucose homeostasis.*

genesis. Thus, insulin decreases the release of glucose from the liver.

Glucagon stimulates glycogenolysis in the liver. It also stimulates the conversion of alanine, lactic acid, and pyruvic acid to glucose (i.e., it enhances gluconeogenesis). In addition, glucagon increases lipolysis in liver and adipose tissue.

Thus, the glucose concentration in the blood is regulated by the following feedback mechanism. When the blood glucose level is high (i.e., after a meal), insulin secretion is stimulated and glucagon secretion is suppressed. As a result, cellular uptake and utilization of glucose is increased, conversion of glucose to glycogen and fat for storage is promoted, gluconeogenesis is suppressed, and incorporation of amino acids into protein is favored. Consequently the blood glucose level is lowered. When the blood glucose level falls (i.e., in the fasting state), insulin secretion declines and glucagon secretion is stimulated. As a result, glycogenolysis, lipolysis, and gluconeogenesis are stimulated and glucose is released from the liver. Protein breakdown is favored, glucose utilization is decreased, and oxidation of fatty acids is increased. These actions raise the blood glucose concentration.

Effects of Other Hormones

Growth hormone promotes an increase in the blood glucose concentration. It decreases the transport of glucose into the cells and acts as an insulin antagonist. Growth hormone also increases the mobilization and utilization of fat and decreases the utilization of carbohydrate for energy. In addition, it increases the transport of amino acids into cells and promotes protein synthesis. Release of growth hormone from the adenohypophysis is influenced by the concentration of glucose in the blood as well as by other factors. A high blood glucose level suppresses growth-hormone release, whereas a low blood glucose level increases secretion of growth hormone.

Glucocorticoids (primarily cortisol) from the adrenal cortex increase the transport of amino acids into hepatic cells and decrease amino-acid transport into muscle cells. In other words, glucocorticoids mobilize amino acids from the peripheral tissues. Metabolism of amino acids in the liver is enhanced: deamination of amino acids, synthesis of proteins (including plasma proteins), and conversion of amino acids to glucose (i.e., gluconeogenesis) are increased. Glucocorticoids also increase lipolysis in adipose tissue and depress lipogenesis in the liver. Thus, the overall effect of increased secretion of glucocorticoids (e.g., in response to stress) is to raise the plasma levels of glucose, free fatty acids, and amino acids. Glucocorticoids increase the release of glucagon by the pancreas; therefore the effects of the glucocorticoids may be partly mediated by glucagon.

The *catecholamines*, epinephrine and norepinephrine, also influence carbohydrate and fat metabolism, but they usually have only short-term effects. Norepinephrine is released from sympathetic nerve endings. Mainly epinephrine, but also a small amount of norepinephrine, is released from the adrenal medullae in response to sympathetic stimulation. Epinephrine has a greater effect on carbohydrate metabolism than norepinephrine does. Both catecholamines, however, appear to increase glucagon release and suppress insulin secretion. Epinephrine stimulates glycogenolysis and consequently the liver releases more glucose into the blood. Lipolysis is also increased.

Thyroxine and T_3, the thyroid hormones, have a general stimulatory effect on most tissues, but also have specific effects on carbohydrate metabolism. They increase the rate of intestinal absorption of glucose, increase the utilization of glucose (i.e., increase the rate of glycolysis), and tend to increase glycogenolysis. Thyroid hormones also stimulate lipolysis.

In addition to the hormones just mentioned, a variety of hormones are secreted by the gastrointestinal tract, and some of them influence glucose homeostasis. The exact physiological role of the intestinal hormones has not yet been determined. Some intestinal hormones may stimulate insulin release, while others may have a direct effect on carbohydrate metabolism. Gastric inhibitory polypeptide, which is secreted by the duodenum in response to glucose, amino acids, and fat, stimulates the release of insulin. A substance that behaves immunologically like glucagon is also secreted by the intestine. Whether this substance, called glucagonlike immunoreactivity, has the same physiological activity as pancreatic glucagon has not yet been determined.

Effects of Exercise

Resting muscles use very little glucose; most of their energy needs are supplied by the oxidation of fatty acids. At the beginning of exercise, muscle glycogen is the major fuel. As exercise continues, uptake of glucose by the muscle cells is increased and glucose becomes a major energy source. Exercise increases the transport of glucose into muscle cells even in the absence of insulin. The glucose that is required comes from hepatic glycogenolysis and gluconeogenesis. With short-term exercise the release of glucose from the liver is accompanied by an increase in the blood glucose concentration, but with prolonged exercise hepatic glycogenolysis and gluconeogenesis cannot keep up with the requirements of the muscles and the blood glucose level falls. The insulin level declines and glucagon, catecholamine, and cortisol levels increase. Lipolysis is stimulated and the muscles use more fatty acids for energy.

DISTURBANCES OF CARBOHYDRATE METABOLISM

Disturbances of carbohydrate metabolism may be due to genetic deficiencies of enzymes involved in carbohydrate metabolism (i.e., inborn errors of metabolism), toxic effects of drugs, or hormonal imbalances. The most common disturbance of carbohydrate metabolism is diabetes mellitus. As stated previously, the blood glucose concentration is a major factor that is regulated. Therefore, disturbances of carbohydrate metabolism are often reflected by changes in the blood glucose level. An abnormally low blood glucose concentration is called *hypoglycemia*. *Hyperglycemia* is an abnormally high concentration of glucose in the blood.

Assessment of Carbohydrate Metabolism

Carbohydrate metabolism is usually assessed by determining the blood glucose concentration, the presence or absence of glucose in the urine, and the response to a glucose load.

Blood Glucose

Values given for the concentration of glucose in the blood depend on the technique used to measure it and whether the measurement is made on arterial, capillary, or venous blood. The values also vary depending on whether whole blood or plasma is used; plasma levels are higher. In the fasting state, differences between arterial and venous glucose concentrations are usually small, but in the nonfasting state the arteriovenous difference is large. The capillary blood glucose level is similar to the arterial glucose concentration. Methods that are based on the reduction of copper ferricyanide, such as the Hoffman method, the Hagedorn-Jensen method, and the Folin-Wu method, measure some other reducing substances as well as glucose. They give values that may be about 10-20 mg/100 ml higher than glucose-specific methods, such as those using glucose oxidase. Therefore, values given for the "normal" range of blood glucose vary from one laboratory to another, depending on the method used.

Using glucose-specific methods, following an overnight fast the blood glucose concentration (arterial, capillary, or venous) in healthy people is usually within the range 50-90 mg/100 ml. A fasting blood glucose level above 110 mg/100 ml is usually considered abnormal. After digestion and absorption of a meal, the blood glucose level rises and then gradually returns to the basal level.

Urine Tests

Under usual conditions, practically all the glucose that is filtered at the glomerulus is actively reabsorbed by the renal tubules. The slight amount of glucose that is present in the urine is not detectable with the usual tests. When the plasma glucose concentration rises above a critical level, called the *renal threshold*, the reabsorptive capacity of the tubules is exceeded and glucose is detectable in the urine (glucosuria). (The presence of any sugar in the urine is called *glycosuria*. The term *glucosuria* refers specifically to glucose in the urine.) The normal renal threshold is between 180 and 200 mg/100 ml.

The renal threshold depends not only on the ability of the tubules to reabsorb glucose, but also on the glomerular filtration rate. Therefore, if the glomerular filtration rate is unusually low, all of the glucose in the filtrate will be absorbed, even though the plasma glucose level may be high (i.e., the renal threshold is elevated). This situation may occur in some people who have had diabetes for many years and have developed glomerulosclerosis (see below under Chronic Complications of Diabetes). Glomerulosclerosis impairs glomerular filtration; therefore these people may have hyperglycemia without glucosuria.

Some people spill detectable amounts of glucose into the urine even though their blood glucose level may be within the normal range; that is, they have an abnormally low renal threshold. This condition is called *renal glycosuria.* It is sometimes due to an inherited defect in renal tubular reabsorption and is not an indication of diabetes. Renal glycosuria may also be caused by damage to the proximal renal tubules.

As with the methods used for determining blood glucose, some reagents used in urine tests are specific for glucose and some are nonspecific. Nonspecific reagents measure other reducing substances, such as fructose, lactose, pentose sugars, and several drugs (e.g., salicylate), as well as glucose. Lactose is often present in the urine of women during late pregnancy and lactation and gives a positive reaction with these reagents.

With ketosis, ketone bodies (acetone, acetoacetic acid, and β-hydroxybutyric acid) are excreted in the urine. Ketosis can occur with diabetes, during starvation, and following alcohol abuse. Most urine tests for ketones are specific for acetoacetic acid; no simple test is available to detect β-hydroxybutyric acid.

Glucose Tolerance Test

Glucose tolerance is the ability of the body to metabolize glucose. The glucose tolerance test (GTT) measures the response to a glucose load. Usually an oral glucose tolerance test is used. The blood (or plasma) glucose concentration is determined after an overnight fast. After the blood sample is taken, a measured amount of glucose (50 to 100 g) is ingested within a few minutes. Blood

samples for glucose are then taken at 30-minute intervals for three hours or occasionally longer. In addition, the urine may be tested for glucose at the beginning of the test and one and two hours later.

As the glucose is absorbed, the blood glucose level rises, reaching a peak within an hour. The increased blood glucose level stimulates insulin release, and the blood glucose normally returns to the basal (i.e., fasting) level within two and one-half to three hours (Fig. 18-2). In a person with diabetes mellitus the fasting blood glucose level is usually elevated (occasionally it is normal) and the entire GTT curve is shifted upward. The insulin response is deficient and/or delayed, with the result that the decline in the blood glucose concentration is slow and takes four to six hours to return to the basal level.

Criteria for an abnormal oral GTT vary. The Wilkerson Point System and the Fajans and Conn criteria are widely used. Table 18-1 lists the values that are considered the upper limit of normal for the blood glucose concentration. In the Wilkerson Point System, values higher than those listed are assigned points, as indicated in the Table. Two or more points are considered diagnostic of diabetes mellitus. According to the Fajans and Conn criteria, blood or plasma glucose concentrations higher than those listed in the Table are indicative of diabetes mellitus in a person under 50 years of age. Glucose tolerance changes with age so that higher limits of normal are set for older age groups.

Many factors can alter the GTT. For example, hypokalemia produces a diabetic type of response. The GTT also shows a diabetic pattern in people with liver disease. Impaired intestinal absorption of glucose, whether due to intestinal disease or hypothyroidism, results in a flat GTT curve.

Two variations of the GTT that are occasionally used are the cortisone GTT and the intravenous GTT. The intravenous GTT may be used in some cases where intestinal absorption is a problem. In the cortisone GTT, cortisone is administered prior to an oral GTT to unmask a diabetic state in a susceptible person. Cortisone, a glucocorticoid,

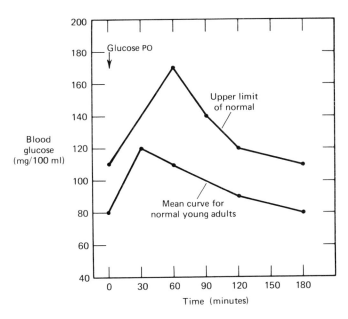

Figure 18-2. *The glucose tolerance curve. Note that the values given here are for blood glucose; values for plasma glucose are higher.*

Table 18-1. Criteria for an Abnormal Glucose Tolerance Test Curve

	Wilkerson Point System		
	Whole Blood Glucose (mg/100 ml)	Serum or Plasma Glucose (mg/100 ml)	Points
Fasting	110	130	1
1 hour	170	195	½
2 hours	120	140	½
3 hours	110	130	1

	Fajans and Conn Criteria	
	Whole Blood Glucose (mg/100 ml)	Serum or Plasma Glucose (mg/100 ml)
1 hour	160	185
1½ hours	140	165
2 hours	120	140

raises the blood glucose level and therefore increases the insulin requirement.

Hypoglycemia

As stated previously, hypoglycemia is an abnormally low blood glucose level (usually less than 50 mg/100 ml). In response to hypoglycemia, the sympathetic nervous system is stimulated and a rapid increase in the level of circulating epinephrine occurs. In addition, secretion of glucagon, cortisol, and growth hormone increases and the levels of these hormones rise (unless the hypoglycemia is due to a deficiency of one of these hormones).

Effects

The effects of hypoglycemia are caused by a lack of glucose to supply the energy needs of the cells, particularly those of the nervous system. When the supply of glucose to the nervous system is inadequate for normal functioning, the condition is called *neuroglycopenia*. Signs and symptoms of hypoglycemia are related to an adrenergic reaction as a result of the outpouring of epinephrine and to a neuroglycopenic reaction. The symptoms depend on individual characteristics and on the rate of fall of the blood glucose level. A rapid reduction in the blood glucose concentration produces more severe symptoms than a slower fall.

The *adrenergic reaction* produces signs and symptoms such as sweating, pallor, tachycardia, palpitations, sensations of hunger and a "sinking" feeling in the stomach, restlessness, and a feeling of anxiety.

The *neuroglycopenic reaction* may produce headache, fatigue, drowsiness, behavioral changes, visual disorders (e.g., inability to focus), and confusion. If the hypoglycemia is severe or remains untreated the confusion can progress to stupor and coma. Convulsive seizures (usually grand mal) may occur. Death may occur if the hypoglycemia is not promptly treated.

When episodes of hypoglycemia occur frequently (e.g., when they are caused by hyperinsulinism), some people may gain weight because they eat in response to the hunger caused by hypoglycemia.

Causes

Hypoglycemia can be exogenous, as a result of injection or ingestion of a hypoglycemic agent, or endogenous, caused by hormonal imbalances, inborn errors of metabolism, gastrointestinal disorders, liver disease, malnutrition, and extreme muscular exercise. The most common cause of hypoglycemia is excessive insulin, whether due to exogenous administration or excessive secretion.

Exogenous causes. In addition to exogenous insulin, oral antidiabetic agents can cause hypoglycemia, particularly in people with impaired metabolism or excretion of the drugs due to renal or hepatic insufficiency. Alcohol inhibits gluconeogenesis in the liver and can cause severe hypoglycemia, especially if it is ingested while fasting. Toxic doses of a variety of drugs, including salicylates, isoproterenol, and monamine-oxidase inhibitors, may cause hypoglycemia.

Insulin-secreting tumors. Neoplasms arising from the β cells of the islets of Langerhans are called *insulinomas*. In most cases these tumors are benign, but in about 15% they are malignant. (See Chapter 20 for a discussion of the characteristics of neoplasms.) Insulinomas secrete insulin and do not respond to the normal physiological controls of insulin release. Consequently insulin secretion is excessive (*hyperinsulinism*) and hypoglycemia can occur, particularly after an overnight fast.

Other tumors, outside the pancreas, are sometimes associated with hypoglycemia. In some cases the tumors may produce insulin or an insulinlike material. In other cases the cause of the hypoglycemia is not known.

Inborn errors of carbohydrate metabolism. Many enzymes are involved in carbohydrate metabolism and genetic defects of several of these enzymes are known. In some cases the inborn error of metabolism can produce hypoglycemia.

Some inborn errors involve enzymes that are required for the conversion of other sugars to glucose; hypoglycemia may accompany these disorders. An example is galactosemia (see Chapter 6 under Inborn Errors Due to Blocked Metabolic Pathways).

Inborn errors of metabolism involving enzymes necessary for gluconeogenesis and glycogenolysis can also produce hypoglycemia. The disorders due to inborn errors of glycogenolysis are referred to as *glycogen storage diseases*, or *glycogenoses* (singular: glycogenosis). Several glycogen storage diseases are known, each one involving a different enzyme. These conditions, which are rare, are characterized by the accumulation of glycogen in one or more tissues, with subsequent impaired functioning of the organ(s) involved. Hypoglycemia accompanies some, but not all, glycogenoses. An example is glucose-6-phosphatase deficiency (Von Gierke's disease; type I glycogenosis).

Glucose-6-phosphatase, which catalyzes the release of free glucose from glucose-6-phosphate, is found mainly in the liver and kidneys. Deficiency of this enzyme affects not only glycogenolysis, but also gluconeogenesis, because the product of both of these pathways is glucose-6-phosphate. With glucose-6-phosphatase deficiency, glucose-6-phosphate cannot be converted to free glucose. As a result, the concentrations of glucose-6-phosphate and intermediate compounds in the gluconeogenesis pathway are relatively high. These substances affect the activity of certain regulatory enzymes, with the result that glycogenolysis is inhibited and glycogenesis is stimulated. (Regulatory enzymes are discussed in Chapter 1 under Homeostatic Control Mechanisms Operate at All Levels.) Consequently glycogen accumulates in the liver and produces liver enlargement (hepatomegaly). Hepatic lipogenesis is also stimulated and the plasma lipid level may be elevated. Since glucose-6-phosphate cannot be converted to free glucose, the liver is unable to respond to the usual stimuli for the release of glucose into the blood and hypoglycemia frequently develops. Ketoacidosis may occur due to increased oxidation of fatty acids. Growth and development are usually retarded. Severely affected infants die in early childhood, but some people appear to be able to adapt to the enzyme deficiency and are less severely affected. The exact mechanisms of the adaptation are not known but may involve decreased sensitivity to insulin and increased activity of enzymes that may be able to circumvent the block in the conversion of glucose-6-phosphate to free glucose.

Reactive hypoglycemia. Hypoglycemia occurring after the ingestion of carbohydrate is called *reactive hypoglycemia.* It is diagnosed on the basis of a blood glucose concentration of 45 mg/100 ml or less after a 100-gram oral GTT. The hypoglycemia usually occurs at some time between two and four hours after glucose ingestion. The pathogenesis of reactive hypoglycemia is not clear and is probably not the same in all cases.

Reactive hypoglycemia often occurs following gastric surgery *(alimentary hypoglycemia).* In this case rapid gastric emptying occurs and the mechanism responsible for the hypoglycemia appears to be overproduction of insulin in response to the rapidly absorbed glucose. Intestinal hormones may also be involved in the pathogenesis of this hypoglycemia. Alimentary hypoglycemia may occur in the absence of gastrointestinal surgery due to an unusually rapid rate of intestinal absorption of glucose.

Reactive hypoglycemia may occur in people with latent (chemical) diabetes (see below). In this case the insulin response to glucose is excessive and the plasma insulin level rises higher than normal.

Reactive hypoglycemia sometimes occurs in obese people. In this case the insulin level is higher than in nonobese people, but not higher than in obese people without reactive hypoglycemia. Some people with renal glycosuria also exhibit reactive hypoglycemia. They do not have a greater insulin response than people who have renal glycosuria without reactive hypoglycemia, but with or without hypoglycemia people with renal glycosuria tend to have a greater than normal insulin response. It is possible that the people who exhibit hypoglycemia have a defective counterregulatory mechanism or are unusually sensitive to insulin.

"Spontaneous" reactive hypoglycemia may occur in people who have not had gastric surgery, are not obese, and do not have renal glycosuria. In some cases an excessive insulin response to glucose appears to be responsible for the hypoglycemia, but in other cases the insulin response is normal. Again, it is possible that those who exhibit hypoglycemia with a normal insulin response may be excessively sensitive to insulin or have an abnormal counterregulatory mechanism.

Diabetes Mellitus

Diabetes mellitus has been defined variously as an absolute or relative deficiency of insulin; as hyperglycemia inappropriate to the existing environmental and nutritional state; and as a disorder of metabolism which, in its fully developed clinical expression, is characterized by hyperglycemia, atherosclerotic and microangiopathic vascular disease, and neuropathy. It is a complex metabolic disorder in which the basic defect is unknown. Since insulin is the only bodily substance known to lower the blood glucose level, however, the existence of hyperglycemia implies an absolute or relative lack of insulin.

An *absolute* deficiency of insulin occurs if the normal requirement for insulin cannot be met. Theoretically, an absolute insulin deficiency can result from destruction or removal of the β cells, from suppression of insulin release, or from inactivation of insulin. A *relative* insulin deficiency occurs if an increased need for insulin cannot be met. A relative insulin deficiency can result from metabolic or endocrine changes that increase the blood glucose level by overproducing glucose or by antagonizing insulin action. Usually the body can compensate for an increased insulin requirement by increasing the rate of insulin secretion and increasing the number of β cells. If the body cannot meet the increased requirement by these means, manifest diabetes may occur.

In the pathogenesis of diabetes, *etiological factors* refer to changes in the pancreatic islet cells or in the availability of insulin. In most cases of diabetes the etiological factors are not known and the condition is referred to as *primary idiopathic diabetes*. It is generally agreed that a genetic susceptibility plays an important role in the development of primary diabetes, but the exact mode of inheritance is not known. Diabetes appears to be a heterogeneous condition and it seems likely that the mode of inheritance is not the same in all cases. In addition to insulin deficiency, increased glucagon release may contribute to the development of this condition. *Secondary diabetes* can result from pancreatitis, pancreatic carcinoma, trauma to the pancreas, and surgical removal of the pancreas.

Promoting or *precipitating* factors are those which increase the insulin requirement and unmask a predisposition to diabetes. They include glucocorticoid excess (Cushing's syndrome), treatment with steroids or ACTH, growth-hormone excess (acromegaly), excess glucagon due to a glucagon-secreting tumor (glucagonoma), obesity, and cirrhosis of the liver.

Natural History of Diabetes

Primary idiopathic diabetes mellitus may be divided into four stages. Progression or regression from one stage to the next may occur very rapidly, very slowly, or not at all.

The earliest stage is *prediabetes,* or *potential diabetes.* Tests of glucose homeostasis are normal, but the person has an increased probability of developing diabetes because of a genetic predisposition (e.g., both parents have diabetes). Large babies are characteristic of women with diabetes, and many women give birth to large babies many years before they develop overt diabetes. Therefore prediabetes is suspected in women who bear big babies.

The next stage is *subclinical diabetes* (latent diabetes by another classification system). The fasting blood glucose level is normal. The oral glucose tolerance test is also usually normal, but it may be abnormal under conditions of stress or during pregnancy. The cortisone-glucose tolerance test is abnormal.

Subclinical diabetes may or may not progress to *latent diabetes* (asymptomatic or chemical diabetes). In this stage the fasting blood glucose level may be normal or elevated. The person has none of the usual clinical manifestations of diabetes, but the glucose tolerance test is abnormal. Some people in this stage may have reactive hypoglycemia.

Overt diabetes (or clinical diabetes) is the most advanced stage. The fasting blood glucose level is elevated and glucose may be detected in the urine if the renal threshold is exceeded. The glucose tolerance test is abnormal. Symptoms or complications of diabetes are evident. The two major types of overt diabetes are maturity-onset diabetes (MOD) and juvenile-onset diabetes (JOD). Juvenile-onset diabetes accounts for only about 5% of cases.

Juvenile-Onset Diabetes

The juvenile-onset type of diabetes usually becomes manifest in childhood or adolescence but occasionally has its onset in adulthood. It is characterized by an abrupt onset of insulin insufficiency with severe symptoms and a tendency to ketoacidosis. Progression from prediabetes to overt diabetes occurs rapidly (i.e., within days or weeks) without recognition of subclinical or latent diabetes. People with this type of diabetes require insulin.

A current hypothesis for the etiology of JOD is that the inherited susceptibility is at least partly conferred by certain immune response genes. These genes are believed to cause a defective T lymphocyte response to some environmental agents (certain viruses and chemicals), leading to β-cell damage directly or through autoimmune mechanisms. (The immune response is described in Chapter 29; autoimmunity is discussed in Chapter 30.)

The essential pathological feature in JOD is a decrease in the functioning β-cell mass due to a reduction in the number of β cells. Not only is the total amount of islet tissue decreased but the proportion of β cells in the remaining islet tissue is also reduced. Consequently insulin secretion is insufficient to meet normal demands and the plasma insulin level is very low.

Intestinal absorption of glucose does not require insulin, but most tissues, with the exceptions of liver, brain, and renal tubular epithelium, require insulin for the transport of glucose into the cells. When insufficient insulin is available, cellular uptake and utilization of glucose is impaired. In addition, the liver releases glucose into the blood. Consequently, the blood glucose level rises (hyperglycemia). The exact role of glucagon in the pathogenesis of diabetes is not known, but the glucagon level may be inappropriately high, thus contributing to the hyperglycemia.

When the blood glucose level exceeds the renal threshold, glycosuria occurs. The glucose in the urine causes an osmotic diuresis (see Chapter 12 under Diuresis), producing an excessive urinary output (polyuria) and loss of electrolytes. Water deficit may occur. Excessive thirst (polydipsia) occurs because the excessive water loss increases the osmolarity of the ECF, which stimulates the thirst center in the hypothalamus. Hunger may be increased (polyphagia) due to the loss of glucose.

The inability to use glucose results in the increased use of fat for energy and in increased breakdown of body protein. The results are weight loss and, in children, failure to grow. The loss of water due to polyuria contributes to the weight loss. Muscle weakness and fatigue occur, partly as a result of inability to use glucose, and partly due to loss of muscle protein. The increased protein catabolism results in increased urea production and increased urinary loss of nitrogen. The increased mobilization of fat results in increased production of ketone bodies and may lead to ketoacidosis (see below).

Blurring of vision may occur because the increased concentration of glucose in the ECF alters the refractive index of the lens and other media of the eye.

The blood lipid level may be elevated (hyperlipidemia). The increased lipids are mainly due to dietary chylomicrons, but endogenous triglycerides (VLDL) may be elevated as well. As mentioned earlier, insulin stimulates the activity of the enzyme lipoprotein lipase, which is involved in the uptake of triglycerides by adipose tissue. With insulin deficiency, removal of triglycerides from the plasma is impaired. Associated with the hyperlipidemia may be yellow-orange papular skin eruptions called *eruptive xanthomas,* or *xanthoma diabeticorum.* They are due to localized collections of macrophages filled with lipid. The retinal blood vessels may appear white, gray, or light pink instead of deep red, because of the excess lipid in the blood. This condition is called *lipemia retinalis.*

Maturity-Onset Diabetes

The maturity-onset type of diabetes usually occurs in adults over 40 years of age, although it can occur in young people. The onset is gradual and the symptoms are mild. In some cases there are no symptoms but glycosuria is detected on a routine examination. In other cases the presenting symptoms are those of vascular or neurological complications (see below). People with MOD are not usually prone to ketoacidosis, although it can occur under conditions of stress (e.g., infection, surgery, trauma).

In MOD the pancreas is still able to secrete insulin. The plasma insulin level may be low or high, but a *relative* insulin deficiency exists. People with MOD do not usually require insulin therapy. In most cases they can be maintained on oral hypoglycemic agents and diet therapy and in some very mild cases on diet therapy alone. Many people with MOD are obese and reversion from overt diabetes to latent diabetes can sometimes be achieved by weight reduction.

Maturity-Onset-Type Diabetes in the Young

A small portion of children and adolescents who develop diabetes have a mild form of diabetes that resembles the maturity-onset type. This form of diabetes is called maturity-onset diabetes of young age (MODY). It is defined as diabetes developing in a person under the age of 25 years in whom fasting hyperglycemia, if present, can be normalized without insulin for more than two years. In contrast to JOD, which has an abrupt onset and severe weight loss, MODY has an insidious onset and weight loss is minimal or does not occur. Insulin secretion in response to a glucose stimulus is retained, but the response is delayed and decreased. Ketonuria does not occur. In most people with MODY the condition shows little or no progression in severity with age. The current belief is that MODY is inherited as an autosomal dominant condition, but the basic genetic defect is not known.

Acute Complications of Diabetes

Three acute, life-threatening complications of diabetes mellitus are hypoglycemia, ketoacidosis (diabetic coma), and hyperosmolar nonketotic diabetic coma.

Hypoglycemia, which was discussed previously, is most likely to occur in a person with diabetes who is taking insulin. The onset of hypoglycemia is typically rapid and sudden. The usual causes are too little food (e.g., a missed meal); too much insulin, usually due to accidental overdosage, but sometimes due to decreased requirement (e.g., after recovery from infection); and exercise that is not balanced by extra food.

Ketoacidosis may occur before diabetes has been diagnosed or if insulin is discontinued for some reason. Stress due to intercurrent infection, trauma, or other illness may precipitate ketoacidosis. Occasionally no precipitating cause is apparent. Insulin deficiency is present, however, and severe hyperglycemia occurs. Lipolysis and fatty-acid oxidation are increased, leading to excessive production of ketone bodies. Excessive hydrogen ions from acetoacetic acid and β-hydroxybutyric acid consume bicarbonate and metabolic acidosis results. Thus, the plasma bicarbonate is decreased, the pH is decreased, and the hydrogen-ion concentration is increased. The anion gap is increased. (See Chapter 15 under Metabolic Acidosis.) Glucosuria occurs and the urine is strongly positive to tests for ketones (unless the renal threshold is elevated due to kidney disease, as discussed earlier). Acetone is volatile and is excreted through the lungs, giving the breath a fruity odor.

The onset of ketoacidotic diabetic coma is gradual, occurring over hours or days. Increasing polyuria and thirst, weakness, lethargy, and drowsiness occur. Gradually the person lapses into stupor. Although the term diabetic coma is used, complete unconsciousness does not necessarily occur, but consciousness is depressed. True coma is a grave prognostic sign. Deep, rapid, sighing (Küssmaul) respirations due to the acidosis are characteristic. Reflexes are depressed and the muscles are hypotonic. Generalized abdominal pain and vomiting may occur, presumably due to gastrointestinal distension as a result of hypotonia. Clinical manifestations are related to water deficit as well as to ketoacidosis (Fig. 18-3). Soft sunken eyes, dry mucous membranes, and loss of skin tur-

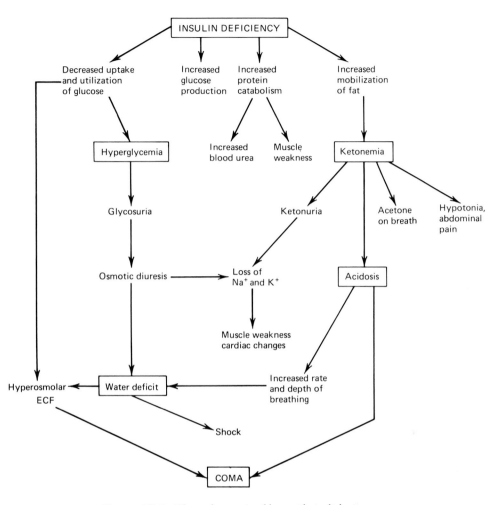

Figure 18-3. *The pathogenesis of ketoacidotic diabetic coma.*

gor may occur as a result of water deficit (see Chapter 12 under ECF Volume Deficit). A degree of shock may be present.

Hyperosmolar nonketotic diabetic coma is characterized by hyperosmolarity of the extracellular fluid, severe hyperglycemia (blood glucose greater than 600 mg/100 ml) without ketoacidosis, and a depressed level of consciousness. This condition occurs most often in older people with mild diabetes. A precipitating factor such as severe infection, myocardial infarction, pancreatitis, burns,

renal failure, hyperalimentation, or administration of drugs (e.g., thiazide diuretics, corticosteroids. diphenylhydantoin) is often present. These precipitating factors are associated either with a decrease in insulin effect due to insulin antagonism (e.g., uremia, corticosteroids) or interference with the release or action of insulin (e.g., various drugs) or with excessive carbohydrate administration to a stressed person (e.g., dialysis, hyperalimentation, treatment of severe burns).

The reason for the absence of ketoacidosis is not

clearly understood. More insulin is required to stimulate transport of glucose into adipose tissue than to inhibit lipolysis. Therefore, when the insulin level declines, glucose uptake is impaired before the adipose tissue is released from the antilipolytic effect of insulin. In people who develop hyperosmolar nonketotic coma it is possible that the amount of available insulin is sufficient to inhibit lipolysis (and therefore the formation of ketone bodies) but not sufficient to stimulate uptake of glucose. Possibly in some cases the ability of the liver to synthesize ketone bodies from free fatty acids is impaired.

The onset of hyperosmolar nonketotic diabetic coma is gradual. It is manifested by increasing thirst, glycosuria, weakness, and lethargy, progressing to somnolence, stupor, and coma. In contrast to people with ketoacidosis, hyperpnea does not usually occur and there is no acetone odor to the breath. As with ketoacidosis, the glycosuria causes osmotic diuresis, which leads to water deficit, hypovolemia, and shock. In addition to the depression of consciousness, other neurological abnormalities such as generalized or focal seizures or hemiplegia may occur. Fever may be present.

The coma and other neurological abnormalities in hyperosmolar nonketotic coma are presumably due to hyperosmolarity of the extracellular fluid (ECF) caused by the high glucose level and the water deficit. The hyperosmolar ECF causes water to move out of the cells and the cells shrink (see Chapter 11 under Movement of Water between ECF and ICF). Consequently brain cell functioning is impaired. In addition, the high glucose concentration increases the viscosity of the blood and alters blood flow. Therefore hypoxia possibly contributes to the condition. In ketoacidosis several factors are likely responsible for the depression of consciousness, including acidosis, hyperosmolarity of the ECF, and cerebral hypoxia.

Chronic Complications of Diabetes

Chronic complications of diabetes include vascular and neurological changes. The development of these complications appears to be related to the duration of the diabetes.

Vascular complications. The vascular changes are atherosclerosis and microangiopathy. Although atherosclerosis is not unique to people with diabetes, it begins at an early age and progresses rapidly in those with diabetes. The reasons for the increased susceptibility to atherosclerosis are not known, but hyperlipidemia and hypertension, which occur commonly in people with diabetes, are probably contributory. One consequence of atherosclerosis is ischemic heart disease; myocardial infarction is the most common cause of death in people with diabetes.

Alterations in the arterioles, capillaries, and venules are called *microangiopathy*. In diabetes the microangiopathy includes arteriolosclerosis and thickening of the capillary basement membranes. The arteriolosclerosis is due to deposition of hyaline material in the walls of the arterioles and hyperplasia of the intimal lining, with resultant thickening and hardening of the walls and narrowing of the lumens. (See also the discussion of arteriolosclerosis in Chapter 13 under Effects of Hypertension.)

Capillary basement membrane thickening occurs in all tissues but is most marked in the muscles, skin, and kidneys. It can lead to local ischemia, increased capillary permeability, local edema, and hemorrhage. The cause of the basement membrane thickening is not known. The basement membrane is a glycoprotein and it is possible that with impaired metabolism of glucose, more glucose is shunted into the formation of the carbohydrate portion of the basement membrane.

Microangiopathy in the eyes gives rise to *diabetic retinopathy*. The changes include thickening of the capillary basement membranes, weakening of the vessel walls with formation of microaneurysms (minute outpouchings), exudation of plasma, hemorrhage, and irregular dilation of veins. Retinal capillaries may become occluded, causing areas of ischemia. New vessels grow into the nonperfused area and may extend into the vitreous.

Bleeding often occurs from these vessels, leading to healing by organization with fibrous tissue. Contraction of the fibrous tissue may cause retinal detachment. Varying degrees of visual impairment result from diabetic retinopathy, depending on the locations of the lesions.

Microangiopathy in the kidneys gives rise to *diabetic nephropathy*. Thickening of the glomerular capillary basement membranes causes glomerulosclerosis. In addition, the afferent and efferent arterioles are affected by arteriolosclerosis, producing glomerular ischemia. The earliest sign of nephropathy is proteinuria, which may be intermittent at first but becomes progressively worse. The plasma protein level falls and edema develops (see Chapter 11). The edema is probably partly due to abnormal permeability of peripheral capillaries. Eventually renal failure occurs, accompanied by uremia and hypertension.

Peripheral vascular disease particularly affects the lower extremities. In some cases narrowing of major arteries due to atherosclerosis causes intermittent claudication. In other cases occlusion of major arteries does not occur but ischemia may result from microangiopathy. Symptoms may include fatigue, weakness, numbness, and pain in the legs and feet at rest. Ulcers or gangrene may develop, particularly in the feet. Neuropathy contributes to these developments.

Neurological complications. Functional and pathological changes in the peripheral nervous system (*neuropathy*) are common complications of diabetes mellitus. Peripheral *polyneuropathy*, with bilateral symmetrical involvement of the lower extremities, is the most common form of diabetic neuropathy. The pathological lesion is degeneration of the myelin sheath. The myelin sheath is formed by Schwann cells and altered metabolism in the Schwann cells is believed to be responsible for this lesion. Sensory function is particularly affected, although motor function may also be impaired. The two major symptoms are pain and paresthesias. The pain may have a dull, aching quality or may be more severe. It is usually worse at night. The skin may be very sensitive and tender to touch; even the touch of clothing may be intolerable. The paresthesias consist of sensations of coldness, numbness, tingling, or burning. Signs include reduced or absent reflex ankle jerks and knee jerks.

Sensory neural impairment is sometimes accompanied by painless degeneration of joints (*Charcot's joints*). In diabetes the ankle joints and tarsal joints are most commonly involved. The foot becomes shorter and wider and the longitudinal arch is flattened. Joint disorganization causes abnormal pressure points and painless perforating ulcers often develop at sites of abnormal pressure.

Mononeuropathies usually involve motor nerves. These lesions are believed to be due to nerve infarction subsequent to microangiopathy of the vessels supplying the nerve. Mononeuropathies are characterized by sudden onset of intense pain and muscle weakness or paralysis occurring unilaterally. Any nerve may be involved, including those supplying the extrinsic eye muscles. The ulnar, femoral, and peroneal nerves are commonly involved. Peroneal nerve involvement produces foot drop.

Autonomic neuropathies affect visceral function. The pupils may be irregular and of unequal size, with diminished reactivity to light. Neuropathy involving the gastrointestinal tract may result in gastric atony, with delayed emptying of the stomach. Altered function of the small intestine produces intermittent bouts of diarrhea, often accompanied by fecal incontinence at night. The diarrhea is usually followed by a period of constipation. In addition to gastrointestinal disturbances, bladder paralysis with urinary retention may occur. Impotence due to autonomic neuropathy is relatively common in men with diabetes.

DISTURBANCES OF LIPID METABOLISM

Lipids are not water soluble, therefore they are transported in the blood in association with protein. The four classes of lipoproteins in the blood are chylomicrons, very-low-density lipoproteins (VLDL), low-density lipoproteins (LDL), and high-density lipoproteins (HDL), as described in Chapter 17 (see under Lipids). The proteins involved in lipid transport are called apolipoproteins. Those associated with the HDL are called apo-A and those in LDL are called apo-B. VLDL and chylomicrons contain apo-B and apo-C. Apo-C is also found in HDL.

Altered metabolism of fat and cholesterol is reflected by changes in the lipoprotein pattern in the blood. In addition, diet influences the blood lipid levels. A diet high in saturated fats and/or cholesterol tends to increase the level of LDL. A high carbohydrate diet increases the level of VLDL. Excessive alcohol ingestion also increases the level of VLDL.

Hyperlipidemia (or hyperlipemia) means an excess of lipids in the blood. An excess of cholesterol in the blood is *hypercholesterolemia;* an excess of triglycerides, *hypertriglyceridemia.* When the levels of both cholesterol and triglycerides in the blood are elevated, the term *combined hyperlipidemia* is sometimes used. An excess of lipoproteins in the blood is *hyperlipoproteinemia.* Since most of the lipids in the blood are in lipoproteins, the terms hyperlipidemia and hyperlipoproteinemia are sometimes used interchangeably. *Hypolipidema* (or hypolipemia) is an abnormally decreased amount of lipid in the blood. *Hypolipoproteinemia* is an abnormally decreased amount of lipoproteins in the blood.

In addition to disturbances of fat and cholesterol metabolism, several disorders of sphingolipid metabolism are known. Sphingolipids occur in membranes and form part of the myelin sheath around nerves. They are found in high concentrations in the brain and nerve tissue. Therefore, disorders of sphingolipid metabolism are associated with neurological disturbances.

Hyperlipoproteinemias

Hyperlipoproteinemia can occur secondarily to several conditions that affect plasma lipid metab-

olism. In many cases, however, an underlying disorder is not apparent and the hyperlipoproteinemia is referred to as primary. Some primary hyperlipoproteinemias are inherited disorders, but the exact nature of the genetic defect is not known in all cases. The increased plasma lipoprotein levels may be due to overproduction of lipoproteins, to impaired degradation and removal of lipoproteins from the plasma, or to simultaneous operation of both mechanisms. Hyperlipoproteinemias have been classified into six abnormal lipoprotein patterns.

Type I Hyperlipoproteinemia

Type I hyperlipoproteinemia is characterized by the presence of chylomicrons in the blood in the fasting state and hypertriglyceridemia. The chylomicrons disappear from the blood if an affected person is placed on a fat-free diet. VLDL may be normal or slightly increased. The primary condition is a rare inherited disorder due to a deficiency or abnormality of the enzyme lipoprotein lipase, which is necessary for uptake of triglycerides by the tissues. Occasionally this abnormal plasma lipoprotein pattern occurs secondarily to uncontrolled juvenile-onset diabetes. Affected people may have episodes of acute abdominal pain. The liver and spleen may be enlarged due to accumulations of foam cells (reticuloendothelial cells filled with lipid). Lipemia retinalis may be seen.

Type IIa Hyperlipoproteinemia

This condition is characterized by an increased LDL concentration. The plasma cholesterol concentration is usually increased but may be normal due to a reciprocal decrease in HDL. The VLDL and triglyceride levels are normal. Type IIa hyperlipoproteinemia is a common blood lipid abnormality. In addition to the primary form it can occur secondarily to the nephrotic syndrome. It is associated with accelerated atherosclerosis and an increased risk of ischemic heart disease. Many people with this condition have *tendon xanthomas,* particularly in the Achilles tendons and in the extensor tendons of the hands. These xanthomas are nodules due to deposits of lipids. *Xanthelasmas* may also occur. These are xanthomas on the eyelids; they appear as soft yellowish plaques.

Type IIb Hyperlipoproteinemia

This abnormal blood lipid pattern is also common. It is characterized by increased concentrations of both LDL and VLDL. The plasma triglyceride level is always increased and the cholesterol level is usually increased. As with type IIa, this condition is associated with an increased risk of premature ischemic heart disease. Tendon xanthomas and xanthelasmas may be present. This pattern of hyperlipoproteinemia sometimes occurs secondarily to hypothyroidism and to the nephrotic syndrome.

Type III Hyperlipoproteinemia

This hyperlipoproteinemia is rare. It is characterized by the accumulation of an abnormal plasma lipoprotein called floating-beta-lipoprotein (broad-beta-lipoprotein; beta-VLDL). This lipoprotein is believed to be an intermediate in the conversion of VLDL to LDL; it normally exists transiently in the plasma and is not usually detectable. Levels of both cholesterol and triglycerides are increased. Chylomicrons may be present in the fasting state. This disorder is associated with increased risks of peripheral vascular disease and ischemic heart disease. Xanthomas also occur. The usual types are linear xanthomas in the creases of the palmar surfaces of the hands and tuberous xanthomas, rounded pink or orange nodules, occurring mainly over the elbows or knees. The liver and spleen may be enlarged. The oral GTT is abnormal in some people with this disorder.

Type IV Hyperlipoproteinemia

This abnormal plasma lipoprotein pattern is common. It is characterized by an increased concentration of VLDL. The LDL concentration is normal and chylomicrons are absent in the fasting state. The triglyceride level is elevated; the cholesterol level may be normal or elevated. People with this disorder are often obese and may have an abnormal oral GTT. They have an increased risk of ischemic heart disease and peripheral vascular disease. Hepatomegaly is fairly common. In addition to the primary disorder, type IV hyperlipoproteinemia may occur in association with diabetes mellitus, hypothyroidism, the nephrotic syndrome, or alcoholism.

Type V Hyperlipoproteinemia

This disorder is characterized by increased VLDL, the presence of chylomicrons in the plasma in the fasting state, and severe hypertriglyceridemia. The cholesterol level may be normal or modestly elevated. This abnormal lipoprotein pattern is uncommon. In most cases it is secondary to uncontrolled diabetes, to alcoholism, or to the nephrotic syndrome. Affected people may have hepatomegaly, splenomegaly, and episodes of acute abdominal pain. Eruptive xanthomas and lipemia retinalis often occur.

Hypolipoproteinemias

Two hereditary disorders result in deficiencies of plasma lipoproteins: abetalipoproteinemia and Tangier disease (HDL deficiency). *Abetalipoproteinemia* is characterized by a lack of chylomicrons, VLDL, and LDL in the plasma. It is believed to be due to a defect in the synthesis of apo-B, but this mechanism has not yet been definitely established. Abetalipoproteinemia is described in Chapter 6 under Inborn Errors Due to Deficient or Abnormal Circulating Proteins.

Tangier disease is characterized by almost complete absence of HDL from the plasma. Cholesterol and phospholipid concentrations are decreased; triglyceride levels are normal or slightly increased. The basic defect in this condition is not known but it is possibly due to defective synthesis of apo-A. The classic sign of Tangier disease is the presence of large orange tonsils due to the accumulation of lipids, especially cholesterol esters, in the tonsils. In addition, the liver and spleen may be enlarged due to accumulations of foam cells.

Disorders of Sphingolipid Metabolism

Three classes of sphingolipids are sphingomyelins, which are phosphosphingolipids, and cerebrosides and gangliosides, which are glycosphingolipids. Normal metabolism of these substances involves a dynamic state of simultaneous synthesis and deposition, and degradation. Genetic defects of a number of enzymes that are necessary for these processes are known. Examples of inborn errors of sphingolipid metabolism are Niemann-Pick disease, which affects sphingomyelin metabolism; Gaucher's disease, which affects cerebroside metabolism; and Tay-Sach's disease, which affects ganglioside metabolism. These disorders have an autosomal recessive mode of inheritance.

Niemann-Pick Disease

Niemann-Pick disease has been classified into five varieties; the most common are type A (classic infantile) and type B (visceral form). The basic defect is very low activity (about 10% of normal) of the enzyme sphingomyelinase, which is necessary for sphingomyelin catabolism. Foam cells filled with sphingomyelin accumulate throughout the body, but especially in lymphoid tissue, bone marrow, liver, and lungs. Degenerative changes occur in the nervous system, manifested histologically by demyelination and ballooning of neurons.

Onset of clinical manifestations occurs in infancy or early childhood with failure to thrive, and mental and motor developmental retardation or loss of previously acquired abilities. Frequent vomiting and poor feeding lead to emaciation. A protuberant abdomen, hypotonic extremities, brownish yellow discoloration of the skin, hepatomegaly, splenomegaly, tremors, and poor coordination soon follow. Destruction of retinal neurons exposes the underlying choroidal blood vessels and produces a cherry-red spot in the retina in many cases. Death usually occurs within three years of the onset of symptoms.

Gaucher's Disease

Gaucher's disease is caused by a deficiency or lack of the enzyme β-glucosidase, which catalyzes the degradation of glucocerebroside derived from senescent erythrocytes. Consequently glucocerebroside accumulates in the reticuloendothelial cells. These cells filled with glucocerebroside are called Gaucher's cells. They infiltrate the parenchyma of the liver, spleen, lymph nodes, and bone marrow, causing secondary leukopenia, thrombocytopenia, and anemia. The liver and spleen are enlarged. Gaucher cells may also infiltrate the lungs and adrenal glands. In some cases the brain is also involved. Neuronal degeneration occurs and the brain becomes smaller than average.

Gaucher's disease occurs in three forms: acute, subacute, and chronic. The acute form is usually manifested in infancy. Hepatic and splenic enlargement and neurological involvement occur. The child fails to thrive. Hypertonicity usually occurs: the upper extremities are flexed and rigid and the lower extremities are scissored. Strabismus, dysphagia (difficulty swallowing), laryngeal spasm, convulsive seizures, and mental retardation may occur. Complete deterioration and death ensue within a few months.

The subacute form has a more insidious course than the acute form and progresses over several years. It may have its onset in infancy or late childhood. Bleeding manifestations due to thrombocytopenia and secondary infections due to leukopenia often occur. The liver and spleen are enlarged and eventually the CNS is involved.

The chronic form usually becomes manifest in adulthood but may be seen in childhood. Bleeding due to thrombocytopenia is the usual presenting sign. Hepatic and splenic enlargement are found and anemia may occur. Neurological involvement does not usually occur and affected people may live for many years.

Tay-Sach's Disease

Tay-Sach's disease (type 1 GM_2 gangliosidosis) is caused by a deficiency of the enzyme hexosaminidase A, which is necessary for the catabolism of one type of ganglioside. The major pathological manifestations of this condition occur in the nervous system. Brain cells accumulate gangliosides and ballooning of the neurons occurs, accompanied by demyelination. The brain may atrophy.

Tay-Sach's disease usually becomes manifest about 6 months of age. Poor tolerance to loud noises is a common early sign. Neurological development is slow and acquired developmental skills may be lost. Mental retardation occurs. A cherry-red spot may be seen on the retina. Anorexia and failure to thrive are common. The child may be apathetic or irritable and may have a feeble cry. The muscles become weak and hypotonic, convulsive seizures occur, and spastic paralysis, strabismus, or nystagmus may develop. Death may occur within a few months and usually occurs within three years of the onset of signs and symptoms.

SUGGESTED ADDITIONAL READING

Lavine RL: How to recognize . . . and what to do about . . . hypoglycemia. Nursing 79 9(4): 52–55, 1979.

McCarthy J: Somogyi effect: managing blood glucose rebound. Nursing 79 9(2): 38–41, 1979.

McFarlane J: Children with diabetes: special needs during growth years. Am J Nurs 73(8): 1360–1363, 1973.

McFarlane J, Hames CC: Children with diabetes: learning self-care in camp. Am J Nurs 73(8): 1362–1365, 1973.

Rancilio N: When a pregnant woman is diabetic: postpartal care. Am J Nurs 79(3): 453–456, 1979.

Schuler K: When a pregnant woman is diabetic: antepartal care. Am J Nurs 79(3): 448–450, 1979.

Vogel M: When a pregnant woman is diabetic: care of the newborn. Am J Nurs 79(3): 458–460, 1979.

Wimberley D: When a pregnant woman is diabetic: intrapartal care. Am J Nurs 79(3): 451–452, 1979.

19
Endocrine Imbalance

A *hormone* is a chemical substance that is secreted into the extracellular fluid (ECF) by a specific organ or cells of an organ and that has a regulatory effect on the activity of other cells (target cells) at some distance from the secretory organ. (Hormones that diffuse only a short distance and exert their actions locally are called *tissue hormones.*) Organs that secrete hormones are called *endocrine glands.* As stated in Chapter 1, the endocrine system and nervous system integrate and coordinate the concerted cellular activities that maintain homeostasis. It follows, therefore, that endocrine dysfunction results in loss of a control mechanism and leads to a disturbance of homeostasis.

The major endocrine glands and the hormones they secrete are listed in Table 19-1. This chapter is mainly concerned with imbalances of adenohypophyseal hormones, adrenocortical hormones, and thyroid hormones. Antidiuretic hormone is discussed in Chapter 12; epinephrine and nor-

Table 19-1. Endocrine Glands and Hormones

Gland	*Main Hormones*
Adenohypophysis (anterior pituitary)	Growth hormone (GH, somatotropin, STH) Adrenocorticotropic hormone (ACTH, corticotropin) Thyroid-stimulating hormone (TSH, thyrotropin) Follicle-stimulating hormone (FSH) Luteinizing hormone (LH, interstitial cell–stimulating hormone, ICSH) Prolactin (lactogenic hormone, luteotropic hormone, LTH)
Neurohypophysis (posterior pituitary)	Antidiuretic hormone (ADH, vasopressin) Oxytocin
Adrenal cortex	Cortisol ⎱ glucocorticoids Corticosterone ⎰ Aldosterone ⎱ mineralocorticoids Deoxycorticosterone ⎰ Androgens Estrogens
Adrenal medulla	Epinephrine Norepinephrine
Thyroid	Thyroxine (thyroid hormone, T_4) Triiodothyronine (T_3) Calcitonin
Parathyroid	Parathyroid hormone (PTH, parathormone)
Islets of Langerhans of pancreas	Insulin Glucagon
Ovary	Estrogens Progesterone
Testis	Testosterone

epinephrine are covered in Chapter 13; parathyroid hormone and calcitonin are considered in Chapter 16; and insulin and glucagon are discussed in Chapter 18.

Endocrine imbalance can result from overactivity (hyperfunctioning) or underactivity (hypofunctioning) of an endocrine gland, with resultant excess or deficiency of one or more hormones. A few endocrine disorders may be the result of altered metabolism or breakdown of hormones. For example, men with cirrhosis of the liver may develop gynecomastia due to failure of the diseased liver to inactivate estrogen.

Endocrine hyperfunction can be due to hypertrophy, hyperplasia, or a tumor of an endocrine gland. In addition, a tumor arising from a nonendocrine tissue may secrete a protein or polypeptide hormone or hormonelike substance. This situation is referred to as ectopic hormone production and it also can cause endocrine imbalance.

Endocrine hypofunction can result from destruction of a gland by hemorrhage, infarction, autoimmunity, a tumor, or trauma, or from surgical removal of a gland. In addition, inherited deficiencies of enzymes necessary for hormone synthesis can cause endocrine dysfunction. Occasionally a gland is congenitally absent or hypoplastic. In some cases a gland may secrete an adequate amount of a hormone but the target tissue fails to respond to the hormone; the effect is the same as hormone deficiency. Theoretically this situation could result from a lack of receptors on the cell surfaces or from an alteration in the hormone or receptor that prevents hormone-receptor binding. An example of unresponsiveness of the target tissue is the failure of the renal tubules to respond to ADH in nephrogenic diabetes insipidus (see Chapter 12).

HORMONE ACTIONS

Hormones can be divided into two classes. The first class includes protein, peptide, and amine hormones which are soluble in water and do not require a carrier molecule for transport in the blood. These hormones have a relatively rapid turnover rate and their concentrations may fluctuate quite widely within seconds or minutes in response to stimuli. Examples are growth hormone, ACTH, TSH, FSH, LH, prolactin, ADH, PTH, calcitonin, insulin, glucagon, and catecholamines. The second class includes steroid hormones (e.g., estrogens, progesterone, testosterone, cortisol, aldosterone) and thyroxine, which are not water soluble and are transported in the blood in combination with a carrier protein. The bound hormone is in equilibrium with a small amount of unbound (free) hormone. The bound hormone cannot diffuse out of the blood, but the free hormone can diffuse throughout the ECF and is the physiologically active form. These hormones have a much slower turnover rate and their concentrations change gradually. The mechanisms of action of these two groups of hormones also differ.

Hormones of the first class are believed to interact with specific receptors on the surfaces of cells, thus altering a membrane-bound enzyme and leading to a change in the concentration of an intracellular "second messenger" (the hormone is the "first messenger"). The second messenger then influences the activity of other enzymes within the cell, bringing about a particular response. In most cases the second messenger is believed to be cyclic adenosine monophosphate (cAMP), but probably other second messengers are involved as well.

Hormones of the second class cross cell membranes relatively easily and bind with an intracellular receptor or receptors. The hormone-receptor complex is believed to then interact with chromatin in the nucleus to influence transcription of messenger RNA from the genes. The hormone-receptor complex may also influence translation of messenger RNA (i.e., protein synthesis) and/or the function of organelles (e.g., mitochondria) directly. In addition, hormones of this class may alter membrane structure and function in some way.

Hormones exert regulatory influences on target

tissues by affecting growth, differentiation, and/or metabolic activity. They can enhance or inhibit the activity of an already differentiated cell; increase the number of active cells by inducing differentiation of precursor cells; increase the number of active cells by stimulating cell division; or act in all of these ways. Some hormones (e.g., tropic hormones of the adenohypophysis) act only on one target organ or gland, while others (e.g., sex hormones) have more general actions in addition to their specific effects on specialized tissues. Several hormones (e.g., growth hormone, thyroid hormone, insulin, and cortisol) exert their effects on most or all of the tissues of the body.

The effects of many hormones interact to regulate various physiological processes. For example, insulin, glucagon, cortisol, epinephrine, growth hormone, and thyroid hormone all influence carbohydrate metabolism (see Chapter 18). Some hormone interactions are antagonistic; for example, parathyroid hormone and calcitonin have opposing effects on the plasma calcium concentration. Other interactions are synergistic; for example, growth hormone and insulin both promote amino acid uptake by cells and growth hormone exerts its maximal protein-anabolic effect only when insulin is present. Some hormones have a permissive effect on the actions of other hormones; for example, glycogenolysis due to epinephrine can only occur when cortisol is present. Consequently, dysfunction of one endocrine gland often affects the function of another gland.

THE HYPOPHYSIS

The hypophysis (pituitary) has been called the "master gland" because its hormones influence the functioning of several other endocrine glands. It is now known, however, that the hypophysis is in turn influenced by the part of the brain called the hypothalamus. The hypothalamus is very important for the coordination of nervous and endocrine responses.

The hypophysis has three sections: the neurohypophysis, pars intermedia, and adenohypophysis. The neurohypophysis (posterior pituitary) is directly connected with the hypothalamus by the hypophyseal stalk (infundibulum). Two hormones, antidiuretic hormone (ADH) and oxytocin, are released from the neurohypophysis in response to nervous stimulation from the hypothalamus. These hormones are actually synthesized in nuclei of the hypothalamus. They travel down nerve fibers as secretory granules and are stored in the nerve endings in the neurohypophysis. The pars intermedia is a small portion of the gland that secretes melanocyte-stimulating hormone (MSH). This hormone has no known function in human beings, although it may be involved in certain conditions of abnormal pigmentation.

The adenohypophysis (anterior pituitary) secretes many important hormones that influence the activity of other endocrine glands. The adenohypophysis receives its blood supply from the hypophyseal portal system, which originates in the hypothalamus. The hypothalamus secretes several releasing factors and inhibiting factors, which are carried in this portal system to the adenohypophysis and influence its activity.

Adenohypophyseal Hormones

The hormones of the adenohypophysis are growth hormone (GH), adrenocorticotropic hormone (ACTH), thyroid-stimulating hormone (TSH), follicle-stimulating hormone (FSH), luteinizing hormone (LH), and prolactin.

Growth Hormone

GH has a direct effect on protein, carbohydrate, and fat metabolism. During childhood and adolescence it stimulates growth of the body, probably as an indirect effect of its influence on metabolism. GH stimulates amino acid uptake and protein synthesis in most tissues. It promotes endochondral bone growth by increasing the number and activity of the cells of the epiphyseal cartilages and by stimulating protein synthesis. GH also stimulates hepatic production of a substance called somatomedin (sulfation factor), which promotes the incorporation of sulfate into cartilage, a process necessary for skeletal growth. GH has no effect on linear growth after closure of the epiphyses. (Epiphyseal closure is influenced by other hormones.)

GH promotes the retention of several minerals and electrolytes in the body, including potassium, sodium, chloride, calcium, phosphate, and magnesium. Potassium and phosphate are incorporated into the increasing cell mass; calcium and phosphate are deposited in the growing bone. Growth hormone actually increases urinary excretion of calcium but it also enhances intestinal absorption of calcium, so that the net effect is usually positive calcium balance.

The effects of GH on metabolism depend partly on whether a person has just eaten or is fasting, and partly on the level of insulin. Following a meal the rise in blood sugar stimulates insulin release and leads to a fall in the level of GH. Uptake of glucose by the cells, glycogenesis, and lipogenesis are stimulated. As the blood sugar level declines, the GH level rises while insulin is still available. Under these conditions maximal protein synthesis is promoted. Uptake of glucose by muscles and adipose tissue diminishes so that available glucose is reserved for the brain. In the fasting state the blood sugar and insulin levels fall and the GH level rises. Lipolysis is stimulated so that fat is available for energy and protein is spared.

GH secretion is influenced by many factors and is under the control of the hypothalamus. The hypothalamus secretes both a GH-releasing factor and a GH-release–inhibiting factor. GH secretion is stimulated by fasting, hypoglycemia, stress, fever, exercise, insulin, glucagon, thyroxine, estrogens, and epinephrine. GH secretion is also stimulated following ingestion of a large protein meal or administration of certain amino acids (e.g., arginine, histidine, and lysine), especially in females. (These amino acids simultaneously stimulate insulin secretion and the two hormones act synergistically to enhance protein synthesis.) Ingestion of carbohydrate or administration of glucose, and high concentrations of cortisol inhibit GH secretion.

Adrenocorticotropic Hormone

ACTH acts on the adrenal cortex to stimulate production of adrenocorticosteroids, particularly glucocorticoids, but also androgens and mineralocorticoids to a slight extent. ACTH also promotes growth of the adrenal cortex. In addition to its effects on the adrenal cortex, ACTH stimulates lipolysis.

Secretion of ACTH by the adenohypophysis is controlled by corticotropin-releasing factor (CRF) from the hypothalamus. In addition, glucocorticoids influence ACTH secretion by a negative feedback mechanism (Fig. 19-1). A high level of cortisol inhibits ACTH secretion, probably by a direct effect on the adenohypophysis as well as an indirect effect on the hypothalamus. Stress causes an increase in ACTH secretion.

Thyroid-Stimulating Hormone

TSH promotes growth of the thyroid gland and stimulates production and release of the thyroid hormones. Secretion of TSH is stimulated by thyrotropin-releasing factor (TRF) from the hypothalamus. Thyroid hormone inhibits TSH secretion by a negative feedback mechanism.

Gonadotropins

Two hormones secreted by the adenohypophysis, follicle-stimulating hormone (FSH) and luteinizing hormone (LH), exert their effects on the gonads and are called gonadotropins. FSH stimulates development of ovarian follicles in females and spermatogenesis in males. LH contributes to the development of ovarian follicles and stimulates ovulation. It is necessary for the formation of the corpus luteum and also stimulates estrogen secretion. In males LH is called interstitial cell–stimulating hormone (ICSH), and it stimulates production of testosterone by the interstitial cells of the testes.

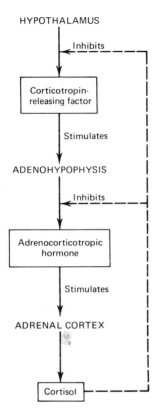

HYPOTHALAMUS

Inhibits

Corticotropin-
releasing factor

Stimulates

ADENOHYPOPHYSIS

Inhibits

Adrenocorticotropic
hormone

Stimulates

ADRENAL CORTEX

Cortisol

Figure 19-1. *Control of ACTH secretion.*

The gonadotropins are secreted in response to a releasing factor from the hypothalamus. In females their secretion is also controlled by estrogen and progesterone levels (see Chapter 1 under Positive Feedback) and varies with the menstrual cycle and with pregnancy and lactation. In males the gonadotropins are secreted at a relatively steady rate. Testosterone inhibits ICSH secretion by a negative feedback mechanism. In infants and children the adenohypophysis secretes very small quantities of gonadotropins. Effective secretion begins just before the onset of puberty.

Prolactin
Prolactin stimulates the secretion of milk. Prolactin secretion is controlled by prolactin-releasing factor (PRF) and prolactin-release–inhibiting factor (PRIF) from the hypothalamus. The prolactin level is high during pregnancy and lactation but at other times very little is secreted. The function of this hormone in males is not known.

Hypofunction

Hypofunction of the adenohypophysis usually affects all of the adenohypophyseal hormones (panhypopituitarism), but in some cases only partial deficiency occurs, usually involving GH and gonadotropins. Primary hypofunction is due to disease or destruction of the adenohypophysis. Failure to secrete GH usually occurs first, followed by gonadotropins, then TSH, and finally ACTH. Decreased hypothalamic stimulation or increased feedback from hormones secreted by target tissues produces secondary adenohypophyseal hypofunction.

Causes
Destruction of the hypophysis by a nonfunctioning tumor such as a chromophobe adenoma or craniopharyngioma is the most common cause of hypofunction in men and in children. As the tumor grows, it compresses the hypophysis against the walls of the sella turcica. In some cases hypophyseal insufficiency in children may be inherited or may be idiopathic. Occasionally only GH is deficient. It is not always possible to determine whether the basic defect is in the adenohypophysis or in the hypothalamus.

In women postpartum ischemic necrosis (*Sheehan's syndrome*) is a frequent cause of adenohypophyseal hypofunction. It is usually a sequela of postpartum hemorrhage but on rare occasions may follow an apparently normal parturition. During pregnancy the hypophysis hypertrophies and this enlargement in a confined space, together with the limited portal venous blood supply, makes the adenohypophysis especially vulnerable to ischemia. It is postulated that hemorrhage and shock result in hypotension and arteriolar spasm, impeding blood flow in the hypophyseal portal system. Thrombosis may then occur in the portal vessels and capillaries of the adeno-hypophysis, causing infarction. The necrotic tissue is subsequently replaced with nonfunctional fibrous scar tissue. The neurohypophysis is rarely affected because it is less dependent on the portal system for its blood supply.

On rare occasions destruction of the hypophysis may be caused by infectious granulomatous disease such as tuberculosis, brucellosis, or fungal infections.

Effects

Clinical manifestations of adenohypophyseal insufficiency usually develop slowly and are due to hormonal deficiencies. In addition, if hypophyseal destruction is due to a tumor, manifestations may include headache due to pressure within the sella turcica or increased intracranial pressure; visual impairment due to pressure on the optic chiasma; and obesity, drowsiness, polydipsia, polyuria, and disturbances of temperature regulation due to pressure on the hypothalamus.

Effects in children. Adenohypophyseal insufficiency occurring in childhood results in growth failure due to lack of growth hormone and in many cases failure of sexual development due to lack of gonadotropins. Thyroid and adrenocortical insufficiency only occur occasionally.

Affected children are usually of normal size at birth. Growth may be normal during the first year or two and then becomes progressively slower. Body proportions are usually normal but the person has a very small stature (i.e., is a *dwarf*). Intelligence is usually normal. Mild obesity may occur because of the absence of the lipolytic action of growth hormone. Hypoglycemic episodes may occur due to deficiency of GH and ACTH.

If the person has an isolated deficiency of GH, sexual development is normal but stature is abnormally short. When gonadotropins are also lacking, adult sexual development is not attained and the person's features remain childlike. With gonadotropin deficiency the pubertal growth spurt

does not occur but closure of the epiphyses is delayed so that growth continues into the third decade. Untreated people usually have an adult height between 100 and 140 cm.

Effects in adults. Menstrual irregularities due to gonadotropin deficiency are usually the first indication of adenohypophyseal insufficiency in women. Menstrual bleeding is scanty and irregular and finally amenorrhea results. The uterus and vagina atrophy and sexual desire diminishes. Pubic and axillary hair disappear. If hypophyseal insufficiency is due to postpartum ischemic necrosis, there may be failure of lactation, rapid involution of the breasts, and failure of pubic hair to regrow (if it was shaved before delivery).

In men, testicular atrophy, loss of libido, and impotency result from gonadotropin deficiency. Facial hair becomes softer and grows slowly.

Deficiency of TSH produces hypothyroidism, which causes dry skin, cold intolerance, constipation, and possibly mental apathy and depression (see below).

ACTH insufficiency results in a deficiency of cortisol. Consequently hypoglycemia may occur and the person withstands stress poorly. Aldosterone secretion is not usually affected.

Loss of skin pigment may occur due to lack of MSH.

Hyperfunction

Hyperfunction of the adenohypophysis is usually due to a hormone-secreting neoplasm. On rare occasions hyperplasia of acidophil cells that secrete GH may result from hypothalamic dysfunction. Loss of negative feedback inhibition due to deficiency of a target-gland hormone can lead to hypersecretion of ACTH, TSH, or gonadotropins.

The effects of excess ACTH are discussed in the section on the adrenal cortex and the effects of excess TSH are discussed in the section on the thyroid. Only hypersecretion of GH and prolactin are considered here.

Growth-Hormone Excess

The effects of GH hypersecretion depend on whether or not the epiphyses have closed. In children and adolescents before epiphyseal closure GH excess produces gigantism (giantism). In adults excess GH produces acromegaly. If the condition is not treated, deficiencies of other adenohypophyseal hormones eventually develop because cells that produce other hormones are displaced by GH-secreting tumor cells.

The characteristic feature of *giantism* is rapid and excessive growth of the skeleton and soft tissues, especially at puberty. The bodily proportions remain normal. Skeletal deformities such as kyphosis and scoliosis may occur. Sexual development is usually normal at first, but hypogonadism and amenorrhea may develop later in life due to gonadotropin deficiency.

Acromegaly usually begins between the ages of 20 and 40, but it has a very insidious onset and may take years to develop fully. It is characterized by proliferation of bony and soft tissues. After closure of the epiphyses linear growth is no longer possible but the excess GH affects the remaining cartilaginous areas and the extremities. The cartilages of the ribs and joints proliferate and have a tendency to ossify.

Endochondral ossification of the costochondral junctions causes elongation of the ribs and an increase on the anteroposterior diameter of the chest. Endochondral ossification occurring at the mandibular condyles causes enlargement of the jaw and separation and malocclusion of the teeth. In addition, new bone is laid down under the periosteum of many bones. This process causes general thickening of the skull and prominence of bony ridges. All bones become thickened where muscles and ligaments attach. Bony overgrowth damages the articular cartilages and leads to arthritis. The intervertebral foramina may be narrowed due to growth of new bone. The result may be pressure on nerve roots, which causes pain and muscle weakness in the limbs.

Growth of soft tissue, together with bony enlargement, causes an increase in the size of the hands and feet. The hands become thick and broad, with blunt fingers. The tongue, lips, nose, and ears also become enlarged and the skin is thickened.

The excess GH may impair glucose tolerance and may precipitate overt diabetes mellitus in susceptible people (see Chapter 18).

Prolactin Excess

Hypersecretion of prolactin causes persistent abnormal secretion of milk (*galactorrhea*) in men as well as women. A reciprocal mechanism appears to control secretion of prolactin and gonadotropins, so that prolactin excess is usually accompanied by gonadotropin deficiency. This deficiency causes amenorrhea in women and impotence in men.

THE ADRENAL CORTEX

The adrenal (or suprarenal) glands have two main components. The inner part, the *adrenal medulla*, is derived embryologically from neural ectoderm and secretes epinephrine and norepinephrine. The outer part, the *adrenal cortex*, surrounds the medulla and is derived embryologically from mesoderm. The adrenal cortex secretes a variety of steroid hormones, the major ones being cortisol (hydrocortisone), corticosterone, aldosterone, deoxycorticosterone, dehydroepiandrosterone, androstenedione, and 11-hydroxyandrostenedione. In addition, small amounts of testosterone are produced and probably very small amounts of estrogens are secreted as well.

The term *corticosteroids*, or *corticoids*, refers to steroid compounds of the adrenal cortex that have 21 carbon atoms. This term includes inactive metabolites as well as hormones that influence carbohydrate and electrolyte metabolism. The term *17-ketosteroids* refers to steroids with 19 carbon atoms that have a ketone group in the 17 position. It includes steroids with androgenic activity and their inactive metabolites.

Adrenocortical Hormones

The hormones of the adrenal cortex can be divided into three groups on the basis of their primary physiological activity. The *glucocorticoids*, cortisol and corticosterone, mainly affect carbohydrate and protein metabolism. The *mineralocorticoids*, aldosterone and deoxycorticosterone, exert their effects mainly on sodium and potassium metabolism. The *androgens*, dehydroepiandrosterone, androstenedione, and 11-hydroxyandrostenedione, are male sex hormones. There is some overlapping of the effects of glucocorticoids and mineralocorticoids. Their actions are not one or the other, but varying degrees of both. Adrenocortical hormones are synthesized from cholesterol and the pathways for their synthesis share common intermediate compounds. Some of the intermediate compounds have weak physiological activity that is not significant in the amounts normally secreted. Overproduction of these intermediates, or of by-products, however, may have clinical significance.

Glucocorticoids

Cortisol is the major glucocorticoid; the activity of corticosterone is much weaker. Cortisone is a commercially prepared steroid that has glucocorticoid activity; it is not synthesized in the body. As mentioned earlier, glucocorticoids are secreted in response to ACTH from the adenohypophysis. Normal secretion cannot be maintained without ACTH.

Glucocorticoids stimulate protein breakdown and promote the conversion of amino acids to glucose (gluconeogenesis). In this respect they antagonize the action of growth hormone. At the same time, glucocorticoids inhibit uptake and use of glucose by the tissues (except the brain). This effect, together with the increased gluconeogenesis, raises the blood glucose level. Therefore glucocorticoids antagonize insulin action (see also Chapter 18).

Glucocorticoids promote the mobilization of fat from adipose tissue, probably as an indirect result of their effect on carbohydrate metabolism. Glucocorticoids also influence deposition of fat. This effect is possibly due to a compensatory increase in insulin secretion as a result of the increased blood glucose level; insulin promotes storage of fat in adipose tissue.

Glucocorticoids have a permissive effect on the activity of catecholamines. Blood vessels are unable to respond to norepinephrine and epinephrine in the absence of glucocorticoids.

Glucocorticoids are important in the body's response to stress (see Chapter 2 under Physiological Responses to Stress) and in large amounts have an antiinflammatory effect. They decrease capillary permeability, decrease the infiltration of phagocytic cells into the area of inflammation, and inhibit the growth of fibroblasts.

Mineralocorticoids

Aldosterone is the major mineralocorticoid. Deoxycorticosterone (DOC) is less potent. Unlike the other hormones of the adrenal cortex, synthesis of aldosterone does not require ACTH. Aldosterone secretion is mainly influenced by the renin-angiotensin system. (See Chaper 12 under Hormonal Mechanisms.)

The major effects of the mineralocorticoids are conservation of body sodium and enhancement of potassium excretion. Mineralocorticoids increase sodium reabsorption by the distal renal tubules, increase intestinal absorption of sodium, and decrease the sodium concentration in sweat. At the same time, they enhance urinary excretion of potassium, decrease intestinal absorption of potassium, and increase the potassium concentration in sweat. Through their effects on sodium metabolism, mineralocorticoids influence fluid balance and are essential for life.

Sex Hormones

The adrenal sex hormones are secreted in response to ACTH rather than gonadotropins. In males the amount of testosterone secreted by the testes is much greater than the quantities of androgens secreted by the adrenal cortex, and the adrenal androgens probably have a very minor physiological role. In females the adrenal androgens are probably responsible for the growth of axillary and pubic hair. In the amounts normally secreted, the adrenal estrogens have no known physiological function.

Hyperfunction: Cushing's Syndrome

Cushing's syndrome is a condition that results from chronically elevated levels of glucocorticoids in the blood. The levels of adrenal androgens and deoxycorticosterone may also be increased. Females are affected more often than males.

Causes
Four basic disturbances can produce Cushing's syndrome. One cause is a cortisol-secreting neoplasm (either an adenoma or a carcinoma) within the adrenal cortex. The tumor does not respond to the normal controls of cortisol secretion and elaborates an excessive amount of cortisol.

A second cause of Cushing's syndrome is overproduction of ACTH due to a disturbance of hypothalamic or hypophyseal function. The excessive ACTH causes hyperplasia and hyperfunction of both adrenal glands. The excessive ACTH secretion may be due to a tumor within the adenohypophysis. Often, however, a tumor is not found and it is believed that the primary disturbance is increased production of CRF by the hypothalamus. The hypothalamus is less sensitive to the inhibitory effect of cortisol (i.e., the set point of the negative feedback control system is set higher) and very high levels of cortisol are required to suppress ACTH secretion. In addition the normal circadian rhythm of ACTH secretion is lost; the usual decline in the evening fails to occur.

A third cause of Cushing's syndrome is secretion of ACTH or an ACTH-like substance by a neoplasm outside of the adenohypophysis, most commonly carcinoma of the lung (*ectopic ACTH syndrome*). The uncontrolled ACTH secretion causes excessive stimulation of the adrenal cortices and overproduction of cortisol.

A fourth, and common, cause of Cushing's syndrome is chronic therapy with pharmacological doses of glucocorticoids such as cortisone.

Effects
Some of the clinical manifestations of Cushing's syndrome can be explained as an exaggeration of the effects of cortisol, but the basis of other manifestations is obscure. A redistribution of body fat is characteristic of Cushing's syndrome, but the underlying mechanism is not known. Fat is deposited in the face, neck, and trunk, but the limbs remain thin. The face becomes rounded (moon face) due to increased deposition of fat in the cheeks (Fig. 19-2). A fat pad over the cervical spine causes a "buffalo hump."

Increased protein catabolism affects the muscles, skin, bone matrix, and capillaries. Muscle wasting occurs particularly in the limbs and causes weakness. The skin atrophies and appears thin, stretched, and shiny. Dark red to purple stripes (striae) develop, especially on the abdomen. Osteoporosis due to loss of protein from the bone matrix may cause backache, spinal deformities, and pathological fractures. Cortisol antagonizes the action of vitamin D in promoting intestinal absorption of calcium, possibly contributing to the osteoporosis. Atrophy of capillary walls causes easy bruising and purpura.

The skin has a florid complexion; the face especially may be very red. The exact basis of this feature is not known. Thinning of the skin together with an increase in the hemoglobin concentration may be partly responsible.

Glucose tolerance is often impaired due to the antagonism between cortisol and insulin. Overt diabetes mellitus may develop.

Sodium retention and hypokalemia may occur because cortisol has some mineralocorticoid activity. DOC may also be secreted in excess and contribute to the altered electrolyte metabolism.

Hypertension is common in people with Cushing's syndrome. It may be partly due to the excess

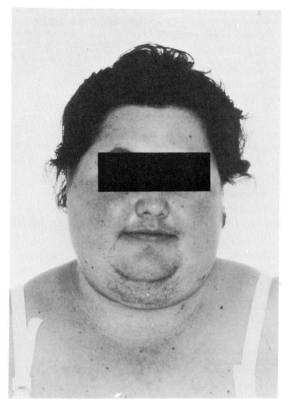

Figure 19-2. *Typical moon face of Cushing's syndrome. Also note excessive facial hair. (Courtesy of Ronald D. Brown, M.D., Endocrine Research Unit, Mayo Clinic, Rochester, Minn.)*

and the testes may atrophy. The basis of these disturbances of sexual function is not known.

Women may develop coarse hair on the face, chest, and limbs (hirsutism), and children may develop pubic hair, probably due to excess adrenal androgens. Acne is common. It may be due to cortisol or androgen excess.

Hyperfunction: Primary Aldosteronism

Hypersecretion of aldosterone (hyperaldosteronism) sometimes occurs without excess secretion of other adrenocorticoids. It is more common in females than males. *Primary aldosteronism (Conn's syndrome)* is usually caused by an aldosterone-secreting adenoma of the adrenal cortex. Secondary hypersecretion of aldosterone is usually due to renin excess. In contrast, the renin level is low with primary aldosteronism.

Effects

Excess aldosterone causes retention of sodium, which leads to expansion of the ECF volume and produces hypertension (see also Chapter 13). Edema does not usually occur because the elevated blood pressure increases the glomerular filtration rate; a new equilibrium is established, limiting the amount of fluid that is retained. Headaches are a common symptom of primary aldosteronism and are presumably due to the hypertension.

Excessive potassium excretion causes hypokalemia (see Chapter 16), which is associated with alkalosis (see Chapter 15). Hypokalemia causes muscle weakness and electrocardiographic changes. In addition, postural hypotension may occur because hypokalemia impairs the baroreceptor reflex.

The distal tubular cells of the kidneys may become distorted and filled with vacuoles. These changes are attributed to loss of potassium, because similar changes have been noted with chronic hypokalemia due to other causes (hypokalemic nephropathy). These lesions impair the urine concentrating mechanism, resulting in an ADH-resistant diuresis. Polydipsia accompanies the polyuria.

cortisol potentiating the vasoconstrictive effect of norepinephrine and partly due to sodium and water retention.

The high levels of cortisol cause a decrease in the size of lymphoid tissue and a decrease in the number of lymphocytes and eosinophils in the blood. The polymorphonuclear leukocyte count may be increased. Wound healing may be impaired due to the antiinflammatory effect of cortisol.

Menstrual irregularities, sterility, and atrophy or cystic degeneration of the ovaries often occur in women with Cushing's syndrome. Affected men usually experience loss of libido and impotence

Hypofunction

Hypofunction of the adrenal cortex may be due to destruction of the adrenal cortex (*primary adrenocortical insufficiency; Addison's disease*) or lack of ACTH (*secondary adrenocortical insufficiency*). Primary adrenocortical insufficiency results in deficiencies of all three classes of adrenocortical hormones. With secondary adrenocortical insufficiency, however, aldosterone secretion is not affected. This section is concerned with primary adrenocortical insufficiency. Lack of ACTH was discussed earlier, in the section on hypofunction of the adenohypophysis.

Chronic Adrenocortical Insufficiency

Causes. Addison's disease is caused by destruction of the adrenal cortex. The adrenal cortex has a very high regenerative capacity; therefore overt signs of chronic adrenocortical insufficiency usually do not occur until more than 90% of the gland has been destroyed.

Formerly infectious granulomatous diseases, especially tuberculosis, were the most common cause of adrenocortical destruction. Now, however, primary atrophy is a more common cause of adrenocortical insufficiency. This condition, which is called primary, cytotoxic, or idiopathic adrenocortical atrophy, is believed to be due to an autoimmune reaction.

Effects. Addison's disease has an insidious onset, and it is not usually possible to determine exactly when the condition starts. Early symptoms are easy fatigability, weight loss, and anorexia.

Lack of aldosterone causes loss of body sodium and water and retention of potassium. Loss of sodium and water results in decreased ECF volume, hypovolemia, and hypotension. Lack of cortisol, which is necessary for the tonic action of norepinephrine on the arterioles, contributes to the hypotension. Sodium deficiency sometimes causes muscle cramps. Some people may have a craving for salt. Hyperkalemia alters cardiac con-

ductivity (see Chapter 16) and is a potentially lethal complication of Addison's disease.

Lack of cortisol alters carbohydrate metabolism. Intestinal absorption of glucose is delayed and hepatic glycogenesis and gluconeogenesis are impaired. Consequently hypoglycemia may occur, especially after an overnight fast. Cortisol deficiency is apparently responsible for the anorexia. Weight loss is caused by fluid loss and decreased intake of food due to anorexia. Muscle weakness results partly from impaired carbohydrate metabolism and partly from electrolyte disturbances.

Inability to concentrate, lack of initiative, and depression are common in people with Addison's disease. These mental disturbances may result partly from electrolyte imbalance and hypoglycemia, but in addition cortisol deficiency probably has a direct effect on nervous function.

Lack of cortisol results in a loss of inhibition of ACTH secretion. MSH appears to be secreted together with ACTH and the two have similar structures. The high levels of MSH and/or ACTH cause increased formation of melanin, resulting in increased skin pigmentation and darkening of the hair. The degree of pigmentation depends on the ability to form pigment; light-complexioned people may notice only an increase in the number and size of freckles.

Women with Addison's disease may lose their pubic and axillary hair due to lack of adrenal androgens. Little effect is noted in men because they continue to secrete testicular androgens.

If a person with chronic adrenal insufficiency is subjected to stress from any cause, acute adrenal insufficiency (*Addisonian crisis*) can occur. For example, acute infectious diseases, physical overexertion, vomiting and diarrhea, or surgery can precipitate life-threatening Addisonian crisis.

Acute Adrenocortical Insufficiency

Causes. In addition to Addisonian crisis, acute adrenocortical insufficiency can be caused by adrenal hemorrhage and infarction. Adrenal hemorrhage sometimes occurs in newborns, possibly due to birth trauma or hypoprothrombinemia. Adrenal hemorrhage may also be a complication of acute sepsis, especially due to meningococci (Waterhouse-Friderichsen syndrome), or a complication of anticoagulant therapy. Bilateral venous thrombosis is another cause of acute adrenal insufficiency. It is rare and mainly occurs postpartum or following severe burns.

Effects. Vomiting is common during acute adrenal insufficiency and severe colicky abdominal pain and diarrhea may occur. These manifestations are possibly due to electrolyte imbalances. A vicious cycle develops because vomiting and diarrhea cause further loss of fluid and electrolytes. The person is irritable and restless at first, but then becomes extremely weak, so that even speech is difficult. Severe shock and coma ensue. The shock is partly due to hypovolemia, but vascular unre-

sponsiveness due to lack of cortisol contributes to the circulatory collapse. Hypoglycemia may occur. Fever is present when the acute adrenocortical insufficiency is due to sepsis. In other cases the body temperature is usually subnormal; development of fever is a terminal sign.

Congenital Adrenal Hyperplasia

Several enzymes are involved in the synthesis of the adrenocortical hormones, as indicated in Figure 19-3. A genetic deficiency of any of these enzymes causes a block in the metabolic pathway, leading to deficiencies of some hormones and excesses of others. (See Chapter 6 under Inborn Errors Due to Blocked Metabolic Pathways.) Lack of cortisol results in loss of the normal negative feedback control of ACTH secretion. Consequently ACTH secretion is increased and the ad-

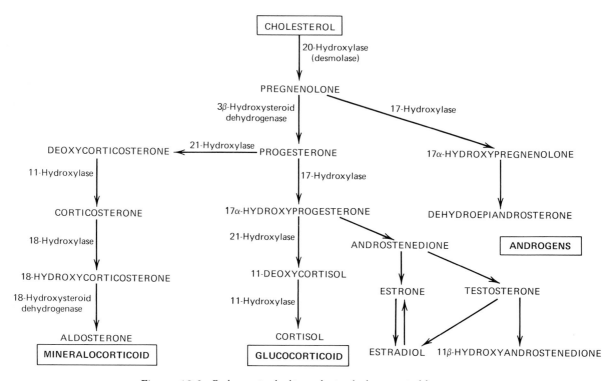

Figure 19-3. *Pathways in the biosynthesis of adrenocortical hormones.*

renal cortex is stimulated, causing adrenal hyperplasia. Therefore these inborn errors of metabolism are grouped under the term *congenital adrenal hyperplasia* (CAH). Six varieties of congenital adrenal hyperplasia are known, each attributable to deficiency of a different enzyme. They appear to have an autosomal recessive mode of inheritance. Some forms of CAH are associated with excessive secretion of adrenal androgens, which causes virilization. The condition may then be referred to as *adrenogenital syndrome.*

20-Hydroxylase Deficiency

The enzyme 20-hydroxylase (cholesterol desmolase) is necessary for the conversion of cholesterol to pregnenolone. This step is believed to be essential for the synthesis of all adrenal steroid hormones. Therefore, when this enzyme is lacking, production of all adrenocortical hormones is impaired. The adrenal glands become very large and filled with cholesterol. This condition is rare and affected infants usually do not survive very long.

This enzyme is probably also involved in the synthesis of sex hormones in the gonads. Affected infants have female genitalia even though they may be genetically male, presumably because the fetal testes are unable to secrete testosterone.

3β-Hydroxysteroid Dehydrogenase Deficiency

Conversion of pregnenolone to progesterone is catalyzed by the enzyme 3β-hydroxysteroid dehydrogenase. Progesterone is the precursor for most of the adrenocortical hormones (see Fig. 19-3). Therefore 3β-hydroxysteroid dehydrogenase deficiency results in a lack of both glucocorticoids and mineralocorticoids, as well as some androgens and estrogens. The synthesis of dehydroepiandrosterone (DHEA) is not blocked, however, and excessive amounts of this weak androgen are produced.

Affected newborns of either sex have ambiguous external genitalia. Excessive secretion of DHEA is probably responsible for the partial masculinization of the external genitalia in female infants.

Synthesis of gonadal steroids also requires 3β-hydroxysteroid dehydrogenase and failure of development of normal external genitalia in male infants is presumably due to inability of the fetal testes to produce androgen.

Infants with this disorder show signs of adrenocortical insufficiency because they are deficient in cortisol and aldosterone. Excessive amounts of salt and water are lost. Weakness, apathy, difficulty feeding, vomiting, and diarrhea occur within the first few weeks of life and death may occur due to circulatory collapse.

17-Hydroxylase Deficiency

The enzyme 17-hydroxylase is necessary for early steps in the synthesis of cortisol, androgens, and estrogens in the adrenal cortex and of sex hormones in the gonads. Therefore normal amounts of these hormones cannot be synthesized when 17-hydroxylase is deficient. Lack of cortisol results in excessive secretion of ACTH. Under the stimulation of ACTH the adrenal cortex produces large amounts of DOC and corticosterone because the pathway for their synthesis is not blocked.

DOC causes sodium retention, which leads to expansion of the ECF volume and produces hypertension. Consequently secretion of renin by the kidneys is suppressed and very little aldosterone is produced because it is not needed. (Recall that the renin-angiotensin system is the major stimulus for aldosterone secretion.)

Male external genitalia fail to develop because the fetal testes are unable to secrete androgens. Therefore affected males are pseudohermaphrodites (i.e., the external genitalia appear female). Affected females fail to menstruate and fail to develop secondary sexual characteristics at the normal age of puberty because of the lack of estrogen secretion by the ovaries.

21-Hydroxylase Deficiency

Deficiency of 21-hydroxylase is the most common form of CAH. Synthesis of all glucocorticoids and mineralocorticoids is impaired. Deficiency of cortisol results in excessive ACTH secretion, which causes adrenal hyperplasia and excessive secretion of adrenal androgens. Two forms of this condition occur. In one form the block in the metabolic pathway is almost complete, causing deficiencies of aldosterone and cortisol and producing the severe manifestations of adrenocortical insufficiency, as described earlier. In the other form the block is only partial, and adrenocortical insuffiency is not manifest.

In the severe form early virilization occurs due to the excess adrenal androgens. Female infants have an enlarged clitoris and varying degrees of fusion of the labial folds at birth (female pseudohermaphroditism), and they may be mistaken for males with undescended testes and hypospadias. In males the external genitalia appear normal at birth, but the penis begins to enlarge within a few weeks. Adrenocortical insufficiency may become evident before that time, however, and can be fatal if the condition is not promptly diagnosed and treated.

Except for clitoral enlargement in some cases, the mild form of 21-hydroxylase deficiency may not be noticed until the child is between 2 and 10 years old. Then the condition is manifested by rapid growth, excessive muscular development, early appearance of pubic and axillary hair, deepening of the voice, acne, and early closure of the epiphyses due to excessive adrenal androgens. Affected females do not menstruate, do not develop normal secondary sex characteristics, and develop facial hair.

11-Hydroxylase Deficiency

Deficiency of 11-hydroxylase impairs secretion of cortisol and aldosterone. Low levels of cortisol result in increased secretion of ACTH, with consequent stimulation of the adrenal cortex and overproduction of adrenal androgens and DOC. The excess androgens cause virilization. (See the discussion of this condition in Chapter 6.) The excess DOC more than compensates for the lack of aldosterone. As a result sodium retention occurs, producing hypertension.

18-Hydroxysteroid Dehydrogenase Deficiency

The enzyme 18-hydroxysteroid dehydrogenase is necessary for the last step in the synthesis of aldosterone. Therefore deficiency of this enzyme results in aldosterone deficiency. This condition is characterized by loss of sodium and water, hypovolemia, and hypotension. Potassium is retained, causing hyperkalemia. The plasma renin level is elevated as a result of the sodium deficit and hypotension.

THE THYROID

The thyroid gland produces three hormones: thyroxine (T_4) and triiodothyronine (T_3), which are secreted by the follicular cells; and calcitonin, which is secreted by the parafollicular (C) cells. Calcitonin is discussed in Chapter 16 with calcium metabolism and will not be considered here.

Thyroid Function

The thyroid follicles are vesicles made up of a single layer of cuboidal epithelial cells surrounding a mass of colloid. Synthesis of thyroxine and triiodothyronine by the follicles requires iodine and the amino acid tyrosine.

Most of the iodine in the diet is in the form of iodide (I^-). The small amount of organic or molecular iodine in food is reduced to iodide during intestinal absorption. The concentration of inorganic iodide in the blood depends mainly on dietary intake. Some of the iodide filtered in the renal glomeruli is reabsorbed by the renal tubules and some is excreted in the urine.

Synthesis and Release of Thyroid Hormones

Iodide from the blood is actively transported into the follicular cells by the "iodide pump." This step is stimulated by TSH. Inside the cells iodide is quickly oxidized to iodine. Tyrosine is present in thyroglobulin, a glycoprotein molecule, and subsequent reactions take place in the matrix of thyroglobulin. Iodine combines with tyrosine at one or two sites to form monoiodotyrosine (MIT) or diiodotyrosine (DIT), respectively. Then two DIT combine to form tetraiodothyronine (T_4, thyroxine) or one DIT and one MIT combine to form triiodothyronine (T_3). The thyroglobulin molecules containing T_4, T_3, and small amounts of DIT and MIT are stored as colloid in the lumen of the follicle. Synthesis of T_3 and T_4 requires energy. TSH stimulates glucose metabolism in thyroid cells and thus more energy is provided for hormone synthesis.

When thyroid hormones are to be released into the blood, stored thyroglobulin is taken back into the follicular cells by pinocytosis. This process is also stimulated by TSH. Inside the cells lysosomes combine with the pinocytic vesicles. Lysosomal proteolytic enzymes break down the thyroglobulin molecules, releasing T_3, T_4, MIT, and DIT. The hormones T_3 and T_4 are secreted into the capillaries around the follicles. An enzyme in the follicular cells removes iodine from the DIT and MIT and the iodine is reutilized for hormone synthesis. The processes involved in synthesis and release of thyroid hormones are summarized in Figure 19-4.

The thyroid gland secretes mostly T_4 and only a small amount of T_3. Both hormones are reversibly bound to plasma proteins for transport in the blood; thyroxine is bound more strongly than T_3. The hormones are combined mainly with thyroid-binding globulin (TBG) and to a lesser extent with thyroid-binding prealbumin (TBPA) and albumin. A very small proportion of the thyroid hormones exists free (unbound) in the plasma. The unbound hormone is the active form.

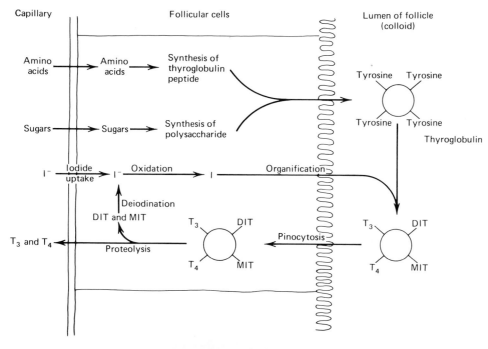

Figure 19-4. Synthesis and release of thyroid hormones.

As T_3 and T_4 are taken up by the tissues, more hormone is released from the binding proteins.

Regulation of Thyroid Activity

Activity of the thyroid gland is stimulated by TSH from the adenohypophysis, as mentioned earlier. High levels of thyroid hormones in turn exert an inhibitory effect on TSH release by a negative feedback mechanism (Fig. 19-5). As stated previously, secretion of TSH is stimulated by TRF from the hypothalamus. TRF production is influenced by emotional factors and environmental temperature. Cold increases TRF production and therefore stimulates TSH secretion; TSH in turn stimulates thyroid function. Thyroid hormone stimulates metabolism and increases body heat production

(see below). Heat inhibits TRF production. Emotional states can either increase or decrease TRF production, which in turn influences TSH production and thyroid activity.

Availability of iodide also influences thyroid activity. Large doses of iodide inhibit binding of iodine with tyrosine and coupling of MIT and DIT. Release of T_3 and T_4 from stored thyroglobulin is also inhibited. These inhibitory effects prevent an excessive increase of hormone synthesis when excessive amounts of iodine are available. An acute iodine deficiency induces increased iodide uptake by the thyroid. The iodide pump is more responsive to TSH when the iodine stores in the thyroid are low than when a large amount of iodine is present in the gland.

Effects of Thyroid Hormones

Both T_3 and T_4 are hormonally active. T_3 is more active physiologically than T_4 and some of the circulating T_4 is converted to T_3 in the tissues. The thyroid hormones affect metabolism in several ways.

Thyroid hormones increase oxygen consumption and heat production, probably by a direct effect on mitochondria to enhance oxidative phosphorylation. This effect occurs in the liver, kidneys, heart, and skeletal muscles, but not in the brain, gonads, or lymph tissues. Consequently, thyroid hormones influence the basal metabolic rate and caloric requirement.

Thyroid hormones increase protein synthesis, probably by a direct effect on the translation process, as well as by increasing the transcription of RNA in the nucleus. Therefore T_3 and T_4 stimulate and support growth.

Carbohydrate and lipid metabolism are affected in several ways. Thyroid hormones increase the intestinal absorption of glucose and tend to increase glycogenolysis. They also stimulate lipolysis. In addition, degradation and excretion of cholesterol is stimulated by thyroid hormones; synthesis of cholesterol is also slightly increased. Thyroid hormones are necessary for the conversion of carotene to vitamin A.

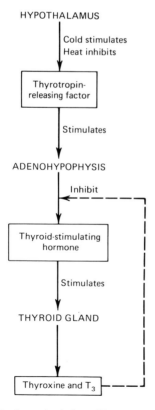

Figure 19-5. *Control of thyroid-hormone synthesis and release.*

Thyroid hormones influence the synthesis of proteins and lipids in the nervous system at various stages of development in the fetus and infant and are necessary for cerebral maturation. In addition, thyroid hormones have a stimulatory effect on nervous system function throughout life. The mechanism responsible for this effect is not known. Possibly T_3 and T_4 act as precursors for adrenergic neurotransmitters. Thyroid hormones enhance the effects of epinephrine and norepinephrine.

Thyroid hormones have a stimulatory effect on bone cells and increase both osteoblastic and osteoclastic activity.

Goiter

A *goiter* is an enlargement of the thyroid gland; it may be barely detectable or may be an enormous enlargement protruding over the chest. A goiter may be associated with normal thyroid function (*simple*, or *nontoxic*, *goiter*), with hyperfunction (*toxic goiter*), or with hypofunction (*hypothyroid goiter*). The thyroid gland may be uniformly enlarged (*diffuse goiter*) or may be irregular due to small protuberant masses of tissue (nodules) in its substance (*nodular goiter*).

Swelling of the neck may be the only manifestation of goiter. Symptoms that may occur in some cases are dyspnea or a choking feeling due to pressure on the trachea, difficulty swallowing due to pressure on the esophagus, or difficulty speaking due to pressure on the laryngeal nerves. Deep veins in the neck may be compressed, resulting in compensatory enlargement of superficial veins. If venous obstruction is severe, the head and neck may be cyanosed. If the goiter is associated with thyroid hypofunction or hyperfunction, signs and symptoms of thyroid hormone deficiency or excess will also be present (see below).

Endemic Goiter

In certain areas of the world large percentages of the population have goiters and the condition is called *endemic goiter* (Fig. 19-6). Iodine deficiency

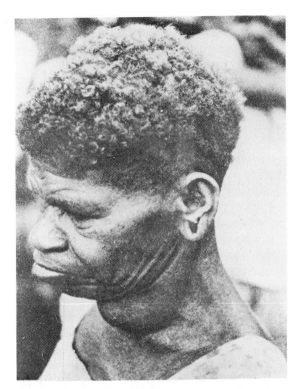

Figure 19-6. *Endemic goiter. (From DeGroot LJ, Stanbury JB: The Thyroid and Its Diseases, ed 5. New York, John Wiley and Sons, Inc., 1979.)*

is the major cause of the goiter although other factors may contribute to the etiology. Endemic goiter occurs mainly in inland and mountainous areas where the soil and water are deficient in iodine. When the iodine deficiency is mild to moderate the goiter is associated with normal thyroid function. In areas where iodine deficiency is severe, hypothyroidism and cretinism occur (see below).

Since not all members of the population in an iodine-deficient area develop goiter, other factors must play a role. It is possible that some people who develop goiters have inherited partial defects of enzymes required for thyroid-hormone synthesis. When iodine is readily available the defect may not be manifested, but in conditions of iodine deficiency the defect predisposes affected people to develop goiter. Substances called goitrogens, which are present in some plants, interfere with thyroid function and produce goiter. Varying intakes of goitrogens may be the reason some people in regions of iodine deficiency develop goiter and others do not. Goiters are more common in females than males. In some cases an increased need for thyroid hormones during puberty, pregnancy, or lactation may unmask a relative iodine deficiency and contribute to goiter formation.

Lack of iodine impairs production of thyroid hormones. Consequently the output of TSH from the adenohypophysis is increased. Under the influence of TSH a compensatory diffuse hyperplasia of the thyroid gland occurs (the evolutionary phase). As a result of this adaptive mechanism the thyroid gland is able to take up more iodine so that the total iodine content of the gland is usually within normal limits but the amount of iodine per gram of tissue is reduced. Initially the follicle cells are increased in height and the amount of colloid is decreased as the gland puts out all the stored hormone that it has. The increased size and increased activity of the gland are able to maintain adequate circulating levels of thyroid hormones. The evolutionary phase is followed by involution of the thyroid gland. The follicular cells decrease in size, and the follicles become dilated and filled with colloid due to the increased production of thyroglobulin. Normal iodination of the thyroglobulin fails to occur, and the thyroglobulin cannot be mobilized for use. Up to this time the thyroid is symmetrically and smoothly enlarged.

Sometimes the sequence of evolution and involution occurs in cycles, presumably caused by alternating periods of increased or decreased need for thyroid hormones, relative sufficiency or insufficiency of iodine, and/or the presence of other goitrogenic factors. The processes tend to become irregular and do not affect the gland uniformly. Areas of hyperplasia may be interspersed with areas of involution and some areas of the gland

may atrophy. As a result, a multinodular goiter is formed.

With iodine deficiency the thyroid gland forms more MIT and less DIT than normal. Consequently more T_3 and less T_4 is produced. Since T_3 is physiologically more active than T_4, this adaptive mechanism maintains a euthyroid state (i.e., normal thyroid function) with the utilization of less iodine.

Hypofunction

A deficiency or absence of thyroid hormones, with resultant lack of the physiological effects of the hormones, is called *hypothyroidism*. Hypothyroidism may or may not be associated with formation of a goiter. Hypothyroidism is usually primary, due to failure of the thyroid tissue itself, but can be secondary, due to TSH deficiency. All hypothyroid states have certain features in common, regardless of the cause of thyroid-hormone deficiency. Some manifestations depend on the age of onset of hypothyroidism.

Adult Hypothyroidism

Causes. The most common cause of primary hypothyroidism is atrophy of the thyroid gland. The atrophy is considered to be the end result of a chronic inflammatory process due to an autoimmune reaction. (The chronic inflammatory disease of the thyroid is called Hashimoto's thyroiditis; it does not always lead to hypothyroidism.) In some cases of thyroid atrophy no autoantibodies can be detected and the condition is idiopathic.

Surgical removal of an excessive amount of the thyroid gland or destruction of the gland by radiation in the treatment of hyperthyroidism can lead to hypothyroidism.

Occasionally hypothyroidism develops as a result of ingestion of goitrogens or antithyroid drugs. In some cases hypothyroidism results from overdosage of antithyroid drugs in the treatment of hyperthyroidism. In other cases hypothyroidism is a side effect of drugs used in other conditions. For example, lithium, which is used in the treatment of manic-depressive illness, inhibits iodide transport in the thyroid gland and can cause hypothyroidism.

Secondary hypothyroidism is usually due to panhypopituitarism. This condition was discussed earlier in the chapter.

Effects. Hypothyroidism is characterized by a general slowing of bodily processes. The onset is usually insidious, except after thyroidectomy or during treatment with antithyroid drugs.

The basal metabolic rate is decreased, resulting in intolerance to cold. Lethargy, fatigue, muscular pains, and stiffness in the arms, thighs, and legs are common. Nervous system function is also impaired. Deep tendon reflexes have a prolonged relaxation time. Mental processes are slowed, as manifested by slow speech, apathy, and drowsiness. Memory may be impaired. Partial deafness occurs quite commonly; the pathogenesis is not clearly understood.

Appetite may be decreased but weight loss does not occur because metabolism is also decreased; weight gain may occur. Decreased metabolism and decreased gastrointestinal motility cause constipation. Fecal impaction or paralytic ileus may occur, causing intestinal obstruction.

Increased amounts of mucoprotein ground substance are deposited in the interstitial space. Fluid adsorbs to the mucoprotein and the total amount of interstitial fluid increases, producing a nonpitting edema called *myxedema*. (Strictly speaking, the term myxedema refers to the edema due to the deposition of excess mucoprotein. Some people, however, use the term interchangeably with hypothyroidism. Others reserve the term for severe cases of hypothyroidism. Myxedema is usually, but not always, present in people with hypothyroidism.) The mechanism responsible for the excessive deposition of mucoprotein is not known. Swelling is particularly noticeable around the eyes and the tongue is thickened. Pericardial or pleural effusions and occasionally ascites develop in some advanced cases.

The skin appears waxy and pale due to myxedema and cutaneous vasoconstriction. It often has a yellowish tinge due to deposition of carotene because conversion of carotene to vitamin A is impaired. In addition the skin is dry and scaly. Scalp hair is coarse, breaks easily, and may fall out. Wound healing is impaired.

The female sexual cycles may become anovulatory and menorrhagia (excessive menstrual flow) is common. This effect is possibly due to decreased ovarian metabolism with resultant decreased estrogen production. Both sexes exhibit decreased libido.

Plasma cholesterol and plasma triglyceride levels are usually elevated, apparently due to a slow rate of removal of lipids from the blood.

Congenital Hypothyroidism

Causes. Congenital hypothyroidism may be caused by thyroid aplasia or hypoplasia due to faulty embryological development (*athyreotic cretinism*). In some cases the rudimentary thyroid tissue fails to migrate to its normal position during embryological development and thyroid tissue is found in an abnormal position (*ectopic thyroid gland*). The most common site is the base of the tongue (*retrolingual thyroid*). In some cases the ectopic thyroid tissue produces adequate amounts of thyroid hormones but in other cases hypothyroidism occurs.

A second cause of congenital hypothyroidism is lack of iodine. In this case the hypothyroidism is associated with goiter. When it occurs in a region where iodine deficiency is severe and goiter is common, the condition is called *endemic cretinism.*

A third cause of congenital hypothyroidism is maternal ingestion of goitrogens (either as drugs or in food) during pregnancy.

Congenital hypothyroidism can also be caused by inherited defects of enzymes required for synthesis of thyroid hormones. The lack of thyroid hormones results in increased TSH secretion and compensatory hyperplasia of the thyroid gland, producing a goiter. Several inborn errors of thyroid hormone synthesis have been recognized. With an iodide-transport defect iodide uptake is impaired and the thyroid gland is unable to concentrate iodine. This defect can be overcome by administration of large doses of iodine. The most common inborn error of thyroid hormone synthesis is an iodide-organification defect. In this case oxidation of iodide and binding of iodine to tyrosine are impaired (i.e., MIT and DIT are not formed). Probably more than one enzyme is involved in organification of iodide, and this defect represents a heterogeneous group of disorders. With iodotyrosyl-coupling defect, conversion of MIT and DIT to T_3 and T_4 is blocked. In another defect, abnormal inactive iodinated peptides are present in the plasma, either as a result of defective thyroglobulin synthesis or abnormal proteolysis of thyroglobulin when thyroid hormones are to be released into the blood. Another inborn error is failure to deiodinate MIT and DIT after they are released from thyroglobulin. In this case the iodine is not available for reutilization and iodine deficiency may result.

Effects.   The syndrome resulting from severe congenital hypothyroidism is called *cretinism* and the affected person a *cretin.* With endemic and athyreotic cretinism hypothyroidism is usually evident at birth. Even with prompt treatment affected infants are incapable of normal intellectual development because of impaired brain development during the fetal period. Infants with inborn errors of thyroid metabolism, however, may appear normal at birth but develop signs of hypothyroidism later. Occasionally a goiter is present at birth but usually it develops during early childhood. In some cases the enzymatic defect is only partial and the hypothyroidism is mild.

The neonate with hypothyroidism occasionally has a large tongue and a puffy red face. Physiological jaundice (icterus neonatorum; see Chapter 26) may last longer than usual. Signs of decreased metabolism become apparent during the first few weeks of life. The baby is very quiet, feeds poorly, and is constipated.

Within the first few months motor and mental retardation become apparent, as manifested by physical inactivity (e.g., lack of kicking), and by later than normal raising of the head and learning to smile. The muscles are flaccid, resulting in protrusion of the abdomen. An umbilical hernia is often present. The hair is dry and grows slowly, the tongue enlarges, and the face becomes puffy. The skin becomes dry and thickened and usually has a yellowish tinge. Temperature and heart rate tend to be low.

Symptoms become very evident from 6 to 12 months of age and gradually increase in severity in subsequent years if the condition is not treated. Mental and physical development are very retarded. The child has a dull expression and slow actions. Faulty skeletal growth and maturation result in dwarfism, with abnormal body proportions. The extremities are short and the head is large in relation to the trunk. The head is short and wide (brachycephalic), with an increased interocular distance and a broad flat nasal bridge. The serum alkaline phosphatase level is often low due to decreased osteoblastic activity (see Chapter 16 under Bone Formation and Resorption). Dentition is delayed and may be defective. Sexual maturation is delayed and may fail to occur, depending on the severity of the hypothyroidism.

The degree of intellectual impairment depends on the severity of the hypothyroidism. In severe cases the cretin may not be able to speak and has vegetative functions only. With less severe hypothyroidism limited speech is possible, and in milder cases the person may be capable of simple manual skills as well.

Juvenile Hypothyroidism

Acquired hypothyroidism is rare during childhood and adolescence. It is usually due to idiopathic thyroid atrophy or hypofunction of the adenohypophysis. Surgical removal of the thyroid or treatment with antithyroid drugs are occasional causes. In some cases hypothyroidism due to inborn errors of thyroid-hormone synthesis in which the defect is only partial becomes apparent in childhood.

When hypothyroidism develops during the first

year of life it is difficult to distinguish from cretinism. The mental impairment is less severe, however, and usually responds well to treatment.

Hypothyroidism with its onset in late childhood or early adolescence is similar to adult hypothyroidism except that skeletal growth is impaired and sexual development is delayed and may be incomplete. Occasionally precocious puberty occurs. This development is believed to be due to an overlap in the feedback inhibition of gonadotropins and TSH by thyroid hormones. Lack of T_3 and T_4 results in increased gonadotropin secretion.

Myxedema Coma

Myxedema coma, or *crisis,* occurs in severe untreated hypothyroidism (or when people with hypothyroidism neglect to take prescribed medication). Metabolism is so slow that body temperature cannot be maintained and hypothermia occurs (see Chapter 24 for a discussion of body-temperature regulation and hypothermia). Usually the condition is precipitated by exposure to cold, infection, or drugs such as barbiturates or phenothiazines. The person becomes very drowsy and progresses into coma.

Alveolar hypoventilation with resultant hypercapnia is an important contributory factor in the development of the coma. The exact cause of the hypoventilation is not clearly understood, but impaired function of the respiratory center, disturbed neuromuscular transmission, and weakness of the respiratory muscles may be involved.

Hyperfunction

An increased concentration of circulating thyroid hormones, with resultant excessive physiological effects of the hormones, is called *hyperthyroidism,* or *thyrotoxicosis.* Hyperthyroidism is relatively rare in children; it occurs most commonly in adult females.

Causes

The most common cause of hyperthyroidism is diffuse hyperplasia and hyperfunctioning of the thyroid gland (*Grave's disease*). The vascularity of the gland is increased, the follicular epithelial cells are increased in height and in number, and the amount of colloid is decreased. It was once thought that the hyperplasia was due to excess TSH, but with the availability of better techniques for the assay of hormone levels in recent years this mechanism has been refuted. The TSH level is in fact low because of negative feedback inhibition of TSH secretion by the excess thyroid hormones. (Hyperthyroidism secondary to excess TSH caused by a tumor of the adenohypophysis can occur, but is very rare.)

The exact etiology of Grave's disease is not known. An immunoglobin of the IgG class (see Chapter 29), which is produced by lymphocytes, has been demonstrated in the serum of some, but not all, people with Grave's disease. This immunoglobulin has the properties of an antibody against thyroid tissue and it stimulates thyroid activity in experimental animals. It has a slower and more sustained effect than TSH and has been given the name long-acting thyroid stimulator (LATS). The exact role of LATS in the etiology of Grave's disease is not known.

A less common cause of hyperthyroidism is hyperfunctioning of single or multiple thyroid nodules. When the condition is due to a single hyperplastic nodule the condition is called *Plummer's disease.* The hyperplastic nodule loses its responsiveness to TSH and produces thyroid hormones without regard to the concentration of T_3 and T_4 in the plasma (i.e., the nodule becomes autonomous). The excessive secretion of thyroid hormones by the hyperplastic nodule inhibits TSH secretion, so that the rest of the gland, which is responsive to TSH, involutes. Thus in a thyroid scan uptake of radioactive iodine by the hyperfunctioning nodule is excessive, causing a region of high radioactivity (a "hot," or toxic, nodule), whereas very little radioactivity is taken up by the rest of the gland. The pathogenesis of Plummer's disease is not understood.

Effects

A goiter is almost always present in people with hyperthyroidism. Grave's disease frequently has a sudden onset and most commonly affects young adults who have not had a previous goiter. Plummer's disease, in contrast, usually has an insidious onset and usually occurs in older people who may have had a goiter for many years.

The excess thyroid hormones stimulate metabolism and enhance the effects of norepinephrine and epinephrine. The basal metabolic rate is increased, resulting in increased heat production and oxygen consumption. The increased metabolism is accompanied by negative nitrogen balance, weight loss, and sometimes increased appetite. Glucose metabolism is altered and hyperglycemia and glycosuria may occur. Increased heat production results in intolerance of heat and causes peripheral vasodilation and increased sweating to dissipate the heat (see Chapter 24 for a discussion of body temperature regulation). Therefore the skin is usually flushed, warm, and moist.

Hypermotility of the gastrointestinal tract occurs, causing an increased frequency of bowel movements and in some cases frank diarrhea.

The heart may undergo hypertrophy due to the increased load imposed by the increased metabolism. In addition, thyroid hormones enhance the effects of the catecholamines and have a direct stimulatory effect on cardiac function, as mentioned earlier. Therefore the heart rate is rapid and the cardiac output is raised, causing an increase in the systolic blood pressure. Diastolic pressure is low due to peripheral vasodilation, however, so the pulse pressure is increased. Abnormal cardiac rhythms and palpitations may occur. In elderly people, cardiac manifestations of hyperthyroidism may be severe, whereas metabolic changes are often mild.

Osteoporosis may develop due to increased activity of bone cells (see Chapter 16 under Metabolic Bone Disease). The plasma alkaline phosphatase level is often increased.

Altered nervous system function may cause irritability, nervousness, insomnia, and tremor. Nervous manifestations depend partly on the severity of the thyrotoxicosis and partly on the basic personality of the affected person. The person is often tense and restless. Anxiety and lability of mood are other manifestations that may occur.

Eye changes are common in people with Grave's disease but rarely occur in those with hyperthyroidism due to nodular goiters. The eye changes are independent of the degree of hyperthyroidism and their pathogenesis is not understood.

The earliest ocular change is usually lid retraction, in which the upper lid is elevated. As a result, the palpebral fissure is widened and the sclera above the cornea is visible, producing a characteristic stare. Lid retraction is probably due to increased sympathetic tone in the superior palpebral muscle.

A second ocular change is *exophthalmos*, an abnormal protrusion of the eyes due to forward displacement of the eyeball (proptosis). The protrusion is caused by increased deposition of fat behind the globe of the eye and between the bundles of the extrinsic eye muscles. In severe cases edematous degeneration of the muscles and lymphocytic infiltration occur and contribute to the forward bulging. The conjunctiva may also be edematous (chemosis).

In severe cases an affected person may not be able to close the eyelids completely because of lid retraction and exophthalmos. Consequently the cornea may become dry and ulcerated.

A third ocular change is *ophthalmoplegia*, or weakness of the external eye muscles. This change occurs in advanced cases and is least common. It is probably caused by the edematous degeneration of the muscles just mentioned. It may cause diplopia or a squint.

Thyrotoxic Crisis

Thyrotoxic crisis, or *thyroid storm*, is an acute exacerbation of all thyrotoxic symptoms. It is potentially fatal and if untreated, death usually occurs within 36 to 48 hours. The exact cause of thyrotoxic crisis is not known, but presumably it is due to a massive release of thyroid hormones into the blood. It is usually precipitated by some stress such as infection, trauma, or surgery. Relative adrenocortical insufficiency may be a contributing factor. Thyrotoxic crisis sometimes occurs on the first day following thyroidectomy, presumably due to excessive release of thyroid hormones into the blood during the operative procedure.

Fever is always present. The skin is flushed and hot and the person perspires profusely. Restlessness, agitation, confusion, or delirium are common. Tachycardia, atrial fibrillation, and shock may occur. Vomiting, abdominal pain, and diarrhea may be the predominant manifestations of thyrotoxic crisis in some people.

SUGGESTED ADDITIONAL READING

Gillie BR: Endemic goiter. *Sci Am* **224** (6): 92–101, 1971.

Tunbridge WMG: Acromegaly. *Nurs Times* **75**(3): 110–112, 1979.

20
Neoplasia

Neoplasia literally means "new growth." It is a process of progressive uncontrolled proliferation of cells with no relation to the physiological needs of the organism. The mass of cells that makes up the abnormal new growth is called a *neoplasm*. The term *tumor*, strictly speaking, means a swelling. In general usage, however, the term has come to be used synonymously with neoplasm and is rarely used to denote swellings due to other causes. The study of tumors is called *oncology*. *Cancer* is a general term that refers to all types of malignant neoplasms.

Other disturbances of growth and differentiation that can occur are hypertrophy, hyperplasia, metaplasia, and dysplasia. These processes differ from neoplasia in that when the inciting stimulus is removed, the tissue reverts to normal; that is, the process is controlled. In the contrast, neoplasia represents an escape from the normal homeostatic controls of cell division.

CELL DIVISION AND DIFFERENTIATION

Growth occurs as a result of an increase in both the size and the number of cells. Some cells divide by mitosis at regular intervals to produce identical daughter cells. During interphase the daughter cells may increase in size until their volume has doubled, then they undergo mitosis. (Mitosis is

described in Chapter 3.) These events can be described by the cell cycle (see below).

In many tissues of the body the destinies of the daughter cells are not identical (e.g., epithelial tissues). Immature precursor cells, or *stem cells*, divide. One of the daughter cells is destined to form more stem cells and completes the cell cycle. The other daughter cell is destined to mature into a functionally and structurally specialized cell. This process of maturation is called *differentiation* and the specialized cell is said to be *differentiated*. Differentiated cells are often nondividing and may be considered as *end cells*. The factors regulating whether a cell will differentiate and how it will differentiate are not clearly understood.

Often tissues contain a group of cells that are intermediate between stem cells and end cells. These cells form a dividing transit population (Fig. 20-1). For example, in erythropoiesis cells that are descended from stem cells and that are committed to give rise to mature red blood cells (committed erythroid precursors) undergo cell division to amplify the number of cells during the differentiation from stem cells to mature erythrocytes. Cells

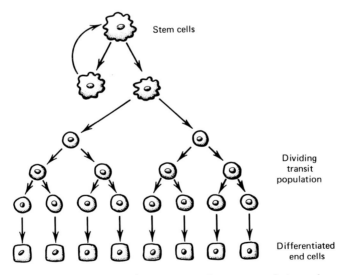

Figure 20-1. *Stem cells divide in order to maintain their own population and to provide cells that will differentiate into end cells. Cells intermediate between stem cells and end cells form a dividing transit population that is committed to differentiate into a particular type of end cell.*

are constantly being fed into the dividing transit population from the stem-cell pool and removed from it as mature end cells are formed.

Each human being is derived from a single cell, the zygote, which initially undergoes a series of divisions to form a ball of cells. During embryonic and fetal development many more cell divisions occur, and many cells differentiate to form the characteristic functional cells of the various organs. At birth or shortly after, some tissues (e.g., nervous tissue) contain most of the cells they need and further growth is achieved mainly by enlargement of existing cells. In other tissues (e.g., bone) growth is achieved by continued cell division and differentiation throughout childhood. In an adult some differentiated cells, such as liver cells, do not normally divide; but if a large part of the liver is destroyed or removed, the remaining cells will undergo cell division to replace lost tissue (see Chapter 8 under Healing of Liver). Some highly differentiated end cells are no longer capable of dividing. Some cells in this category (e.g., neurons) have long lives, and when they die they are not replaced. Other cells in this category (e.g., erythrocytes, some epithelial cells) have short lives. Throughout life as these cells die or are shed from the body they are replaced by cells from the dividing transit population.

The Cell Cycle

Dividing cells proceed through a characteristic cycle (Fig. 20-2). Before cell division can occur, the genetic information must be duplicated. Synthesis of chromosomal DNA occurs during a specific period of interphase called the S phase. The period between the previous cell division and the beginning of S phase is called G_1 (the first gap). During the last part of the G_1 phase, just before the cell enters the S phase, specific substances and enzymes that are required for DNA replication are produced. The period following the S phase is called G_2 (the second gap). During this time the cell produces some of the proteins required for mitosis. The cell then enters the M, or mitotic, phase of the cell cycle and divides.

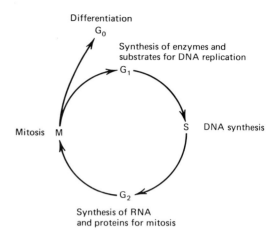

Figure 20-2. *The cell cycle.*

The length of time spent in each period of the cell cycle varies according to the cell type and environmental conditions (e.g., adequacy of nutrition; hormonal factors). Some cells may complete the cell cycle in 8 to 10 hours, whereas others may take several days. As mentioned earlier some differentiated cells, such as liver cells, do not normally divide but are capable of undergoing cell division in response to certain stimuli. Such nondividing differentiated cells are arrested at some stage of the cell cycle, most commonly in the G_1 phase. The prolonged nondividing state of differentiated cells is usually considered as a special alternative to G_1, which is called the G_0 phase. The addition of an appropriate stimulatory substance or the removal of tissue-specific inhibitory substances called chalones cause the cells to return to G_1 and continue through the cell cycle. The exact nature of the stimulatory and inhibitory substances is not known. Potential arrest points also occur in other phases of the cell cycle.

Nonneoplastic Disturbances of Growth and Differentiation

Hypertrophy

Hypertrophy is an enlargement of an organ or part due to an increase in the size of its constituent cells. The number of cells does not increase. Hypertrophy occurs mainly in muscles in response to an increased work load. In some cases hypertrophy occurs in response to a normal physiological stimulus. For example, the uterus hypertrophies during pregnancy. In other cases hypertrophy is an adaptive response to a pathological situation. For example, the wall of a duct or hollow organ hypertrophies when outflow of the luminal contents is obstructed (see Chapter 21).

Hyperplasia

Hyperplasia is an increase in the number of normal cells in a normal arrangement in a tissue or organ. It usually causes enlargement of the part and is accompanied by increased functional activity. Hyperplasia may be physiological, for example, the increase in glandular epithelium of the breast during pregnancy and lactation. In some cases hyperplasia is compensatory. For example, after removal or destruction of one kidney, the other kidney enlarges. The number of nephrons does not increase, but the size of each nephron increases due to an increase in the number of tubular epithelial cells, possibly accompanied by hypertrophy of the cells. In addition the glomerular capillaries may enlarge as a result of proliferation of endothelial cells. In some cases hyperplasia is pathological, for example, thyroid hyperplasia producing hyperthyroidism (see Chapter 19). Pathological hyperplasia is sometimes induced by excessive hormonal stimulation. For example, excessive amounts of estrogen (e.g., due to an ovarian tumor) cause abnormal endometrial hyperplasia. Pathological hyperplasia occasionally transforms to neoplasia.

Metaplasia

Metaplasia is the replacement of one type of fully differentiated cells by another type of fully differentiated cells in a part of the body where the second cell type does not normally occur. That is, the stem cells differentiate into end cells that are not normally found in that area of the body. (Epithelial stem cells always differentiate into some type of epithelium, however, and connective tissue

precursors into some type of connective tissue. Epithelial stem cells do not differentiate into connective tissue.) An example of metaplasia is the replacement of mucus-secreting columnar epithelium by stratified squamous epithelium in response to irritation or inflammation, as in the gallbladder when gallstones are present. In this case metaplasia may be considered an adaptive response to stress; a delicate tissue is replaced by tissue that is more capable of meeting the demands of the situation. Replacement of columnar epithelium by keratinizing stratified squamous epithelium occurs in vitamin A deficiency. This situation is also metaplasia.

Dysplasia

Dysplasia is an alteration in the size, shape, and organization of differentiated cells. It occurs most often in epithelial tissue and is associated with chronic irritation or inflammation. The cells lose their regularity and show variable sizes and shapes (pleomorphism). In addition, the cells lose their usual architectural orientation. For example, in a normal stratified squamous epithelium mitosis occurs only in the cells of the basal layer and there is progressive maturation of cells from the basal layer to the surface. In a dysplastic stratified squamous epithelium mitosis may occur in cells at any level and there may be a disordered mixture of cells of varying stages of differentiation at each level. Dysplasia may occur, for example, in the respiratory passages of people who smoke cigarettes and the cervix of women with chronic cervicitis. The dysplastic tissue usually reverts to normal when the inciting stimulus is removed, but in some cases neoplastic transformation occurs.

CLASSIFICATION AND CHARACTERISTICS OF NEOPLASMS

On the basis of behavior, neoplasms are classified as benign or malignant. *Benign neoplasms* remain localized and are usually relatively innocent, although they can sometimes have serious effects (see below). *Malignant neoplasms* invade and destroy surrounding tissues, can spread to distant sites in the body, and can cause death. Within these two main categories, tumors are classified according to the tissue type from which the tumor arises; that is, according to their *histogenesis*. In addition, neoplasms may be classified histologically as well, moderately, or poorly differentiated according to the degree of maturation of the tumor cells. When the tumor cells are completely undifferentiated and bear no resemblance to the cells of the tissue of origin, the neoplasm is said to be *anaplastic*. The cells of an anaplastic tumor vary in size and shape and have large nuclei.

Tumors are made up of two parts: the neoplastic cells proper (parenchyma) and a stroma derived from normal tissues. The stroma is the supporting connective tissue and vasculature.

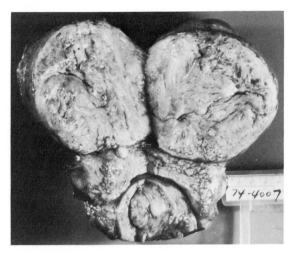

Figure 20-3. *A uterine fibroid (leiomyoma). (Courtesy of Dr. J. Burton, Vancouver General Hospital, Vancouver, B.C., Canada.)*

Benign Neoplasms

Nomenclature

Benign tumors are usually named according to the tissue of origin, followed by the suffix *-oma*. In some cases, however, the name may be derived from the appearance of the neoplasm.

A benign tumor arising from fibrous tissue is called a *fibroma;* one arising from adipose tissue is called a *lipoma*. Fibromas are uncommon. Lipomas are relatively common and usually arise during middle age as soft, movable, spherical masses underneath the skin. A *chondroma* arises from cartilage and an *osteoma* from bone. A benign neoplasm of the meninges is a *meningioma*.

A benign tumor formed of blood vessels is called an *hemangioma*. Hemangiomas may be present at birth and are sometimes referred to as strawberry marks or birthmarks. In some cases they form dark red patches and are referred to as port-wine stains. A *lymphangioma* is a benign tumor of lymph vessels.

Rhabdomyomas are benign tumors of skeletal muscle; they are rare. Tumors of smooth muscle,

which are called *leiomyomas,* are much more common. They often occur in the uterus, where they are commonly referred to as *fibroids* (Fig. 20-3).

Benign tumors arising from glandular epithelium are called *adenomas*. Some adenomas may secrete fluid that cannot escape, but collects inside the tumor, forming a cyst. Such tumors are called *cystadenomas*. Benign tumors that arise from surface epithelium and have fingerlike projections are called *papillomas*.

Benign skin tumors that produce melanin pigment are called *nevi* (singular: *nevus*). They are commonly known as moles. Nevi are usually congenital but may not be apparent at birth. They tend to grow slowly and often become stationary or regress after reaching a certain size. Occasionally nevi transform into malignant melanomas.

Structure and Growth

Benign tumors are usually well differentiated, and the tumor cells closely resemble the cells of origin. They usually grow very slowly and enlarge by *expansion*. That is, they grow from the center and push adjacent tissues aside. As benign tumors grow and compress the surrounding tissue, most develop a fibrous capsule. Therefore they are usually sharply demarcated from the normal host tissue. The capsule is probably derived partly from the tumor stroma and partly from the surrounding tissues. Pressure on the tissues causes necrosis and subsequently they undergo fibrosis.

When a benign tumor arises near or out of a surface epithelium a projecting mass of tissue, or *polyp,* tends to be produced. The polyp may be broad-based (*sessile*) or hanging on a stalk (*pedunculated*). Adenomatous polyps have a smooth surface; polyps formed by papillomas have an irregular surface. When a benign tumor arises out of a deep tissue, the pressure of the surrounding tissue causes it to take on a spherical or ovoid form. It may be solid or cystic.

Malignant Neoplasms

Nomenclature

Malignant tumors arising from mesenchyme and its derivatives are called *sarcomas.* Mesenchyme is the meshwork of embryonic connective tissue in the mesoderm. It gives rise to connective tissues, blood vessels, and lymph vessels in the body. Sarcomas are further designated according to their histogenesis. Thus a malignant neoplasm of fibrous connective tissue is a *fibrosarcoma* and one of adipose tissue a *liposarcoma.* A *chondrosarcoma* is a tumor of cartilage and an *osteosarcoma* (or osteogenic sarcoma), a tumor of bone. A malignant neoplasm of blood vessels is an *angiosarcoma.* Malignant tumors of muscles are also called sarcomas. Muscles are not derived from mesenchyme but are derived from mesoderm, as is the mesenchyme. Smooth muscle tumors are *leiomyosarcomas* and skeletal muscle tumors are *rhabdomyosarcomas.*

Malignant neoplasms of hematopoietic tissue that cause proliferation of leukocytes and/or their precursors are known as *leukemias.* Hematopoietic tissue includes myeloid tissue (red bone marrow), which produces granular leukocytes (neutrophils, eosinophils, and basophils) as well as red blood

cells and platelets; and lymphoid tissue, which produces nongranular leukocytes (lymphocytes and monocytes). When the abnormal proliferation of cells involves granular leukocytes (usually neutrophils) and their precursors, the condition is called *granulocytic, myelocytic,* or *myelogenous leukemia.* When the cancer arises in lymphoid tissue and involves lymphocytes and their precursors, with resultant flooding of the circulation with neoplastic cells, the condition is called *lymphocytic, lymphatic,* or *lymphogenous leukemia.* When immature precursors of lymphocytes predominate the condition is called *lymphoblastic leukemia.* Leukemias are also classified as acute or chronic, depending on the clinical course. When the neoplasm remains localized in the lymph tissue to give rise to solid tumor mass without involving the peripheral blood, it is called a *lymphoma,* or *lymphosarcoma.*

Malignant neoplasms arising from epithelial tissue are called *carcinomas.* Tumors arising from glandular epithelium or growing in a glandlike pattern are called *adenocarcinomas.* Neoplasms arising from stratified squamous epithelium are called *squamous cell,* or *epidermoid, carcinomas.* *Basal cell carcinoma* is a form of skin cancer that arises from the basal layer of the epidermis or hair sheath. *Malignant melanomas* are pigmented neoplasms derived from the melanocytes of the basal layer of the epidermis. Cancer arising from the epithelium lining the respiratory tract is *bronchogenic carcinoma.* Malignant tumors involving liver cells are referred to as *hepatic cell carcinomas* or simply *hepatomas.* *Transitional cell carcinoma* arises from transitional epithelium lining the urinary tract (renal pelves, ureters, bladder, and urethra). Malignant neoplasms of renal tubular epithelium are called *renal cell carcinomas.*

Malignant neoplasms arising in the nervous system include gliomas, which are derived from neuroglia in the CNS, and *neuroblastomas,* which are derived from embryonic precursors of nerve cells. Neuroblastomas usually affect children before the age of 10 years and most arise in the adrenal medulla or sympathetic chain (*sympatheticoblas-*

toma). Those developing in the retina are called *retinoblastomas.*

Most tumors are composed of one type of cells, but some are composed of more than one cell type. When the cells represent tissues derived from a single germ layer, the neoplasm is referred to as *mixed.* An example is *Wilm's tumor,* a kidney tumor made up of embryonal elements. It usually affects children before the age of 5 years. A *teratoma* is a neoplasm made up of several tissues representing derivatives of more than one embryonic germ layer. Teratomas arise from totipotential cells (i.e., cells that can give rise to any cell type) and may be benign or malignant. They usually develop in the ovary or testis but occasionally arise in other sites.

Structure and Growth

Malignant neoplasms show variable degrees of differentiation, but in general all show some degree of anaplasia. They usually grow rapidly and progressively, but the rate of growth may be erratic. It is often assumed that division of neoplastic cells occurs at a faster rate than in normal cells, but this assumption is not true in all cases. Cell division occurs more rapidly in normal hematopoietic tissue and gastrointestinal epithelium than it does in some tumors. The rate of increase in the size of a tumor depends not only on the rate of cell division but also on the fraction of tumor cells that are actively dividing and the number of cells lost from the tumor. In some tumors, especially the more differentiated ones, cell division may occur in only one fraction (the growth fraction), which corresponds to dividing transit-cell populations in normal tissues. The nongrowing fraction consists of two groups: one cell population incapable of further division and another cell population composed of cells in G_0 that can reenter cell division and give rise to a new growth fraction. Cells may be lost from a tumor as a result of necrosis due to inadequate nutrition, destruction by host defenses, or being shed from the tumor mass.

Cancers grow by *infiltration.* That is, they grow from the periphery, so that strands of cells invade and destroy the surrounding tissue. They are not encapsulated. Consequently malignant tumors usually have an irregular shape and their borders are not sharply defined. Rapidly developing malignant tumors also grow by expansion and may appear encapsulated because of compression of the surrounding tissues. The surrounding tissues are always infiltrated with strands of neoplastic cells, however.

The vasculature of the tumor stroma is derived by growth of new blood vessels from preexisting blood vessels of the host (angiogenesis). The neoplastic cells apparently secrete a substance called *tumor angiogenesis factor* that acts on capillary endothelium to induce the growth of blood vessels into the tumor. A neoplasm cannot grow more than 2 to 3 mm in diameter without angiogenesis. Rapidly developing tumors may outgrow their blood supply, with resultant necrosis and hemorrhage at the center of the tumor.

The amount and nature of the stroma varies from one tumor to another. Some tumors, particularly rapidly growing sarcomas, have very little fibrous connective tissue in their stroma but are highly vascular. Such tumors are soft and fleshy. (Sarcoma literally means "fleshy tumor.") Other tumors stimulate the formation of excessive amounts of fibrous connective tissue in the stroma. Such neoplasms are hard and are referred to as *scirrhous.*

Carcinomas may appear as nodular or papillary outgrowths of tissue from a surface, or as fissures or ulcers. In some cases they may be cystic structures forming masses beneath the surface. Some carcinomas that are highly infiltrative may cause diffuse hard masses in the tissues. Fibrosis may accompany diffuse carcinomas of the alimentary tract, producing strictures. When a neoplasm is still contained within the epithelium of origin and has not invaded the basement membrane, the lesion is referred to as *carcinoma in situ,* or preinvasive cancer. Most of these lesions, which can occur in the uterine cervix, epidermis, lung, prostate, and breast, eventually progress to invasive carcinoma.

Sarcomas tend to be larger than carcinomas. They are generally more invasive than carcinomas and form diffuse sheets in which the neoplastic cells merge closely with the surrounding tissues. Fibrosarcomas may elaborate collagen, osteosarcomas may produce bone, and chondrosarcomas may form cartilaginous matrix.

Spread

Malignant neoplasms are characterized by their ability to spread, not only locally, but to distant sites in the body. This feature distinguishes malignant neoplasms from benign tumors. Local spread, or *invasion,* occurs by direct infiltration of surrounding tissues. Invasion by neoplastic cells tends to occur along the lines of least resistance, such as tissue planes.

The ability of malignant neoplasms to spread from a primary site and set up secondary foci of disease at distant sites throughout the body is called *metastasis.* The secondary foci of neoplastic growth are referred to as *metastases* (singular: metastasis). The degree to which different cancers metastasize varies widely. Some tumors, such as basal cell carcinomas and gliomas, invade local tissues extensively but rarely metastasize. At the other end of the scale are neoplasms such as melanomas and lung carcinomas, which metastasize widely but may not be very invasive at the primary site. Dissemination from the primary site may occur by way of lymph channels, through the bloodstream, or by implantation (Fig. 20-4).

Carcinomas have a predilection for spreading *through the lymph system.* After invading the lymphatic vessels, clumps of neoplastic cells may detach and become emboli. The emboli are carried to the nearest lymph nodes and become lodged there, forming a metastatic growth. Eventually the entire lymph node becomes involved and the cancer may spread to the next group of lymph

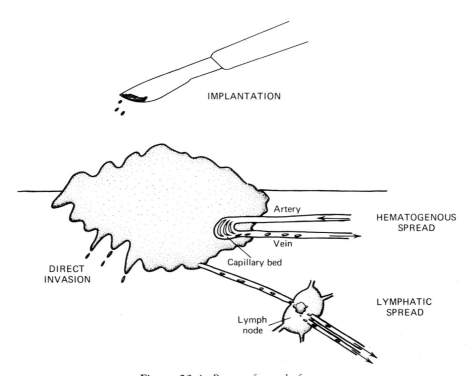

Figure 20-4. *Routes of spread of cancer.*

nodes. Alternatively, cancer cells may invade the lymph channels around the carcinoma and proliferate as a continuous growth within a lymph vessel. This type of spread is called lymphatic permeation. When lymph containing neoplastic cells enters the blood the cancer can be spread further.

Sarcomas tend to metastasize mainly *by way of the blood.* Carcinomas also spread through the blood, but usually at a later stage. Cancer cells may enter the blood by infiltrating small veins or capillaries or by way of the lymph, as already mentioned. The neoplastic cells are carried in the bloodstream either singly or in clumps held together by fibrin strands. Probably most of these cells do not survive. Clumps of cells (enboli) that lodge in small vessels at a distant site give rise to a secondary tumor only when the cancer cells infiltrate the blood vessel wall and enter the surrounding tissue.

The site of metastasis depends mainly on the venous drainage of the primary tumor. Carcinomas of the gastrointestinal tract usually first invade the tributaries of the hepatic portal vein and usually metastasize to the liver. Cancer of an organ that drains into the systemic veins (e.g., the kidney) tends to metastasize to the lungs because tumor emboli lodge in the pulmonary vascular bed. Clumps of neoplastic cells from a lung carcinoma may be carried in the blood to the brain and set up metastases there. Tumor emboli from cancers arising in the midline and in close proximity to the vertebral column (e.g., cancers of the prostate and thyroid) tend to be carried through the paravertebral system of veins and cause metastases in the vertebral column.

Spread by implantation, or transplantation, refers to the dissemination by mechanical means of clumps of cells detached from the surface of a neoplasm. This type of spread occurs in serous cavities. For example, carcinoma of the breast may invade the pleural cavity or carcinoma of the colon may invade the peritoneal cavity. Cancer cells that detach from the primary tumor are then conveyed mechanically by the serous fluid to other parts of the serous cavity, where they lodge and set

up metastases. Neoplastic cells may also be transported and implanted by surgical instruments or the surgeon's gloved hands to other sites in an operative wound.

Cancer cells possess certain properties that appear to be related to their ability to spread. Compared with normal cells, cancer cells show *decreased adhesiveness, increased motility,* and *loss of contact inhibition.* In addition, cancer cells may secrete toxins that injure normal cells or enzymes (e.g., hyaluronidase) that break down the ground substance in the tissue matrix, thus facilitating invasion.

The surface membranes of cancer cells are altered and the anchors by which normal cells are held together may fail to develop between cancer cells. In addition, the negative surface charge is increased on cancer cells, so that adjacent cells tend to repel each other. Calcium permits binding of cells by ionic bonding (see Chapter 16 under Calcium Imbalance), but tumors contain less calcium than normal tissues and cancer cells may not bind calcium. All these factors contribute to make cancer cells less cohesive than normal cells. As a result of this decreased adhesiveness, cancer cells may be shed from the surface of a tumor or into secretions. (This fact forms the basis of the Papanicolaou smear test and the examination of various secretions for the detection of cancer.)

Migration of cells occurs during embryonic development, and presumably all cells contain the genetic information that permits mobilization. With the exception of cells such as leukocytes and macrophages, however, expression of this characteristic is limited in postembryonic cells. (Cell migration does occur in wound healing, however. See Chapter 8 under Healing of Surface Wounds.) Regulation of expression of this characteristic is lost in cancer cells, and they migrate with little restraint.

Contact inhibition refers to the cessation of cell division and migration by normal cells when they make contact with other cells. For example, during healing of a surface wound epithelial cells at the margin of the wound undergo cell division and migrate across the surface of the wound. When the surface of the wound is covered, however, cell division and mobility cease. It is hypothesized that further cell proliferation is inhibited by the interchange of signals (e.g., electrical currents) or substances at cell contact points. Cancer cells do not exhibit contact inhibition, and this characteristic is considered important in the invasiveness of malignant tumors.

Grading and Staging of Cancer

Grading of cancer is an attempt to estimate the degree of malignancy of a neoplasm based on histological criteria. Usually the degree of differentiation of the tumor cells and the estimated rate of growth of the tumor are considered. The degree of differentiation is estimated from the resemblance of the tumor to the normal tissue of origin. For example, a squamous cell carcinoma that forms considerable keratin and intercellular bridges is considered well differentiated. The estimate of growth rate is based on the number of mitoses per unit of tissue. A rapidly growing tumor has more mitotic figures than a slowly growing tumor.

Cancers are usually classified into three or four grades designated by Roman numerals. The higher numbers indicate a greater degree of anaplasia (i.e., undifferentiation) and a greater degree of malignancy. The criteria for each grade varies for different types of cancer. Along with other considerations, grading is a useful prognostic indicator and is sometimes useful for determining the type of therapy, but it is more valid when applied to groups of cases than for predicting the behavior of individual cases. Generally the higher the grade the poorer the prognosis, but the greater the radiosensitivity of the tumor.

Staging is an evaluation of the extent of a cancer based on clinical findings. For most malignant neoplasms the choice of treatment (i.e., surgery, radiotherapy, chemotherapy, or combined therapy) is based on this evaluation. According to the TNM system devised by the International Union Against Cancer, the stage is based on the extent (i.e., size) of the tumor (T); the presence and extent of regional lymph node involvement (N); and the presence or absence of distant metastases (M). Cancer in situ is designated Tis and T1, T2, T3, and T4 indicate increasing size of the tumor. No involvement of lymph nodes is represented by N0; increasing degrees of involvement are designated N1, N2, and N3. Absence of metastases is indicated by M0; M1 indicates their presence.

TUMOR-HOST INTERACTIONS

Effects of Benign Neoplasms on the Host

Although benign tumors are generally regarded as innocent, they can produce serious effects in some cases. By virtue of their *position*, benign tumors may impair the functioning of vital organs. For example, when they impinge on the lumen of a duct or hollow organ such as the trachea, intestinal tract, or ureter, benign neoplasms can cause obstruction, with serious consequences (see Chapter 21). Tumors such as meningiomas, growing within the confined space of the skull, damage normal brain tissue by compression and eventually cause death if they are not removed.

Benign tumors can have significant systemic effects by *secreting hormones*. Adenomas often secrete the hormone(s) normally produced by the tissue of origin but do not respond to the normal feedback control of hormone secretion. Consequently these benign tumors are often responsible for hormone excess (see Chapter 19).

Development of *complications* may produce clinical effects. For example, benign tumors may compress blood vessels or nerves and thus impair functioning of an organ. A benign tumor may cause pressure on overlying epithelium and erode through the surface, producing an ulcer. The ulcer may become infected or hemorrhage may occur if a blood vessel is ruptured.

Effects of Malignant Neoplasms on the Host

Malignant tumors can have all the effects of benign neoplasms, but the effects are accentuated. As with benign tumors, cancers can cause obstruction of ducts and hollow organs. In addition they can impair organ function by compression and destruction of normal tissue (Fig. 20-5). As with benign tumors, ulceration, infection, or hemorrhage can occur. In addition, cancer can produce a variety of systemic effects, not all of which are specific for cancer. The mechanisms producing some of these effects are poorly understood.

Hormone Production

A well-differentiated adenocarcinoma may secrete the hormone normally secreted by the gland in which the tumor arises and may produce hormonal excess. Very anaplastic tumors, however, are usually nonfunctional and may cause hormone

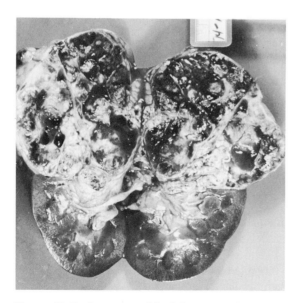

Figure 20-5. *Carcinoma of the kidney. Note destruction of normal tissue by the neoplasm in the upper portion of the kidney. (Courtesy of Dr. J. Burton, Vancouver General Hospital, Vancouver, B.C., Canada.)*

deficiency due to destruction of the normal endocrine tissue.

In addition to hormone secretion by tumors arising in endocrine glands, some undifferentiated malignant neoplasms arising in nonendocrine tissues secrete hormones or hormonelike substances. This ectopic hormone secretion can be the cause of hormone excess (see Chapter 19). For example, some carcinomas of the lung secrete adrenocorticotropic hormone (ACTH) and produce Cushing's syndrome. Presumably the undifferentiated tumor cells are expressing genes that are normally repressed.

Hematological Effects

Anemia often accompanies cancer. Known contributing factors in some cases are blood loss; neoplastic infiltration of the bone marrow; or deficiencies of iron, vitamin B_{12}, and/or folic acid. The nutritional deficiencies may be due to malabsorption or may be due to lack of intake as a result of anorexia. In some cases anemia is a side effect of treatment; both chemotherapy and radiotherapy can affect bone-marrow function. In some cases no specific factor can be found to account for the anemia and it is assumed to be due to suppression of bone marrow function by an unknown mechanism.

Disorders of coagulation often occur with cancer. Many of the factors that cause anemia can also lower the platelet count, producing a hemorrhagic tendency in some people with malignant neoplasms. Disseminated intravascular coagulation may also accompany cancer (see Chapter 7 under Deficient Clotting Factors). Some cancers, particularly those of the pancreas and stomach, are associated with increased coagulability of the blood, resulting in multiple venous thromboses.

The leukocyte count is variable. In addition to the elevated white blood cell count that occurs in leukemia, leukocytosis may occur as a result of intercurrent infection. In other cases the leukocyte count is low due to depression of bone marrow function, with the result that resistance to infection is decreased.

Changes in the concentrations of plasma proteins and protein-bound carbohydrates may also occur. Serum glycoprotein levels increase. In addition, abnormal tumor-associated proteins may appear in the blood.

Hypercalcemia may accompany cancer (see Chapter 16). In some cases it may be related to immobilization (see Chapter 22). In most cases it results from bone destruction by the neoplasm. Occasionally it may be due to ectopic secretion of parathyroid hormone by the tumor.

Dermatological Effects

A variety of skin changes may accompany cancer, although they are not specific to cancer. The mechanisms producing these changes are not understood. People with various types of malignant neoplasms may develop dermatomyositis. This condition is a nonsuppurative inflammation of the skin, subcutaneous tissue, and muscles. Erythema (redness) and pruritus (itching) are two other nonspecific skin manifestations of cancer. Acanthosis nigricans (diffuse hyperplasia and thickening of the prickle-cell layer of the epidermis with gray to black pigmentation) may accompany carcinoma, particularly of the stomach. Herpes zoster also occurs with cancer in some cases.

Musculoskeletal Effects

As already mentioned, dermatomyositis may accompany cancer, but in some cases myositis occurs alone. This condition is an inflammatory reaction in muscle, which produces muscle necrosis. It is manifested by muscle weakness and elevated plasma levels of lactic dehydrogenase and creatine kinase (two enzymes from muscle cells).

Osteoporosis can occur with cancer, but the skeletal effects of malignant neoplasms are mainly related to bone destruction due to metastases. The affected bone may fracture.

Clubbing of the fingers (pulmonary osteoarthropathy) accompanies some cancers, particularly those of the lung. This condition is not specific for cancer but also occurs with some chronic lung disorders (see Chapter 21 under Mucoviscidosis). The mechanism responsible for the clubbing is not known.

Neurological Effects

Degenerative changes in the CNS may occur without metastases to the CNS. The reasons for these changes are not known. Various tracts are affected by progressive demyelination. Cerebellar degeneration may occur, manifested by ataxia, instability of gait, and difficulty speaking. In other cases the clinical picture may be that of peripheral neuritis, with sensory and motor disturbances.

Pain

The early stages of cancer are usually painless, but with advanced cancer pain is common. Tumors do not contain nerves, but pain is produced indirectly, usually as a result of pressure or tension on nerves in surrounding tissues. For example, when bone is involved pain is caused by stretching of the periosteum. When a neoplasm causes ulceration pain may result from irritation of the exposed tissue. Necrotic tissues liberate chemicals that stimulate nerve endings and produce pain. In other cases pain may be secondary to obstruction of a duct or hollow organ (see Chapter 21).

Cachexia

Cachexia is a vague term encompassing the progressive weakness, weight loss, emaciation, and malnutrition that commonly occurs with advanced cancer. Untimately it leads to death. The direct causes are obscure. Hemorrhage, infection, and necrosis of tissues with release of toxins may contribute.

Anorexia often accompanies cancer and is probably significant in producing the malnutrition and wasting. Anorexia is a side effect of most cancer therapies. In addition, however, the disease itself induces anorexia by an undnown mechanism. Altered taste sensations may be at least partly responsible.

Malignant tumors are said to act as "nitrogen traps" because their cells concentrate large amounts of the amino acids alanine, methionine, histidine, and isoleucine in competition with the liver and other normal body tissues. Eventually negative nitrogen balance occurs and normal tissues are catabolized, contributing to the cachexia.

Complications

Infection, hemorrhage, and obstruction are frequent complications associated with malignant neoplasms and are common causes of death. For example, with pelvic cancers death may be caused by urinary tract obstruction and anuria. Fulminating hemorrhage occurs particularly with cancers of the esophagus, upper digestive tract, upper airways, or bronchi.

Intercurrent infection is a common complication of cancer. Often the infection is localized, but fatal septicemia can develop. Infection is particularly common with cancer of the lungs, gastrointestinal tract, or hematopoietic system. When cancer is present the defense barriers of the respiratory mucosa or gastrointestinal epithelium are breached, providing portals of entry for infectious agents (see Chapter 28). Skin lesions and intravenous sites are other common portals of entry. With leukemia, the white blood cell count is elevated but the neoplastic cells are not functionally competent, so that affected people are susceptible to infection. In addition, chemotherapy and radiation therapy for cancer depress the immune system, causing increased susceptibility to infection. Gram-negative bacilli are frequently responsible for septicemia, but gram-positive cocci, fungi, or other infectious agents can also be the cause of overwhelming infection in people with cancer.

Effects of the Host on the Tumor

Neoplasms are affected by several host factors. Tumors derive their blood supply from the host, as previously mentioned. If an adequate blood supply is not established, tumor necrosis can occur.

Hormones secreted by the host influence some cancers. Since hormones affect growth and differ-

entiation, this effect is not surprising. Some breast cancers, for example, are dependent on estrogen and regress when sources of estrogen secretion are removed or androgens are administered. Prolactin may also influence breast cancer. Sex hormones also influence cancer of the prostate. Tumors in other tissues, including the kidney, bladder, liver, skin, and lymphatic tissue can be influenced by the hormonal environment.

In rare cases spontaneous regression and disappearance of a malignant tumor occurs, implying an active defense reaction by the host. Spontaneous cure has been observed mainly with neuroblastoma in children, bladder and renal cell carcinoma, and malignant melanoma. The nature of the host defense reaction is not well understood but it is believed to be an immunological response. The immune reaction appears to be primarily of the cellular type (see Chapter 29). The surfaces of cancer cells are altered, giving them new antigenic properties that provoke an immune response. The *immunological surveillance theory* proposes that neoplastic cells arise quite often but are destroyed by an immunological reaction before they can develop into a clinically detectable tumor. People with immunodeficiency diseases and those receiving immunosuppressive therapy after transplant operations have a high incidence of cancer.

CAUSES OF CANCER

In 85% to 90% of cases, the cause of human cancer is not known. In some cases, however, the development of cancer in a person can be linked to exposure to a particular environmental agent. Most epidemiologists are convinced that environmental agents play a major role in the causation of most cancers.

An environmental agent that can produce cancer is called a *carcinogen*. Many chemicals, ionizing radiation, ultraviolet radiation, and some viruses are known carcinogens. Although it is known that these agents can produce cancer, the basic mechanism underlying the development of cancer is not known.

Mechanisms of Carcinogenesis

All neoplasms, both benign and malignant, have the capacity for uncontrolled proliferation. In addition, malignant neoplasms have the capacity to invade and metastasize. Therefore, the changes that occur to transform normal cells into cancer cells not only permit uncontrolled growth but also permit active migration. The basic factor underlying the development of cancer is the loss or alteration of a normal control mechanism or mechanisms. The exact nature of normal control mechanisms controlling cell proliferation and the expression of genetic information are not clearly understood, however, and it is not known how these controls are altered in cancer cells. Whatever change or changes occur in cells to make them cancerous, the changes are transmitted to progeny cells (i.e., the changes are heritable).

Although any tissue in the body may become cancerous, cancer is most likely to develop in tissues made up of actively dividing cell populations. This fact is consistent with experimental observations that whether neoplastic transformation is induced by chemicals, radiation, or viruses, cell proliferation is required for carcinogenesis. It appears likely that cell division is required to firmly fix the cancerous state in the cells.

Although the basic mechanism responsible for carcinogenesis is not known, various theories have been proposed based on three mechanisms. It is quite conceivable that a single mechanism is not responsible for all cases of cancer; one mechanism may be operating in some cases and a different one in other cases.

Theories based on an *epigenetic mechanism* propose that all the genetic information required to produce the cancer phenotype is present in normal cells but is not expressed. (See Chapter 3 for a discussion of control of gene expression.) A change in the intracellular environment in which the DNA functions may allow expression of malignant neoplastic behavior. Earlier it was stated that the cancerous change is heritable. A heritable change need not require a change in the genetic information, however, as evidenced by the fact that liver cells give rise to liver cells and epithelial cells give rise to epithelial cells, yet both presumably contain the same genetic information. Somehow the "packaging" of the DNA in the chromosomes controls the expression of a specific part of the genetic information and this packaging can be maintained from one cell generation to another.

Another possible mechanism of carcinogenesis is a change in the genetic information of the cells as a result of chemical changes in the DNA. *Somatic mutation* theories are based on this mechanism. (Mutations are discussed in Chapter 3.) The nature of the genetic changes that are necessary to produce the cancer phenotype are not known. They could possibly involve alteration of enzymes necessary for differentiation of the cell or alteration of a regulator gene. Another possibility is that the mutant genes affect the structure of the cell membrane, resulting in functional changes.

The third mechanism involves *addition of new genetic information* to the cells as a result of viral infection (see Chapter 27). Just how the addition of the viral genome to the cell causes neoplastic transformation is not known. The viral nucleic acid possibly codes for specific proteins that are responsible for establishing and maintaining the neoplastic state. Alternatively, products of viral genes may activate normal host genes that are not usually expressed.

Carcinogens

Chemicals

Many chemicals are known to be carcinogenic. Several polycyclic aromatic hydrocarbons derived from coal tar can cause cancer. Some of them require metabolic conversion to more active compounds before exerting their carcinogenic effect. These compounds can bind to proteins and nucleic acids in the cells. Several azo dyes and aromatic amines also bind to proteins and nucleic acids and are carcinogenic. Alkylating agents, such as nitrosamines, react with both RNA and DNA and can produce cancer.

Aflatoxins are chemical carcinogens produced by a fungus, *Aspergillus flavus*. This fungus contaminates several vegetable products, particularly peanuts, cottonseed flour, soybeans, maize, wheat, and rice, especially during storage under warm, moist conditions. The refining process destroys the aflatoxins in peanuts.

Some carcinogens in small (subthreshold) amounts may not immediately give rise to a tumor but do cause some change in the cells. Subsequent exposure to another chemical that does not in itself produce cancer, stimulates active tumor growth. The carcinogenic agent is sometimes referred to as the *initiator* and the second substance as the *promoter,* or *cocarcinogen.*

Excesses of some hormones, especially estrogens, are associated with the development of some types of cancer. It is not known whether hormones act as initiators or promoters.

The exact mechanism of chemical carcinogenesis is not known. Binding of the chemicals to cellular proteins could alter proteins that are involved in the regulation of gene expression and produce cancer by an epigenetic mechanism. Binding to DNA could cause a somatic mutation.

Radiation

Both ultraviolet radiation and ionizing radiation can cause cancer (see Chapter 23). Both types of radiation cause damage to DNA as well as to other cellular components.

The fact that ionizing radiation can be carcinogenic and yet is used in the treatment of cancer may seem paradoxical, but it is not. Ionizing radiation has its greatest effect on actively dividing, undifferentiated cells (i.e., cells such as cancer cells). The effects depend on the dose, the degree of damage to the cells, and whether or not the cells can repair the damage. In some cases damage to cell components may be repaired. In other cases cellular damage may not be repaired, but the cell is still able to survive. In this case the damage may cause a somatic mutation. In still other cases, cells are damaged so severely that they die. The aim in radiation therapy is to kill the cancer cells but cause minimal damage to normal cells.

Viruses

Several viruses are known to cause certain types of cancer in various animals. These tumor-producing viruses are called *oncogenic viruses.* To date, no virus has been proven as a cause of human cancer, but circumstantial evidence points to a possible viral etiology for Burkitt's lymphoma, leukemia, and breast cancer. Two benign human neoplasms, the common wart and mucosal papilloma, do have a proven viral etiology.

SUGGESTED ADDITIONAL READING

Bingham CA: The cell cycle and cancer chemotherapy. *Am J Nurs* **78**(7): 1200–1205, 1978.

Croce CM, Koprowski H: The genetics of human cancer. *Sci Am* **238**(2): 117–125, 1978.

Nicolson GL: Cancer metastasis. *Sci Am* **240**(3): 66–76, 1979.

Old LJ: Cancer immunology. *Sci Am* **236**(5): 62–79, 1977.

Winters WD: Viruses and cancer. *Am J Nurs* **78**(2): 249–253, 1978.

UNIT FIVE

PHYSICAL STRESSORS

21
Foreign Bodies and Obstruction

A foreign body represents the intrusion of an un-wanted mass into a part of the body. Some foreign bodies may be fairly innocuous, but other foreign bodies can seriously impair the functioning of an organ and therefore disrupt homeostasis. Foreign bodies are a frequent cause of obstruction. Obstruction of a duct or hollow organ may lead to severe, life-threatening consequences if the obstruction is not removed.

FOREIGN BODIES

A *foreign body* is a mass or particle of material that is not normal to the place in which it is found.

Particulate matter that enters the body from outside is an *exogenous*, or *extrinsic*, foreign body. Nonliving particulate material formed within the body constitutes an *endogenous*, or *intrinsic*, foreign body.

Types of Foreign Bodies

Exogenous Foreign Bodies
Exogenous foreign bodies may be large objects such as coins, buttons, pins, or animal bones that are accidentally swallowed or aspirated. In addition to large objects, fine particulate material such as soot, asbestos, silica, or any other type of dust

may be inhaled into the lungs. Inhalation of oil may occur when cod liver oil or mineral oil is administered to infants or people with impaired swallowing or cough reflexes.

Any objects inserted into body orifices represent foreign bodies, whether they are urinary catheters or other drainage tubes inserted for therapeutic purposes, or small objects pushed into the ear canals or nares by young children.

Foreign bodies may also penetrate the skin and become embedded in the tissues. These exogenous foreign bodies may be penetrating objects such as bullets, glass splinters, or wooden slivers. In addition, fine particles such as sand may be driven into the skin during an injury. Another source of fine particulate material that may be implanted into tissues is talc used on surgical gloves.

Endogenous Foreign Bodies

Endogenous foreign bodies may be free fat or lipid substances released into adjacent tissue following injury or destruction of adipose tissue. Following injury to adipose tissue that is in close contact with large veins, droplets of fat may enter the blood (fat embolism). Fat embolism may result from the release of yellow marrow following extensive fractures.

Other products of the body may accumulate in body tissues. Examples are hairs in the walls of dermoid cysts and urate crystals in gout.

By far the most common endogenous foreign bodies are calculi (Fig. 21-1). A *calculus* (stone) is a solid mass formed by precipitation from a secretion and deposited in a hollow organ or excretory duct. Urinary, biliary, salivary, pancreatic, or prostatic calculi may occur. Primary, or metabolic, calculi occur as a result of an increase in the concentration of a substance in a secretion. Examples are calcium oxalate stones, uric acid stones, or cystine stones in urine. Cystine stones, which are rare, occur as a result of an inborn error of metabolism called cystinuria (see Chapter 6). Secondary, or concretion, calculi occur when a solid mass such as a foreign body, fibrin, sloughed epithelial cells, or clumps of microorganisms are present and

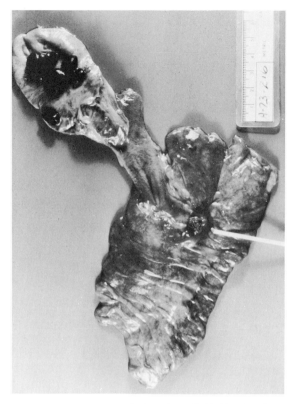

Figure 21-1. *Biliary calculi. The gall bladder has been opened, showing several stones. Also note bulge where a stone is lodged at the ampulla of Vater (arrow). (Courtesy of Dr. J. Burton, Vancouver General Hospital, Vancouver, B.C., Canada.)*

act as a nucleus, or nidus, around which substances from the secretion precipitate. For example, with bacterial inflammation of the gallbladder, bile pigments, cholesterol, and calcium salts may precipitate around a nidus of bacteria or epithelial cells. Another example is the precipitation of phosphates from alkaline urine around a nidus of inflammatory exudate, bacteria, or a primary calculus.

Not all the many factors that may influence stone formation are known. The solubility of a substance is influenced by pH, therefore fluctuations in the pH of a secretion may contribute. For example, an alkaline urine, which occurs with some types of urinary tract infections, favors the precipitation of calcium phosphate and stone formation. On the other hand, uric acid is relatively insoluble at a low pH and a persistently very acid urine contributes to the formation of uric acid stones. Stasis of a secretion is another factor in the development of calculi. When secretions are pooled substances of low solubility have time to settle out. In addition, stasis results in retention of desquamated epithelial cells, clumps of mucus, and other substances that can act as a nidus for the formation of a calculus.

The solubility of some substances in a secretion is influenced by the concentrations of other substances in the fluid. Therefore, alterations in the relative amounts of various substances can influence stone formation. For example, phospholipids (e.g., lecithin) and bile salts enhance the solubility of cholesterol in bile. When the concentrations of bile salts and phospholipids are decreased proportionate to the amount of cholesterol, gallstones may form.

Diet can influence the composition of secretions such as bile and urine; therefore diet can play a part in the development of calculi. Inherited metabolic factors also appear to contribute to the development of stones, but the exact genetic factors are not known. Racial and sexual differences have been noted in the types of calculi formed.

Effects of Foreign Bodies

The general response to a foreign body is to eliminate it from the body if possible. The specific response and effects depend partly on the nature of the foreign body and partly on the specific site.

Foreign Bodies
in the Gastrointestinal (GI) Tract

Small undigestible foreign bodies often pass through the GI tract without any difficulty and are eliminated in the feces, but larger foreign bodies may cause obstruction. An accidentally swallowed large foreign body, such as a denture, lodges in the pharynx or esophagus. Other swallowed objects, such as coins or spoons, may reach the stomach but often are too large to pass through the pylorus. They remain in the stomach and may cause obstruction.

Foreign Bodies
in the Respiratory Tract

Entry of a foreign body into the respiratory tract initiates a cough reflex in an attempt to expel the foreign substance. Inhalation of fine particulate material produces irritation which causes coughing and stimulates mucus production. Aspiration of larger foreign bodies or fluid substances immediately causes choking, gagging, coughing, respiratory distress, wheezing, and temporary loss of voice. Brief laryngospasm often occurs. The foreign body may be expelled by coughing, but frequently it causes obstruction.

Large inhaled objects may become impacted in the larynx or trachea, but often they enter the bronchial tree and become lodged either in a main bronchus or one of its branches. Since the right main bronchus is oriented more vertically and is wider than the left main bronchus, foreign bodies enter the right main bronchus more often than the left. The foreign body itself may cause only partial obstruction, but it incites an inflammatory reaction. Obstruction may then become complete as a result of mucosal swelling. Organic foreign bodies, such as peanuts, cause a much more severe inflammatory reaction than more inert foreign bodies, such as mineral objects.

Inhalation of oil may cause *lipid pneumonia*. An acute inflammatory reaction occurs and the oil droplets are ingested by macrophages. Often a secondary bacterial infection develops. The inflammation may lead to fibrosis.

Any pathological condition caused by inhalation and deposition of fine particulate material in the lungs is called *pneumoconiosis*. Specific types of pneumoconiosis are anthracosis, due to carbon; silicosis, due to silica; siderosilicosis, due to iron oxide and silica; asbestosis, due to asbestos (largely composed of magnesium silicate); bagassosis, due to crushed sugar cane fibers ("bagasse"; mainly cellulose but about 1% protein and 5% silica); and byssinosis, due to cotton dust. The most serious degrees of anthracosis occur in coal miners, but people living in industrial areas inhale some soot, which is carbon. Most cases of pneumoconiosis, however, result from occupational exposure to various types of dust.

Coarse particles are trapped in mucus in the larger bronchi. The trapped particles are swept upward by the cilia and subsequently coughed up. Fine particles that reach the terminal air passages are ingested by macrophages. Some of the macrophages are subsequently coughed up in the sputum, but others migrate through the alveolar walls and enter the lymphatics. The dust particles are then deposited in lymph nodes in the lungs and pleura, as well as the mediastinal and cervical lymph nodes.

Carbon particles incite very little reaction in the tissues, but silica and silicates incite active fibrosis with granuloma formation (see Chapter 8). Silica produces inflammation and fibrosis as a result of its chemical action as well as mechanical irritation. Silica very slowly dissolves in the tissue fluids and forms silicic acid, which is very irritating. Tissue necrosis and fibrosis result. Granulomas develop not only throughout the lungs, but also in the regional lymph nodes where silica particles have been deposited (Fig. 21-2). Gradually as silicosis progresses, the granulomas enlarge and coalesce. As a result, large areas of the lungs become solid and lose their distensibility, thus interfering with pulmonary function.

Foreign Bodies Embedded in Tissues

The effects of a foreign body embedded in the tissues depend on the size, digestibility, and chemical reactivity of the particle. In addition, the effects depend on whether or not the foreign body carries pathogenic microorganisms with it.

A large, undigestible foreign body is surrounded by cells that form a fibrous capsule around the foreign body and isolate it (i.e., "wall it off"). Relatively inert, sterile objects such as bullets, shrap-

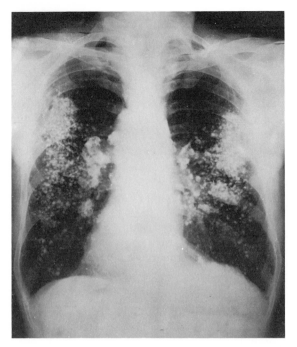

Figure 21-2. *Chest roentgenogram of a person with chronic silicosis. Granulomas and hilar lymph nodes have calcified. (Courtesy of Environmental Sciences Laboratory, Mount Sinai School of Medicine of the City University of New York, New York, New York. By permission.)*

nel, and surgically implanted metal plates or prostheses incite very little reaction and are surrounded by only a very thin fibrous capsule. Organic foreign bodies, such as pieces of clothing carried into penetrating wounds or splinters of wood, are not inert and cause a much more severe reaction. Even if an organic foreign body is sterile, extensive formation of fibrous tissue occurs if the foreign body is not removed. Unsterile objects will cause secondary infection, which may result in abscess formation. If the foreign body is embedded near the body surface (e.g., a wooden splinter) it may be pushed out along with the pus when the abscess ruptures.

Fine particulate matter, such as sand or talc, is treated in essentially the same way as a large foreign body. Inert substances are surrounded by a thin fibrous capsule. Talc or sand particles containing silica are not inert and incite granuloma formation.

Large or small digestible foreign bodies (e.g., catgut sutures) are surrounded by many large, multinucleated foreign-body giant cells formed by the fusion of macrophages. In addition, lymphocytes, plasma cells, and fibroblasts may be present. Enzymes from the phagocytic cells digest the foreign substance and it is absorbed. The phagocytic cells then disperse, leaving behind a small amount of fibrous tissue.

Very small particles are taken up by phagocytic cells and digested if possible. Indigestible particles may be carried to the lymph nodes.

Calculi

Small stones may pass through excretory ducts and be eliminated. Occasionally a stone may be passed with only slight discomfort, but usually the passage of a stone is accompanied by severe cramping pain (colic) due to spasmodic contractions of the smooth muscle in the walls of the duct. Passage of a renal calculus may be accompanied by waves of excruciating pain beginning in the lumbar region and radiating around the side to the groin. In males the pain may then pass to the scrotum or penis; in females, to the labia. With passage of a gallstone the pain is usually referred to the midepigastric region. It may radiate along the costal margins and through to the back. The pain usually increases in intensity in a crescendo fashion until it is quite severe and then may remain constant for hours.

Calculi may cause obstruction of a duct or hollow organ (see below). In addition, they may cause inflammation due to mechanical irritation. The irritation due to a stone in the urinary tract may cause hematuria (blood in the urine).

OBSTRUCTION

Obstruction of the lumen of a duct or hollow organ may result from: (1) external pressure or constriction (*extramural*); (2) a pathological change in the wall (*mural*); or (3) the presence of a mass within the lumen itself (*intraluminal*).

Examples of obstruction due to extramural causes are compression of the right middle-lobe bronchus by enlarged mediastinal lymph nodes and obstruction of the urethra by an enlarged prostate gland. Examples of mural causes of obstruction are tumors of the wall that project into the lumen of a duct or hollow organ, swelling of the mucosal lining of a duct, or strictures caused by contraction of scar tissue around a hollow organ or duct. Paralysis of the muscular wall (e.g., paralytic ileus) may prevent the normal luminal contents from being carried forward, causing accumulation of the normal contents and obstruction. Foreign bodies and plugs of mucus are common intraluminal causes of obstruction. Swelling of the mucosa due to inflammation frequently accompanies an intraluminal mass and contributes to the obstruction.

Obstruction of a Hollow Organ or Excretory Duct

Obstruction of a hollow organ or excretory duct produces several general effects. Strong muscular contractions occur in an attempt to push the luminal contents past the point of obstruction. The forceful contractions may cause severe cramping pain. As a result of the increased work the muscles of the wall hypertrophy. The normal fluid or semifluid contents of the lumen accumulate above the point of obstruction, causing increased intraluminal pressure and dilatation. The increased pressure and distension may also cause pain. Stagnant secretions in a blocked organ or duct provide a fertile medium for bacterial growth. Therefore infection is a frequent complication of obstruction. Inflammation of the wall may occur from infection or from mechanical irritation if the obstruction is caused by a mass in the lumen. Accumulated secretions in an excretory duct cause a backpressure in the secretory organ, impairing the function of glandular cells. If the pressure is not relieved the secretory cells atrophy. Eventually they may die and be replaced with fibrous scar tissue.

Biliary Obstruction

The most common causes of biliary obstruction are gallstones (biliary calculi; cholelithiasis), tumors of the gallbladder or bile ducts, and tumors of adjacent structures that compress the ducts.

Most gallstones form within the gallbladder; stones present in the ducts usually arise from that source. Stones remaining in the gallbladder rarely cause problems; if they enter the ducts, however, they may cause obstruction.

If a stone obstructs the cystic duct or the neck of the gallbladder, flow of bile into and out of the gallbladder is blocked. The blocked duct becomes swollen and may compress blood vessels, causing ischemia. Inflammation of the gallbladder (cholecystitis) occurs, initially from chemical irritation and later frequently from infection as bacteria invade and multiply in the stagnant contents of the gallbladder.

The obstruction is accompanied by pain. The initial pain is caused by spasmodic forceful contractions of the ducts and gallbladder and is usually referred to the midepigastric region. Later pain occurs in the right upper quadrant due to inflammation of the gallbladder and irritation of the parietal peritoneum. Often the pain of cholecystitis is referred to the right scapula or interscapular area. With acute cholecystitis, tenderness and muscle guarding over the area of the gallbladder may be present and fever and leukocytosis may occur. When the cystic duct is blocked bile can still flow directly into the duodenum from the liver via the hepatic ducts and common bile duct. Occasionally, however, the swollen cystic duct may compress the common bile duct and cause partial occlusion of the lumen.

Calculi entering the common bile duct often become lodged at the point where the common bile duct crosses the duodenal wall, just before the ampulla of Vater (see Fig. 21-1). The common bile duct crosses the duodenal wall obliquely to open into the duodenum. This portion of the duct is the narrowest and least distensible. Passage of stones and impaction of stones in the bile duct cause pain due to muscular contractions, as already mentioned. Nausea and vomiting often accompany the pain, presumably due to reflex stimulation of the vagus nerves.

As a result of obstruction of the common bile duct, bile will not be able to enter the duodenum. Consequently digestion and absorption of fat will be impaired, resulting in bulky loose stools. Deficiencies of fat-soluble vitamins due to impaired fat absorption can occur if the obstruction is prolonged. Deficiency of vitamin K leads to a bleeding tendency, which may be manifested by ecchymoses (see Chapter 7). The stools may be pale due to a lack of bile pigments and urobilinogen. Urobilinogen is formed by bacterial action on bile pigments in the intestine. Some urobilinogen is absorbed and subsequently excreted in the urine. With biliary obstruction, therefore, the amount of urobilinogen excreted in the urine will decrease.

Since the flow of bile into the intestine is blocked, bile accumulates in the bile ducts and gallbladder, causing distension of these structures. (If chronic cystitis is present, as it often is, the gallbladder may be contracted due to fibrous scar tissue and therefore does not become distended.) The liver may also be slightly enlarged. Impaired excretion of bile causes elevated levels of bile salts and bilirubin in the blood. The bile salts may cause pruritus (itching), while the elevated bilirubin level causes jaundice (obstructive jaundice). The plasma level of conjugated (direct) bilirubin is elevated because of the inability to excrete it in the bile. In addition, the level of unconjugated (indirect) bilirubin may be elevated because the backpressure impairs hepatic cell metabolism. (See Chapter 26 for a discussion of bilirubin metabolism.) If the obstruction is prolonged, damage to hepatic cells may occur. As a result, enzymes from the liver cells will leak into the blood. Therefore, serum alkaline phosphatase and serum glutamic-oxaloacetic transaminase (SGOT) levels may be elevated.

Gastrointestinal Obstruction

Many disorders can cause obstruction in the GI tract. In infants and young children the most common causes are congenital pyloric stenosis, intussusception, and swallowed foreign bodies. In older children and adults the usual causes are hernias, adhesions, tumors, and volvulus.

In *congenital pyloric stenosis,* the pylorus is narrowed by hypertrophy and spasm of the muscular coat. The condition is more common in males than females, and usually becomes manifest when the infant is 2 to 3 weeks old, although obstruction may occur at any time between 10 days and 4 months of age.

Intussusception is the telescoping of one portion of the intestine into the lumen of the immediately distal segment (Fig. 21-3). Intussusception is most common in infants and occurs more often in males than females. In infants the condition usually occurs in an otherwise healthy bowel, unassociated with any structural lesion. When intussusception occurs in older children or adults, usually some intraluminal mass or lesion is present, which acts as a point of traction. The telescoped segment is carried further into the distal segment by peristalsis

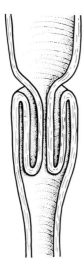

Figure 21-3. *Intussusception. One portion of the intestine telescopes into the immediately distal segment.*

and its mesentery is pulled along with it. As a result, the mesenteric blood vessels are compressed and infarction of the telescoped segment of bowel may occur.

A *hernia* is the protrusion of a pouch of peritoneum through a weakness or defect in the peritoneal wall. Loops of bowel, omentum, or other viscera may become trapped in the pouch. Common sites for hernias are the inguinal canal, the femoral canal, the umbilicus, and weak surgical scars. Intestinal obstruction occurs when a loop of bowel is constricted by the neck of the hernial sac. The constriction impairs venous outflow from the loop of bowel, causing swelling. A vicious cycle may then be established because the swelling causes greater constriction, which in turn causes further vascular obstruction. If the hernia is not quickly reduced, infarction of the trapped loop of bowel may occur (*strangulated hernia*).

Adhesions are bands of fibrous tissue that may develop after inflammation of the peritoneum (peritonitis) or after abdominal surgery. The adhesions extend from one organ to another organ or from an organ to the peritoneal wall and can form closed loops. A bowel segment may become trapped in one of these loops, with resulting partial or complete intestinal obstruction. Infarction of the trapped bowel segment may occur, just as occurs in a strangulated hernia.

Volvulus is the complete twisting of a loop of intestine, with resultant obstruction.

Intestinal obstruction usually causes intermittent abdominal pain. As already mentioned, the pain is caused by forceful peristaltic contractions and by distension. Quite severe pain lasting a few minutes is followed by a brief absence of pain and then the pain recurs. If infarction occurs, the pain may become constant. With paralytic ileus the pain is usually constant and is caused by distension only, not by muscular contractions.

Intestinal obstruction causes vomiting. With congenital pyloric stenosis, projectile vomiting following a feeding is characteristic. Vomiting is more frequent and occurs earlier when the obstruction is high in the small bowel than when it is in the distal portions of the intestine. The vomiting is presumed to be a reflex response to distension of the intestine. When the obstruction is high in the bowel, vomiting may temporarily relieve the distension and decrease the severity of the pain. The vomiting results in fluid loss and electrolyte disturbances.

Constipation or diarrhea may occur with intestinal obstruction. Usually constipation occurs, but diarrhea is common with a partial obstruction of the large bowel. The liquid stools flow past the site of partial obstruction.

With prolonged obstruction abdominal distension may be quite severe. The upward pressure on the diaphragm may cause difficulty in breathing.

The increased pressure in the lumen of the obstructed bowel interferes with movement of sodium and water from the intestinal lumen into the blood. In addition, venous drainage is impaired because of the increased intraluminal pressure. The impaired venous drainage causes edema of the intestinal wall, and some of the fluid may exude into the peritoneal cavity and into the intestinal lumen. As a result of this fluid loss, together with the fluid loss due to vomiting, hypovolemic shock may occur (see Chapter 14).

Fever and tachycardia may occur if a loop of bowel becomes strangulated. With strangulation, fluid containing blood, bacteria, and bacterial toxins leaks into the peritoneal cavity. Absorption of these substances can lead to septic shock (see Chapter 14).

Urinary Obstruction

Many conditions can obstruct the flow of urine and the obstruction can occur at any level of the urinary tract. Usually obstruction is partial, but sometimes it is complete. Obstruction in the renal pelvis or at the junction of the pelvis and ureter is commonly caused by a calculus, a tumor, or tuberculosis. Obstruction of a ureter may result from a stone that has become impacted during its descent from the kidney, compression by an extramural tumor or mass, or strictures. The strictures may be congenital or may be acquired as a result of

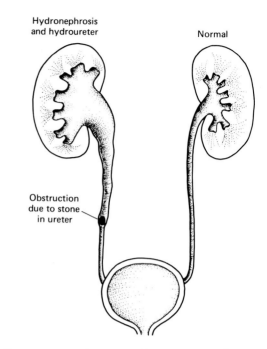

Figure 21-4. *Obstruction of a ureter causes hydroureter and hydronephrosis.*

inflammation. Obstruction at the neck of the bladder or in the urethra is frequently caused by enlargement of the prostate gland, but strictures, a tumor, or occasionally a stone may cause obstruction here. Urethral strictures are commonly caused by gonorrheal infection. Paralysis of the bladder due to spinal-cord injury or disease (neurogenic bladder) may cause retention of urine and produce the same effects as obstruction.

Obstruction to the flow of urine causes dilatation of the pelvis and calyces of the kidney and atrophy of the kidney parenchyma. This condition is called *hydronephrosis*. When the obstruction occurs in a ureter, the ureter is also dilated above the point of obstruction (*hydroureter*). Hydronephrosis and hydroureter are shown in Figure 21-4. When obstruction is sudden and complete the kidney soon stops excreting urine because the intrapelvic pressure rapidly rises above the glomerular filtration pressure. Therefore, only slight distension of the renal pelvis occurs. With partial or intermittent obstruction, which is the usual case, the kidney continues to produce urine and the pelvis gradually enlarges until it reaches a massive size. Pressure on the renal blood vessels causes ischemia, which contributes to parenchymal damage. If the obstruction is removed early, the damage to the kidney is reversible, but with prolonged obstruction the changes become irreversible.

Urinary stasis predisposes to calculus formation and to infection. If the infection produces pus in the dilated renal pelvis the condition is called *pyonephrosis*. Extension of the infection to the renal tubules causes *pyelonephritis*, which contributes to the renal damage. Infection causes flank pain, fever, and pus in the urine. Septicemia is a possible complication of pyelonephritis.

If infection does not intervene, unilateral hydronephrosis may be asymptomatic. If the other kidney is normal, it will enlarge (compensatory hypertrophy) and take over most of the renal function. Symptoms that do occur are often due to the underlying cause of the obstruction (e.g., renal calculi or a tumor).

Obstruction below the level of the ureters causes bilateral hydronephrosis. If unrelieved, this condition can lead to renal failure with consequent oliguria (or anuria), fluid and electrolye imbalances, and retention of metabolic end products such as urea and uric acid. Severe reduction in renal function causes life-threatening uremia. (Uremia is discussed in Chapter 26.)

Obstruction at the neck of the bladder or in the urethra causes dilatation of the bladder and hypertrophy of its muscular wall. Backflow of urine and backpressure in the ureters and kidneys does not occur immediately because the nature of the opening of the ureters into the bladder prevents backflow. Eventually backpressure does develop, however, and bilateral hydroureter and hydronephrosis result.

Partial obstruction of the urethra or neck of the bladder causes difficulty in initiating micturition and the person may strain to void. The size and force of the urinary stream is diminished. Urine is retained and the person may feel a sensation of incomplete emptying of the bladder. As a result of urinary retention the effective bladder capacity is reduced and the bladder refills more quickly. Consequently frequency of voiding and nocturia occur. Stasis of urine predisposes to infection; development of infection in the bladder causes burning and discomfort on voiding (dysuria) and urgency. The urine is usually cloudy and may contain blood.

Complete obstruction of the urethra or the neck of the bladder results in an absence of urine outflow and painful overdistension of the bladder. Eventually some urine may be forced through the urethra due to the excessive pressure in the bladder (retention with overflow).

Airway Obstruction

Acute airway obstruction usually results from inhalation of a foreign body or from inflammation. The inflammation is usually due to viral or bacterial infection; obstruction occurs because of swelling and excess mucus in the airways. Several conditions can cause chronic airway obstruction; chronic obstructive pulmonary disease is discussed in Chapter 10. The effects of airway obstruction depend on the nature of the obstruction and its position in the tracheobronchial tree.

A partial obstruction may act like a bypass valve, in which case air can still move past the obstruction during inspiration and expiration but the airway is narrowed. As a result, resistance to airflow is increased and breathing requires more effort. Airways are more widely open during inspiration than expiration because during expiration the pressure outside the bronchi is greater than the intraluminal pressure and tends to compress the airways. Therefore resistance to airflow is greater during expiration when the airway is narrower and the lung may become overdistended distal to the obstruction.

Some types of partial obstruction (e.g., from a tumor attached to the bronchial wall by a stalk) act like a check-valve. In this case air flows past the obstruction during inspiration, but as the bronchus narrows during expiration the lumen becomes completely blocked. As a result, air is trapped in the portion of the lung distal to the obstruction and the alveoli become overinflated.

When obstruction is complete, no air moves into or out of the portion of the lung distal to the obstruction. Complete obstruction of the upper airway quickly causes asphyxia and death if the obstruction is not immediately removed or bypassed by means of a tracheotomy. Complete obstruction of a bronchus or bronchiole causes collapse of the alveoli (atelectasis) distal to the obstruction as the alveolar gases are gradually absorbed into the blood. If the condition does not last too long, the alveoli usually re-expand when the obstruction is removed.

Manifestations
of Airway Obstruction

With partial obstruction of the upper airway inspiration is prolonged. The increased effort necessary to draw air into the lungs may require use of accessory muscles of respiration and may cause supraclavicular, suprasternal, substernal, and/or subcostal indrawing. Partial obstruction of the upper airway causes a harsh crowing sound (stridor), which may occur only on inspiration or during both inspiration and expiration. Laryngeal obstruction also causes hoarseness and a cough.

The only manifestation of a gradually developing obstruction of a large bronchus may be a cough. Sudden obstruction of a large bronchus usually results in intense dyspnea (a subjective feeling of shortness of breath and difficulty in breathing). The manifestations of obstruction in small bronchi and bronchioles depend on the extent of involvement. Obstruction of only a few small bronchi may not produce symptoms. Generalized involvement of small bronchi and/or bronchioles (e.g., as in asthma or bronchiolitis) may produce severe dyspnea. Suprasternal, intercostal, and subcostal indrawing may occur.

All types of bronchial obstruction are usually associated with a cough. The amount of coughing

increases with the degree of obstruction. In addition, a bypass type of partial obstruction is associated with a wheezing sound (rhonchus). The wheezing sound results from vibrations caused by turbulence and eddies in the air currents at the site of obstruction. Turbulence increases when the airway is narrowed, and the airway is narrower during expiration than inspiration. Therefore wheezing primarily occurs during expiration but may also occur during inspiration. If the obstruction is due to secretions, the wheezing sound may disappear after coughing.

Bronchial obstruction interferes with the drainage of secretions and the retained secretions provide a good medium for bacterial growth. Therefore, if infection was not already present, it may soon develop as a consequence of obstruction. Signs of infection, such as fever and leukocytosis, will then occur in addition to the primary manifestations of obstruction. Infection increases the production of secretions, which results in increased coughing.

Obstruction at any level of the respiratory tract can lead to varying degrees of hypoventilation, depending on the location and degree of obstruction and the ability to compensate by increased respiratory effort. As a result hypoxia, with its related signs such as cyanosis and increased heart rate, may occur (see Chapter 10). Carbon dioxide retention may also occur.

Mucoviscidosis

Mucoviscidosis (cystic fibrosis) is an autosomal recessive genetic disorder involving the exocrine glands of the body. Extremely viscous secretions cause obstruction in several organs. The exact cause of the secretory abnormality is not known, but the sweat glands, bronchial glands, pancreas, mucosal glands of the small intestine, and bile ducts of the liver may all be involved to varying degrees.

The earliest sign may be *meconium ileus*, which occurs in about 10% of newborns with mucoviscidosis. The meconium is extremely viscous due to abnormal secretions of the intestinal glands and causes obstruction, usually in the terminal part of the ileum. The infant fails to pass meconium and has a distended abdomen. A possible complication of this condition is perforation of the bowel.

The exocrine portion of the pancreas secretes very viscous fluid. The enzyme content of the pancreatic secretion may or may not be normal, but thick mucus blocks the pancreatic ducts and prevents the enzymes from reaching the small intestine. As a result, digestion and absorption are seriously impaired. The enzyme deficiency is rarely complete in the early stages, so that the infant may appear normal at birth. Between the fourth and sixth weeks the condition may become manifest by failure to thrive. The fat deposited in utero gradually disappears and the child becomes emaciated. The abdomen is distended. Several bulky, foul-smelling stools containing undigested food are passed each day. The stools are often loose and pale. Vitamin K deficiency may occur, leading to a bleeding tendency and easy bruising. Evidences of other vitamin deficiencies may become apparent later.

The pancreatic ducts and acini become dilated and filled with inspissated mucus, forming cysts. The acinar cells atrophy and stop secreting. Eventually fibrous tissue replaces the pancreatic tissue (hence the term cystic fibrosis).

Some degree of respiratory involvement occurs in most cases and is usually manifest by 2 years of age. The size of the bronchial glands is normal at birth, but the glands rapidly hypertrophy and excessive production of thick, tenacious mucus occurs. The thick mucus causes either partial or complete obstruction of small bronchi and bronchioles in various parts of the lungs. Complete obstruction causes areas of atelectasis. Infection frequently develops, usually from *Staphylococcus aureus* or *Pseudomonas aeruginosa*. As the disease progresses, destruction of lung tissue and multiple abscess formation occur. Further progression results in respiratory failure with carbon dioxide retention and hypoxia, pulmonary hypertension, and right ventricular failure.

A dry, hacking cough is the first pulmonary symptom; it usually develops when the infant is a few months old. Later the cough sounds loose and productive. Dyspnea, wheezing, and cyanosis may occur at times. The child fatigues easily and is irritable. Clubbing of the fingers and toes develops. (Clubbing is a painless enlargement of the terminal phalanges of the fingers and toes caused by an increase in the amount of fibroelastic tissue, dilation and engorgement of small blood vessels, and edema. Clubbing accompanies a variety of pulmonary and heart conditions, and occasionally develops in people with diseases of the liver or GI tract. The underlying mechanism in the development of clubbing is not known.)

Evidence of obstructive lesions in the liver develops later and may not be seen. Plugs of mucus block bile ducts, resulting in focal areas of liver cell atrophy and fibrosis. New bile ducts grow adjacent to the blocked ones. In rare cases, if the child lives long enough, cirrhosis may develop.

The sweat glands and salivary glands are also involved. Diminished reabsorption of electrolytes in these glands results in secretions with higher than normal sodium and chloride concentrations. The increased chloride concentration in the sweat is the basis of a diagnostic test for mucoviscidosis. The excessive loss of sodium and chloride in the sweat makes the child susceptible to heat exhaustion (see Chapter 24 under Hyperthermia).

SUGGESTED ADDITIONAL READING

Gault PL: How to break the kidney stone cycle. *Nurs 78* 8(12): 24–31, 1978.

Stahlgren LH, Morris NW: Intestinal obstruction, *Am J Nurs* 77(6): 999–1002, 1977.

Vogel CH: Keeping patients alive in spite of postobstructive diuresis. *Nurs 79* 9(3): 50–56, 1979.

22

Position
and Activity

Human beings have many adaptive mechanisms to meet the demands of an upright posture, changes in position, and varying degrees of activity. A certain degree of activity is necessary to maintain optimal functioning of the body. Tissues and organs develop increased functional ability (within limits) in response to increased physiological demands (i.e., use). Lack of activity, as in prolonged bedrest, can lead to deterioration of structure and function in various parts of the body. Abnormal or inadequate adaptive mechanisms can lead to inappropriate responses to position changes,

RESPONSES TO POSITION

The Upright Posture

To maintain an erect posture, the human body has to resist the force of gravity. Muscular work must be done to prevent the body from "crumpling up" and falling forward. In addition, the weight of the column of blood in the blood vessels exerts a pressure that, together with the distensibility of the veins, tends to cause pooling of blood in the legs and feet when a person is standing. Therefore, compensatory mechanisms are necessary to maintain adequate circulation.

Antigravity Muscles

To maintain an upright posture, the vertebral column must support the upper part of the body. Standing erect also involves full extension of the hip and knee joints. The force of gravity holds these joints in extension because the center of gravity of the head, arms, and trunk is slightly behind the center of motion of the hips and the line of gravity falls anterior to the knees. Initially when a person stands the knee joints are usually locked in extension, but after a few moments the knee joints may unlock and the person may stand with the knees slightly flexed. Standing with the knees flexed requires considerable muscular effort, however, to support the weight of the body against the force of gravity. Therefore, people with weak thigh muscles or those who must remain standing for a long period of time tend to stand with the knees locked in extension.

The erector spinae, the gluteal muscles, the quadriceps femoris, and the calf muscles are the principal muscles working to hold the body upright. These muscles have several special characteristics that adapt them to support the body against gravity. They have slower contractions than other muscles and not only do they usually contract to the appropriate length to maintain posture, but they are able to remain contracted at that length for long periods of time.

Circulatory Mechanisms

When a person is standing erect, the blood pressure at a given point will be determined not only by the cardiac output and peripheral resistance, but also by the weight of the vertical column of blood above the point of measurement. The *weight* of a substance is the gravitational force exerted on the substance. *Pressure* is a force exerted per unit area. Because of its weight (i.e., because of the gravitational force acting on it), a substance or object exerts a pressure on an underlying surface. The greater the mass of a substance, the greater

the pull of gravity on it, the greater its weight, and the greater the pressure. Therefore, the higher the column of blood in the blood vessels (i.e., the greater the mass of blood), the greater will be the hydrostatic pressure of the blood. Thus for an adult of average height, mean arterial pressure may vary from 90 mm Hg at heart level, to 40 mm Hg at the wrist if the arm is held above the head, to 175 mm Hg at the ankle (Fig. 22-1). Similarly, venous pressure may vary from zero at a level just above the heart to about 85 mm Hg at the ankle if a person stands relaxed and motionless.

Since the veins are not rigid tubes, they collapse whenever the external tissue pressure equals the venous pressure. The effective venous pressure at this point is zero. When a person is standing the effective venous pressure is zero in the extracranial veins above the level of the heart. Blood can still flow through the collapsed veins, however.

Within the rigid confines of the skull the venous pressure drops below atmospheric pressure when a person is standing. A principle of physics (Pascal's principle) is that if the pressure of a fluid enclosed in a rigid chamber is changed at one point, the pressure changes by an equal amount at all points in the fluid. Therefore, within the skull the drop in intravascular hydrostatic pressure is balanced by an equal change in extravascular tissue pressure, so that the intracranial veins and venous sinuses do not collapse. As long as the arterial pressure change equals the venous pressure change, the arteriovenous pressure gradient will remain constant and tissue blood flow will not change. If the decline in arterial pressure is greater than the drop in venous pressure, however, the arteriovenous gradient will decrease and tissue perfusion will be reduced.

In the lower parts of the body, increased hydrostatic pressure in the capillaries results in increased movement of fluid from the capillaries into the interstitial space. (See Chapter 11 for a discussion of the factors influencing movement of fluid across the capillary membrane.) Consequently, swelling of the feet may occur after prolonged standing. As a result of the loss of fluid to the interstitial spaces

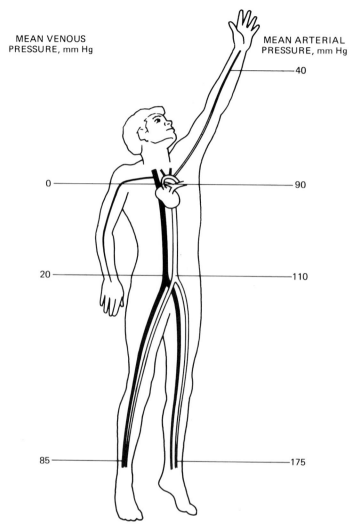

MEAN VENOUS
PRESSURE, mm Hg

MEAN ARTERIAL
PRESSURE, mm Hg

40

0 ——————————— 90

20 ————————— 110

85 ——————————— 175

Figure 22-1. *Effect of gravity on blood pressure when a person is standing.*

in the lower extremities, total plasma volume may decrease by about 15% after 40 minutes of standing.

In addition, the increased hydrostatic pressure in the lower parts of the body tends to cause distension of the blood vessels. The veins are very distensible; as the vein walls are pushed out by the increased hydrostatic pressure the venous capacity increases, resulting in pooling of blood in the lower extremities. Consequently venous return is decreased, which in turn decreases the stroke volume of the heart, and reduces cardiac output. On the arterial side the blood vessels have a thicker muscular coat and are therefore less distensible, although the high hydrostatic pressure still tends to cause passive vasodilation. Fortunately, the body has several mechanisms to counteract these tendencies, otherwise the reduced cardiac output together with peripheral vasodilation would cause a severe drop in systemic arterial blood pressure. As a consequence of decreased arterial pressure, blood flow through the brain would diminish and consciousness would be lost.

A sympathetic reflex response is elicited immediately upon standing. As a result, the heart rate increases slightly and vasoconstriction occurs. Thus systemic arterial pressure is maintained. Vasoconstriction also decreases the amount of blood flowing through the capillaries in the dependent portions of the body. This effect helps to decrease capillary hydrostatic pressure and prevent excessive loss of fluid to the tissues. The increased sympathetic activity also increases venomotor tone so that the veins are less distensible.

Other mechanisms promote venous return and prevent pooling of blood in the legs and feet. Many valves are located along the veins of the extremities (Fig. 22-2). These valves are designed to allow blood to flow only toward the heart and pre-

vent backflow. Contraction of skeletal muscles in the legs compresses the veins and reduces their capacity. Blood flows away from the area of compression and, since the valves prevent backflow, blood is forced toward the heart. The muscular contraction produces momentary complete emptying of veins in the thigh and interrupts the column of blood. Thus the venous and capillary hydrostatic pressures in the lower leg are reduced, because now the height of the column of blood extends only from the foot to the knee, not from the foot to the heart. As the muscles relax and as blood flows through the capillaries into the veins, the collapsed veins refill and the venous pressure in the foot rises once more. If muscular contractions occur again before the veins in the thighs are refilled (e.g., by repetitive movements, as in walking), the venous pressure remains at the lower level. Capillary pressure is also decreased and so less fluid is lost to the interstitial space. Skeletal muscle contractions also assist lymph flow and thereby help prevent accumulation of excessive fluid in the interstitial space.

Venous insufficiency. Venous insufficiency is an impairment of the mechanism of venous return from the legs. It commonly produces varicosities of the superficial veins, but not all people with venous insufficiency have varicose veins. *Varicose veins*, or *varices* (singular: varix), are abnormally distended, tortuous veins.

Several factors may be involved in the development of venous insufficiency, but the basic cause is valvular incompetence. The number and distribution of venous valves, the structural and biochemical properties of the vein wall, and the degree of development of the muscles and fascia all influence the development of venous insufficiency and varicose veins. The more valves there are, the greater the number that can be damaged before venous insufficiency occurs. Variations in the structure of the vein wall determine whether or not abnormal pressure will cause varices. The strength of the surrounding muscles and fascia will influence the pressure abnormalities resulting from

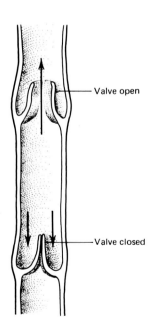

Figure 22-2. *Normal venous valves prevent backflow of blood.*

Valve open

Valve closed

valvular incompetence. Deep leg veins rarely develop varices because surrounding muscles provide them with a firm support.

Some people develop varicose veins at a relatively young age due to a familial predisposition. Inherited differences in biochemical and structural properties of the vein walls presumably contribute to this condition. Individual variation in the number of venous valves may also be inherited. Degenerative changes and loss of tissue tone occur with aging and may contribute to the development of varicose veins in older people.

Valvular incompetence may be primary or secondary. Primary valvular incompetence results from irreparable damage of the venous valves, usually caused by thrombophlebitis. Secondary valvular incompetence is caused by distension of the veins. The valve cusps are normal but cannot close completely due to the increase in diameter of the veins (Fig. 22-3). Distension of the veins results from a prolonged increase in pressure, such as occurs when a person stands most of the time or when venous flow is obstructed (e.g., due to thrombosis). Compression of the iliac veins (e.g., due to a pelvic tumor or pregnancy) also increases the venous pressure in the legs.

The lower part of the leg is particularly liable to minor trauma, which may damage veins and venous valves. Valvular incompetence of the communicating veins commonly occurs at this site.

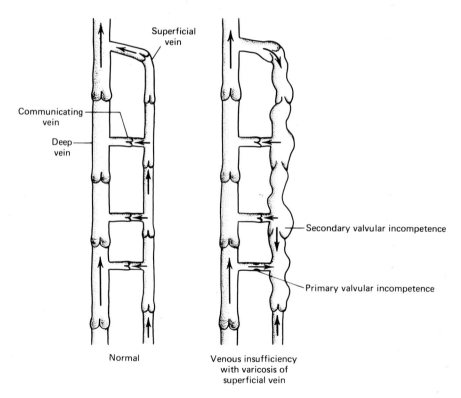

Figure 22-3. *Venous insufficiency. Primary valvular incompetence results from destruction of the venous valves. Secondary valvular incompetence is produced by venous distension. Arrows indicate direction of blood flow. Note that normally blood flows from the superficial vein into the deep vein.*

Consequently high pressure developing in the deep veins is transmitted directly to the superficial veins and the poorly supported superficial veins dilate.

When the venous valves are incompetent backflow of blood occurs. Consequently venous pressure rises and causes further distension of the veins. Thus a vicious cycle is established.

As a result of the increased venous pressure capillary hydrostatic pressure also rises, producing edema (see Chapter 11). The circulatory impairment and edema interfere with tissue nutrition and removal of wastes. Therefore the muscles may become weak and painful and the skin over the lower legs may become thin and eventually ulcerate. In addition, venous stasis predisposes to thrombosis (see Chapter 7).

Orthostatic hypotension. Some people are unable to maintain an adequate arterial pressure when they change from a recumbent to an erect position. This fall in arterial pressure on standing is called *orthostatic,* or *postural, hypotension.* It is accompanied by dizziness and possibly syncope.

Many conditions can cause postural hypotension, but basically two mechanisms are responsible. In some cases, cardiac output may be so diminished that arterial pressure falls in spite of reflex sympathetic stimulation. As a result of this mechanism, hypotension can occur secondarily to conditions that interfere with venous return (e.g., incompetent venous valves), diminish blood volume (e.g., Addison's disease), or interfere with cardiac functioning (e.g., myocarditis). The other mechanism responsible for postural hypotension is failure of the sympathetic response at some point along the reflex arc. The failure of the sympathetic reflex may occur secondarily to diseases that cause neurological dysfunction of the afferent sympathetic limb (e.g., tabes dorsalis), diseases of the central nervous system (e.g., Parkinsonism and Wernicke's syndrome), or diseases affecting the efferent sympathetic limb (e.g., polyneuritis). In some cases the sympathetic reflex is impaired due to administration of drugs that either act in the central nervous system (e.g., meprobamate) or affect the efferent limb (e.g., adrenergic blocking agents). Orthostatic hypotension can also occur following sympathectomy.

Sometimes neurogenic orthostatic hypotension occurs as a primary disorder rather than secondary to some other disease. The exact cause of the failure of the sympathetic reflex is not known and the condition is referred to as idiopathic orthostatic hypotension. Some people with idiopathic orthostatic hypotension have other neurological disorders as well (the Shy-Drager syndrome) and the defect appears to be in the central nervous system. The peripheral sympathetic nervous system appears to be intact in these people but they are unable to activate the sympathetic nerves appropriately in response to exertion or a change in posture. In other people the orthostatic hypotension is not associated with other neurological disorders, and the defect appears to be in the peripheral sympathetic nerves.

Changing from Erect to Recumbent

Many immediate physiological changes occur when a person lies down. Some of these changes result from redistribution of the blood volume and alterations of blood flow. When a person remains in a recumbent position for a prolonged period of time further changes occur. These subsequent changes are discussed later in this chapter in the section on decreased physical activity.

Musculoskeletal Changes

In the supine position the muscles that are important for maintaining the upright posture can relax. Other muscles, however, have to work harder when a person is lying down. For example, the pectoralis major has to contract to keep the shoulder girdle from falling backwards when a person lies supine.

In the erect position the head is held up by the erector spinae. Gravity assists neck flexion when the erector spinae relax. In the supine position the weak anterior neck muscles must contract to flex the neck and raise the head against the force of gravity.

When a person is in an upright position the upper arm hangs vertically during most hand movements. In the supine position, however, the upper arm is horizontal and has to be raised up to permit a reasonable degree of hand movement.

When a person is standing the foot is in the plantigrade position at a 90-degree angle with the leg. When a person is lying prone the foot is plantarflexed unless there is enough space between the end of the mattress and the bed frame for the toes to project down and maintain the plantigrade position of the foot. In the supine position the pull of gravity tends to cause plantarflexion. Contraction of dorsiflexor muscles is necessary to keep the foot in the plantigrade position.

Thus, when a person lies down for a few hours, many muscles have to perform unaccustomed work and may become fatigued, especially if the person is performing activities such as eating or using a bedpan while lying down. If the person does not change position, the neck, arms, and legs may ache.

Joint alignment is altered when a person lies down. The hip joints, which are locked in extension when standing, are slightly flexed, abducted, and externally rotated when a person is supine. The spine is straighter when lying down than when standing up. Extension of the thoracic spine, elevation of the chest, and forward tilting of the pelvis cause the anterior abdominal wall to be stretched when a person is lying supine.

Circulatory Changes

When a person is lying down all the blood vessels are at or near the level of the heart, and the hydrostatic pressure differences due to gravity are eliminated. Blood no longer tends to pool in the leg veins, so that circulating blood volume and venous return increase. Consequently stroke volume and cardiac output increase. The increased stroke volume activates the aortic and carotid sinus baroreceptors, bringing about a reflex slowing of the heart and vasodilation. The vasodilation decreases peripheral resistance. Although heart rate decreases, cardiac output remains higher when lying down than when standing erect because of the increased stroke volume. Thus, the work load on the heart is greater when a person is lying down than when standing up.

Reabsorption of tissue fluid increases when a person lies down, with the result that blood volume is increased and the blood is slightly diluted.

Blood flow through the kidneys increases, resulting in increased glomerular filtration. In addition, secretion of antidiuretic hormone (ADH) is decreased because of baroreceptor stimulation due to the increased circulating blood volume. (See Chapter 12 for a discussion of the factors influencing ADH secretion and urine volume.) Therefore water reabsorption decreases and urine volume increases over a period of about one hour after lying down. (Although this change occurs with lying down when awake, urinary excretion exhibits diurnal variation and during sleep urine volume is usually decreased.)

Vasodilation and increased blood flow through the skin cause a rise in skin temperature when a person lies down. Consequently an increased amount of heat is lost from the body and the rectal temperature may decrease. (See Chapter 24 for a discussion of body-temperature regulation.)

Pulmonary Changes

When a person lies down, some of the blood that was pooled in the legs while standing is shifted to the thorax, and the volume of blood in the lungs increases. The distensibility of the pulmonary vessels prevents any great fluctuation in pulmonary blood pressure, however, despite the change in blood volume.

Vital capacity is slightly less when a person is lying down than when standing erect. This decrease is primarily due to the increased volume of blood in the thorax, which reduces the space available for air. In addition, when a person lies down the shape of the chest changes in a way that decreases its maximum capacity, and the diaphragm rises because the abdominal viscera push up against it.

Compliance (i.e., the distensibility of the lungs as indicated by the change in volume per unit change in pressure) is lower when a person is in the supine position than when sitting. Mechanical resistance (i.e., resistance to airflow and to tissue deformation) is higher when in the supine position than in the sitting position. Compliance and mechanical resistance are usually intermediate when a person is in the prone position as compared to the other two positions. Therefore it requires more work to breathe when lying down than when in an upright position. These positional differences are probably related to changes in hydrostatic pressure, which influence physical properties of the lungs as well as the distribution of pulmonary blood flow.

Normally a person automatically compensates for positional changes in the mechanics of breathing, and the changes have little significance. These differences can be important, however, in people with cardiopulmonary disease. Such people often have difficulty breathing when lying down (*orthopnea*), but their distress is lessened if they sit up or stand. Also, in people with predominantly unilateral lung disease, compliance is generally higher and resistance lower (i.e., the work of breathing is less) when lying on the healthy side than when lying on the diseased side.

Both the distribution of inspired air (ventilation) and the distribution of blood flow in the lungs are affected by gravity and therefore affected by body position. The distribution of blood flow is influenced in the same direction as the distribution of ventilation, however, so that in the normal lung ventilation and perfusion are relatively well matched regardless of position and arterial gas levels are not seriously affected.

In the erect position (sitting or standing) pleural pressure shows a gradient from the top to the bottom of the lung, the pressure being more negative in the apex than the base because of the weight of the lung. In the supine position, the pleural pressure gradient between the apex and base of the lung is abolished, but a gradient in pleural pressure exists between the upper (ventral) and lower (dorsal) parts of the lung. Similarly, in the lateral position the upper lung regions have a more negative pleural pressure than the dependent lung regions.

The degree of inflation of lung units depends on the elastic properties of the lung tissue and on the transpulmonary pressure (i.e., the difference in pressure between the alveolar space and the pleural space). As a result of the pleural pressure gradient, the transpulmonary pressure is greater for lung units in the upper part of the lung than for those in the lower part. Therefore, the upper lung units are expanded more than those in the lower parts. This situation influences the distribution of inspired air. The compliance of lung tissue is affected by the volume of air in the lungs at the start of inspiration. Near maximum inflation, compliance decreases. Thus, lung units that are most inflated are least compliant (i.e., will undergo a smaller volume change for the same change in pressure) than less fully inflated units, and will receive a smaller portion of the tidal air. Since the alveoli in the upper regions of the lung are more expanded than those in the lower regions, when a person takes a breath the ventilation per alveolus is less in the uppermost lung units than in the lower (dependent) regions of the lung. In other words, for the range of lung volumes that occur during normal breathing, ventilation is distributed preferentially to the lower lung regions. (At low lung volumes the distribution of ventilation is reversed due to airway closure in the dependent portions of the lungs.) The difference in ventilation per alveolus between the uppermost and lowest parts of the lung is less in the supine and prone positions than in the sitting or the lateral position, however. In the supine and prone positions the vertical lung distance is less and therefore the difference in pleural pressure between the upper and lower parts is less.

Just as the weight of the column of blood affects pressures in the systemic circulation when a person is standing, pulmonary blood pressure varies from the top to the bottom of the lung. This pressure difference influences blood flow through the pulmonary capillaries. In the systemic circulation blood flow is determined by the gradient between arterial and venous pressure. In the pulmonary circulation, however, alveolar pressure also influences capillary blood flow. When alveolar pressure is greater than arterial pressure the capillaries are compressed, and no blood flows through (alveolar dead space). This situation exists in the apex of the lung in the erect position. When arterial pressure is greater than alveolar pressure, blood will flow through the capillaries. If alveolar pressure is greater than venous pressure, the amount of blood flowing through the capillaries will be determined by the difference between arterial pressure and alveolar pressure. This situation exists in the middle portions of the lung. If venous pressure is greater than alveolar pressure, blood flow is determined by the arteriovenous pressure gradient. This situation exists in the basal regions of the lung in the erect position.

In the supine and prone positions apical and basal blood flow is more even, but again the lower (dependent) regions have greater blood flow than the uppermost regions. This situation also exists when a person is in a lateral position. The difference in blood flow between the uppermost and dependent parts of the lungs is least when a person is in a supine or prone position.

Thus, both ventilation and perfusion are greater in the lower parts of the lungs. The gradient in blood flow, however, does not exactly match the gradient in ventilation. In the upright position the alveoli are relatively overventilated in relation to perfusion in the upper parts of the lungs and relatively underventilated in relation to perfusion in the lower parts of the lungs. The degree of matching of ventilation and perfusion is not the same for every position, however, and in general ventilation and perfusion are better matched when a person is lying down than in an upright posi-

tion. In addition, it has been noted that arterial oxygen tension is higher when a person is in the lateral position than in the supine position.

Although arterial oxygen *tension* (PO_2) may be affected by position, under normal conditions the oxygen *content* of the blood is not significantly altered. Oxygen tension reflects the amount of dissolved oxygen in the blood, but most of the oxygen in the blood is carried by hemoglobin. Because of the shape of the oxygen-hemoglobin dissociation curve (see Chapter 10 under Decreased Oxygen-Carrying Capacity of the Blood), changes in arterial oxygen tension do not significantly alter hemoglobin saturation until the PO_2 falls below 60 mm Hg. In people with lung disease, however, the normal ventilation-perfusion distribution is often disturbed. In these people, postural differences may have an effect on oxygenation of the blood.

RESPONSES TO ACTIVITY AND INACTIVITY

The maximal physiological potential of any organ is genetically determined, but its actual functional capacity at any time is largely determined by the intensity and frequency of its previous activity (as well as by a person's nutritional status). The functional capacity of an organ, under normal conditions, is its maximal metabolic rate. By increasing the rate of metabolic activity of the organ, the functional capacity can be increased. Functional capacity, however, cannot exceed the maximal physiological potential. Maximal activity of the organ is required to bring about a maximal increase in functional capacity. Functional capacity can be maintained at a particular level by moderate activity, but will not increase. It decreases if activity is restricted. Complete inactivity of an organ results in a rapid decline of functional capacity.

For example, frequent contractions that produce tension are necessary to maintain the strength of muscles. Contractions that produce maximal tension of short duration, occurring several times each day, will increase the strength of a muscle. Muscle strength is just maintained by contractions of 20% to 30% maximal tension performed each day. Contractions of less than 20% maximal tension are not sufficient to maintain strength and the muscle weakens. When no tension is produced each day, strength declines very rapidly.

Exercise

Exercise not only affects the development of skeletal muscles, but affects cardiovascular and pulmonary functions because muscles require more oxygen during exercise and produce more carbon dioxide, which must be eliminated. Under normal conditions exercise capacity is determined by the ability of the circulatory and respiratory systems to deliver increased amounts of oxygen to the contracting muscles, because less oxygen is stored in the tissues than any other substance in relation to rate of utilization.

Musculoskeletal Effects

Not all muscle fibers are the same. Three types have been described, according to their structural and functional properties: high-oxidative slow-twitch fibers, low-oxidative fast-twitch fibers, and high-oxidative fast-twitch fibers. The makeup of skeletal muscles in different parts of the body varies according to the type of activity usually performed by the muscle. Muscles that primarily perform one type of activity (e.g., the antigravity muscles, which must remain contracted for prolonged periods of time to maintain posture) may contain predominantly one type of fiber. Most often, however, a muscle must perform high-intensity strength activity of short duration on some occasions and endurance-type activity at other times. Therefore, most muscles are composed of varying numbers of all three types of fibers.

High-oxidative slow-twitch fibers are relatively small in diameter. They do not contain as much actin and myosin as the other fiber types; therefore they produce less tension and use adenosine triphosphate (ATP) at a slower rate. High-oxidative slow-twitch fibers contain many mitochondria and have a high rate of oxidative phosphorylation to produce the ATP needed for contraction. These fibers appear red because they contain myoglobin, an iron-containing protein that can combine reversibly with oxygen, similar to hemoglobin. Myoglobin enhances the diffusion of oxygen into the muscle cell and also provides a means of intracellular storage of small amounts of oxygen. High-oxidative slow-twitch fibers contain very little stored glycogen but are surrounded by many capillaries. Therefore they have a relatively high rate of blood flow, so that oxygen and nutrients are delivered at a fast enough rate to keep up with the relatively slow rate of ATP utilization. Consequently high-oxidative slow-twitch fibers do not fatigue very easily.

Low-oxidative fast-twitch fibers are large-diameter fibers that contain more actin and myosin and therefore are capable of producing greater tension. They use ATP at a rapid rate. Very few capillaries surround these fibers and they contain very little myoglobin. The lack of myoglobin gives them a white appearance.

They have few mitochondria and produce most of their ATP by anaerobic glycolysis. Low-oxidative fast-twitch fibers contain large amounts of glycogen, which serves as an immediate source of glucose. These fibers fatigue quickly because anaerobic glycolysis produces a low yield of ATP per molecule of glucose (see Chapter 10 under Cellular Respiration) and their high rate of ATP utilization depletes their glycogen stores very rapidly.

High-oxidative fast-twitch fibers have characteristics intermediate between the other types.

When the amount and/or type of activity performed by a muscle is altered, the composition of the muscle changes. The changes that occur adapt the muscle for the particular type of activity it is required to perform. Therefore, exercise of one type will not necessarily improve muscle performance of a different type. Exercises that are of high intensity and short duration, such as weight lifting, cause an increase in the size of the muscle fibers (*hypertrophy*). This increase in size is associated with an increase in the amount of actin and myosin and an increase in muscle strength. Exercise of endurance, such as swimming or jogging, performed on a regular basis, does not produce much increase in muscle mass or strength, but is associated with biochemical changes that adapt the muscles for activity of low intensity and long duration. Low-oxidative fast-twitch fibers are transformed into high-oxidative fast-twitch fibers, while the number of mitochondria (i.e., the capacity to produce ATP) in the high-oxidative fibers increases. The number of capillaries surrounding the fibers also may increase.

Muscle activity also influences the size and shape of bone. Increased muscular activity causes the bones to become thicker and heavier. Trabeculae in the center of a bone are laid down according to the lines of stress on the bone. The stress on a bone is determined by weight-bearing and by the pull of the muscles on the bone. Osseous tissue is constantly being laid down by osteoblast cells and resorbed by osteoclast cells. The factors influencing the turnover of bone are not well understood, but it has been noted that blood flow influences osteogenesis and bone resorption. It is quite probable that activity of surrounding muscles influences the blood flow within a bone.

Pulmonary Effects

During exercise, the demand for oxygen and the amount of carbon dioxide to be eliminated increase. Accordingly, ventilation increases. The factors that bring about the increase in ventilation during exercise are not well understood, but several seem to be acting together. Activation of joint receptors plays a part in initiating an increase in ventilation, as discussed in Chapter 1 (see under Use of Disturbance Detectors). Psychogenic conditioned responses probably play a role: the breathing pattern may be changed in anticipation of exercise. As exercise continues, the increased amount of carbon dioxide produced by the muscles

acts as a stimulus to breathing. An increase in the hydrogen-ion concentration due to production of lactic acid by the muscles also contributes.

During light exercise, increased ventilation occurs mainly as a result of an increase in the depth of breathing (i.e., tidal volume). With heavier exercise the rate of breathing is also increased.

Pulmonary arterial pressure increases during exercise. As a result, the distribution of blood flow throughout the lungs is more uniform. Blood flow increases through capillaries that were previously perfused but not fully dilated; capillaries that were previously closed are opened. Therefore the amount of alveolar dead space decreases and ventilation and perfusion are better matched. The result is an improvement in gas exchange. In addition, the opening up of more pulmonary capillaries increases the surface area for gas exchange and so pulmonary diffusing capacity increases.

In people with normal, healthy lungs these mechanisms are adequate to maintain arterial oxygen saturation and eliminate the excess carbon dioxide produced during exercise near sea level. For people living at high altitudes, however, the rate of diffusion of oxygen into the blood is decreased because of the low oxygen content of the inspired air. At rest this decrease in oxygen usually presents no problem, but maximal oxygen uptake is reduced and therefore exercise capacity is limited. Similarly, in people with pulmonary disease, gas exchange is impaired and maximal oxygen uptake and exercise capacity are decreased.

Circulatory Effects

During exercise, the increased demand for oxygen by the contracting muscles is met by increased transport of oxygen to the muscles and by increased extraction of oxygen from each increment of blood. At rest the muscles extract only about 25% of the oxygen in the blood flowing through them. During exercise, however, the active muscles extract almost all of the oxygen.

Several mechanism are responsible for the increased oxygen extraction. The P_{O_2} within the muscle cells approaches zero as oxygen is used by the contracting muscle. As a result of the low intracellular PO_2 the diffusion gradient between the capillaries and the cells increases and more oxygen diffuses from the blood to the cells. Therefore the plasma PO_2 decreases and more oxygen is released from the hemoglobin. In addition, the increase in muscle metabolism results in a local decrease in pH and an increase in temperature. These two factors shift the oxygen-hemoglobin dissociation curve to the right and facilitate the release of oxygen from hemoglobin (see Chapter 10 under Decreased Oxygen-Carrying Capacity of the Blood). Also, during exercise a greater number of muscle capillaries are perfused so that the surface area for diffusion increases. All these factors contribute to an increase in extraction of oxygen from the blood during exercise.

Oxygen transport depends on tissue blood flow and the oxygen content of the blood. As previously mentioned, in normal people at sea level, pulmonary function is able to increase adequately to maintain arterial oxygen saturation. Blood flow is increased by circulating the blood more rapidly (i.e., increasing cardiac output) and by redistributing the blood so that an increased portion of the cardiac output goes to the active muscles.

Vasodilation occurs in the exercising muscles, partly from local chemical changes and partly from increased activity of sympathetic vasodilator nerves. This vasodilation lowers vascular resistance and therefore increases blood flow. At the same time, vasoconstriction occurs in other tissues, such as the GI tract, liver, and kidneys. Blood flow is therefore reduced in these areas and blood is shunted instead to the active muscles. Ultimately, however, the extent to which blood flow can be increased depends on the cardiac output and under usual conditions cardiac output is the limitation in a person's capacity to perform exercise of endurance.

Cardiac output can be increased by increasing stroke volume and/or heart rate. During exercise, the increase in cardiac output is mainly brought about by an increase in heart rate resulting from sympathetic stimulation. For a normal adult the heart rate may increase to about 100 beats/minute during light exercise, to 130 beats/minute during moderate exercise, and to almost 200 beats/minute during heavy exertion. In general, the heart rate of an untrained person increases to about two to three times the resting rate. A trained endurance athlete, however, usually has a lower resting heart rate and can increase the heart rate about fourfold during exercise.

Stroke volume increases by varying amounts during exercise. The increase in stroke volume with exercise is less when a person is in the supine position than in the upright position. As mentioned previously, stroke volume at rest is greater when a person is lying down than when upright. Several factors are responsible for the increase in stroke volume during exercise. Venous return is increased from increased activity of the skeletal muscle pump, increased respiratory movements, and venoconstriction brought about by sympathetic stimulation. Increased venous return results in an increase in the end-diastolic ventricular volume. Consequently the force of contraction increases as a result of the Frank-Starling mechanism. In addition, myocardial contractility is increased by sympathetic stimulation. Therefore a greater amount of blood is ejected with each beat. As the heart rate increases, however, diastolic filling time decreases and end-diastolic volume is reduced. Therefore, at very rapid heart rates diastolic filling time becomes the limiting factor and stroke volume decreases.

Total peripheral resistance decreases during exercise due to vasodilation in the skeletal muscles and the skin. (Vasodilation occurs in the skin to dissipate some of the heat produced during exercise. See Chapter 24.) Systemic blood pressure rises during exercise, however, as a result of the increased cardiac output. As already mentioned, pulmonary blood pressure also rises during exercise.

Cardiovascular function and exercise capacity are influenced by a person's usual level of physical activity and can be altered by changes in activity. Long-term physical training involving endurance-type exercise performed on a regular basis can improve cardiovascular function. With training, heart rate decreases and stroke volume increases for a given work load. The maximum heart rate does not increase, but there is an increase in the amount of work that can be performed at any given heart rate. In other words, the work of the heart is decreased for a given level of exercise. People who have a slow heart rate and low arterial pressure at rest, minimal changes due to a specific amount of exercise, and a rapid return of heart rate and blood pressure to basal levels following exercise are generally considered to be "physically fit."

Cardiovascular Reserve

Depending on a person's state of physical fitness, systemic blood flow can be increased by three to five times the resting value to meet the varying requirements of the body. The potential degree to which cardiovascular function can increase above the functional level at rest is called the *cardiovas-*

cular reserve. During extreme exercise, cardiovascular reserve is utilized to the limit. Cardiovascular reserve depends on the venous oxygen reserve and the cardiac reserve (Fig. 22-4).

The blood entering the systemic capillaries normally contains approximately 19 ml of oxygen per 100 ml of blood. The amount of oxygen extracted from the blood depends on the metabolic activity of each tissue. At rest only about 25% of the oxygen is extracted from the blood as it flows through the capillaries. The amount of oxygen left in the blood that can still be extracted represents the *venous oxygen reserve.* Although some active tissues may extract nearly all the oxygen from the blood, some residual oxygen always remains in the mixed venous blood. Conditions that reduce the oxygen-carrying capacity of the blood, such as anemia (see Chapter 10), decrease the venous oxygen reserve and therefore decrease exercise capacity.

Cardiac reserve is the extent to which cardiac output can be increased above the resting level by

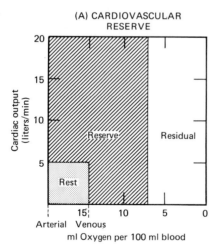
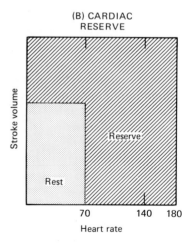

Figure 22-4. *(A) Oxygen delivery to the tissues at rest is determined by the product of the cardiac output and the AV oxygen difference. Maximum oxygen delivery is achieved by increased cardiac output and greater oxygen extraction, corresponding to the cardiovascular reserve for oxygen delivery. Residual oxygen remains in the mixed venous blood even at maximal levels of oxygen transport. (B) Cardiac reserve refers to the extent to which cardiac output can be increased by greater stroke volume and acceleration of the heart rate. (Modified from Rushmer: Cardiovascular Dynamics, ed 4. © 1976 by the W.B. Saunders Co., Philadelphia.)*

increasing the stroke volume and heart rate. As already mentioned, stroke volume can be increased by increasing the end-diastolic volume and/or decreasing the end-systolic volume (i.e., ejecting a larger fraction of the end-diastolic volume). The maximum effective heart rate is approximately 180 beats/minute. As mentioned previously, at very rapid heart rates diastolic filling time is decreased and stroke volume diminishes. Therefore, although higher heart rates may be possible, they do not contribute effectively to increasing cardiac output. In addition, extremely rapid heart rates may interfere with coronary blood flow.

In one sense, the maximal cardiac output that can be sustained is determined by the cardiac efficiency and the coronary blood supply. *Cardiac efficiency* is the amount of useful work performed by the heart relative to the total energy expended. The useful work performed by the heart is the potential and kinetic energy transferred to the blood as it is ejected from the ventricles during systole. Cardiac efficiency is quite variable, but averages about 23%. In other words, about 77% of the energy expended during ventricular contraction is not used to circulate the blood. A small amount of the energy is expended in maintenance and repair of myocardial cells and in propagating the wave of excitation through the heart. Considerable energy is lost as heat from friction and chemical reactions.

Since the heart must beat continually to support life, the energy expended during systole must be restored during the next diastole. Oxygen and metabolic fuels must be continuously delivered in sufficient amounts to provide the energy necessary for myocardial contraction. The amount of oxygen available to the myocardium depends on the arterial oxygen content and coronary blood flow. Even when a person is resting, the myocardium extracts about 74% to 80% of the oxygen from the blood. Consequently the venous oxygen reserve of the coronary blood is very small and increased requirements must be met by increasing coronary blood flow.

Most types of heart disease reduce the cardiac reserve. Some of the reserve capacity is being used at rest to compensate for the deficit caused by the disease so that the amount of reserve available for use during stress and exercise is decreased and exercise capacity is limited. Cardiac reserve can be decreased in various ways. For example, complete atrioventricular block seriously limits the heart rate and thus increased cardiac output can only be achieved by increasing the stroke volume. With valvular insufficiency the stroke volume reserve is decreased because in order to maintain adequate systemic blood flow the stroke volume at rest must increase to compensate for the amount of blood that regurgitates through the valve. Myocarditis, heart failure, and various metabolic diseases decrease cardiac efficiency. Consequently a greater amount of oxygen is required to perform the same amount of work and maximal stroke volume is restricted. Coronary artery disease restricts coronary blood flow and therefore limits the transport of oxygen to the myocardium. Thus cardiac reserve is diminished.

Exercise and Heart Disease

The role of exercise in the prevention of coronary heart disease is still controversial. Physical inactivity is but one of many factors associated with the development of coronary artery disease. Other risk factors, such as hypertension and blood lipid abnormalities, are thought to be more significant than physical inactivity in predisposing a person to heart disease. It appears, however, that physical training involving endurance-type exercise performed on a regular basis may reduce the risk of coronary heart disease. Elevated levels of serum lipids are associated with the development of coronary heart disease and exercise can reduce serum lipid levels.

A person with heart disease may have a normal heart rate, cardiac output, and oxygen consumption at rest because some of the cardiac reserve capacity is being utilized, but as mentioned previously, exercise capacity is limited. Standard exercise tests are therefore useful to evaluate the degree of cardiac disability. In an exercise test, various cardiovascular measurements are made while the subject exercises against a progressively increasing work load (e.g., walking or running on an inclined treadmill on which the speed and/or incline are increased every two or three minutes). The person continues until fatigued. The degree of cardiac impairment is given by the percent difference between the subject's maximal oxygen uptake and that predicted from normal standards on the basis of age, sex, and activity status. Maximal oxygen uptake is equal to maximal cardiac output (i.e., blood flow) times maximal arteriovenous oxygen difference (i.e., oxygen extraction).

In addition, exercise stress testing is a useful diagnostic and prognostic tool in the evaluation of people with chest pain. The use of exercise ECG testing in screening asymptomatic people to identify those with a high risk of developing coronary heart disease is controversial. People with coronary artery disease, however, may have a normal ECG at rest but show an abnormal ECG response during exercise. An abnormal ECG response occurring at a relatively low level of physical effort may indicate significant coronary artery disease. Also, the duration of exercise that can be tolerated and the maximum heart rate achieved during exercise are useful prognostic indicators in people with known coronary artery disease. Those with a low exercise capacity or low maximum heart rate (less than 120 beats/minute) generally have a poorer prognosis than those who are able to exercise longer or achieve a maximum heart rate greater than 160 beats/minute.

Physical training has a beneficial effect in people suffering from angina pectoris or convalescing after myocardial infarction. These people generally experience a subjective feeling of enhanced well-being following physical training. The maximal effort they are able to achieve after physical training is greater than before training. In addition, the amount of work done by the heart for a given amount of physical effort is less after training, indicating an improvement in the circulation. No direct effect of physical training on the heart (either beneficial or detrimental) has been demonstrated and it has been suggested that the beneficial effect of exercise is in the peripheral vascular system and in tne muscles. Probably there is less stress on the myocardium as a result of the peripheral improvement.

Decreased Physical Activity

Physical activity may be curtailed in a variety of ways and to varying degrees. The functional impairment that occurs depends on the duration and degree of limitation of physical activity. Body movement is produced when contracting muscles pull on a part of the skeleton. The stimulus for muscle contraction comes from nerve impulses. Therefore, a loss or decrease of motor function may occur as a result of disease or trauma involving the nervous, muscular, or skeletal systems.

Damage to the central or peripheral nervous system can impair motor function. For example, when consciousness is lost, no voluntary motor activity is initiated. Localized cerebral lesions (e.g., due to cerebrovascular accident) may result in a loss of voluntary movement on the opposite side of the body. Paralysis of one side of the body is called *hemiplegia*. Damage to the spinal cord above the level of C4 can result in complete paralysis of the trunk and all four limbs (*quadriplegia*). Spinal-cord lesions as low as T1 may cause complete paralysis of the trunk and legs as well as some limitation of movement of the upper extremities. Damage occurring at lower levels of the spinal cord can cause paralysis of the lower part of the trunk and legs (*paraplegia*). Damage or disease affecting peripheral nerves or neuromuscular junctions may involve varying numbers of muscles and consequently limit movement.

Damage to the muscles and skeleton can also limit movement. Muscle function may be impaired as a result of disease that affects the muscles directly (e.g., muscular dystrophy) or as a result of muscle fibers being cut, either surgically or accidentally. Movement may also be restricted as a result of injury to a tendon or ligament. Activity may be curtailed as a result of fracture of a bone or painful joint disease (e.g., arthritis).

Activity may also be limited due to diseases of the circulatory or respiratory systems. As stated previously, the ability of the respiratory and circulatory systems to deliver adequate oxygen to the muscles limits exercise capacity. As a result of pulmonary disease, decreased oxygen-carrying capacity of the blood, or heart disease, the normal demand for oxygen may not be met and activity is limited due to fatigue.

Physical activity may be restricted as a result of therapeutic measures. For example, bedrest may be prescribed when the body is unable to meet normal metabolic demands (e.g., during acute myocardial infarction). Casts, traction, monitoring devices, respirators, and other clinical devices mechanically restrict movement.

From the examples just given, it is obvious that limitation of activity may involve one limb or the whole body to varying degrees. This section is primarily concerned with the effects of prolonged bedrest. Several aspects of limitation of activity are involved when a person is confined to bed: total body movement decreases; body position remains constant in relation to gravity; and sensory stimulation is decreased. Since many movements occur in response to sensory stimulation, this sensory deprivation leads to decreased physical activity. In addition, depending on the reason that the person is confined to bed, musculoskeletal activity may be restricted or limited, for example, due to paralysis or therapeutic devices such as casts or traction.

Musculoskeletal Effects

Whether one limb is immobilized or total activity is decreased, lack of use results in muscle atrophy. *Atrophy* is a decrease in the size of a cell, tissue, or organ. Muscle atrophy involves a reduction in the diameters of individual fibers. If a muscle is im-

mobilized in the shortened state during growth, the number of sarcomeres in series along the lengths of the muscle fibers is decreased and therefore the muscle fibers are shorter.

Disuse atrophy is associated with a loss of muscle protein, including actin and myosin as well as enzymes. In addition, the number of capillaries in the muscle may decrease. As a result of this atrophy, muscle strength and endurance decrease. With prolonged bedrest, impairment of circulation contributes to the decline of endurance. Muscle atrophy due to bedrest begins after a few days in bed and primarily affects the antigravity muscles.

The pattern of nerve-impulse activity to a muscle influences the development of muscle fibers. When motor nerves are cut or destroyed, muscles not only atrophy, but muscle fibers degenerate and the number of fibers decreases.

Another effect of limitation of activity is the development of contractures. Contractures, in turn, further restrict motion—a vicious cycle. A *contracture* is a shortening of the muscle fibers, or a condition of high resistance to passive stretch of a muscle, usually due to fibrosis of the tissues supporting the muscles or the joints. When motion is restricted due to contractures more muscular energy is required in order to perform physical activity and muscular fatigue occurs more rapidly.

In the normal maintenance of the body, a constant turnover of connective tissue occurs. Collagen fibers are continuously being removed, replaced, and reorganized. In parts of the body where considerable motion occurs, such as around joint capsules and in muscle sheaths, randomly oriented fibers of collagen are laid down as a loose meshwork (loose areolar connective tissue), which permits a considerable range of motion. The collagen meshwork shortens after it is laid down. Under usual conditions this shortening process is opposed by movement of the body parts so that the degree of shortening is determined by the length to which the connective tissue is frequently stretched.

If a part of the body is immobilized, connective tissue continues to be laid down and to shorten without opposition. As a result, instead of loose areolar tissue being laid down dense connective tissue is formed. This formation of dense connective tissue (fibrosis) in the joint capsules, fascia, and muscles can occur within a week and cause loss of motion. Fibrosis occurs even more quickly in the presence of an impaired blood supply, trauma, or edema. Contractures can be prevented by performing full range-of-motion exercises every day during the period of bedrest.

Contractures around the knees, hip joints, or ankles interfere with normal standing and walking. Normal standing and walking require full extension of the hips and knees. If a person is unable to fully extend the hips or knees due to flexion contractures, considerable muscular effort is required to support the weight of the body for standing and walking and fatigue may occur rapidly. Consequently, anyone with muscular weakness may not be able to stand or walk without support following the development of contractures.

Osteoporosis is another consequence of prolonged bedrest. Osteoporosis represents an imbalance in the process of bone turnover. The chemical composition of the bone remains normal, but a net loss of bone occurs because of an increase in bone resorption (osteoclastic activity). The rate of bone formation (osteoblastic activity) is usually normal, but occasionally it is slightly decreased.

Increased bone resorption begins within a few days of immobility. In this process the matrix and collagen fibrils of the osseous tissue are degraded and resorbed and the bone minerals (primarily calcium and phosphorus) are released into the blood. As a result of the increased bone resorption the bone becomes thin and porous and fractures easily. The loss of bone tissue does not necessarily occur uniformly throughout the skeleton. Bones that normally bear weight, such as the bodies of the vertebrae, the leg bones, and the os calces (heel bones) may be affected more than other bones. Increasing the amount of calcium in the diet does not prevent the development of osteoporosis and merely adds to the load of calcium being excreted by the kidneys (see below under Metabolic and Endocrine Effects).

Circulatory Effects

Although plasma volume may be slightly increased immediately after lying down, when a person remains recumbent the plasma volume decreases. The largest decrease occurs during the first few days in bed, then the rate of decline slows. The loss of plasma appears to be due to a loss of water, since the concentrations of plasma proteins, protein-bound carbohydrate, and some other plasma solids increase. In addition, the hematocrit may increase as a result of the decreased plasma volume (i.e., hemoconcentration occurs). Consequently, blood viscosity is slightly increased. These increases are transient; as the body adapts to bedrest, regulatory mechanisms gradually restore the concentrations to normal, although plasma volume remains below normal. The loss of body water during bedrest is possibly due to increased sodium excretion (see below), although decreased ADH secretion may be a contributing factor. When a person is recumbent, left atrial volume is greater than when standing, which results in stimulation of atrial volume receptors and brings about a decrease in ADH secretion.

Some researchers report that the resting heart rate progressively increases during prolonged bedrest, but others do not observe any significant change. An increase indicates deconditioning of the heart and a decreased cardiac reserve. Following bedrest the heart rate for a given work load is greater than for the same work load prior to bedrest. The cardiovascular deconditioning, together with the loss of skeletal muscle strength and endurance, leads to a decrease in exercise capacity. Consequently a person fatigues very easily when reambulation occurs following a period of bedrest. Carefully prescribed exercises during bedrest can prevent this deconditioning.

A person confined to bed frequently involuntarily performs the Valsalva maneuver while moving about, for example while getting on or off a bedpan. The *Valsalva maneuver* consists of a forced expiration against a closed glottis, with a resultant increase in intrathoracic pressure. The increased intrathoracic pressure interferes with venous return and decreases the filling pressure of the heart. Consequently the cardiac output and coronary blood flow decrease. If the increase in intrathoracic pressure lasts more than five seconds the heart rate increases. At the end of the maneuver, when the glottis is opened, intrathoracic pressure falls and venous return is suddenly increased. As a result, cardiac output and blood pressure increase and the heart rate slows. The changes occurring during and immediately following a Valsalva maneuver do not have any adverse effect on a normal heart but may embarrass a failing heart.

When a person remains in bed in a horizontal position for more than a day or two, the normal adaptive response to the upright posture is impaired. This decreased ability to adapt to the circulatory changes that occur on standing has no significance while the person remains in bed, but results in orthostatic hypotension when she or he attempts to get up. Consequently the person feels dizzy and may faint on standing. Pallor and sweating are characteristic during the reaction. The mechanism responsible for the orthostatic hypotension that occurs as a result of prolonged bedrest is not well understood. It may be due to increased beta-adrenergic sympathetic activity, which causes vasodilation in skeletal muscles and decreases peripheral resistance. Decreased plasma volume may be a contributing factor.

Thrombosis in the deep leg veins is a possible complication of bedrest, particularly in older people. The reason for the increased risk of venous thrombosis in the elderly is not known. The calf veins are the commonest sites for thrombosis, although thrombosis may also occur in the femoral and iliac veins. A possible serious consequence of venous thrombosis is pulmonary embolism (see Chapter 7).

Swelling and pain may occur in the leg, especially if the thrombus obstructs blood flow. In the majority of cases, however, deep venous thrombo-sis is asymptomatic. A thrombus may be quite extensive and yet not cause obstruction if it is floating freely in the middle of the venous stream with only a few attachments at valve cusps and vein junctions. Often the first indication of thrombosis appears following bedrest when the person is sitting in a chair or walking about. Presumably when the leg is horizontal in bed the thrombus is elongated and blood is able to flow past it. When the person gets up, however, the leg veins are in a vertical position and the thrombus becomes shorter and wider due to the force of gravity. In this position the degree of obstruction to venous flow may be greater and swelling of the leg occurs as a result of increased venous pressure.

As discussed in Chapter 7, the factors predisposing to thrombosis are slowing of blood flow, changes in the wall of the blood vessel, and hypercoagulability of the blood. Venous stasis is believed to be the major factor in the development of deep vein thrombi secondary to immobility. Blood flow is slowed without the activity of the skeletal muscle pump. For example, during general anesthesia when the muscles are completely relaxed, venous flow in the legs is slowed. Also, following cerebrovascular accidents deep venous thrombosis is common in the paralyzed leg but occurs much less frequently in the nonparalyzed leg. The slight increase in blood viscosity from hemoconcentration during bedrest might also contribute to slowing of blood flow.

Bedrest per se does not necessarily cause venous stasis, however, because usually some muscle contractions occur while a person is in bed. Various researchers report that no decrease in venous flow rate or circulation time occurs when healthy young men are confined to bed. Some researchers, however, have found evidence of decreased flow in the clinical situation. During bedrest pockets of venous stasis may occur, especially around the cusps of venous valves, at vein junctions, and in venous sinuses within the muscles. Also, in the clinical situation other factors that increase the risk of venous thrombosis are frequently present in the people who are likely to be confined to bed. For example, a hypercoagulable state exists following surgery, accidental trauma, and myocardial infarction. The platelet count rises and platelet adhesiveness increases, the concentrations of some clotting factors increase, and fibrinolytic activity decreases in these situations.

Pulmonary Effects

As mentioned previously, the work of breathing is greater when a person is lying down than when standing or sitting. In addition, the pressure of the bed against the chest offers resistance to chest expansion. Also, when a person lies in bed the stimulatory effect of exercise on ventilation is lacking. As a result of these factors, a person confined to bed tends to breathe shallowly.

Prolonged recumbency does not affect pulmonary function in healthy young people. When ill or debilitated people remain immobilized in bed, however, hypostatic pneumonia may develop. Secretions are moved out of the lungs by coughing and by ciliary action. In addition, changes in position aid the drainage of secretions by the effect of gravity. An ill person lying in bed may not have the strength to cough well or with some conditions coughing may be painful. The cough reflex may be depressed as a result of drugs or some other factor. People who are paralyzed or unconscious cannot change position by themselves. These conditions favor stasis of secretions and pooled secretions form a fertile medium for bacterial growth.

A horizontal position also favors pooling of secretions and hinders ciliary action. With the exception of the middle-lobe bronchioles, when a person is in an upright position most of the bronchioles have their long axes vertically oriented and the layer of mucus lining the bronchioles is evenly distributed around the bronchiolar lumen. Under these conditions the cilia of the respiratory epithelium work very efficiently, sweeping the mucus and any trapped particles away from the lungs. When a person is in the supine position, however, most of the bronchioles are oriented horizontally and the mucus is no longer evenly distributed. Gravity draws the mucus downward,

so it tends to pool on the lower side, while on the upper side the mucous layer is very thin and the epithelium may become dried out. The dry mucosa is more vulnerable to bacterial invasion than a normal moist mucous membrane. The cilia on the lower side of the bronchiole may not be able to clear the mucus away as fast as it is being formed and a buildup of secretions may occur, especially if mucus production is increased. If the person is dehydrated the mucus tends to be thicker and more tenacious; in this situation it is more difficult to move the mucus out of the lungs. These factors may all contribute to the development of hypostatic pneumonia in debilitated people during bedrest.

Gastrointestinal Effects

Anorexia (loss of appetite) often accompanies prolonged rest in bed. Prolonged bedrest per se does not appear to affect the digestive functions of the GI tract or intestinal motility but these functions may be altered for other reasons when a person is ill. Absorption of nutrients may be altered, partly reflecting the internal state of the body. For example, with the development of osteoporosis calcium absorption may decrease.

When people are confined to bed in hospital their bowel habits may change. This change in habits is usually a result of changes in diet and environment, as well as decreased exercise. Constipation is often a problem.

Metabolic and Endocrine Effects

Inactivity decreases the energy requirements of the body and alters metabolism. Since endocrine activity is involved in the regulation of metabolism, bedrest also influences endocrine activity. Not only the levels of some hormones but also their circadian rhythms are altered by prolonged bedrest. Endocrine activity and the regulation of body energy stores are greatly influenced by the hypothalamus and one group of researchers has suggested that hypothalamic or hypophyseal function is impaired by prolonged bedrest.

Basal metabolic rate decreases slightly with

prolonged bedrest because of the decreased energy requirements. Mean daily body temperature also decreases, reflecting the decreased metabolism.

The mean daily concentrations of thyroxine (T_4) and triiodothyronine (T_3) increase during bedrest, possibly due to decreased cellular uptake and utilization. The T_3 level remains elevated but after about 10 days of bedrest the T_4 level reverts to normal. A large increase in thyroxine concentration occurs on reambulation, however.

Both T_3 and T_4 show circadian rhythmicity but the amplitude of the variation is very low. With usual activity, the plasma level of T_3 is highest in the early morning and gradually decreases during the day and evening. Plasma T_4 concentration shows two peaks, one occurring in the early morning and a smaller peak occurring in midafternoon. During prolonged bedrest this pattern is altered and different people show wide individual variation in the occurrence of the peaks. The normal rhythm is promptly reestablished when activity resumes.

Inactivity alters glucose metabolism. (See Chapter 18 for a discussion of glucose metabolism.) Glucose tolerance is decreased during bedrest, at least partly due to reduced uptake of glucose by the cells. The mean daily glucose concentration in the blood is not altered by 30 days of bedrest, but the amplitude of the diurnal variation is increased (i.e., fluctuations at different times throughout the day are more pronounced). With bedrest continued beyond 30 days, mean glucose concentration decreases, dropping to very low levels at some times during the day.

The mean daily plasma insulin concentration and the amplitude of the diurnal variation increase during the first 30 days of bedrest. With more prolonged bedrest the insulin level decreases toward the level observed during ambulation. Not only is the plasma insulin concentration affected by bedrest but the circadian pattern also changes. During normal activity insulin levels reflect the pattern of food intake, with large increases following breakfast and the midday meal and a smaller but more prolonged increase after the eve-

ning meal. During the first 10 to 20 days of bedrest peak insulin levels continue to occur in the early part of the day, but as bedrest continues beyond this time the peak gradually shifts until the highest concentrations of insulin occur in the late evening.

Growth hormone (GH) levels are also altered during bedrest. During normal activity GH shows diurnal variation, with peak plasma hormone concentrations occurring about 0400 h and 2000 h. After 10 days of bedrest the amplitude of the variation is greatly diminished and the mean daily GH level is decreased. During the next 10 days, however, the GH level increases. Both amplitude of the variation and the mean daily GH level are significantly increased after 20 to 30 days of bedrest. With a longer period of bedrest the circadian rhythm almost completely disappears and the mean daily level of GH decreases significantly.

The circadian rhythm of plasma cortisol is not altered by bedrest. The peak cortisol level occurs consistently at about 0800 h. With very long periods of bedrest (longer than 30 days), however, the amplitude of the variation is decreased and the mean daily cortisol concentration is decreased.

The large diurnal fluctuations that occur in the levels of glucose, insulin, and growth hormone suggest that prolonged bedrest causes an instability of the homeostatic mechanisms that regulate glucose metabolism.

Mineral and electrolyte metabolism are also altered by immobility, as reflected by urinary excretion of various substances. Sodium excretion increases during bedrest, resulting in negative sodium balance. The greatest loss of sodium occurs during the first week of bedrest. No significant changes in aldosterone secretion have been observed to account for the increased sodium excretion. It is possibly related to the increased calcium excretion (see below), since calcium and sodium excretion are linked (see Chapter 16). Negative potassium balance also occurs during prolonged bedrest. Consequently the plasma potassium level decreases slightly.

The mean daily aldosterone concentration is

not significantly altered by bedrest, although the circadian variation is affected, reflecting changes in the plasma renin level. (Recall that the renin-angiotensin system is the major factor influencing aldosterone secretion. See Chapter 12.) With normal activity the plasma renin level (and that of aldosterone) is usually maximal at about noon and then decreases later in the day and in the evening. During bedrest this pattern is altered: the level is highest in the early morning and declines during the day.

Urinary excretion of nitrogen and sulfur increase, reaching a peak during the second week of bedrest. Nitrogen excretion exceeds nitrogen intake (i.e., negative nitrogen balance occurs). Gradually, however, the body adapts to the situation and after three or four weeks of immobility nitrogen intake and output become balanced. A person swings into positive nitrogen balance when activity resumes following a period of bedrest. Both nitrogen and sulfur are constituents of protein; the increased amounts of these substances in the urine during bedrest presumably result from the breakdown of muscle protein.

A progressive increase in urinary calcium excretion occurs during bedrest. The greatest rate of increase appears to occur during the first two weeks of inactivity and the amount of calcium in the urine reaches a peak after about four weeks of bedrest. The increased urinary excretion of calcium reflects the release of calcium from the bones due to the excessive bone resorption. The increased excretion of calcium usually maintains the plasma calcium concentration within the normal range despite the excessive mobilization of calcium from the bones, although the plasma calcium may increase slightly.

Phosphorus excretion also increases during bedrest. This increase results from the loss of muscle and bone, since phosphorus is a constituent of both these tissues.

Urinary Effects

As just mentioned, urinary excretion of many substances is altered during bedrest. The high concentrations of calcium and phosphorus in the urine present a potential hazard of calcium phosphate stone formation (see Chapter 21 under Endogenous Foreign Bodies). Calcium phosphate stones are particularly likely to occur if the urine is alkaline. In addition, the supine position favors stasis of urine in the kidney pelves and stasis in turn favors the formation of urinary calculi.

Urine flows from the collecting ducts into the calcyces of the kidney. Active contractions of the calyces, renal pelvis, and ureter move the urine along the urinary tract. If the contractions of the calyces are weak, urine may pool in them (Fig. 22-5). In the upright position, stasis is likely to occur only in the lower calyx because gravity assists drainage from the other calyces. Since the ureters leave the kidneys medially, urine drains easily from the ventral portions of the calyces when a person is in the supine position, but stasis is likely to occur in the dorsal parts of all the calyces. Stasis of urine not only favors stone formation, but also favors infection. Urinary infection causes an alkaline urine, which favors precipitation of calcium phosphate, as already mentioned.

Integumentary Effects

When a person is on bedrest, unrelieved pressure on the skin can lead to the development of *pressure sores* (also called decubitus ulcers or bedsores).

The skin and subcutaneous tissue of the soles is adapted to withstand the pressure imposed on the feet by the weight of the body when a person is standing. The skin of the soles is much thicker than the skin covering other parts of the body; it is three to four times thicker than the skin of the back. The skin of the feet is also tougher because of increased thickness of the keratinous layer. The subcutaneous layer of the soles is composed of a dense network of connective tissue fibers containing small pockets of fat. This tissue can withstand the pressure from the weight of the body without being flattened.

In other areas of the body, however, the skin is much thinner and the subcutaneous tissue is com-

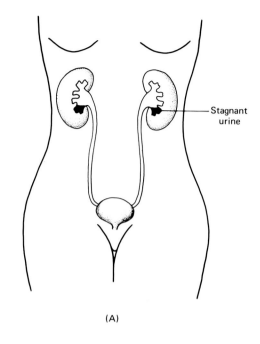

(A)

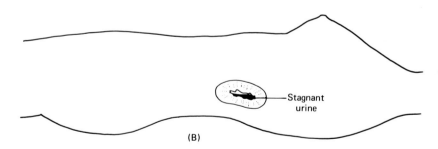

(B)

Figure 22-5. *(A) A frontal section through the kidneys showing stasis of urine in the lower calyces in the upright position. (B) A sagittal section through the kidney showing stasis of urine in the dorsal parts of the calyces in the supine position.*

posed of loose areolar connective tissue containing large soft fat globules. This subcutaneous tissue is easily flattened. Fortunately the weight of the body is spread over a large surface area when a person is lying down so that the pressure on any one point is less than the pressure on the soles of the feet when a person is standing. Unfortunately, the weight is not distributed evenly; bony protuberances support more of the weight than other areas. Consequently the skin and subcutaneous tissue covering these bony prominences is subjected to considerable pressure. The subcutaneous tissue is flattened and blood vessels in the area are compressed, blocking blood flow and causing local areas of ischemia. If the pressure is unrelieved tissue necrosis occurs. Eventually the tissue sloughs and an ulcer is formed.

Normally the part becomes painful due to ischemia or numbness and tingling occur from pressure on nerves. As a result, a person automatically alters position to relieve the pressure. Some people, however, such as those with neurological disorders, may not feel the discomfort and so remain in one position for a long time. Others may feel the discomfort but are unable to change position by themselves. For example, debilitated people may be too weak to move without assistance; those who are paralyzed are unable to change position. Some people, for example those who are unconscious, neither feel the pain nor are they able to move themselves. People who do not feel the discomfort or who are unable to respond to it are particularly likely to develop pressure sores.

Psychosensory Effects

Experiments with healthy young people have shown that a variety of psychosensory changes may occur during bedrest. Bedrest and even the anticipation of bedrest produce increased degrees of depression, hostility, and anxiety.

The EEG pattern is altered during bedrest. This change is believed to be at least partly due to decreased kinesthetic and proprioceptive stimulation as a result of decreased muscular activity. EEG sleep patterns show that the percentage of total sleep time spent in deep sleep increases with prolonged bedrest, with a resultant decrease in the proportion of light sleep. The proportion of REM sleep does not change significantly.

A variety of sensory disturbances may occur, even with short periods of bedrest. The occurrence of visual, auditory, tactile, or olfactory distortions and hallucinations has been reported. Another possible disturbance is disorientation for time or space.

SUGGESTED ADDITIONAL READING

Ciuca R, Bradish J, Trombly SM: Active range-of-motion exercises: a handbook. Nurs 78 8(8): 45–49, 1978.

Conlee RK, Fisher AG: Skeletal muscle adaptations to growth and exercise. Nurse Practitioner 4(3): 34–35, 1979.

Downs FS: Bedrest and sensory disturbances. Am J Nurs 74(3): 434–438, 1974.

Ennis S, Harris TR: Positioning infants with hyaline membrane disease. Am J Nurs 78(3): 398–401, 1978.

Kinnear GR, Bently K: Fitness and you. Can Nurse 74(6): 11–14, 1978.

Schwaid MC: Advice to arthritics: keep moving. Am J Nurs 78(10): 1708–1709, 1978.

23

Electromagnetic Radiation

All living organisms are constantly exposed to electromagnetic radiation. *Electromagnetic radiation* is composed of a system of electric and magnetic fields that travels at the speed of light. Scientists have been struggling for a long time to understand the nature of electromagnetic radia-tion; for many years physicists argued over whether it consisted of particles or waves. Scientists today accept that electromagnetic radiation has charac-teristics of both particles and waves. The smallest unit of electromagnetic radiation is called the *photon*, or *quantum*.

NATURE AND SOURCES
OF ELECTROMAGNETIC RADIATION

Electromagnetic radiation is characterized by its frequency and wavelength. The electric and magnetic fields that make up electromagnetic radiation oscillate. In other words, the intensity of the fields fluctuates between one extreme and another. The intensity builds up in one direction until it reaches a maximum; the polarity of the field then reverses and the intensity builds up in the opposite direction. The oscillating electric and magnetic fields are perpendicular to and in phase with each other. They are also perpendicular to the direction of propagation of the radiation (Fig. 23-1). The *frequency* of electromagnetic radiation is the number of oscillations, or cycles, per unit time. Just as with sound waves, the frequency is expressed as cycles per second, or hertz (Hz). The *wavelength* is the distance in the direction of propagation between two successive points that are in the same phase of oscillation. Wavelength is expressed in meters, centimeters (cm; 10^{-2} meter), millimeters (mm; 10^{-3} meter), micrometers (μm; 10^{-6} meter), or nanometers (nm; 10^{-9} meter). Sometimes wavelengths are given in Angstrom units (10^{-10} meter), but these units are not commonly used now.

Frequency and wavelength are reciprocally related, which means that as frequency increases, the wavelength decreases. Stated in another way, as the wavelength increases, the frequency decreases. The amount of energy per quantum is directly proportional to the frequency. In other words, energy increases with increasing frequency, so that the higher the frequency, the greater the energy of the electromagnetic radiation. Thus, short waves have a high frequency and high energy, whereas longer waves have a lower frequency and lower energy content.

The Electromagnetic Spectrum

Electromagnetic radiation of varying wavelengths and frequencies forms the *electromagnetic spectrum* (Fig. 23-2). The electromagnetic spectrum ranges from electrical waves many kilometers in length (waves longer than those used in radio broadcasting) to cosmic rays with wavelengths less than one billionth of one billionth of a meter (i.e., less than 10^{-18} meter). The electromagnetic radiation that is visible to human beings as light is from a very narrow region of the spectrum with wavelengths ranging from 7.5×10^{-7} to 3.8×10^{-7} meter.

The basic nature of all electromagnetic radiation is the same, but the interaction of the radia-

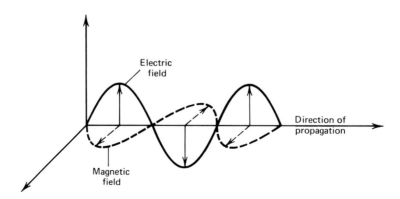

Figure 23-1. *Electromagnetic radiation is made up of oscillating electric and magnetic fields that are perpendicular to and in phase with each other.*

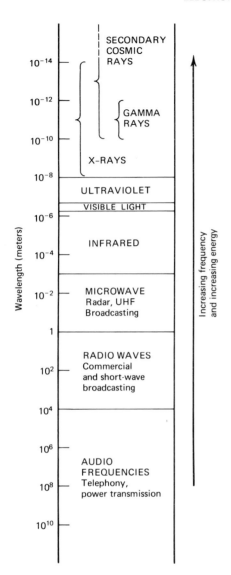

Figure 23-2. *The electromagnetic spectrum.*

different names, as indicated in Figure 23-2. For example, the region of the spectrum next to visible light but with longer wavelengths is called infrared radiation. Radiation with shorter wavelengths than visible light, but similar properties, is called ultraviolet (UV) light. The boundaries between different spectral regions are not sharp and overlap considerably. Therefore the limits of the different regions are set arbitrarily.

Natural Sources

The sun is a major source of electromagnetic radiation. Solar radiation covers the entire electromagnetic spectrum, but the earth's atmosphere acts as a screen that prevents much of the radiation, such as gamma rays and some of the UV rays, from reaching the earth. The radiation that reaches the earth is mainly infrared, visible, and UV light.

In addition to the electromagnetic radiation that reaches the earth from the sun, the earth itself emits electromagnetic radiation. Any warm object or body, including the earth, radiates infrared light. Also, certain substances within the earth (e.g., uranium and radium) spontaneously emit high-energy electromagnetic radiation.

Radioactive Isotopes

Isotopes are atoms of a single element that differ from each other in mass. For example, three isotopes of carbon exist. The most common carbon isotope has a mass of 12 atomic mass units (amu), but isotopes of carbon with 13 amu and 14 amu also exist. The difference of mass is due to a difference in the number of neutrons in the nuclei of the atoms. The number of neutrons in the nucleus does not affect the chemical properties of an atom, but does affect its physical properties. (Chemical reactivity is determined by the configuration of electrons in an atom.) Some isotopes are unstable and their nuclei tend to spontaneously break down to more stable forms, emitting highly energized particles and radiation in the process. These unstable isotopes are said to

tion with substances in terms of emission, absorption, scattering, and transmission through and around obstacles differs for electromagnetic radiation of different wavelengths. Therefore, radiation from different regions of the spectrum is used for different purposes. Also, electromagnetic radiation from different regions of the spectrum is given be *radioactive*. The process by which the unstable nuclei break down is called *radioactive decay*. Carbon-14 is an example of a radioactive isotope. Radium and uranium are also radioactive. (In addition to natural radioactivity, radioactivity can be induced by bombarding stable isotopes with highly energized particles.)

Not all radioactive isotopes decay in the same manner. Some radioactive nuclei emit alpha particles while others emit beta particles. In addition, most radioactive-decay processes are accompanied by the emission of a quantum of radiant energy called a gamma ray.

An *alpha particle* is identical to the nucleus of a helium atom: it is composed of two protons and two neutrons and carries a double positive charge. Alpha particles emitted during radioactive decay travel at a high speed, but because of their relatively large mass they do not travel very far; they are easily absorbed by a few centimeters of air. Clothing or a sheet of paper will stop the transmission of alpha particles and those striking the skin cannot penetrate past the stratum corneum. An example of an alpha emitter is radium. A radium nucleus also emits a gamma ray when it undergoes radioactive decay.

A *beta particle* has the same mass as an electron, which is much, much less than the mass of an alpha particle. (An alpha particle has more than 7000 times the mass of a beta particle.) Beta particles may be associated with negative charge, in which case they are identical to electrons; or they may be associated with positive charge, in which case they are positrons. Beta particles are ejected from radioactive nuclei at speeds close to the speed of light and can travel several meters in the air. They are more penetrating than alpha particles but can be stopped by a sheet of aluminum foil. Beta particles can penetrate about 1 cm into soft tissue. Carbon-14 is an example of a radioactive isotope that undergoes decay by emitting an electron. Phosphorus-30 emits a positron.

As already stated, *gamma rays* are quanta, or photons, of radiant energy. They have no mass; that is, they are not particles. Following emission of an alpha or beta particle by a radioactive nucleus, the residual nucleus is often in an unstable, excited state. It changes from this unstable state to a more stable state with lower energy by emitting a photon of radiant energy (i.e., a gamma ray). Gamma rays are much more penetrating than alpha or beta particles because they have no mass. Gamma rays can travel very long distances. Large masses of lead, concrete, earth, or water are required to stop their transmission.

A few radioactive isotopes (e.g., californium-252) decay by emitting neutrons. Neutrons have no charge, but have a relatively large mass (approximately one-fourth the mass of an alpha particle).

Radioactive isotopes are used for many purposes in research and industry. They are also used in health care for diagnosis and treatment. For example, radioactive iodine (^{131}I) is used to assess thyroid function and also to treat certain thyroid disorders. Radioactive isotopes are also used in the treatment of cancer. They may be implanted in the body to provide a high dose of radiation to a localized area, or they may be used as a source of radiation in external beam therapy.

Although people who work with radioactive isotopes usually take precautions to avoid exposure, some exposure to very high-energy electromagnetic radiation is inevitable. Not only people who work with radioactive isotopes in industry, research, and health care but also people who mine and mill substances such as uranium are exposed to this high-energy radiation.

Technological Sources

With modern technology and electronic devices, electromagnetic radiation from all regions of the spectrum is produced daily. Long-wavelength (low-energy) radiation is produced in radio and television broadcasting. Microwave radiation is produced for radar and communications purposes. In addition, microwave ovens are used commercially and in homes. In the health care field, microwave diathermy units are used to produce heating of deep tissues for therapeutic purposes.

Moving to shorter wavelengths, infrared radiation is emitted by hot objects such as the elements of toasters and electric stoves. Visible radiation comes from electric light bulbs and many other sources. Mercury-vapor lamps are commonly used to produce UV radiation. In addition to research purposes, UV radiation is used in the health care field for sterilization and other purposes.

At the very short-wavelength (high-energy) end of the spectrum, x rays are produced whenever a beam of high-energy electrons strikes matter. X rays are identical to gamma rays of the same wavelength. X rays are used for a number of industrial purposes, such as examining metal structures for defects. The diagnostic use of x rays in the health care field is an everyday occurrence. Color television tubes produce x rays, and many early color television sets emitted these x rays. Now, however, product safety standards in most countries require that adequate shielding be built into television sets to prevent the emission of x rays.

Everybody is exposed to electromagnetic radiation. The amount and kinds of electromagnetic radiation to which different people are exposed varies according to each person's occupation and life-style.

EFFECTS OF ELECTROMAGNETIC RADIATION

The physical, chemical, and biological effects of electromagnetic radiation depend on the amount of energy per quantum. Therefore, electromagnetic radiation from different regions of the spectrum has different effects. Radiation must be absorbed before it can exert an effect on the body. The physiological effects of electromagnetic radiation are determined not only by the energy of the radiation but also by the length of time of exposure,

the dose absorbed, and the ability of the body to repair any damage that is done.

Thermal and Photochemical Effects

The effects of electromagnetic radiation may be thermal or photochemical. When a substance absorbs electromagnetic radiation, the energy of the radiation can increase the motions of the molecules in that substance. Heat is a manifestation of the motions of molecules; therefore, when a substance absorbs electromagnetic radiation, heating can occur. In other words, the radiation has a *thermal effect*. For example, people feel warm when they sunbathe because they absorb infrared radiation from the sun.

The electrons in atoms and molecules have various discrete amounts of energy. By absorbing a packet of energy (i.e., a photon) of just the right amount, an electron may be raised a step up to a higher energy level. An electron in this higher energy level is said to be in an excited state. Atoms and molecules containing excited electrons are very reactive chemically. As a result, reactions occur that ordinarily would not proceed at the temperatures compatible with life. When the energy of absorbed electromagnetic radiation produces chemical reactions in this manner, it is said to exert a *photochemical effect*. The chemical changes that occur in the pigments of the rod and cone cells when light strikes the retina are examples of photochemical reactions. Photosynthesis—that is, the formation of carbohydrates from carbon dioxide and water by green plants when they are exposed to light—is another photochemical effect of electromagnetic radiation.

Gamma rays and x rays can produce photochemical effects. Electromagnetic radiation in the visible and ultraviolet regions produces mainly photochemical, but also thermal, effects. On the longer-wavelength (i.e., lower-energy) side of the spectrum, infrared and microwave radiation mainly produce thermal effects. Very long-wavelength radiation, such as used in radio broadcasting, is not appreciably absorbed by the body.

Ionization

Electromagnetic radiation of very short wavelengths has so much energy that it can cause an electron to be ejected from an atom or molecule, leaving behind a positive ion. (An *ion* is an atom or group of atoms carrying an electric charge.) The free electron may subsequently be recaptured by the parent positive ion, creating an excited molecule. Alternatively, the electron may be captured by a neutral molecule to produce a negative ion. Decomposition of the excited molecule may give a stable product or a free radical. Similarly, the negative ion may decompose to form a more stable ion or a free radical. A *free radical* is an atom or group of atoms containing an unpaired electron in its outer orbital. Electrons have a tendency to form pairs and they can become paired by forming a chemical bond. Therefore, free radicals are very reactive.

Very high-energy electromagnetic radiation that is capable of producing ions when it passes through matter is referred to as *ionizing radiation*. Ionizing radiation does not cause ionization every time it strikes an atom or molecule. Often it causes excitation, as described previously. Therefore, as it passes through matter, ionizing radiation leaves behind a trail of very reactive excited molecules, ions, and free radicals. Alpha particles, neutrons, beta particles, gamma rays, and x rays are types of ionizing radiation. Alpha particles have the greatest potential to cause ionization, but as mentioned previously, they are the least penetrating. Neutrons also cause considerable ionization when they pass through matter, but not quite as much as alpha particles. Beta particles have less ionization potential. Gamma rays and x rays have the least potential to cause ionization but are the most penetrating. When gamma rays or x rays strike a person, some are absorbed, some are transmitted (i.e., pass right through), and some are scattered.

Effects of Microwave Radiation

The main hazard of microwave radiation is overheating of susceptible tissues; the eyes and the testes are particularly vulnerable. These tissues have a limited flow of blood and therefore a limited capacity to remove the heat produced by absorption of microwave radiation. Exposure of the testes to microwave radiation reduces the number of maturing spermatocytes and can cause testicular degeneration. The part of the eye that is most susceptible to microwave radiation damage is the lens. Overheating causes disruption of the cells of the lens. As a result, the lens becomes opaque; that is, a *cataract* is formed.

For many years it was believed that the only biological effects of microwave radiation were thermal effects. More recent research, however, has indicated that excessive exposure to microwave radiation may interfere with nerve-impulse transmission and cause behavioral effects such as depression and difficulty in concentrating. In addition, microwave radiation can alter endocrine activity; in particular, increased thyroid activity has been reported. Microwave radiation can also cause bradycardia (slowing of the heart).

A potential hazard of the clinical use of microwave radiation is electromagnetic interference with medical electronic equipment. For example, microwave radiation can interfere with the function of electronic cardiac pacemakers. New pacemakers are manufactured with increased shielding to overcome this problem, but many older pacemakers are still in use.

Effects of Infrared Radiation

Heating is the primary effect of infrared radiation; in fact, infrared radiation is sometimes called thermal radiation. The effects of heat on the body are discussed in Chapter 24.

Like microwave radiation, long-wavelength infrared can cause cataracts. The cornea and aqueous humor are essentially transparent to the longer wavelengths of the infrared region of the spectrum, but the lens is not. The lens absorbs the longer wavelengths and heating occurs as a result. The lens is more transparent to the short wavelengths of infrared radiation and so the short wavelengths are less likely to cause cataracts.

Effects of Visible Light

Photochemical Effects

Electromagnetic radiation in the 390 nm to 780 nm wavelength region of the spectrum has many photochemical effects and is very important to human beings. As already mentioned, photochemical effects in the eye permit vision. Visible radiation also provides the energy for plant photosynthesis and therefore is the basic source of food for all animals and human beings.

One photochemical effect of light that is useful for therapeutic purposes is the breakdown of bilirubin on exposure to blue light. Bilirubin is a lipid-soluble substance derived from the breakdown of hemoglobin. It is not readily excreted from the body until it has been altered (conjugated) by the liver cells. Bilirubin easily crosses the blood-brain barrier in neonates and can cause brain damage. (Bilirubin metabolism and toxicity are discussed more fully in Chapter 26.) Exposure of the skin to sunlight or artificial illumination causes decomposition of bilirubin to a more water-soluble product, which is more readily excreted by the kidneys. In addition, this water-soluble product does not cross the blood-brain barrier as easily as bilirubin and so is less toxic. Clinically, artificial illumination of high intensity in the 420 nm to 480 nm region of the spectrum (usually cool blue fluorescent light) is used to prevent hyperbilirubinemia in newborns. This treatment takes several hours to have any effect and therefore is not very useful in cases where the serum bilirubin concentration is rising rapidly.

As already indicated, the photochemical effects of light on the eye are normal physiological events. The eye is capable of adapting to a wide range of light intensities, but extremes of light intensity may cause damage to the eye. The eye may possibly be damaged by prolonged complete darkness. If an infant's eye is covered during the critical phase of central nervous system development in the first few weeks after birth, the result may be a permanent visual defect in that eye.

Retinal Burns

At the other extreme, very intense levels of illumination can cause retinal burns (i.e., light can have a thermal effect). The cornea, aqueous humor, lens, and vitreous humor are relatively transparent to visible radiation, but pigments in the retina and choroid absorb nearly all the visible electromagnetic radiation that strikes them. Some of the energy of the radiation is converted to heat. The eye focuses light on the retina. Therefore, energy from very intense light sources is concentrated on a small area of the retina and can produce enough heat to damage retinal cells. The resulting retinal burns can produce blind spots or permanent defects of the visual field. If these defects are in the periphery of the visual field, no serious visual impairment occurs. When a person looks directly toward the source of intense light, however, the radiation is focused on the fovea centralis, which is in the center of the visual field. The fovea centralis normally is the area of greatest visual acuity. Therefore, damage to this part of the retina by intense light can result in serious impairment of vision. This mechanism is the cause of eclipse blindness, which occurs when people view solar eclipses through inadequate filters.

Effects of Ultraviolet Radiation

Ultraviolet light includes electromagnetic radiation ranging in wavelengths from about 100 nm to 390 nm. Ultraviolet radiation of wavelengths shorter than 290 nm does not reach the earth from the sun because it is absorbed by the earth's atmosphere. People can, however, be exposed to the shorter wavelengths from artificial sources.

Ultraviolet radiation has several photochemical effects. A beneficial effect of UV radiation is the conversion of provitamin D (7-dehydrocholesterol) to vitamin D_3 when the skin is irradiated. Other effects of UV radiation are harmful.

Damage to Protein and Nucleic Acids

The harmful biological effects of UV radiation result from its photochemical effects on the protein and nucleic acid constituents of cells. Certain of the amino acids in proteins can be altered by UV radiation. These alterations can change the three-dimensional conformation of a protein and influence its functioning. For example, if the protein is an enzyme, the enzyme may be inactivated. The most damaging effect of UV radiation, however, is disruption of deoxyribonucleic acid (DNA), the genetic material of the cell. Ribonucleic acid (RNA) can also be altered as a result of photochemical effects of UV radiation.

Ultraviolet radiation is absorbed by the purine and pyrimidine bases in nucleic acids and can produce structural alterations of the bases, particularly the pyrimidines. An individual base may be altered or two adjacent bases may be linked together. Structural alterations of the bases can disrupt the hydrogen bonds that hold the two strands of DNA together. Alterations of the bases in DNA can also change the genetic code and lead to the production of faulty proteins (see Chapter 3). The consequence of such changes may be only a minor functional impairment of the cell or may be cell death. Ultraviolet irradiation of cells can also interfere with DNA replication.

The germicidal effectiveness of UV light is due to its damaging effect on DNA. Ultraviolet radiation not only can kill bacteria, but also can inactivate some viruses.

Damage to DNA can be repaired, although the repair may not be complete. DNA may be repaired by photoreactivation or by the action of cellular enzymes. Several enzymes are involved in DNA repair and the process, which is complicated, is not completely understood. *Photoreactivation* is the reversal of the biological effects of UV radiation by subsequent exposure to radiation of longer wavelengths. This process may involve activation of some repair enzymes by light. In some cases photoreactivation may result from a second photochemical reaction that is the reverse of the first reaction. It is not known to what extent photo-

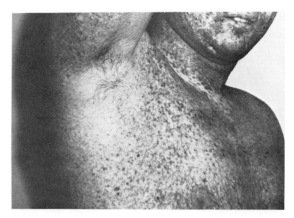

Figure 23-3. *Xeroderma pigmentosum. Axillary skin is normal because it has not been exposed to sunlight. (From Braverman IM: Skin Signs of Systemic Disease. Philadelphia, W.B. Saunders Co., 1970. By permission.)*

reactivation occurs in human cells, but it can occur in some bacteria.

Xeroderma pigmentosum is an inherited condition characterized by extreme sensitivity to sunlight. It appears that people with xeroderma pigmentosum are lacking an enzyme required for DNA repair. Following initial exposures to sunlight, affected children develop erythema (redness), freckling, and increased pigmentation of the skin. These manifestations are soon followed by dryness and scaling. The skin atrophies and fine telangiectasia develop. (*Telangiectasia* are abnormal dilations of arterioles, capillaries, or venules in the skin.) Multiple skin cancers develop after a few years and can cause death in severely affected people. Photophobia, keratitis (inflammation of the cornea), and eversion of the eyelids often occur. Blindness may result. In areas of the body not usually exposed to sunlight, the skin remains relatively normal (Fig. 23-3).

Sunburn

Sunburn is one effect of UV radiation that is familiar to many people. Caucasians are most susceptible, but Negroes can also experience sunburn. Sunburn represents the reaction of skin to

PRE IRRADIATION   POSTIRRADIATION

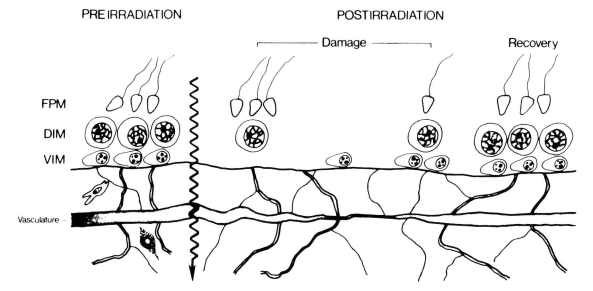

Figure 23-4. *Mechanism of damage in a radiosensitive organ (testis). The wavy arrow indicates irradiation. After irradiation the number of parenchymal cells decreases with time, resulting in damage. Regeneration of VIM cells may occur and restore the organ to its preirradiated condition. Although the vasculature may become occluded, stromal damage is not the primary cause of damage to the parenchyma. (From Travis EL:* Primer of Medical Radiobiology. *Copyright © 1975 by Year Book Medical Publishers, Inc., Chicago. Used by permission.)*

spermatocytes and spermatids (DIM cells), and spermatozoa (FPM cells). Hematopoietic tissue, the intestinal tract, and the skin also contain more than one category of cells in their parenchyma. Where this situation exists, cells move from the stem cell section (VIM) to the intermediate differentiating section (DIM) to the end cell section (FPM) as required. In these organs that contain a series of developing cells, the most sensitive cell will determine the sensitivity of the organ. Also, in these organs the parenchyma is more radiosensitive than the stroma. Radiation damage is therefore a result of destruction of the radiosensitive parenchymal cells. After irradiation, the number of all types of parenchymal cells decreases with time. For example, following irradiation of the testes sterility occurs because the immature spermatogonia are destroyed, with subsequent de-

pletion of mature spermatozoa (Fig. 23-4). The organ may be partially or completely restored to its preirradiated condition by regeneration of VIM cells, provided that some undamaged VIM cells remain. Although higher radiation doses may also cause damage to the stroma, such as narrowing and occlusion of blood vessels, stromal damage is not the primary cause of damage to the parenchyma in radiosensitive organs.

The parenchyma of some organs is composed of only RPM or FPM cells; for example the liver, muscles, brain, and spinal cord. In these radioresistant organs the stroma is more sensitive to radiation than the parenchyma. Therefore, damage to the parenchyma of these organs usually occurs secondarily to stromal damage. Damage to vascular cells may cause narrowing and occlusion of blood vessels, with subsequent ischemia. Paren-

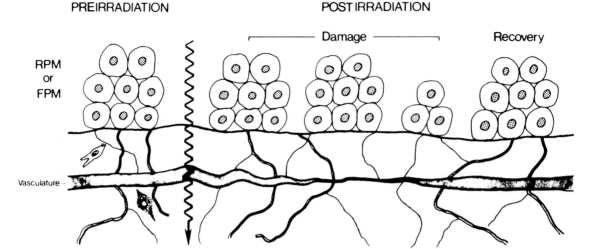

Figure 23-5. *Mechanism of damage in a radioresistant organ. Damage occurs indirectly, mainly through vascular damage. Compared to radiosensitive organs, a decrease in parenchymal cells occurs at a later time postirradiation. (From Travis EL:* Primer of Medical Radiobiology. *Copyright © 1975 by Year Book Medical Publishers, Inc., Chicago. Used by permission.)*

chymal cells will then be damaged as a result of the decreased blood supply (Fig. 23-5). Compared with radiosensitive organs, a decrease in the number of parenchymal cells occurs at a later time following irradiation.

Effects on Tissues and Organs

This section describes the effects of ionizing radiation when individual tissues and organs are irradiated (i.e., only a part of the body is exposed to radiation). Effects of total-body irradiation are discussed in the next section. Low doses refer to less than 100 rads; moderate, 100 to 1000 rads; and high doses, more than 1000 rads received in a single dose.

In most cases the visible effects of ionizing radiation on tissues and organs are no different than the changes produced by other agents that damage tissue. Inflammation, edema, and hemorrhage are the usual early changes in most organs. Healing occurs by regeneration or repair, as discussed in Chapter 8. Tissues and organs that are capable of

regeneration may be partially or completely restored to their preirradiated state, both structurally and functionally. If damage has been too great, however, regeneration may not be possible. When regeneration is not possible, healing is by repair. Repair results in the formation of a fibrous scar; therefore normal structure and function are not restored. When damage is very extensive healing may not occur and the result is tissue necrosis.

Blood and hematopoietic tissue. Hematopoietic tissue includes red bone marrow and lymphoid organs (lymph nodes, spleen, and thymus gland). It contains the stem cells for mature circulating blood cells. Hematopoietic stem cells are very radiosensitive. Low doses of ionizing radiation produce a slight decrease in the number of stem cells, but the normal number of stem cells is replaced within a few weeks by division of surviving cells (i.e., recovery occurs). A more severe depletion of stem cells occurs following moderate and high doses of radiation. In these cases recovery takes a longer time and may not be complete (i.e., stem cell numbers may be permanently decreased).

Radiation damage to hematopoietic tissue will be reflected in decreases in the number of circulating blood cells. Except for lymphocytes, which are very radiosensitive, circulating blood cells are resistant to radiation damage. They have a limited life span, however, and as they die they must be replaced by cells from the hematopoietic tissues. Therefore, following irradiation of bone marrow and lymphoid tissue, blood cell counts will be decreased. The length of time required before decreases in the number of circulating blood cells become apparent will depend on the varying sensitivities of the different stem cells and the life span of each type of cell in the circulating blood. The lymphocyte count decreases first; doses as low as 10 rads can cause a decrease. Neutrophils are affected next, but 50 rads are necessary to decrease the count. Decreased numbers of lymphocytes and neutrophils will make a person vulnerable to infection. Platelets and red blood cells are decreased at a later time and recovery also begins later. Doses greater than 50 rads are required to bring about a decrease. Hemorrhage results when the platelet count is decreased. Depression of the red blood cell count due to radiation damage to bone marrow, together with the hemorrhage, produces anemia.

Doses of radiation used for diagnostic procedures are unlikely to produce noticeable changes in the blood. Doses used for radiation therapy, however, can cause a decrease in circulating blood cells, especially leukocytes.

Gastrointestinal (GI) tract. The mucous membrane lining the GI tract consists of some differentiated, nondividing cells that are radioresistant and some undifferentiated, dividing cells that are radiosensitive. As mature surface epithelial cells die they are shed into the lumen and are replaced by cells from the dividing cell population. Different parts of the GI tract vary in their sensitivity to radiation.

The esophagus and the rectum are the most resistant portions. Moderate to high doses of radiation cause inflammation of the mucosa. High doses can result in atrophy and fibrosis; fibrosis may cause strictures. The stomach is more sensitive. Repeated small doses may cause decreased secretion of hydrochloric acid and pepsin. Moderately high doses can cause atrophy or ulceration. Healing is by repair.

The small intestine is the most radiosensitive portion of the GI tract. Epithelial cells at the tips of the villi in the small intestine do not divide. As they are sloughed each day, these cells are replaced by cells arising from the crypts of Lieberkühn at the bases of the villi. The crypts contain undifferentiated, dividing cells, which are damaged by moderate doses of radiation. Consequently the villi are shortened because there are not enough cells from the crypts to replace the surface cells as they are shed. Shortening of the villi impairs the absorptive function of the small intestine. Regeneration of the crypt cells can occur, however, and gradually the villi are restored to normal. High doses of radiation will kill so many crypt cells that not only will the villi become shortened and flattened but the intestine may also become denuded because the surface cells cannot be replaced as they are shed. The consequences are ulceration and hemorrhage. Regeneration will be minimal. Healing will be by repair or may not occur.

The large intestine is less sensitive to radiation than the small intestine. Radiation will decrease the number of epithelial cells and produce inflammation. Complete denudation is rare, however, unless very high doses are received. Serious infection may be a consequence of radiation damage to the intestine. The intestinal epithelium normally forms a barrier between the internal and external environments. Damage to the epithelium disrupts this barrier and the bacteria that normally inhabit the intestine can easily gain entrance to the blood.

The doses of radiation used in diagnostic procedures are not large enough to produce the degrees of damage just described. Therapeutic doses can cause inflammation of irradiated portions of the GI tract. Therapy involving irradiation of the abdomen often causes nausea, vomiting, and diarrhea as a result of damage to the small intestine.

Skin.   The skin is relatively sensitive to radiation because cells in the basal layer of the epidermis divide regularly to replace surface cells as they are lost. Moderate doses of radiation produce inflammation, erythema, and desquamation. Healing of the epidermis occurs by regeneration. Damage to the hair follicles causes temporary epilation (loss of hair); hair starts falling out about one week postexposure. Following high doses of radiation epilation is permanent and damage to the epidermis is more severe. Mild erythema develops a few hours after exposure but subsides within a day. A second, more severe erythema develops about a week later and is accompanied by edema. As the edema fluid accumulates it lifts the superficial layers of the skin off the basal layer, producing blisters. Enlargement of the blisters distends the skin and it cracks, producing hemorrhagic ulcers. Re-epithelialization occurs slowly and the new epidermis is thinner than the original. High doses of radiation can also cause atrophy and fibrosis of sebaceous and sweat glands, with resultant loss of function.

Very high doses can kill most of the cells of the basal layer and may also cause necrosis of underlying connective tissue. The blood vessels are blocked by thrombi and consequently the necrotic tissue is not easily eliminated. Although the necrotic tissue may become infected, little suppuration occurs because few neutrophils reach the area. Sometimes healing does not occur; when it does the process is one of repair, producing scarring and disfiguration.

Radiation doses used in therapy can cause the skin changes just described for moderate and high doses. Necrosis as produced by very high doses rarely occurs as a result of therapy with present techniques, but sometimes occurred in the past.

Gonads.   The testes are radiosensitive, but other tissues of the male reproductive system are radioresistant. As mentioned previously in the discussion of radiosensitivity, ionizing radiation destroys the spermatogonia. As a result, the number of mature spermatozoa is depleted. The spermatozoa present at the time of radiation are relatively radioresistant, therefore sterility does not occur immediately. As the sperm are lost from the testes, however, they are not replaced and sterility results. A dose of 250 rads produces temporary sterility lasting about 12 months. A dose of 500 to 600 rads can cause permanent sterility. Although ionizing radiation can cause sterility, it does not cause impotency. Exposure of the testes to ionizing radiation is always hazardous, because even if the radiation dose is not high enough to cause sterility, it can produce genetic changes that may be passed on to succeeding generations.

In females, the developing ova are contained within follicles in the ovaries, and only one mature ovum is released per month. The radiosensitivity of the follicles varies according to their stage of development. Small follicles are relatively radioresistant, but intermediate follicles are very sensitive; mature follicles are moderately sensitive. Moderate doses of radiation do not destroy the mature follicles, therefore an initial period of fertility may follow irradiation of the ovaries. The radiosensitive intermediate follicles are damaged, however, preventing maturation and release of an ovum. Therefore, the fertile period is followed by temporary or permanent sterility. Fertility may be restored as the radioresistant small follicles mature. A higher dose of ionizing radiation is required to produce permanent sterility in young women than in older women, because the ovaries of young women contain more undeveloped follicles. Regardless of age, however, a dose greater than 625 rads usually produces sterility. Follicular damage and sterilization caused by ionizing radiation may produce menopause with its associated effects on the genitalia and secondary sexual characteristics. Although low doses and some moderate doses of radiation do not produce permanent sterility, they can produce chromosome damage in the functional ova. As a result, an irradiated woman may bear an abnormal child. Even if chromosome damage does not occur, some of the bases in the DNA may be altered, resulting in genetic changes that can be transmitted to succeeding generations.

The doses of radiation used in diagnostic procedures are not large enough to produce sterility in males or females, but may cause genetic changes. Doses used in radiation therapy can cause sterility.

Eyes. Moderate doses of ionizing radiation can produce cataracts. Lens cells that are damaged by ionizing radiation cannot be removed and so they form an opacity. As a result, vision is impaired.

Heart and blood vessels. As stated previously, radiation damage to blood vessels may be responsible for parenchymal damage in radioresistant organs and can contribute to the damage in radiosensitive organs. Blood vessel endothelial cells are moderately sensitive to ionizing radiation. Following damage to these cells thrombosis may occur, with subsequent occlusion of the blood vessel. (Thrombosis is discussed in Chapter 7.) Damaged endothelium is replaced by regeneration through division of undamaged cells. In some cases too many new endothelial cells may be formed, resulting in occlusion. Damage to blood vessels may later result in petechial hemorrhages, telangiectasia, or sclerosis (hardening and loss of elasticity of the vessel wall).

The heart is not structurally damaged by low or moderate doses of ionizing radiation, but these doses can produce functional changes that are detectable on an electrocardiogram. High radiation doses can produce inflammation of the pericardium (pericarditis) or the entire heart (pancarditis).

Bone and cartilage. Mature bone and cartilage are resistant to radiation, but growing bone and cartilage are moderately radiosensitive. Growing bone and cartilage contain mature osteocytes and chondrocytes as well as rapidly dividing, undifferentiated bone-forming cells (osteoblasts) and cartilage-forming cells (chondroblasts). Moderate doses of radiation cause death of some osteoblasts and chondroblasts and temporarily inhibit cell division in others. As a result, bone growth is slowed, but recovery does occur and residual damage is minimal. High radiation doses, however, may produce permanent damage. As a result, bone growth stops. Damage is manifested later as an alteration in the size and shape of the bone.

Radiation doses used in diagnosis do not cause bone changes, but radiation therapy in children may produce bone abnormalities. Radioactive isotopes such as radium or strontium-90 that are deposited in bone following accidental absorption or following administration for nuclear medicine procedures can cause bone damage if they are not removed.

Liver. Hepatic cells are relatively resistant to radiation, but because of its large blood supply the liver is moderately radiosensitive. Damage to hepatic cells is believed to occur secondarily to radiation injury to the blood vessels and does not become manifest until several months postexposure. Liver fibrosis and possibly necrosis occur, with concomitant functional impairment and jaundice.

Lungs. Although the lungs are relatively radioresistant, moderate doses of ionizing radiation produce transient inflammation. High doses produce inflammation and exudation starting 10 to 60 days after irradiation, progressing to fibrosis in six months to a year. If both lungs are involved death is the usual outcome.

Kidneys. The kidneys also are relatively radioresistant and damage appears to be secondary to vascular injury. High doses of radiation produce a slight swelling of the kidneys initially. Damage to the tubules becomes apparent after about four months and progresses over the years. Atrophy and fibrosis of kidney parenchyma may result in proteinuria, uremia, and hypertension. The volume of tissue irradiated is important in determining the outcome. Involvement of both kidneys may lead to death. If only one kidney is affected, removal of the damaged kidney will correct the hypertension. The unirradiated kidney can function adequately to support life.

Brain and spinal cord.   Nervous tissue is the most radioresistant tissue in an adult. Although high doses are required to produce structural changes, functional changes may occur following low doses of radiation. Doses greater than 2000 rads produce inflammation and later necrosis and fibrosis in the brain and spinal cord. The damage appears to be a consequence of vascular injury.

Effects of Total-Body Irradiation

Acute exposure (i.e., total dose received in a matter of minutes) of most or all of the body to external penetrating radiation such as x rays, gamma rays, and neutrons produces the *total-body radiation syndrome*. The syndrome reflects the combined response of all body systems to ionizing radiation. Since different organs differ in their sensitivity to ionizing radiation, the syndrome is primarily determined by the effects of radiation on the most sensitive organs.

The syndrome can be divided into three stages: the prodromal stage, the latent stage, and the stage of manifest illness. The time of onset of signs and symptoms and the length of time in each stage depends on the dose received. The severity of the clinical manifestations and the time of survival are also dose dependent.

Following doses of less than 150 rads most people are asymptomatic, but some may have nausea and vomiting occurring a few hours postexposure and subsiding within 24 to 48 hours.

With doses from 150 to 400 rads prodromal manifestations of nausea and vomiting occur within an hour of exposure and subside within 24 to 48 hours. A latent period of two to three weeks follows, during which time the only symptoms are weakness and fatigue. In the stage of manifest illness chills, fever, weight loss, and in some cases epilation, occur. Other manifestations reflect damage to hematopoietic tissue: secondary infections of the upper respiratory tract, melena, he-

maturia, gingival bleeding, and mild purpura. Weakness and fatigue persist. Within six to eight weeks postexposure some people may succumb, but with adequate therapy most people survive and clinical manifestations begin to subside. Recovery usually occurs within six months.

Doses of 400 to 600 rads produce prodromal nausea, vomiting, and diarrhea within an hour postexposure. Prodromal manifestations reach their maximum intensity in six to eight hours and include weakness and fatigue, conjunctivitis, sweating, and paresthesias (abnormal sensations such as burning or prickling) as well as the nausea and vomiting. Signs and symptoms gradually subside after 48 hours and an asymptomatic latent period of 5 to 14 days follows. The stage of manifest illness begins with manifestations of hematopoietic damage as just described. In addition, within one month postexposure, hematemesis, abdominal pain, and severe diarrhea with blood in the stools occur as a result of damage to the GI tract. Hypovolemia and electrolyte imbalances are consequences of the diarrhea and vomiting. The person goes into severe shock and coma. Death may occur in spite of vigorous therapeutic measures.

A rapid onset of prodromal manifestations follows doses of 600 to 1400 rads. Signs and symptoms of the prodromal period are as just described, but more severe. A latent period of a few days may occur or the prodromal period may merge directly into the stage of manifest illness. Manifestations of GI damage predominate following irradiation with doses in this range; some people may not survive long enough for hematopoietic damage to become manifest. Gastrointestinal hemorrhage begins about eight or nine days postexposure. As mentioned previously, damage to the lining of the GI tract allows bacteria to gain access to the bloodstream. Just as this bacterial invasion is happening, the number of circulating leukocytes is decreased as a result of damage to hematopoietic tissue. The consequence is overwhelming infection, shock, coma, and death within two weeks postexposure.

Radiation doses greater than 2000 rads produce death within a few days as a result of damage to the central nervous system. Within minutes postexposure sweating, nausea, vomiting, diarrhea, paresthesias, nervousness, and confusion are manifested. Convulsive seizures, coma, and death soon follow. The nature of the damage to the central nervous system is not completely known. Death is believed to be due to increased intracranial pressure as a result of edema following damage to blood vessels.

Effects on the Embryo and Fetus

A newborn child is made up of millions of cells that have been derived from one cell, the fertilized ovum, as a result of repeated cell divisions and differentiation. Consequently, the embryo and fetus are extremely sensitive to ionizing radiation. Radiation may be lethal or it may produce gross abnormalities of the fetus. Specific effects depend on the time of gestation when irradiation occurs.

Prior to implantation (i.e., from conception to about the seventh day postconception) the fertilized ovum undergoes cleavage to produce a ball of cells. Since the few cells present at this stage are the progenitors of many other cells, damage to one cell has a high probability of producing lethal effects. Low to moderate doses of radiation at this time, therefore, often result in prenatal death. If the embryo survives, usually no abnormalities are present at birth.

The period from the second through the eighth weeks postconception is the stage of major organogenesis in the embryo. During this time rudiments of all the organs and limbs are differentiating. Not surprisingly, irradiation during this stage has a high probability of producing gross abnormalities. The likelihood of prenatal death is less at this stage than before implantation, but neonatal death may occur as a result of congenital anomalies.

The developing nervous system and sense organs are particularly sensitive to radiation. In contrast to the adult nervous system, which is composed mainly of nondividing, highly differentiated, radioresistant cells, the neuroblasts (stem cells of the nervous system) in the embryo and fetus are undifferentiated, actively dividing cells that are radiosensitive. Exposure of the embryo to ionizing radiation may produce abnormalities such as microcephaly (abnormally small head and brain), hydrocephaly (excessive accumulation of cerebrospinal fluid in the ventricles of the brain), microphthalmia (small eyes), or mental retardation.

Exposure to ionizing radiation can also damage the developing musculoskeletal system, although it is not quite as radiosensitive as the nervous system. Irradiation of the embryo may cause limb abnormalities or stunting of growth.

During the fetal stage, from the ninth week until term, cells are more differentiated than at earlier stages of development. From the 9th to 20th weeks ionizing radiation still may produce gross abnormalities, but after the 20th week the fetus is more radioresistant. Irradiation of the fetus between 20 and 40 weeks gestation is less likely to produce obvious structural abnormalities or death (i.e., higher doses are required to produce these effects), but may produce functional defects that become manifest shortly after birth or later in life (e.g., sterility). Irradiation during this stage may also produce malignant changes, particularly leukemia, later in life.

Late Effects of Ionizing Radiation

People who survive acute low doses of radiation may have incurred damage that does not become manifest until many years later. Similarly, people exposed to chronic low doses of radiation may manifest signs of radiation damage after many years. Chronic low doses means low doses of radiation repeated many times over a long period, such as received by people who are occupationally exposed to ionizing radiation or those who are exposed to many diagnostic procedures utilizing ionizing radiation.

Cancer is one possible late effect of ionizing radiation. Skin cancers were common on the hands of radiologists and people working with radioactive isotopes before this danger was realized and adequate precautions taken (Fig. 23-6). Leukemia is another malignancy commonly produced as a result of radiation exposure. Bone cancer is a

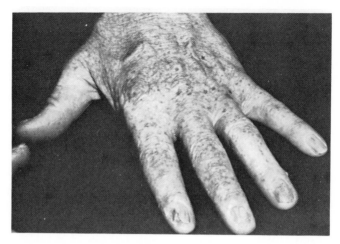

Figure 23-6. *Radiodermatitis with nail dystrophy in a dental technician. (From Braverman IM: Skin Signs of Systemic Disease. Philadelphia, W. B. Saunders Co., 1970. By permission.)*

late effect of absorption and deposition of radioactive isotopes in bone. Many cases of thyroid neoplasia have been reported as late sequelae to irradiation of the neck and chest.

Another possible effect of ionizing radiation is decreased longevity. This effect is difficult to prove because so many factors influence life span. When the longevity of people occupationally exposed to chronic low doses (e.g., radiologists) is compared with the longevity of people not so exposed, however, the average life span of those who are chronically exposed is shorter.

EFFECTS OF ELECTRICITY

Current electricity refers to a continuous movement of electric charges through a conducting medium. A complete circuit (i.e., a continuous loop), with a source of electrical energy, is required in order for current to flow. Current is expressed in units called amperes (A); one ampere corresponds to the movement of one coulomb of charge past some point in an electric circuit in one second. Current can also be expressed in milliamperes (mA); 1000 mA equals 1 A.

The amount of current that will flow through a conductor is determined by the voltage difference between two points in the circuit and by the resistance of the circuit to the flow of charge. Increasing the voltage and/or decreasing the resistance will increase the current. When the resistance is high, very little current flows. As electric charges move through a material that offers resistance, some of the electrical potential energy is dissipated and appears as heat.

Current may be direct or alternating. *Direct current* (DC) means the movement of electric charges is always in the same direction. Batteries are examples of sources of direct current. *Alternating current* (AC) periodically reverses direction. The usual current provided to homes from generating stations is alternating current. Alternating current is actually a form of electromagnetic radiation with very long wavelengths. The usual frequency of alternating current produced by generators in North America is 60 Hz.

Physiological effects of electricity are mainly determined by the amount of current flowing through the body, not by voltage. The amount of current entering the body, the path taken by the current, and the duration of the current are the main factors that determine the harmful effects of electricity. In general, the amount of direct current required to produce a certain effect is greater than the amount of alternating current that is required.

The amount of current that enters the body will be determined by the electrical characteristics of the part that is exposed to the source of electricity. For example, dry skin offers a high resistance to current flow, but wet skin offers little resistance. Therefore, if the skin is dry less current will enter than if the skin is wet. The path taken by the current will be determined by the conductivity of the tissues (i.e., the current will take the path of least resistance). The amount of resistance offered by the tissues will also determine how much energy is dissipated as heat. The body fluids are electrolytic solutions, which are fairly good conductors; the skin has a much higher resistance. As a result, serious skin burns often occur at the points where the current enters and leaves the body. Electrical current tends to travel along the paths of nerves and blood vessels, which have low resistance. Passage of electrical current causes blood to coagulate. Blood vessels may therefore be occluded, resulting in ischemic necrosis of tissue. Neurological complications may occur as a consequence of nerve damage due to heat or ischemia.

With 60 Hz alternating current the threshold for perception of current entering the hand is less than 1 mA. With direct current about 5 mA are required to produce a sensation. Slightly more than this amount causes pain. About 6 to 9 mA AC (40 to 60 mA DC) will cause involuntary muscle contractions that are so strong a person cannot let go of the source of current.

Current entering through a hand and leaving the body through any other extremity must cross the chest and can cause ventricular fibrillation. If immediate treatment is not available, death results. If the electric shock is brief, the phase of the cardiac cycle when the shock is received is critical in determining whether fibrillation will occur. Fibrillation will only occur if the current passes through the heart during repolarization of the ventricles, which is represented by the T wave on an ECG. With a heart rate of 72 beats/minute, one cardiac cycle is completed in less than a second. Therefore, about 100 mA AC crossing the chest for one second or longer will usually cause ventricular fibrillation. About 500 mA DC are required to produce fibrillation. When the current is delivered directly to the heart (e.g., by internally implanted electrodes or cardiac catheters), extremely small amounts of current can produce fibrillation. Even if fibrillation does not occur, electrically shocked people may develop other cardiac arrhythmias or nonspecific electrocardiographic abnormalities.

Electric shock can cause fibrillation, yet electric shock is also employed to defibrillate the heart. The rationale for this seemingly paradoxical situation is that an electric shock of high enough intensity momentarily depolarizes most of the heart muscle fibers. The uncoordinated contractions are thus halted and the sinus node can be reestablished as the cardiac pacemaker.

Electric current passing through the body from head to toe can cause respiratory arrest as a result of disrupted functioning of the respiratory center in the brainstem. Usually such a passage of current does not cause other injury so that affected people may eventually recover, although they require assisted ventilation for a long time.

In electroconvulsive therapy, 60 Hz alternating current of several hundred milliamperes is passed across the cerebrum. The results are brief respiratory arrest, convulsions, unconsciousness, and amnesia.

SUGGESTED ADDITIONAL READING

Deering RA: Ultraviolet radiation and nucleic acid. *Sci Am* **207**(6): 135–144, 1962.

Guimond JH, Wilson SG: Postirradiation thyroid disorders. *Am J Nurs* **79**(7), 1256–1258, 1979.

Pryor WA: Free radicals in biological systems. *Sci Am* **223**(2): 70–83, 1970.

Scott E: Radiation protection for nurses. *Nurs Times* **75**(11): 441–445, 1979.

24
Heat and Cold

Normally the body temperature is kept within a narrow range, because even slight changes in temperature can alter the rates of chemical reactions and many physiological processes are the results of biochemical reactions. At low temperatures functioning is impaired because biochemical reactions are slowed. At high temperatures reaction rates are increased, altering function. In addition, enzymes can be denatured and become nonfunctional at high temperatures. Therefore several homeostatic mechanisms exist to regulate the body temperature. Failure of these mechanisms can result in a severe disruption of homeostasis. In addition to systemic effects, heat and cold can cause serious local damage in the form of burns and frostbite.

REGULATION OF BODY TEMPERATURE

Body temperature is not uniform. The center, or *core* of the body, which has a temperature maintained within narrow limits, is surrounded by an outer shell of variable temperature (Fig. 24-1).

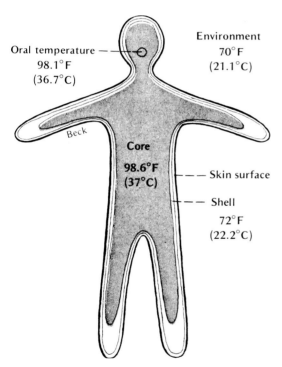

Oral temperature —
98.1°F
(36.7°C)

Environment
70°F
(21.1°C)

Beck

**Core
98.6°F
(37°C)**

— — Skin surface

— — Shell
72°F
(22.2°C)

Figure 24-1. *The skin and subcutaneous tissues form an insulating shell around the body's core. The core temperature is maintained relatively constant, whereas the temperature of the skin surface fluctuates according to the amount of cutaneous blood flow and the environmental temperature. The shell temperature varies between that of the core and that of the skin surface. (From Landau BR: Essential Human Anatomy and Physiology. Copyright © 1976 by Scott, Foresman and Company. Reprinted by permission.)*

The shell is an insulating layer of variable thickness consisting of the skin, subcutaneous tissue, and variable amounts of deeper tissues of the extremities. Heat from the body's core is carried to the surface by the blood and the temperature of the skin surface is determined by cutaneous blood flow as well as by the temperature of the external environment. Usually the surface temperature is lower than the core temperature. Rectal temperature gives the best indication of core temperature.

Although 37 °C (98.6 °F) is often stated as the "normal" body temperature, different people have different temperatures and the variation among healthy people may be as much as 1.5°C (3°F). The normal range of body temperatures and the body temperatures under various conditions are shown in Figure 24-2. Not only are there interindividual variations in body temperature, but for a given person the body temperature varies throughout the day. The temperature is usually lowest in the early morning and highest in the evening, although this pattern may be altered in people who work night shift or who travel by jet across time zones. In women the body temperature also varies with the menstrual cycle. It is usually higher during the postovulatory phase of the cycle, probably because of an effect of progesterone on the hypothalamus.

To maintain thermal balance (i.e., a constant body temperature), heat gain must equal heat loss. The major source of body heat is cellular metabolism. When the external environment is warmer than the body, however, heat may also be gained from the surroundings. In this circumstance, the only way that heat can be lost from the body is by evaporative cooling. When the external environment is cooler than the body, heat can be lost in several ways.

Heat Production

Heat is a by-product of the metabolic reactions in the body and therefore is produced continuously. At rest most of the body heat comes from metabolism in the brain and viscera (especially the liver)

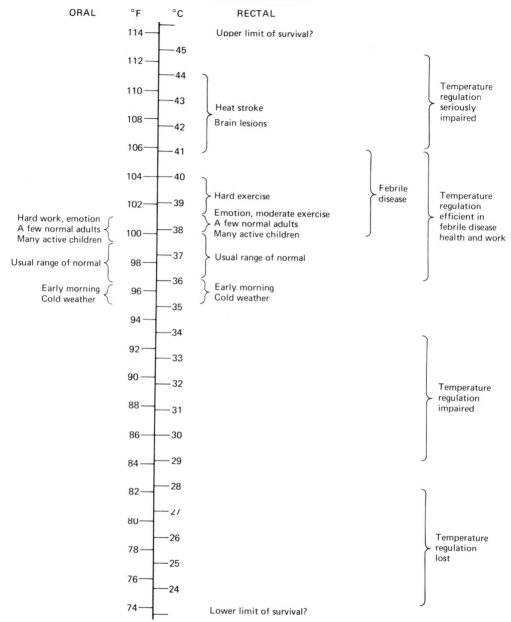

Figure 24-2. *The body temperature under various conditions, including the usual range of normal. (Adapted from DuBois EF:* Fever and the Regulation of Body Temperature. *Springfield, Ill, Charles C Thomas, 1948. Courtesy of publisher.)*

and approximately one-fifth comes from metabolism in the skeletal muscles. During physical exertion, however, the muscles may produce as much as three-quarters of the total heat. After meals heat production is increased by the specific dynamic action of foods, especially protein.

Muscular Activity and Shivering

The major mechanism for increasing heat production to maintain thermal balance is increased skeletal muscular activity. This increased activity may be brought about by voluntary movement or by *shivering*. Shivering is an involuntary act involving rhythmic muscle contractions initiated by impulses from an area of the hypothalamus. The impulses are transmitted to motor neurons and initially cause a progressive increase in muscle tone, which greatly increases heat production. Shivering begins when the muscle tone increases above a critical level and consists of synchronous contractions of small groups of motor units out of phase with other groups and coinciding with antagonists so that gross limb movements do not occur.

Although muscular activity greatly increases heat production, it also increases heat loss. During activity the body core is extended toward the body surface (i.e., the size of the shell decreases) because the skeletal muscles are close to the surface and they are generating heat as well as receiving increased blood flow. Therefore the insulating layer is thinner and more heat is lost by conduction. In addition, muscular activity involving limb movement increases convection and therefore increases heat loss (see below). Less heat is lost with shivering than with voluntary activity because shivering does not increase convection to as great a degree.

Nonshivering Thermogenesis

In addition to heat production by skeletal muscular activity, heat can be produced by nonshivering thermogenesis. *Nonshivering thermogenesis* refers to an increase in metabolism that does not come from muscle contraction but occurs in response to cold. An immediate short-term increase in metabolism is probably mediated by increased sympathetic activity and increased levels of circulating epinephrine and norepinephrine. Cold also stimulates the release of thyrotropin-releasing factor (TRF) from the hypothalamus, which stimulates the release of thyroid-stimulating hormone (TSH) from the adenohypophysis. TSH in turn stimulates the synthesis and release of thyroxine (T_4) and triiodothyronine (T_3) by the thyroid gland. T_3 and T_4 stimulate metabolism and increase heat production (see Chapter 19). This stimulation of the thyroid gland in response to cold does not occur immediately in adults and is probably significant only when exposure to cold is prolonged. Infants and children however, have a prompt increase in the plasma TSH level in response to cold.

Brown fat is a major site of nonshivering thermogenesis in newborns and young infants. Brown fat differs from ordinary adipose tissue in that brown fat cells contain many mitochondria and have numerous small fat droplets suspended in the cytoplasm. The brown color is due to the iron-containing cytochromes in the mitochondria. The large number of mitochondria give brown fat cells a high capacity for oxidative metabolism. Ordinary white adipose tissue cells contain few mitochondria and have a single large fat droplet surrounded by a thin rim of cytoplasm. Norepinephrine from sympathetic nerves stimulates metabolism in the brown fat cells. Triglycerides are split into glycerol and free fatty acids, but in contrast to white fat cells, the brown fat cells do not release the fatty acids. Instead, some of the fatty acids are oxidized within the cell and some are resynthesized to triglycerides. This biochemical cycle converts chemical energy to heat energy. Brown fat has a very rich blood supply to distribute the heat to the rest of the body.

Brown fat is located in subcutaneous deposits between the scapulae and around major blood vessels in the thorax and neck. Deep deposits are located beneath the sternum and around the spine, aorta, and kidneys. Therefore brown fat is strategically located to warm the blood supplying vital organs.

Exchange of Heat with the External Environment

Radiation

All things emit heat by *radiation* in the form of infrared electromagnetic waves, which can pass through a vacuum and travel at the speed of light (see Chapter 23). Therefore heat is transferred from the sun and surrounding objects to the body by radiation and at the same time heat is radiated from the body to the surroundings. The amount of infrared radiation emitted by a mass is proportional to the temperature of the mass. Therefore, if the surroundings are warmer than the body, more heat is radiated to the body than is radiated from it and the body has a net gain of radiant heat. If the surroundings are cooler than the body (the usual situation), more heat is radiated from the body than is radiated to it and the body has a net loss of heat. The amount of heat lost will depend on the temperature gradient between the skin surface and the surroundings. The greater the temperature difference, the more heat will be lost.

Conduction

Conduction is the direct transfer of heat from one atom or molecule to another by transfer of kinetic energy. All atoms and molecules are constantly in motion (i.e., they have kinetic energy). Heat is a manifestation of this motion and represents a quantity of energy. When atoms or molecules collide, kinetic energy can be transferred from one to another (i.e., heat is conducted). For conduction to occur a temperature gradient must exist between two objects or masses and the direction of heat transfer is always from the mass at the higher temperature to the mass at the lower temperature. When the temperatures are equal, no heat will flow.

Thus, for example, heat is conducted from the body to a cold chair or object in contact with the body. The amount of heat lost this way is usually minimal, however, because the object soon warms up to the body temperature and no further heat transfer occurs. On the other hand, heat can also be conducted from a warm object (e.g., a hot water bottle or an electric blanket) to the body.

Specific heat is the amount of heat required to raise the temperature of one gram of a substance by one degree Celsius. Air has a relatively low specific heat. When the air is cooler than the body, heat is conducted from the body to the air, but because of the low specific heat of air the layer of air immediately surrounding the body reaches skin temperature with a minimal loss of body heat.

Water has a much higher specific heat than air and is more dense than air, which means that much more heat is required to raise the temperature of a given volume of water by one degree than is required to raise the temperature of the same volume of air by one degree. Therefore, if the body is immersed in water at a lower temperature, a large amount of heat is conducted to the water before the water temperature reaches body temperature and heat transfer stops. (If a person is immersed in a cold lake or ocean, or course, the water temperature will remain colder than the body temperature and heat loss will continue. If a person is wearing clothing or a wet suit, however, a layer of water is trapped next to the skin. This layer will warm up to body temperature and act as an insulating layer, which slows the rate of heat loss from the body.) Water also has a higher conductivity than air. *Thermal conductivity* is the rate of heat transfer (i.e., the amount of heat that flows per second) per one degree Celsius difference in temperature between two objects or between an object and its surroundings. Therefore the body loses heat much more rapidly when immersed in cold water than in air of the same temperature. Conversely, heat can be rapidly transferred to the body by immersion in a warm bath. (Although water has a relatively high thermal conductivity relative to air and substances such as fat, it has a very low thermal conductivity compared to substances such as metals.)

Convection

Convection is the transfer of heat from one place to another by the motion of a heated fluid (either a gas or a liquid). *Natural convection* results from the change in density that occurs when a fluid is heated. For example, when the surrounding air is cooler than the body, the air next to the body is warmed by conduction and radiation from the body. The heated air is less dense, therefore it rises and is replaced by cooler air, setting up a flow of air known as a *convection current*.

As stated earlier, in order for heat to flow, a temperature gradient must exist. When the layer of air next to the body reaches body temperature, heat conduction stops. When the warmed air is replaced by cooler air as a result of convection currents, however, the thermal gradient is maintained and more heat is lost from the body. When the air is calm, the amount of heat lost by conduction and convection usually represents only a small portion of the total heat loss from the body.

The movement of a fluid by fans or pumps is referred to as *forced convection*. Wind may also be considered as forced convection. When a wind is blowing the air next to the body is replaced with cooler air at a faster rate and may not have time to reach body temperature. Therefore a larger temperature gradient is maintained between the body and the surrounding air and a considerable amount of heat can be lost. Convection is also an important factor in heat loss from the body when a person is immersed in water.

Skin Surface Temperature and Surface Area

As mentioned previously, the exchange of heat between the body and the external environment depends on the presence of a temperature gradient between the skin surface and the surroundings. Therefore, the skin temperature is an important determinant of the rate of heat loss from the body. Since most of the body's heat is produced in the body core, heat must be transferred from the core to the skin before it can be lost from the body. This heat transfer takes place by conduction through the tissues and by the flow of warm blood from the core to the skin.

Transfer of heat to the skin surface by conduction from the center of the body occurs at a slow rate because the subcutaneous tissues act as an insulating layer. The subcutaneous fat is especially important as an insulator because fat has a much lower thermal conductivity than other tissues. The thicker the fat layer, the more effective the insulation. Thin people lose body heat by conduction at a faster rate than obese people. This factor may influence the length of time a person can survive in cold water.

Blood flow through the skin is much more important than conduction in determining surface temperature and heat loss from the body. Unlike the thermal conductivity of the tissues, which is constant, skin blood flow can be varied over a wide range and can be regulated (see below). In addition to the usual capillary beds, the skin and subcutaneous tissue contain venous plexuses that are connected to arterioles by arteriovenous anastomoses. When the anastomoses are open (i.e., dilated), blood is shunted from the arterioles to the superficial venous plexuses, greatly increasing skin blood flow and bringing more heat to the surface. When the anastomoses are closed (ie., constricted), blood flow through the venous plexuses may almost cease and very little heat escapes to the surface.

The amount of heat radiated and conducted from the body is also influenced by the surface area that is exposed to the external environment. Curling up is an innate behavioral response to cold which serves to decrease the exposed surface area and reduce heat loss.

Evaporative Cooling

In addition to heat loss by radiation, conduction, and convection, heat is lost from the body by evaporation of water from the skin surface and the

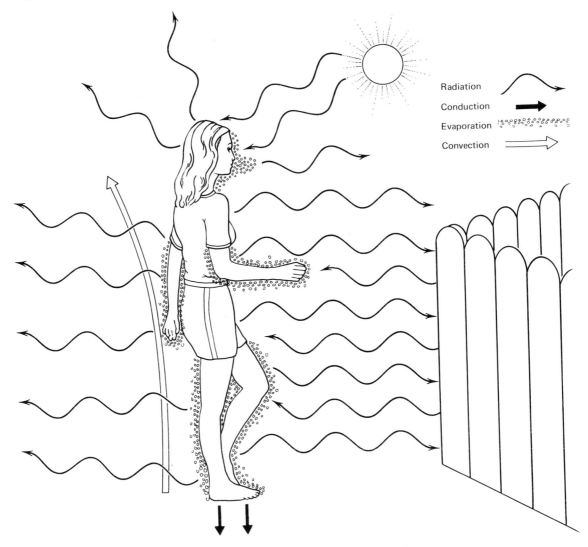

Radiation	
Conduction	
Evaporation	
Convection	

Figure 24-3. *Mechanisms of heat exchange with the external environment.*

lungs (Fig. 24-3). Heat is required to convert a substance from the liquid to gaseous state. Whenever water vaporizes from the body surface, the heat that is necessary for this process is provided by the body and the body surface is cooled. When the external environment is warmer than the body, heat is gained from the surroundings by radiation and conduction and the only mechanism for heat loss is evaporative cooling.

The skin is not completely watertight and water vapor continuously diffuses through the skin. This water loss is referred to as *insensible perspiration* because a person is not aware of it. The amount of insensible perspiration increases with increased skin temperature. Insensible water loss also occurs as a result of vaporization of water from the lungs. The amount of water vapor lost from the lungs is influenced by the rate and depth of breathing and by the temperature and water vapor content of the inspired air. The amount of insensible water loss cannot be controlled by the body for purposes of temperature regulation and heat is always being lost by this route.

When heat production increases due to exercise or when the temperature of the external environment reaches a point at which heat loss by other means is no longer adequate, *sweating* occurs to increase heat loss by evaporative cooling. Sweat is also referred to as *sensible perspiration*. The apocrine sweat glands, which are located mainly in the axillae and pubic regions, do not have a thermoregulatory function. The eccrine sweat glands, which are distributed over the entire skin surface, function in the control of body temperature and are innervated by sympathetic cholinergic fibers. (Most sympathetic fibers are adrenergic.) The eccrine sweat glands can also be activated by emotion or stress, unrelated to the need for body cooling. This response is presumably due to a generalized increase in sympathetic activity.

Sweating is effective as a means of heat loss only if the sweat evaporates. Sweat that drips off the skin has no cooling effect. When the air is saturated with water vapor, sweat cannot evaporate and evaporative cooling does not occur. Therefore, sweating is a much more effective mechanism for cooling the body under warm dry conditions than under hot humid conditions.

Convection currents increase the effectiveness of evaporative cooling. When the air is still, the layer of air immediately next to the skin becomes saturated with water vapor and further evaporation cannot take place. Convection currents move the saturated air away from the skin surface and replace it with unsaturated air.

Nervous Control of Body Temperature

Regulation of body temperature is coordinated by the hypothalamus. The hypothalamus acts as a "thermostat" that compares the actual temperature with a reference, or set-point, temperature and activates the appropriate effector mechanisms to maintain the body temperature at the desired level. (See the discussion under Components of Negative Feedback Control Systems in Chapter 1.) Two areas of the hypothalamus are involved in temperature regulation. Heat loss is controlled by an area in the anterior, or preoptic, region. An area in the posterior portion of the hypothalamus controls heat production.

The hypothalamus receives input from peripheral temperature-sensitive receptors in the skin, from central temperature sensors in the anterior hypothalamus, and possibly from other receptors in the body core. Thermoreceptors in the anterior hypothalamus sense the temperature of the blood flowing through the hypothalamus and provide information about the core temperature. Two types of receptors in the skin provide input regarding the surface temperature. One group of receptors (cold receptors) responds to lower temperatures, and the other group (warm receptors) responds to a higher range of temperatures. The rate of firing of these receptors is influenced not only by the actual temperature at the body surface but also by temperature changes.

The peripheral receptors provide afferent input to the cerebral cortex as well as to the hypothalamus. In addition, impulses from the hypothalamus are relayed to the cerebral cortex. The impulses reaching the cerebral cortex are responsible for conscious sensations of heat or cold. Efferent impulses from the cerebral cortex initiate conscious voluntary behaviors such as putting on warmer clothing in response to cold.

When the core temperature rises above the set point, effector mechanisms are activated to increase heat loss from the body (Fig. 24-4). Sympathetic nerves to skin blood vessels are inhibited, resulting in vasodilation. As a result more heat is delivered to the body surface for dissipation by radiation, conduction, and convection. If this mechanism is not adequate to bring the body temperature back to the desired level, active sweating is stimulated.

In addition to activating heat-loss mechanisms, mechanisms that decrease heat production are also

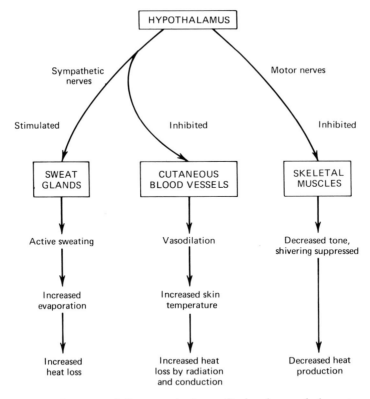

Figure 24-4. *Summary of effector mechanisms utilized to decrease body temperature.*

instituted. Heat production cannot decrease below a minimal level due to basal metabolism, but in response to heat muscle tone decreases and a person usually decreases voluntary activity. In addition, appetite is decreased. (Recall that heat production increases following a meal due to the specific dynamic action of food.)

In response to cold, mechanisms to conserve body heat are activated first. Sweating is inhibited. Sympathetic nerves to the skin blood vessels are stimulated, causing vasoconstriction. Therefore the skin cools and less heat is lost by radiation and conduction. If these mechanisms are not adequate to maintain the core temperature, heat production is increased. Nonshivering thermogenesis is stimulated, muscle tone increases, and shivering may occur as described previously. Voluntary ac-

tivity may increase and the appetite increases. These mechanisms are summarized in Figure 24-5.

HEAT STRESS

Hyperthermia

Whenever heat gain exceeds heat loss the body temperature rises. An elevation of the body temperature above the normal range is called *fever*, *pyrexia*, or *hyperthermia*. The term fever is also used to denote any disease characterized by fever (e.g., typhoid fever, yellow fever). *Hyperpyrexia* means a highly elevated body temperature.

Three basic mechanisms can produce an eleva-

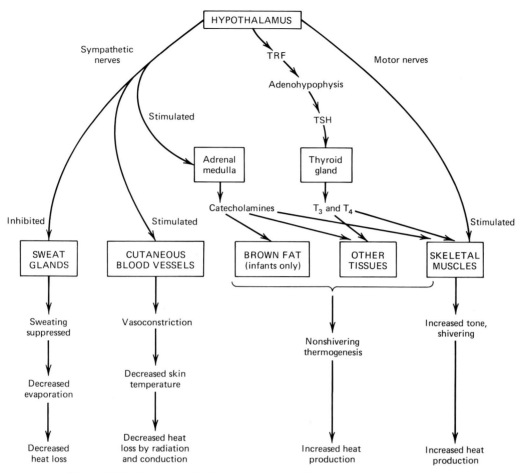

Figure 24-5. *Summary of effector mechanisms utilized to raise body temperature.*

tion of the body temperature above the normal range: (*1*) elevation of the set point; (*2*) heat production and/or gain of heat from the external environment exceeding the body's capacity for heat loss; or (*3*) primary failure of temperature regulation.

Fever Resulting from Altered Set Point

Fever due to inflammation or infection appears to result from an increase in the set point. In other words, the "thermostat" is set higher. The body temperature is then regulated at the higher level. Substances that induce fever by this mechanism are called *pyrogens*. Pyrogens from the external environment, such as infectious agents, are called *exogenous pyrogens. Endogenous pyrogen* is produced within the body. It is a small protein that is released from leukocytes and probably also from reticuloendothelial cells such as Kupffer cells in the liver. Exogenous pyrogens probably act by causing the release of endogenous pyrogen. Endogenous pyrogen acts on the preoptic region of the hypothalamus and raises the set point.

When the set point is first raised a person feels cold because of the discrepancy between the actual body temperature and the set-point temperature.

Heat-conservation and heat-production mechanisms are activated to raise the body temperature to the new set point. Sweating ceases. Vasoconstriction occurs, so that the skin is cold and pale. Metabolism increases, muscle tone increases, and shivering may occur. This stage of fever is often referred to as *chills.*

When the body temperature reaches the new set point, heat production and heat loss are regulated to maintain the temperature at the elevated level. At this point the person has no subjective feeling of being cold or hot, but the skin may feel warm to touch. The metabolic rate is high to maintain the higher temperature. In addition, however, the increase in temperature itself causes biochemical reactions to speed up and increases metabolism. The increase in metabolism increases oxygen consumption by the cells. Therefore the rate and depth of breathing and the heart rate increase to deliver more oxygen to the tissues. Insensible water loss increases due to the increased body temperature and increased ventilation. Therefore water deficit may occur, with its associated signs and symptoms (see Chapter 12). The elevated body temperature affects neurological function and may cause drowsiness, restlessness, or delirium. Convulsive seizures may occur, especially in young children (see Chapter 9). Headache may occur due to dilation of meningeal blood vessels.

Anorexia often occurs during fever. Decreased food intake together with the increased caloric requirement due to increased metabolism results in increased utilization of fat and increased breakdown of body proteins for energy, especially if the fever is prolonged. Ketosis may occur due to the increased fat catabolism. The increased protein catabolism causes increased urinary excretion of nitrogen, muscle wasting, and weakness.

When the cause of the fever is removed, the hypothalamic thermostat is reset to the normal level. The person enters the stage of *defervescence* and the fever "breaks." Now the body temperature is higher than the set point. Therefore the person feels hot and mechanisms to decrease heat production and increase heat loss are instituted. Shivering is inhibited. Cutaneous vasodilation occurs, the skin is warm and flushed, and sweating is profuse. These mechanisms lower the body temperature to the normal level.

Excessive Heat Gain

Heat gain in excess of the body's capacity to dissipate heat will cause the body temperature to rise. Excessive heat gain can occur when heat production is increased, when the temperature of the external environment is warmer than body temperature, or when both factors are operating.

An abnormal increase in metabolism due to hormonal imbalance can cause excessive heat production and produce fever. Fever accompanying hyperthyroidism is usually mild, but life-threatening hyperpyrexia can occur with thyrotoxic crisis (see Chapter 19). Excessive release of epinephrine and norepinephrine due to pheochromocytoma (a tumor of the adrenal medulla) can also produce fever.

Intense physical activity at moderate ambient temperatures or moderate work in a hot environment will cause an increase in body temperature as heat production exceeds the capacity for heat loss. During activity vasodilation occurs in the skeletal muscles. In addition, cutaneous vasodilation occurs to increase skin blood flow to dissipate the heat and to provide water to the sweat glands. Vasoconstriction occurs in the splanchnic circulation, but this mechanism is not sufficient to offset the decrease in peripheral resistance due to vasodilation in the muscles and skin. Therefore cardiac output increases to maintain the blood pressure and to maintain increased blood flow to the skin for heat dissipation. In unacclimatized people the increase in cardiac output is brought about mainly by an increase in heart rate. At very rapid heart rates, however, stroke volume decreases and eventually cardiac output falls. (See Chapter 22 under Exercise.) When an adequate cardiac output can no longer be maintained, weakness, dizziness, and possibly syncope occur.

As acclimatization occurs, a person is able to work more comfortably in a hot environment, and a smaller rise in body temperature occurs with a given amount of exercise. Three cardiovascular adaptations are important in heat acclimatization: (1) maximal cardiac output increases: (2) peak heart rate decreases; and (3) stroke volume increases for a given unit of heat stress. Therefore delivery of heated blood from the muscles to the skin is more efficient, and heat dissipation is facilitated. In addition, during the first two weeks of heat exposure a greater quantity of sweat is produced in response to a given amount of heat, and the sodium concentration of the sweat decreases. The decrease in sodium concentration is brought about by increased secretion of aldosterone. After longer periods of time in a hot environment sweat production declines, probably because physical conditioning results in increased metabolic efficiency so that the amount of endogenous heat production for a given work load is less. Decreased endogenous heat production and more efficient heat dissipation are responsible for the smaller rise in body temperature for a given amount of exercise in an acclimatized person.

Heat stress produces three types of disorders: heat cramp, heat exhaustion, and heat stroke.

Heat cramp.   This condition is characterized by brief, painful, intermittent skeletal muscle cramps following intense physical activity in a hot environment. The precise mechanism responsible for heat cramps is not known, but it is believed to be caused by acute sodium depletion. Heat cramps occur especially in people who are in good physical condition and acclimatized to heat. These people produce large quantities of sweat in response to hard muscular activity. Cramps typically occur when water intake is adequate to replace sweat losses, but sodium replacement is inadequate.

Heat exhaustion.   This condition occurs not only in those engaging in physical activity in a hot environment, but also in inactive people under hot, humid conditions. Heat exhaustion is the most common disorder resulting from heat stress and

two forms occur. One form is primarily due to sodium depletion and the other form is primarily due to water depletion.

Heat exhaustion due to sodium depletion occurs mainly in unacclimatized people and results from replacing sweat losses with water only. It differs from heat cramp in that it is accompanied by systemic effects. Hypotension and rapid heart rate are characteristic findings. Body fluid volume is not usually significantly decreased, therefore urine volume and sweat volume remain normal. The body temperature is usually normal or subnormal. As a result of the sodium deficit the extracellular fluid is hypoosmotic and water shifts into the cells. (See also Chapter 11 under Movement of Fluid Between Compartments and Chapter 12 under Sodium Deficit.) Signs and symptoms caused by sodium depletion include profound weakness, fatigue, headache, anorexia, nausea, vomiting, diarrhea, and muscle cramps. Affected people are not usually thirsty.

Heat exhaustion from water depletion occurs when the volume of water lost by sweating is not replaced. This form of heat exhaustion usually occurs when water is unavailable or the supply is limited. It also occurs in infants and debilitated adults who are unable to express their desire for water and unable to obtain water for themselves. Signs and symptoms of water deficit occur (see Chapter 12). The body temperature is elevated and thirst is intense. Other symptoms include weakness and impaired judgment. Eventually central nervous system dysfunction may cause muscle incoordination and hyperventilation. The hyperventilation produces respiratory alkalosis and tetany. This form of heat exhaustion may progress to heat stroke.

Heat stroke.   This condition is characterized by a rectal temperature greater than 41.1 °C (106 °F), delirium, coma, and lack of sweating (*anhidrosis*). The skin is hot and dry. At the body temperatures occurring with heat stroke, hyperthermia may be considered as an endogenous systemic burn. When the high temperature is maintained over a period of hours, cellular damage occurs (see the discussion under Burns).

Heat stroke typically occurs when the environmental temperature and the relative humidity are high for several days and nights. People with cardiovascular disease, the elderly, and the chronically ill are especially at risk. People with heart disease may not be able to increase cardiac output to maintain adequate skin blood flow for heat dissipation and sweat production. When high temperature and humidity is sustained for several days, sweat production is continuous at first, but eventually the sweat glands fail and the body temperature rises. A vicious cycle is then established because the high body temperature increases the rate of biochemical reactions (i.e., increases metabolism) and produces more heat. When sweating fails the body is unable to dissipate the heat because heat loss due to radiation and conduction can only occur when the temperature of the external environment is lower than the body temperature. As the body temperature rises, cells are damaged and nervous system function is impaired. Heat stroke is lethal unless effective cooling measures are promptly instituted. Even with treatment, some people do not survive.

The first manifestation of heat stroke may be sudden collapse, but some people have prodromal symptoms of nausea, weakness, dizziness, headache, and a feeling of excessive body heat. Other people may have signs and symptoms of water-depletion heat exhaustion before heat stroke occurs. Those who survive heat stroke often have a persistent inability to tolerate heat, possibly due to injury to the sweat glands.

Heat stroke can also be induced by physical exertion in a hot environment, when endogenous heat production exceeds the capacity to dissipate the heat. In this case heat stroke can occur after a few hours, even though sweating does not cease and the skin is moist rather than dry. Heat stroke induced by physical exertion usually occurs in otherwise healthy young people such as athletes and military recruits. It may also occur in people who are occupationally exposed to high temperatures (e.g., boiler-room workers).

Failure of Temperature Regulation

Hypothalamic lesions (e.g., from traumatic injury or tumors) may impair the functioning of the temperature-regulating center and produce hyperthermia. In this case the regulating center is unable to respond appropriately to afferent input and fails to initiate heat-loss mechanisms. Anhidrosis may occur. As with heat stroke, a vicious cycle is established, and lethal temperatures may be reached if effective treatment measures are not promptly instituted.

Burns

Heating of tissues above a critical temperature at which they are damaged produces a burn. Overheating of tissues may be caused by hot air, flames, steam, hot liquids, or hot objects in contact with the skin. Water is the main component of tissues and like water, tissues have a relatively high specific heat and low thermal conductivity. Therefore tissues become overheated slowly but also cool slowly. Consequently the duration of overheating of tissues is longer than the time that the tissues are actually in contact with the agent causing the burn. The degree of damage caused by thermal injury is determined by the temperature and its duration of action. For example, necrosis of epidermal cells occurs after one second at 70 °C or three minutes at 50 °C. A temperature of 42 °C (107.6 °F) acting for six hours can cause total necrosis of the skin. (Thus the danger of applying hot water bottles or heating pads to unconscious people.)

Threshold overheating of tissues causes inapparent, reversible cell damage. With a greater degree of overheating, foci of irreversibly damaged cells are scattered in living tissue. Above a critical threshold of overheating, necrosis of the entire tissue occurs. Colliquative necrosis occurs at temperatures below 58 °C; temperatures above 65 °C cause coagulative necrosis. With colliquative necrosis the tissue initially appears normal histologically. After a period of time, however, nuclear changes are apparent and nuclei and cytoplasm of the cells disintegrate due to the digestive action of cellular enzymes. Consequently the necrotic tissue becomes liquified. With coagulative necrosis changes are immediately apparent in the cell nuclei and further changes to not occur. The basic cell outline is preserved, but the cytoplasm is clumped and opaque, presumably due to denaturation of cellular proteins. (When a protein is denatured the polypeptide chains become randomly oriented and the specific three-dimensional conformation of the protein is lost. As a result, the protein becomes nonfunctional and some of its properties are altered.) The thick coagulated crust, or slough, which develops as a result of a burn is called an *eschar*.

With deep burns there is no sharp demarcation between necrotic skin and healthy tissue, but a gradual transition with a wide range of intermediate injuries. Thus regeneration of the skin proceeds from partly damaged tissue, not from healthy tissue. This fact is one reason why burns do not heal as quickly as wounds of the same depth that are produced by mechanical trauma.

Factors Determining the Severity of Burn Injuries

The main determinants of the local and systemic responses to a burn are the extent of the burn and its depth. Other factors influencing the severity of a burn injury are the person's age and prior state of health, and the part of the body affected.

The *extent*, or size, of a burn is expressed as a percentage of the total body surface area. Several methods using charts and tables are available for estimating the extent of a burn. A widely used and easily remembered method for determining the size of a burn in an adult is the "rule of nines" (Fig. 24-6). This rule divides the body into areas of 9% or multiples of 9% of the total surface area. A child has different body proportions than an adult and body proportions change as a child grows. Therefore the rule of nines is not accurate for determining the extent of burns in children.

Several classifications of the *depth* of burns have been proposed at different times. The traditional classification of burns into first-, second-, or third-degree categories is now largely being re-

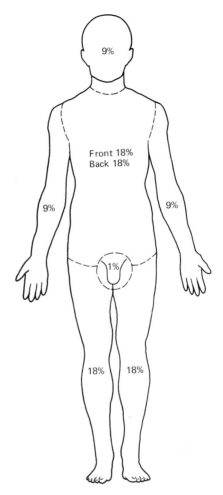

Figure 24-6. *The "rule of nines" for estimating the extent of a burn.*

placed by their classification as partial- or full-thickness burns. *First-degree burns* involve damage to the superficial layers of the epidermis (Fig. 24-7). An inflammatory reaction produces erythema, but accumulation of interstitial fluid is minimal or absent. First-degree burns heal by regeneration in a relatively short period of time. *Second-degree burns* involve destruction of the entire epidermis, including the germinal layer, and part of the dermis. The skin appears red and thick-walled blisters form. Despite the destruction

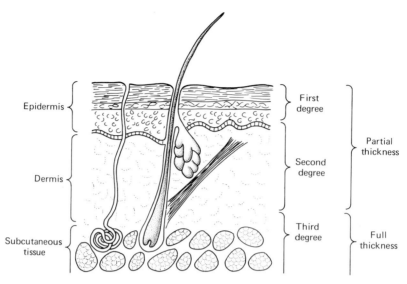

Figure 24-7. *Classification of the depth of a burn.*

of the germinal layer of the epidermis, regeneration is possible because parts of hair follicles, sweat glands, and sebaceous glands that lie deeper in the dermis are not destroyed and can provide epithelial cells to form a new epidermis. Healing is slow, however. A *partial-thickness burn* is equivalent to a first- or second-degree burn.

Third-degree burns involve the entire thickness of the skin; both the epidermis and dermis are destroyed. A *full-thickness burn* corresponds to a third-degree burn. In some cases deeper tissues may also be damaged or destroyed. These burns require grafting because regeneration of the skin is impossible. Full-thickness burns usually have a leathery texture and may appear white, brown, black, or red. If they are red, pressure does not cause blanching. In contrast, the redness of partial-thickness burns blanches with pressure. With full-thickness burns the nerve endings in the dermis are destroyed, therefore no pain or temperature sensation is felt. In contrast, with partial-thickness burns sensitivity to pain and temperature is normal or increased.

The part of the body affected also influences the severity of a burn. Burns of the perineum are espe-cially prone to infection. Burns of the head and neck are frequently accompanied by burning of the airway, although involvement of the respiratory tract may occur even in the absence of skin burns. Inhalation of flames or very hot air produces laryngeal edema, which can cause asphyxia. When noxious fumes and smoke are inhaled they act on the lower respiratory tract and may cause a severe tracheobronchitis. Death may occur from acute pulmonary edema.

Age influences the severity and prognosis of a burn. Infants and young children have a thinner epidermis than adults and consequently are more prone to full-thickness burns, especially from hot liquids. Also, the mortality rate is higher for children under 2 years of age and adults over 60 years old than it is for people of other ages with burns of similar extent. Infants and elderly people have a weaker immune response and therefore are more prone to develop fatal infections. In addition, elderly people often have preexisting cardiovascular disease which is exacerbated by the stress resulting from a burn.

Previous health status influences the prognosis following a burn. An active disease process may be made worse or a latent disease may be activated by the stress resulting from the burn. For example, the prognosis is more serious for people with heart disease or diabetes mellitus than for those who were previously healthy. Excessive tissue loss can occur following a burn in those with severe peripheral vascular disease or diabetes.

Partial-thickness burns covering less than 10% of the body surface are considered *minor*. Partial-thickness burns covering more than 20% of the body surface or full-thickness burns exceeding 10% of the surface area are considered *major*. A burn is also considered major if it involves the face, hands, feet, or perineum; when the burn victim is under 2 years of age or over 60 years; or when other traumatic injuries or preexisting disease are present.

Systemic reactions to minor burns are minimal and systemic therapy is rarely required. Therapy is directed at cleanliness and comfort of the local burn wound. A minor wound usually heals within a few weeks. With major burns, however, every system of the body is affected, a variety of complications can occur, and affected people are *acutely* ill for weeks or even months until grafting is completed and the burn wound has healed.

Systemic Effects of Burns

Hypovolemia.   Depending on the temperature and duration of heat, variable amounts of tissue are actually destroyed, as mentioned previously. The tissues surrounding and immediately underneath the destroyed tissue are still viable, but are damaged. The capillaries in the damaged tissue dilate and their permeability increases from an inflammatory reaction. Consequently, *fluid shifts from the plasma into the interstitial space* (see Chapter 11 under Plasma-to-Interstitial-Fluid Shift). With a minor burn the fluid is returned to the circulation by the lymphatics and little or no edema develops. When the burn is large, however, the amount of fluid that leaks from the capillaries exceeds the capacity of the lymph system. In addition, the lymphatics may have been damaged by the burn.

Consequently fluid collects in the interstitial space, producing edema and swelling. Most of the fluid collects in the subcutaneous tissue spaces, but some may leak into the skin and appear as blisters or be lost as exudate.

Not only water and electrolytes but also plasma proteins shift to the interstitial space as a result of the increased capillary permeability. More albumin than globulin leaks out of the capillaries, presumably because of the smaller size of albumin molecules. Therefore the albumin-to-globulin ratio is decreased. The total amount of circulating *plasma protein is decreased* because of this shift, but a transient hyperproteinemia may occur because the loss of plasma water is usually relatively greater than the loss of plasma protein. Hypoproteinemia usually follows, although the nature and amount of fluid therapy will influence the actual plasma protein concentration. The plasma protein level returns to normal in about a week when the extent of the burn is less than 10% to 15% of the body surface area. The hypoproteinemia is more prolonged and severe in people with more extensive burns, however.

As a result of the shift of fluid to the interstitial space, blood volume is decreased and *hypovolemic shock* may occur. Pain and fear may cause neurogenic shock immediately following a burn, but the major cause of shock in burned people is hypovolemia. (Shock is discussed in Chapter 14.) Sodium loss may contribute to the hypovolemia (see below).

Burned skin is more permeable to water than normal skin. Therefore *insensible water loss is increased.* If the burn area is large, this insensible water loss can contribute to the hypovolemia.

Red blood cells circulating in the skin are hemolyzed by a direct effect of the heat at the time of burning. Therefore, if the burn area is large, a significant *reduction in red blood cell mass* can occur and contributes to the decrease in blood volume. Despite the loss of erythrocytes, the hematocrit usually rises immediately after a severe burn because the decrease in plasma volume is proportionately greater than the decrease in blood cell volume. After a few days, however, the hematocrit decreases as fluid shifts back into the vascular compartment. In addition to the immediate destruction of some red blood cells, others are sublethally damaged and have increased fragility, resulting in delayed hemolysis. Loss of red blood cells produces acute *anemia* (see Chapter 10). Hemoglobin that is released into the plasma from hemolyzed red blood cells combines with a plasma protein called haptoglobin. When all the haptoglobin is bound with hemoglobin, excess free hemoglobin is present in the blood (*hemoglobinemia*), and hemoglobin may appear in the urine (*hemoglobinuria*). Hemoglobinuria may produce kidney damage, but the mechanism by which it does so is not understood.

Several compensatory responses occur in response to the hypovolemia (see Chapter 14 under Hypovolemic Shock). Interstitial fluid from the unburned area shifts to the vascular compartment, heart rate increases, and vasoconstriction occurs in the splanchnic area and unburned areas of the skin. Decreased blood flow as a result of hypovolemia and vasoconstriction produces additional effects. *Gastrointestinal absorption is decreased.* Gastrointestinal ischemia plus decreased motility due to the stress response (see Chapter 2) may produce *paralytic ileus. Vomiting* may occur if food or fluids are ingested. Decreased renal blood flow causes a decrease in the glomerular filtration rate. In addition, secretion of aldosterone and ADH are stimulated to promote renal conservation of sodium and water. Therefore *oliguria* or even anuria may occur.

Reabsorption of edema fluid. With partial-thickness burns the inflammatory reaction and shift of fluid to the interstitial space continue for 12 to 14 hours. With more severe burns the plasma-to-interstitial-fluid shift continues for 36 to 48 hours or sometimes longer. Then as capillary tone and permeability return to normal and the tissue pressure rises to equal the capillary pressure, fluid shifts back into the intravascular compartment. This *shift of fluid from the interstitial space to the plasma* may cause *circulatory overload,* with its associated danger of pulmonary edema, if fluid intake is not carefully monitored and controlled. The increase in blood volume from the reabsorption of edema fluid results in increased urine output. The diuresis may last as long as two weeks.

Electrolyte imbalances. After a burn, potassium ions are released from the damaged cells. If renal function is adequate, the potassium is excreted in the urine. If renal function is impaired, however, *hyperkalemia* may occur in the immediate postburn period (see Chapter 16). By the second week postburn, potassium deficit and *hypokalemia* may occur from increased urinary losses as a result of increased aldosterone secretion and from gastrointestinal losses, especially if vomiting has occurred. Increased protein catabolism is a contributing factor (see below). Lack of intake can also contribute, if intravenous fluids are not supplemented with potassium.

As a result of altered permeability, the damaged cells not only release potassium ions but also take up an abnormal amount of sodium ions. In addition, sodium ions may be lost from the body in burn exudate and gastrointestinal drainage. Consequently *hyponatremia* may occur during the first few days postburn. (See Chapter 12 under Sodium Deficit for a discussion of the manifestations of this imbalance.)

Acid-base imbalances. In the early postburn period mild respiratory alkalosis may occur due to hyperventilation. The hyperventilation is believed to be caused by pain and anxiety.

If significant hypovolemia or shock occur, metabolic acidosis results. The poorly perfused tissues produce lactic acid from anaerobic glycolysis (see Chapter 10). In addition acidic substances are released from the damaged tissue and contribute to the metabolic acidosis. (The manifestations of acid-base imbalances are discussed in Chapter 15.)

Metabolic effects. The *metabolic rate increases* considerably after a burn. The hypermetabolism is accompanied by weight loss from increased catabolism of protein and fat and loss of body water. In some cases the weight loss may be related to decreased intake as well as to increased metabolism. All the factors underlying the derangement of metabolism following a burn are not understood. Increased need for heat production to offset evaporative cooling resulting from increased insensible water loss may contribute, but is not the essential cause of the hypermetabolism. Infection may also contribute. Increased sympathetic nervous activity and increased secretion of catecholamines, cortisol, and growth hormone as a result of the stress caused by the burn are believed to be major factors responsible for the altered metabolism. (See Chapter 2 under Physiological Responses to Stress.)

Hyperglycemia occurs within a few hours after burn injury. It usually lasts several hours but may last several days. It is accompanied by decreased glucose tolerance and a relative insulin resistance. These effects are presumably caused by the increased secretion of epinephrine, which stimulates hepatic glycogenolysis; by increased cortisol, which promotes gluconeogenesis; and by increased growth hormone, which decreases cellular uptake of glucose and antagonizes insulin action (see Chapter 18). *Glucosuria* may occur as a result of the hyperglycemia.

Catecholamines, cortisol, and growth hormone also stimulate lipolysis and the plasma level of free fatty acids may rise. The fatty acids appear to be completely oxidized in most cases, but occasionally ketonemia and ketonuria may occur. (See the discussion of utilization of lipids in Chapter 17.)

The outpouring of cortisol from the adrenal cortex in response to stress causes excessive protein catabolism, particularly in the skeletal muscles. During the first day postburn, nitrogen may be retained if oliguria occurs, but beginning about the second day postburn, nitrogen excretion is increased. In addition, protein is lost in exudate from the burn wound. The person is in a state of *negative nitrogen balance* that may last for days or weeks. Immobilization following a burn contributes to the protein catabolism (see Chapter 22). The increased protein catabolism is associated with a release of potassium, magnesium, phosphorus, calcium, and sulfur from the cells and increased excretion of these substances. Consequently deficits of these minerals may occur. With burns involving less than 10% to 15% of the body surface the duration of negative nitrogen balance is short and the loss of protein is small. In people with more extensive burns the loss is much greater and more prolonged. Age, sex (males lose more nitrogen than females), previous nutritional status, intake of carbohydrate and protein, and presence or absence of infection can all influence the amount and duration of excess nitrogen loss.

Infection

During the first day or two postburn, hypovolemic shock is the major threat to life. After this period, however, infection is a major cause of death. All burn wounds become contaminated with microorganisms, but whether or not serious infection occurs depends on the virulence of the organisms and the defenses of the burned person. (See Chapters 28 and 29 for a discussion of the factors influencing infection.)

Immediately after the burn accident the wound may become contaminated by bacteria that survive in the hair follicles and sweat glands underneath the burned tissue, by dirt from the accident site, or by microorganisms on the clothing. Later, microorganisms from the perineal area or from the nose and throat may spread to the burn wound. In hospital, cross-contamination from other patients and from hospital personnel can occur.

A wide variety of microorganisms can infect burns. Common culprits are the gram-negative bacteria *Pseudomonas aeruginosa* (*pyocyanea*), *Proteus vulgaris,* and *Escherichia coli;* the gram-positive bacterium *Staphylococcus aureus,* and the fungus *Candida albicans.* Infection of the burn wound may delay local healing, may convert a partial-thickness injury to a full-thickness defect from destruction of remaining epithelial cells by bacteria and/or their products, and may cause failure of grafts to take. Infection can also cause prolonged loss of protein and water from the burn wound and contribute to the metabolic derangement and anemia that accompanies severe burns. Significant infection depends not merely on the presence of organisms in the wound but also on the *number* of organisms. When the number is large enough to overwhelm host defenses, microorganisms and/or their toxins may enter the blood stream and produce *septicemia*. Fatal septic shock may result. (Septic shock is discussed in Chapter 14.) Pneumonia and urinary tract infections can also be serious problems in burned people.

Other Complications of Burns

In the early postburn period edema may cause problems. Laryngeal edema may cause *airway obstruction*, as mentioned previously. With circumferential burns of the neck or chest, edema developing under the constricting eschar may cause pressure on the trachea or rib cage and produce *respiratory distress.* Linear incisions may have to be made in the eschar (escharotomy) to relieve the constriction. Edema developing under the constricting eschar of circumferential burns on the arms or legs may produce enough pressure to occlude veins and arteries. Ischemic necrosis of the distal part may result.

As mentioned previously, hyperglycemia often occurs in the early postburn period. This condition is usually transient, but occasionally it persists or recurs and becomes more severe. When hyperglycemia persists the condition is called *pseudodiabetes*, or *burn diabetes*. It appears to be related to the same factors that cause hyperglycemia and insulin resistance in the early postburn period. It may culminate in *hyperosmolar nonketotic coma* (see Chapter 18 under Acute Complications of Diabetes). High-carbohydrate feedings appear to be the precipitating cause, but degenerative changes in the pancreatic islet cells may occur in some cases.

Acute duodenal or gastric ulceration (*Curling's ulcer*) is a fairly common complication of severe burns. Microscopic or gross hemorrhage occurs from these ulcers and contributes to the anemia following a burn. The etiology of Curling's ulcer is not well understood, but stress appears to be an important pathogenetic factor (see Chapter 2 under The General Adaptation Syndrome).

Thromboembolism may occur following burns, particularly in elderly people. (Thrombus formation and embolism are discussed in Chapter 7.) Immobility, preexisting cardiovascular disease, and prolonged intravenous infusion through a cutdown in a deep vein are predisposing factors.

Hypertension may develop as a complication of severe burns, particularly in children. The cause of this hypertension is unclear, but it may be related to excessive catecholamine secretion.

COLD STRESS

Hypothermia

Whenever heat loss exceeds heat production, the body temperature falls. A decrease in body temperature below the normal range is called *hypothermia*. When the body temperature falls, the rate of biochemical reactions slows (i.e., the metabolic rate decreases). Therefore the cells require less oxygen. For this reason, hypothermia is sometimes therapeutically induced (e.g., during heart surgery).

Causes

Three basic mechanisms produce hypothermia: (*1*) decreased heat production; (*2*) excessive heat loss; and (*3*) impairment of temperature-regulating mechanisms.

Decreased heat production. Metabolic heat production requires oxygen and an energy supply in the form of carbohydrates or fat. When the fuel for metabolism is in short supply, heat production is limited. Therefore the body temperature is usually subnormal in people with severe malnutrition (see Chapter 17) and those with conditions that impair delivery of oxygen and nutrients to the tissues (e.g., shock).

Thyroid hormones are important regulators of metabolism. People with hypothyroidism have a low basal metabolic rate and intolerance of cold. Severe hypothermia occurs in people with myxedema coma (see Chapter 19).

Heat production is minimal when a person is inactive, therefore immobility (e.g., due to paralysis) can predispose to hypothermia. An elderly person living alone may become hypothermic after falling and lying on a cold floor for several hours before being found.

Excessive heat loss. Excessive heat loss as a result of accidental exposure to cold is a common cause of hypothermia. People who for any reason are stranded outdoors during cold weather may suffer from hypothermia if they are unable to maintain heat production at a sufficient rate to offset heat loss. In addition, infants and elderly people living in inadequately heated homes during cold weather are prone to develop hypothermia.

Hypothermia may occur during hiking expeditions if hikers are not adequately clothed, especially under conditions of wind and rain or snow. If the clothing becomes soaked through heat is lost from the body at a faster rate. Wind acts as forced convection and increases the rate of heat loss, as mentioned previously. The need for increased metabolic heat production together with the exertion of hiking may cause exhaustion, after which the person may be unable to maintain adequate heat production to offset the loss of body heat.

Immersion in cold water (e.g., as a result of boating accidents) leads to a rapid loss of heat from the body, as discussed previously. When the water temperature is below 25 °C, swimming produces a faster decline in body temperature because it increases heat loss. When people who are not wearing lifejackets are immersed in cold water their body temperatures fall rapidly, coordinated activity becomes impaired, and they are unable to swim. Their struggles then lead to inhalation of water and drowning. On the other hand, people wearing lifejackets do not need to swim or make other movements to stay afloat and lose heat more slowly. If rescue is not prompt, however, hypothermia leads to death.

Impairment of temperature regulation. Hypothermia may be precipitated by intracranial lesions such as cerebrovascular occlusion, neoplasms, or traumatic injuries that impair the functioning of the temperature-regulating center. A variety of drugs can also impair temperature regulation. For example, ethanol causes cutaneous vasodilation, which increases heat loss. It also decreases shivering and depresses the temperature-regulating center. Therefore people who are exposed to cold after ingesting ethanol are prone to develop hypothermia.

Effects

Death can result from severe hypothermia, but the exact cause of death is not always known. Hypothermia by itself does not appear to cause death of tissues, but alterations in physiological processes during cooling and rewarming are probably responsible for most deaths. Survival appears to be determined mainly by the circumstances of cooling and resuscitation. There are many reports of people being revived after they had been severely hypothermic for many hours and appeared to be dead. The lower limit of body temperature at which survival is possible is not known. People have been successfully resuscitated after induced hypothermia during which the core temperature fell as low as 5 °C. With accidental hypothermia people rarely survive core temperatures below 24 to 26 °C, but occasionally people with temperatures as low as 16 to 18 °C have been revived.

As the core temperature falls the body institutes mechanisms to conserve heat and increase heat production. Intense cutaneous vasoconstriction and shivering occur, although shivering may not be visible in elderly people. If these mechanisms are not adequate, the body temperature falls further and tissue metabolism progressively slows. At core temperatures below 33 to 32 °C temperature regulation is impaired. Vasoconstriction is still intense but shivering usually stops and the muscles become increasingly stiff as the body temperature falls. Below 24 °C vasoconstriction can no longer be maintained and the body temperature drops further as more heat is lost to the external environment.

A person is usually alert and well oriented at body temperatures above 34 to 33 °C, but as the core temperature falls mental responses become slower and the person becomes drowsy. Voluntary movements gradually become slower as the body temperature decreases. When the core temperature reaches 34 to 32 °C movements become uncoordinated and speech becomes difficult. As the body temperature declines further, consciousness is depressed. At core temperatures between 29 and 27°C a person's eyes may still be open and limb movements may occur in response to noxious stimuli, but spontaneous movements and speech do not occur. When the core temperature reaches about 26 °C a person usually does not respond to any stimulus.

During the early stages of hypothermia the heart rate increases due to sympathetic stimulation in response to the need for increased heat production and in response to the fear and pain associated with exposure to cold, especially in cases such as immersion in cold water. The blood pressure also tends to rise initially due to the increased heart rate and vasoconstriction. As the body temperature falls to about 33 to 30 °C myocardial function is depressed. The heart rate gradually decreases and may become very slow. The blood pressure also tends to fall, but may be maintained near its usual level due to vasoconstriction and usually does not become seriously depressed until the core temperature falls below 28 °C. Hypotension often does not occur until rewarming is instituted, when loss of vasoconstriction may occur before cardiac output has increased. A variety of cardiac arrhythmias, especially atrial fibrillation, may occur as the body temperature falls below 30 °C. Ventricular fibrillation is the most serious hazard. The exact mechanism responsible for the ventricular fibrillation is not understood, but hypoxia, acidosis, or abnormal plasma calcium levels may be precipitating factors. It is most likely to occur in people with heart disease.

The initial respiratory response to cold is increased ventilation. Sudden immersion in cold water, especially, causes hyperventilation, which may produce respiratory alkalosis. As the body temperature falls, however, ventilation decreases and respirations tend to be slow and shallow. At body temperatures below 32 °C hypercapnia and respiratory acidosis may occur due to decreased ventilation and increased solubility of carbon dioxide in the body fluids.

Hypoxia may also occur with hypothermia because shivering causes an increased need for oxygen and ventilation may not be adequate to meet this increased need. Tissue hypoxia can also occur for other reasons. Tissue cooling is not uniform, therefore the need for oxygen is not the same for all tissues. In addition, decreased cardiac output and vasoconstriction reduce perfusion in some tissues more than others. Capillary blood flow is also slowed because blood viscosity increases at lower temperatures. Also, at low temperatures oxygen is not as readily released from hemoglobin. (See the discussion of the oxygen-hemoglobin dissociation curve under Decreased Oxygen-Carrying Capacity of the Blood in Chapter 10.) Consequently anaerobic metabolism occurs in the tissues and excess lactic acid is produced. In addition, hepatic metabolism of lactic acid and other organic acids is decreased during hypothermia. Therefore metabolic acidosis may develop. The acidosis may be exacerbated during rewarming because acid metabolic products in the tissues are carried to the general circulation as tissue perfusion improves and shivering at this time increases the production of lactic acid.

Renal function and fluid balance are also altered during hypothermia. Exposure to cold often causes diuresis, possibly because cutaneous vasoconstriction shifts the blood centrally and secretion of ADH decreases as a result of increased central blood volume (see Chapter 12 under Hormonal Mechanisms). As the body temperature falls renal blood flow and glomerular filtration rate decrease. Tubular transport of sodium is decreased, however, and reabsorption of water is suppressed by hypothermia. These changes offset the reduction in glomerular filtration rate and a large volume of dilute urine may be produced. In some cases, however, oliguria occurs and occasionally renal failure occurs during rewarming. The reason for the oliguria is not always known, but in some cases it may be due to structural damage.

Severe hypothermia results in increased capillary permeability, probably due to the accumulation of metabolites caused by sluggish blood flow. Therefore fluid shifts from the plasma to the interstitial space, producing edema and hypovolemia.

Frostbite

When tissues actually freeze as a result of exposure to very low temperatures, the condition is called *frostbite*. Frostbite and hypothermia sometimes occur together, but frostbite can occur without any decrease in the core temperature.

Mechanisms of Damage

Slow freezing of tissues causes formation of ice crystals in the extracellular fluid (ECF). Consequently the osmolality of the ECF increases and draws water out of the cells. Therefore the osmolality of the intracellular fluid also increases and cell function is altered. The exact mechanism by which increased osmolality damages cells is not known, but it may denature protein. With rapid cooling, ice crystals form inside the cells and disrupt them, causing cell death. It has also been postulated that below certain temperatures (possibly 22 to 24 °C) the liquid phase of membrane lipids solidifies, resulting in disruption of membrane-bound enzymes and causing cell death.

Damage also occurs as a result of impaired circulation. Arterial and venous constriction in response to cold result in decreased capillary perfusion. In addition, blood viscosity increases due to the cold, resulting in sludging and possibly thrombus formation. Therefore obstruction of small vessels may occur. After a period of exposure to cold, vasodilation occurs, probably because arteriolar smooth-muscle function is impaired by the cold. This vasodilation results in shunting of blood through arteriovenous anastomoses and slight warming of the tissue, but precapillary sphincters may remain closed so that capillary flow is not improved. Damage to capillary endothelial cells results in increased permeability and loss of fluid to the interstitial space, producing edema.

Manifestations of Frostbite

The feet, hands, cheeks, ears, and nose are the parts most commonly affected by frostbite. The degree of frostbite depends on the intensity and duration of exposure. *Superficial frostbite* involves only the skin and sometimes the subcutaneous tissue. With *deep frostbite*, muscles, tendons, and bone are also affected.

Usually as frostbite develops the part initially feels cold, then a pricking or burning painful sensation is felt. Finally sensation is lost. In some cases, however, the onset of frostbite is not accompanied by any particular sensation. The frozen part usually appears white, although it may appear mottled purple due to subcutaneous hemorrhages. When rewarming occurs the part is very painful. Disturbances of sensation may persist for a long time after the pain subsides. Frequently following recovery there is a permanent increase in vascular tone and an abnormal sensitivity to cold.

With mild degrees of frostbite the affected part is red, warm, and swollen after rewarming. No tissue necrosis occurs, however, and the edema gradually subsides. With more severe degrees of frostbite blistering, edema, and tissue necrosis occur. As the part is warmed it becomes blue, then later turns red or black. The edema eventually subsides and the necrotic tissue is gradually sloughed. With superficial frostbite new epidermis regenerates under the necrotic tissue. With deep frostbite however, larger amounts of tissue are lost and spontaneous separation of the part may occur (e.g., a toe may separate at the metatarsophalangeal joint). Infection may supervene, impairing healing. In some cases amputation of the part may be necessary.

SUGGESTED ADDITIONAL READING

Dawkins MJR, Hull D: The production of heat by fat. *Sci Am* **213**(2): 62–67, 1965.

Ewars D: Smoke inhalation: assessment and management. *J Emerg Nurs* **5**(1): 4–9, 1979.

Kessler RL: Care of a scalded child. *Nurs Times* **75**(15):619–624, 1979.

Minar V: Fluid resuscitation of the burn patient. *J Emerg Nurs* **4**(5): 39–43, 1978.

Ozuna JM, Foster C: Hypothermia and the surgical patient. *Am J Nurs* **79**(4): 646–648, 1979.

Porth CM, Kaylor LE: Temperature regulation in the newborn. *Am J Nurs* **78**(10): 1691–1693, 1978.

UNIT SIX

CHEMICAL STRESSORS

25

Interaction of Chemicals with the Body

EXPOSURE AND ABSORPTION

Local Effects

General Factors Influencing Absorption
Solubility
Movement Across Biological Membranes

Ingested Chemicals

Absorption Through the Skin

Inhaled Chemicals

FATE OF ABSORBED CHEMICALS

Transport and Distribution
Binding to Plasma Proteins
Factors Influencing Distribution
of Chemicals
Sequestering of Chemicals

Metabolism of Foreign Chemicals
Degradation Reactions
Conjugation Reactions

Excretion
Urinary Excretion
Biliary Excretion

MECHANISMS OF ACTION OF TOXINS

Interference with Enzyme Action
Irreversible (Noncompetitive)
Enzyme Inhibition
Reversible (Competitive)
Enzyme Inhibition

Interference with Cellular Respiration

Interference with Oxygen Transport

Interference with Neurotransmission
Synaptic Transmission
Interference with Synaptic Transmission

Alteration of Cell Membranes
Accumulation in Cell Membranes
Interaction with Membrane Components

Alteration of DNA

Hypersensitivity Reactions

Every day people are exposed to a wide variety of nonfood chemicals, including drugs, industrial chemicals, pesticides, household cleaning agents, cosmetics, and food additives such as preservatives, binding agents, coloring agents, and flavoring agents. Substances that are not normally found in the body (i.e., foreign compounds) are called *xenobiotics*. A *poison*, or *toxin*, is a substance that is harmful to the body because of its chemical action.

461

The dose of a substance is very important in determining whether it causes harmful effects. Every substance, even pure water, is toxic if taken in large enough quantities (see Chapter 12 for a discussion of water intoxication). Generally the word poison is used in reference to chemicals that cause harm when they are taken in relatively small amounts. On the other hand, some chemical agents that are usually considered harmful may be present in the body in minute quantities without causing harm. In other words, a potentially toxic substance may be present in the body without the occurrence of poisoning. The *toxicity* of a substance is sometimes expressed as the dose that produces a specific harmful effect in 50% of the people (or experimental animals) receiving that dose (TD_{50}). Relative toxicity is also expressed in terms of *lethal dose* (LD_{50}); that is, the dose that causes death of 50% of the experimental animals receiving it. (For obvious reasons, LD_{50} cannot be determined for humans, although estimates can be made from deaths that occur due to accidental poisoning.) The LD_{50} of a specific substance is not the same for all animals and results from animal experiments cannot be directly extrapolated to human beings because of species differences in metabolism. Data from animal experiments, however, can give an indication of whether a substance is highly toxic (i.e., toxic in very small amounts), moderately toxic, or only slightly toxic. For example, for rats the LD_{50} of orally administered arsenic trioxide is 13 mg/kg body weight; the LD_{50} of orally administered acetylsalicylic acid (aspirin), is 1750 mg/kg body weight.

As just mentioned, any substance can be toxic if present in large enough amounts. It follows, therefore, that even substances that are normally present in the body can be toxic. An *endogenous toxin* is a normal body constituent that is present in excessive amounts and causes harmful effects. Endogenous toxins are discussed in Chapter 26. An *exogenous toxin* is a substance that is not normally found in the body, but enters from the external environment.

EXPOSURE AND ABSORPTION

An exogenous substance can exert a systemic toxic effect only after it has been absorbed into the body. Some substances are not absorbed in appreciable amounts but can exert a harmful effect locally on the tissues with which they come in contact. Various properties of the substance, as well as characteristics of the body surface with which it comes in contact, influence the absorption of a chemical compound. Therefore, the absorbed dose is not necessarily the same as the dose to which a person is exposed. Following absorption, only a fraction of the substance reaches tissues with which it can interact (target tissues) and the specific molecular sites within the tissues where reaction occurs. The distribution of the substance within the body, the metabolic handling of the substance, and its rate of excretion will determine the amount of active drug or toxin that is available for interaction with target tissues. Intoxication will only occur when the chemical agent is absorbed into the body at a faster rate than the body can inactivate and excrete the substance. The longer a substance remains in the body in an active form, the greater the risk of harmful interactions at target sites.

Also, if a chemical is excreted slowly, repeated exposure can lead to accumulation of the substance within the body. Thus, a person may be exposed to a low dose of a substance with no effect, but if the substance is not readily eliminated from the body and the person is exposed repeatedly, the concentration of the substance in the body eventually reaches toxic levels and exerts a harmful effect.

The routes of entry for chemicals into the body are the lungs, the skin and mucous membranes, and the gastrointestinal tract. Air pollution results in absorption of chemicals through the lungs. Chemicals encountered as a result of occupational exposure are most commonly absorbed through the lungs and the skin. Occupational exposure may also lead to ingestion of chemicals, however, if contaminated fingers, cigarettes, or other objects are placed in the mouth or if food is prepared and eaten with contaminated hands. In addition to occupational exposure, absorption of chemicals through the skin may result from the use of cosmetics, sprays, and topical drug preparations. Foreign chemicals enter the gastrointestinal tract as a result of ingestion of contaminated food and water; as a result of accidental ingestion of drugs, household cleaners, polishes, paints, and the like by children; or as a result of deliberate ingestion of substances such as alcohol and drugs.

Local Effects

Some caustic, or corrosive, chemicals are destructive to living tissue and cause chemical burns whenever they come into contact with a body surface. Strong acids (e.g., hydrochloric acid, sulfuric acid, and nitric acid) and strong bases (e.g., sodium hydroxide, calcium hydroxide, and ammonium hydroxide) are corrosive. These and a number of other substances such as phenol, denature tissue proteins and exert a harmful effect locally. When a protein is denatured, it becomes nonfunctional and some of its properties are altered. Proteins can be denatured by heat, as well as by extremes of pH (see Chapter 24 under Burns).

The denaturation, or coagulation, of tissue protein by caustic chemicals results in structural and functional changes. Structurally, the tissues lose their elasticity and flexibility and are easily friable. The slightest mechanical stress can cause perforation of the tissue. (For example, after alkali ingestion passage of a gastric tube is contraindicated because it could rupture the esophagus.) Functionally, the affected tissue is biologically inert and its permeability is altered. Healing occurs by repair with formation of a fibrous scar. Subsequent scar contraction can cause strictures in the case of a hollow organ such as the esophagus.

General Factors Influencing Absorption

Solubility is important in the absorption of a chemical agent. The nature of the chemical determines its solubility. Size also influences the rate of absorption; generally, small molecules are taken up faster than large molecules.

Solubility

Water is a *polar* molecule (Fig. 25-1). In other words, the charges on the molecule are not evenly distributed, but one part of the molecule is relatively negative and the rest of the molecule is relatively positive. (The overall molecule, however, is neutral.) Other polar substances and ions are able to orient themselves around the polar water molecule and therefore dissolve easily in water. Such substances are said to be *hydrophilic* (literally, "water loving"). Ionized substances, strong acids, strong bases, and compounds that contain many hydroxyl (–OH) groups (e.g., sugars) are very hydrophilic.

Lipids are nonpolar molecules and are not soluble in water, but are soluble in organic solvents such as chloroform or carbon tetrachloride. Nonpolar substances that dissolve easily in organic solvents are said to be *lipophilic* ("lipid loving") or *hydrophobic* ("water hating"). Octane, toluene, benzene, and nitrobenzene are examples of very lipophilic substances.

Some organic compounds contain both moderately hydrophilic groups, such as hydroxyl or amino (–NH$_2$) groups, and moderately lipophilic groups, such as aromatic rings or small aliphatic groups (carbon chains). When the hydrophilic and lipophilic groups are more or less in balance, the substance is relatively soluble in both water and organic solvents. Examples of such substances are phenols, aniline, benzoic acid, and some alcohols.

The solubility of weak organic acids (e.g., benzoic acid) and weak organic bases (e.g., aniline) is influenced by pH. In an acid environment weak organic bases are strongly ionized and are more water soluble. They are undissociated in a basic environment and therefore are more lipid soluble. The situation is reversed for weak organic acids.

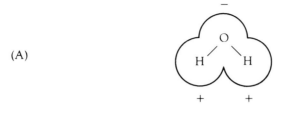

(A)

(B)

Figure 25-1. (A) Water is a polar molecule. (B) Dissolution of ions in water.

Movement Across Biological Membranes

Biological membranes are composed of lipids in association with proteins. At intervals along the membranes are minute pores filled with water. Substances can cross the membranes by filtration, by passive diffusion, by facilitated diffusion, or by active transport. In some cases substances may be taken into a cell by the process of pinocytosis.

Passive diffusion is the movement of atoms, ions, or molecules from a region of high concentration to a region of lower concentration. Facilitated diffusion and active transport require carrier molecules that assist substances across membranes. Facilitated diffusion does not require the expenditure of energy by the cell and the movement of substances is always in the direction of a concentration gradient (i.e., from a region of high concentration to a region of lower concentration). Active transport involves the movement of substances across a membrane against a concentration gradient and requires the expenditure of energy by the cell.

A carrier molecule is specific for a particular compound or group of compounds that are struc-

turally similar. Since the number of carrier molecules in a membrane is limited, the transport system can become saturated. Therefore, when a substance requiring carrier-mediated transport is present in high concentrations, the rate at which the substance crosses the membrane is limited by the maximum capacity of the transport system. In addition, when two or more substances that use the same carrier molecule are present at the same time they will compete with each other. Consequently, one chemical compound may interfere with the passage of another compound across a membrane.

Figure 25-2 illustrates the means by which various substances cross biological membranes. Lipophilic substances can dissolve in the lipid of the membrane and cross by passive diffusion. Inorganic ions and small hydrophilic molecules (e.g., urea) diffuse through the pores in the membranes or are carried through along with water. Larger hydrophilic molecules, such as sugars and ionized acids and bases, require carrier molecules in order to cross cell membranes but can pass easily through capillary membranes.

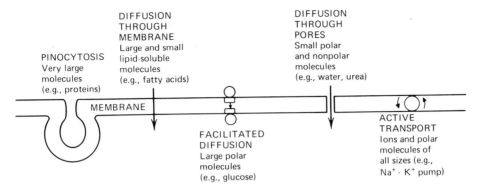

Figure 25-2. *Mechanisms by which substances cross biological membranes.*

Movement of substances into and out of a cell involves passage across a single cell membrane. Movement of substances into the body, however, involves crossing an epithelial surface. In this case substances must cross several membranes. Usually substances pass through the epithelial cells and the greatest barrier is the cell membrane. For example, consider the absorption of a substance from the intestine. From the intestinal lumen the substance must cross the cell membrane lining the lumen, move through the cell, and cross the cell membrane on the other side to enter the interstitial fluid. Then the substance must cross the capillary membrane to enter the blood. If one or more of the steps involved in crossing an epithelial membrane is active (i.e., requires the expenditure of energy), the overall epithelial transport process is considered to be active. Differences exist among epithelial membranes in different parts of the body. For example, it appears that very little passage of substances occurs through the junctions *between* the cells lining the gastrointestinal tract; substances must go *through* the cells. In the respiratory tract, however, some substances may pass between the cells.

Unlike other membranes, active transport of substances does not occur across capillary walls. With the exception of very large molecules, such as the plasma proteins, both lipophilic and hydrophilic substances are rapidly exchanged between the plasma and interstitial fluid. Lipophilic molecules and gases such as oxygen and carbon dioxide probably diffuse through the capillary endothelial cells. Other substances are believed to pass through pores between the endothelial cells. (Anatomically, electron micrographs have failed to reveal the existence of pores, but functionally the capillary membrane behaves as if it has pores. Probably substances pass through the intercellular cement.) In addition, capillary permeability is not the same in all parts of the body. For example, capillaries in the liver are more permeable than capillaries in other parts of the body and permit the passage of some proteins. On the other hand, the capillaries of the brain are more restrictive than those of other parts of the body.

Ingested Chemicals

Most ingested chemicals are absorbed through the small intestine, although they can be absorbed throughout the length of the alimentary canal. Most foreign substances cross by passive diffusion, with the rate of absorption being greatest for nonpolar (i.e., lipophilic) molecules. Organic ions also appear to diffuse across the membrane, but their rate of absorption is much slower. Large, very hydrophilic molecules are poorly absorbed. If a xenobiotic has a chemical structure similar to a compound that is normally absorbed by active transport, the foreign substance may also be actively transported across the intestinal membrane.

As mentioned previously, pH influences the dissociation of weak acids and weak bases and therefore influences their solubility and absorption. Weak organic acids (e.g., salicylic acid) are relatively undissociated (and therefore more lipid soluble) in the acid environment of the stomach and are absorbed through the gastric mucosa. Weak organic bases, in contrast, are more highly dissociated in an acid environment and are not appreciably absorbed from the stomach, but are absorbed to a greater extent from the small intestine.

The presence of food in the gastrointestinal tract can influence the solubility of a foreign chemical and therefore influence its absorption. The xenobiotic may react with a food substance to form an insoluble complex that cannot be absorbed or the chemical agent may adsorb to the surface of particulate material in the gastrointestinal tract.

Passive diffusion requires a concentration gradient. Liquids in the gastrointestinal tract will dilute the foreign substance and therefore decrease its rate of absorption by decreasing the concentration gradient.

Lipophilic substances, such as DDT (1,1-bis-(p-chlorophenyl)-2,2,2-trichloroethane), are practically insoluble in the aqueous environment of the gastrointestinal lumen. They can be emulsified and absorbed along with dietary lipids, however, with the help of bile salts. Therefore, absorption of very lipophilic substances is enhanced in the presence of a fatty meal.

Gastrointestinal motility also influences absorption. Hypomotility allows more time for absorption to occur. On the other hand, hypermotility leads to rapid elimination of intestinal contents without allowing much time for absorption.

Some foreign chemicals may be altered in the gastrointestinal tract before absorption occurs. Substances may be degraded or modified either by digestive enzymes or by the action of intestinal bacteria. The resulting products may be less toxic than the original compounds, but in some cases they are more toxic. For example, as a result of bacterial action azo compounds may be reduced to aromatic amines, which are usually more toxic.

With the exception of some lipids, which enter the lymphatics, most substances absorbed through the gastrointestinal tract enter the hepatic portal system and are carried to the liver. Therefore systemic effects may be modified because a foreign compound may be altered in the liver and/or excreted into the bile before having a chance to enter the general circulation.

Absorption Through the Skin

Although an intact skin provides an effective barrier against the entry of many substances from the external environment into the internal environment, some chemical substances can penetrate the skin. The greatest resistance to passage of substances across the skin appears to be in the epidermal layer; the dermis behaves as a highly porous membrane and is freely permeable to many substances. The epidermis behaves as a lipoid barrier, with nonpolar molecules such as carbon tetrachloride passing through it most easily. Substances such as phenol, which are both water soluble and lipid soluble, are also absorbed quite easily through the skin. In addition, some gases may pass directly through the skin. Inorganic ions, high molecular weight compounds, and particulate material cannot cross an intact epidermal layer. Toxic chemicals of any nature, however, may easily enter the body if the skin is cut or broken.

Inhaled Chemicals

The pulmonary surface area is very large and affords a good portal of entry for gases, fumes, and mists. In addition, irritating gases can cause local damage to the respiratory epithelium.

Very water-soluble caustic gases, such as hydrochloric acid or ammonia, dissolve in the mucus of the upper respiratory tract and cause irritation. As a result, mucus secretion increases and a "scrubbing out" effect occurs. Therefore, small doses of very soluble irritating gases usually do not enter the lungs. Their main effect is erythema and discomfort of the nose and throat and also of the conjunctivae. The scrubbing capacity of the upper respiratory tract is limited, however, and cannot cope with large amounts of such gases. Therefore, with large doses some of the irritant gas reaches the lungs. The resulting chemical burns produce pulmonary edema. On the other hand, gases that are relatively insoluble in water (e.g., phosgene) reach the lungs quite easily because they do not produce very much irritation of the upper respiratory tract and so are not "scrubbed out."

Most gases are absorbed very rapidly through the lungs. Transfer across the alveolar epithelium is by diffusion and the rate of diffusion depends on the difference in the partial pressure of the gas between the alveolar air and the blood. If a person is moved to an uncontaminated environment after exposure to a noxious gas, the partial pressure of the gas in the alveoli decreases (provided that ventilation is maintained) and the gas can be rapidly excreted through the lungs if it is not bound to tissue components.

With mists (liquid droplets suspended in air) and dusts (particles suspended in air) the size of the droplet or particle will determine the depth of its penetration into the respiratory tract. Large particles or droplets settle out in the nose, trachea, and bronchi. The cilia of the respiratory epithelium then sweep the particles toward the throat and they are usually swallowed. Subsequently the substance may be absorbed from the gastrointestinal tract. Smaller particles reach the small bronchi, bronchioles, and alveoli, although very fine particles and droplets may be trapped in turbulent air currents and exhaled. For those particles and droplets reaching the alveoli, absorption will depend on the solubility of the substance. Insoluble liquid substances (e.g., hair-spray resins) and insoluble particles (e.g., coal dust) are not appreciably absorbed and act as foreign bodies (see Chapter 21). Soluble particles (e.g., starch dust), however, are readily absorbed into the blood.

The rate of absorption of substances through the lungs is influenced by ventilation and by pulmonary blood flow. If ventilation and blood flow are increased, for example, due to increased physical exertion, absorption will occur more rapidly.

As mentioned previously, substances absorbed through the gastrointestinal tract are carried first to the liver, where they may be altered or excreted before having a chance to enter the systemic circulation. The body does not have this protection when substances are absorbed through the lungs. Xenobiotics can be carried directly to the brain and other vital organs, thus enhancing the effective dose available for interaction at target sites.

FATE OF ABSORBED CHEMICALS

The absorption of a foreign substance, its distribution within the body, metabolic handling, and excretion are referred to as the *toxicokinetic phase* of toxicological action. (In the case of drug action these processes are called the *pharmacokinetic phase*.)

Transport and Distribution

Following absorption, xenobiotics are carried to various parts of the body by the blood. Very water-soluble substances are simply dissolved in the blood. Compounds that are weakly to moderately water soluble (i.e., relatively lipophilic substances) are mainly bound reversibly to plasma proteins, particularly albumin. Very lipophilic substances entering through the gastrointestinal tract are usually associated with dietary lipids in the chylomicrons.

Binding to Plasma Proteins
With substances that bind to plasma proteins, a small amount of the chemical remains in the free (unbound) form in equilibrium with the bound chemical. Protein binding decreases the amount of

a substance that is available to the tissues, since plasma proteins cannot cross the capillary membrane. The concentration of the particular substance in the interstitial fluid and target tissues is determined by the concentration of the unbound chemical, which is freely diffusible. Protein binding does not prevent metabolism or excretion of the substance, however. In organs where the substance is metabolized or actively secreted the concentration of the free chemical decreases, causing more to be released from the plasma proteins.

Binding of substances to plasma proteins is relatively nonspecific. Therefore a chemical can be displaced from the plasma proteins by a second substance that competes for the same binding site. Consequently, the amount of the first chemical in the tissues will increase. For example, bilirubin, an endogenous substance, is normally bound strongly to plasma proteins, but can be displaced from plasma proteins by sulfonamides. Consequently, if premature infants with jaundice are treated with sulfonamides, the amount of bilirubin entering the brain is increased and may cause serious damage. (See Chapter 26 under Bilirubin Toxicity.)

Factors Influencing Distribution of Chemicals

A chemical agent must cross capillary membranes and cell membranes to enter body cells. The distribution of a substance will be affected by its ability to traverse these membranes. As mentioned previously, passage across cell membranes is restricted to lipophilic compounds and small substances that can enter through pores, but capillary membranes are freely permeable to most substances except very large molecules such as plasma proteins. The penetration of substances into the central nervous system is an exception to this generalization. Either the capillary walls or the surrounding layer of glial cells form a tight barrier to the passage of many substances into the brain and cerebrospinal fluid (the *blood-brain barrier*). Lipophilic substances that can diffuse across cell membranes enter the brain and cerebrospinal fluid

more readily than hydrophilic chemicals, but molecular size is also a factor in determining penetration of substances into the brain. All relatively large molecules, including lipids, polysaccharides, and polypeptides, are restricted. Some substances, such as glucose, some amino acids, and some inorganic ions enter the brain and cerebrospinal fluid by carrier-mediated transport.

High-molecular-weight substances and chemicals bound to plasma proteins will remain in the plasma and will not enter other body tissues. Substances that can cross capillary membranes but are unable to penetrate cell membranes will be distributed throughout the extracellular fluid. Some large hydrophilic substances bind to acid mucopolysaccharides (intercellular ground substance) in connective tissue.

Substances that can penetrate cell membranes will be distributed intracellularly and extracellularly (e.g., urea, ethanol). If binding to a cellular component occurs, a substance will be preferentially distributed within the cells. Very lipophilic substances will be preferentially deposited in body fat. They may also enter the brain because the brain has a high lipid content.

Blood flow also influences the distribution of chemical agents. Chemicals that can diffuse freely across membranes will tend to be concentrated in tissues with a high blood flow. High concentrations of xenobiotics generally occur in the liver and kidneys, probably because these organs are the main sites for metabolism and excretion of the substances.

Sequestering of Chemicals

Some foreign chemicals are preferentially deposited in certain tissues and remain there for a long time (i.e., the substances are *sequestered*) without necessarily causing harmful effects. For example, very lipophilic substances such as DDT and its metabolite DDE (1,1-bis(*p*-chlorophenyl)-2,2-dichloroethylene) are sequestered in adipose tissue, where they are relatively innocuous. Heavy metals, such as strontium and lead, are deposited in bone. Here they do not cause toxic effects.

(Radioactive metals sequestered in bone can be carcinogenic, however. See Chapter 23.) Lead is also sequestered in the gums and gives rise to a dark line along the gingival margin. Silver can also be sequestered in the gums. Tetracyclines bind to teeth and bones and can be held there for a long time.

As a result of sequestration, prolonged absorption of small doses can lead to the accumulation of high concentrations of potentially toxic agents within the body without harmful effects being manifested. Unfortunately, under some circumstances sequestered substances can be mobilized from body depots and cause acute intoxication. For example, with a rapid weight loss lipids are mobilized from adipose tissue and substances such as DDT and DDE are released. These substances may subsequently enter the central nervous system and cause harm.

Metabolism of Foreign Chemicals

The metabolism of xenobiotics requires the presence of genetically determined enzymes to catalyze the biochemical reactions. Foreign compounds are often metabolized by pathways that exist for the metabolism of natural body substances. Enzymes vary in their specificity and many enzymes can act on several related compounds, therefore xenobiotics can be metabolized by virtue of their structural similarity to food molecules or other substances that normally occur in the body. Often a foreign compound is metabolized by more than one pathway. Some people have a genetic lack of certain enzymes that are involved in the metabolism of foreign substances. Consequently these people have a decreased tolerance for certain substances and usual doses of some drugs may provoke toxic effects. (See Chapter 6 under Inborn Errors of Drug Metabolism.)

In some cases a particular enzyme is not present in the cells or is present only in small amounts, although the cells contain the genetic information necessary to produce the enzyme. When the substrate for the enzyme (i.e., the substance that the enzyme acts upon) is present the cells may respond by producing the necessary enzyme(s) to metabolize the substance. This process is called *enzyme induction*. (See also Chapter 4 under Control of Gene Expression.) Foreign compounds sometimes cause enzyme induction. Consequently a person may develop a tolerance for a particualr substance because of an increased ability to metabolize the substance following enzyme induction. In some cases enzyme induction results in an alteration in the way the body metabolizes a second foreign compound or an endogenous substance.

Some enzyme systems involved in the metabolism of foreign compounds are found in the plasma, but most are intracellular. Different tissues vary in their ability to metabolize foreign substances; the liver is the most important organ involved, but other organs, such as the kidneys, intestines, skin, and lungs also play a part. Infants are much more sensitive than adults to many foreign chemicals due to immaturity of the liver. Newborns lack the enzyme systems required for the metabolism of many substances. Also, people with liver disease have decreased tolerance for many drugs and other foreign compounds due to impaired hepatic cell function.

Although metabolism of foreign compounds is often thought of as "detoxification," the metabolic transformation of a xenobiotic does not necessarily produce a less toxic substance. In some cases a relatively innocuous foreign compound is transformed into a more toxic substance. This situation is called *biotoxification*. With some substances given as drugs, the compound administered may be inactive or relatively inactive and the pharmacological effects are due to a metabolic product of the drug. In this case the process is called *bioactivation*.

Two categories of processes are involved in the metabolism of foreign substances: degradation reactions (phase I) and conjugation reactions (phase II). Degradation reactions include hydrolytic cleaving, oxidation reactions, and reduction reactions. As a result of these reactions, relatively lipophilic substances are converted to smaller, more hydrophilic molecules with hydroxyl groups, carboxyl groups, or amino groups. In some cases the products of phase I reactions are readily excreted from the body, but often degradation reactions are followed by phase II. In phase II, endogenous molecules are joined (conjugated) to foreign substances to form hydrophilic products that are very water soluble and readily excreted.

Degradation Reactions

Hydrolytic cleavage, or *hydrolysis,* involves the splitting of a molecule by the addition of water across a bond. For example, an ester may be hydrolyzed to form an alcohol and a carboxylic acid (Fig. 25-3). The enzyme that catalyzes this reaction is called an esterase. A second example is the splitting of an amide, catalyzed by an amidase, to yield a carboxylic acid and an amine.

Oxidation is the loss of electrons from an atom or molecule (see Chapter 10). In biological systems oxidation is usually accompanied by the loss of the proton in hydrogen (i.e., biological oxidation involves the loss of a hydrogen atom). The hydrogen atom is usually transferred to a coenzyme. In the oxidation of foreign substances the coenzyme is usually nicotinamide adenine dinucleotide phos-

phate (NADP), although nicotinamide adenine dinucleotide (NAD) may also be involved. Ultimately the electrons are accepted by molecular oxygen. In some reactions an oxygen atom derived from molecular oxygen is inserted into the foreign compound. Most, but not all, of the oxidation reactions involved in the metabolism of xenobiotics are catalyzed by iron-containing enzymes associated with the endoplasmic reticulum (referred to as the microsomal fraction) of cells.

Oxidation is one of the most common mechanisms for biotransformation of foreign substances. Alcohols, aldehydes, organic acids, compounds with unbranched carbon chains, and organic amines can undergo oxidation. Various types of oxidation reactions are shown in Figure 25-4.

The enzyme systems involved in the oxidation of xenobiotics are also involved in the oxidation of endogenous steroids and so are found in tissues such as the adrenal cortex as well as the liver. Some foreign compounds induce increased amounts of these enzymes in the liver. Consequently, steroid metabolism is increased following absorption of these compounds. For example, after phenobarbital administration the turnover rate of several steroids, including cortisol and testosterone, is increased.

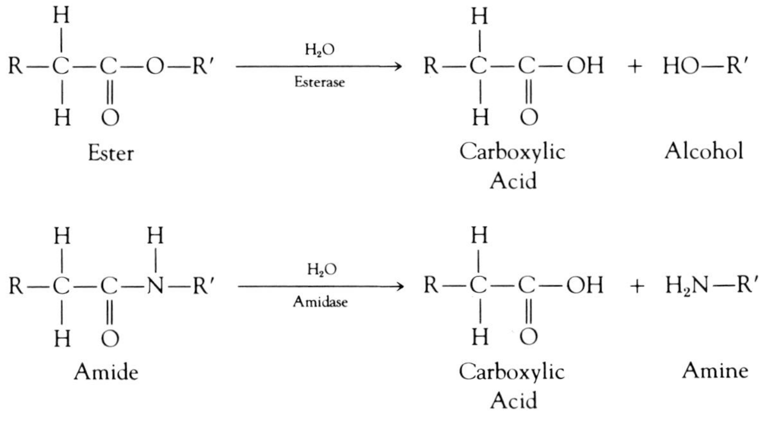

Figure 25-3. *Hydrolysis reactions. R and R' represent different alkyl groups.*

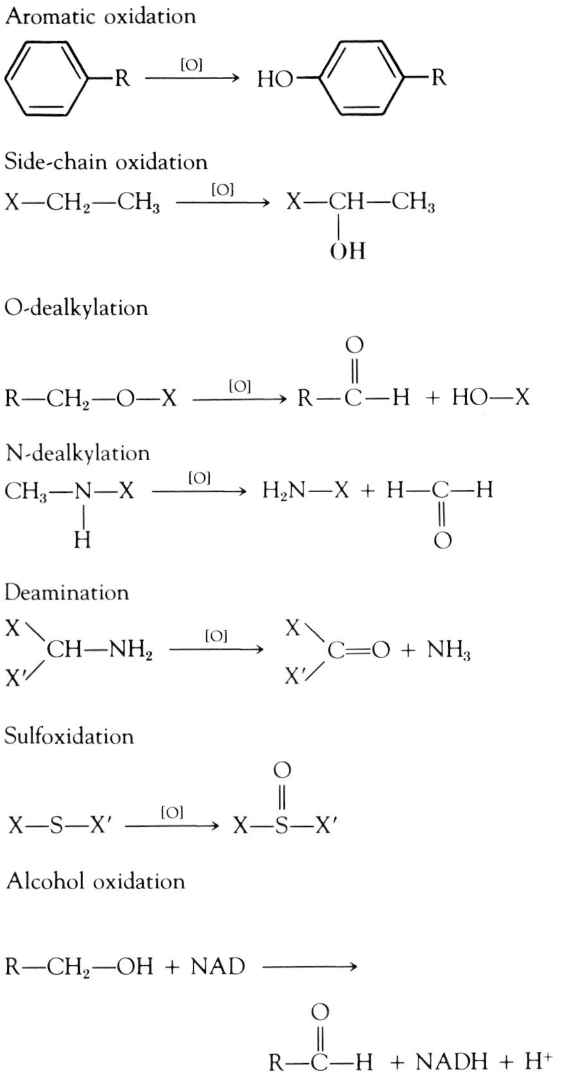

Aromatic oxidation

Side-chain oxidation

$$X-CH_2-CH_3 \xrightarrow{[O]} X-CH-CH_3$$
$$\overset{|}{OH}$$

O-dealkylation

$$R-CH_2-O-X \xrightarrow{[O]} R-\overset{\overset{\displaystyle O}{\|}}{C}-H + HO-X$$

N-dealkylation

$$CH_3-\overset{\overset{\displaystyle}{|}}{\underset{H}{N}}-X \xrightarrow{[O]} H_2N-X + H-\overset{\overset{\displaystyle}{\|}}{\underset{O}{C}}-H$$

Deamination

$$\begin{matrix} X \\ \ \ \ \diagdown \\ \ \ \ \ \ \ \ \ CH-NH_2 \\ \diagup \\ X' \end{matrix} \xrightarrow{[O]} \begin{matrix} X \\ \ \ \ \diagdown \\ \ \ \ \ \ \ \ \ C=O + NH_3 \\ \diagup \\ X' \end{matrix}$$

Sulfoxidation

$$X-S-X' \xrightarrow{[O]} X-\overset{\overset{\displaystyle O}{\|}}{S}-X'$$

Alcohol oxidation

$$R-CH_2-OH + NAD \longrightarrow$$

$$R-\overset{\overset{\displaystyle O}{\|}}{C}-H + NADH + H^+$$

Figure 25-4. *Oxidation reactions. R represents any alkyl group; X represents any cyclic structure.*

Oxidation reactions sometimes result in biotoxification. For example, methanol (wood alcohol) is oxidized to formaldehyde, which denatures protein and causes cellular damage. The enzyme alcohol dehydrogenase, which catalyzes the biological oxidation of alcohols, is present in retinal cells as well as liver cells. Permanent liver damage does not follow the ingestion of methanol because the liver is capable of regeneration. Retinal cells are not capable of regeneration, however, so that blindness is often a sequela of methanol intoxication. Methanol is also metabolized to formic acid, which gives rise to acidosis and is probably responsible for the lethal effect of methanol ingestion. Another example of biotoxification is the conversion of the organophosphorus pesticide parathion, which is only slightly toxic, to a very toxic substance called paraoxon. Paraoxon inhibits the enzyme acetylcholinesterase, with drastic results (see later under Mechanisms of Action of Toxic Substances).

Reduction is the gain of electrons (or in biological systems a hydrogen atom) by an atom or molecule. Reduction of foreign substances does not occur very often. The hydrogen atom required for the process usually comes from the coenzyme NADPH (i.e., reduced NADP). Nitrobenzenes and certain other organic compounds that contain an aromatic ring structure with an attached nitrogen (e.g., sulfanilamide) may be metabolized by reduction. Some ketones and aldehydes resist oxidation and may be reduced instead to produce the corresponding alcohols. In addition, compounds that contain two sulfur atoms linked together (dithio compounds) are reductively cleaved to give compounds with sulfhydryl (–SH) groups. Reduction reactions are shown in Figure 25-5.

$$\underset{\text{Dithio compound}}{R-S-S-R'} \longrightarrow \underset{\text{Mercaptans}}{R-SH + R'-SH}$$

$$\underset{\text{Nitro compound}}{R-NO_2} \longrightarrow \underset{\text{Amine}}{R-NH_2}$$

$$\underset{\text{Aldehyde}}{R-\overset{\overset{\displaystyle O}{\|}}{C}-H} \longrightarrow \underset{\text{Alcohol}}{R-CH_2-OH}$$

Figure 25-5. *Reduction reactions. R and R' represent different alkyl groups.*

Conjugation Reactions

Conjugation reactions are illustrated in Figure 25-6. The most common substances used in conjugation reactions are glucuronic acid, amino acids (particularly glycine), sulfuric acid, and acetic acid, although conjugation with other substances may also occur. The addition of a strong acidic group to the foreign compound makes the compound much more hydrophilic. Not only foreign chemicals but also some normal body substances are conjugated before being excreted (e.g., bilirubin).

Alcohols that contain branched carbon chains (i.e., secondary and tertiary alcohols) are not rapidly oxidized and are conjugated with glucuronic acid. Phenols and molecules with carboxyl groups or amino groups may also be conjugated with glucuronic acid.

Some carboxylic acids cannot be further oxidized and are conjugated with glycine. For

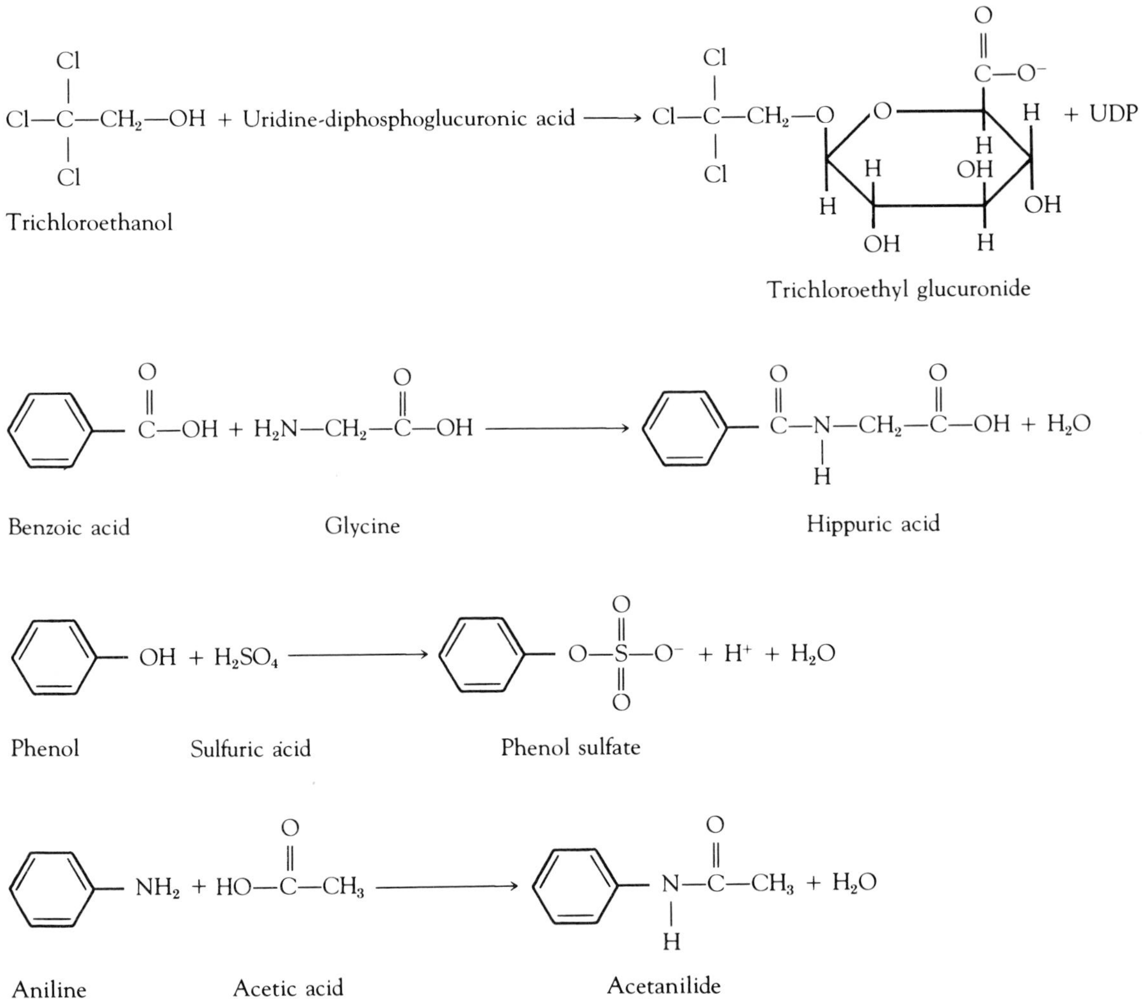

Figure 25-6. *Conjugation reactions.*

example, benzoic acid is converted to hippuric acid by conjugation with glycine, and salicylic acid is conjugated with glycine to form salicyluric acid.

Phenols in particular are conjugated with sulfuric acid. The conjugates that are formed are very hydrophilic because sulfuric acid is a strong acid (i.e., it is almost completely dissociated to give sulfate ions and free hydrogen ions).

Some xenobiotics that contain an amino group cannot undergo oxidative deamination. When the amino group is attached to an aromatic ring or to a carbon atom where a branch occurs in a carbon chain the oxidative deamination reaction is hindered. Such compounds are conjugated with acetic acid (i.e., undergo acetylation) instead. For example, sulfonamides are acetylated. Acetylation makes a substance less hydrophilic and therefore less water soluble. As a result, crystals may precipitate out in the urine when the substance is excreted. Despite this possible side effect, acetylation usually results in decreased toxicity because conjugation with acetic acid masks the amino group and the amino group is usually important in exerting toxic effects.

Excretion

Foreign substances and/or their metabolic products are usually excreted in urine or bile. Other routes of elimination from the body are possible, however. For example, gases and volatile substances can be eliminated through the lungs, as already mentioned. A number of substances (e.g., bromides) are excreted in sweat, although this route is not the major one for most compounds. Some substances bind to keratin (e.g., heavy metals such as arsenic, mercury, and lead) and are gradually lost from the body in hair and nails. Often a particular substance is excreted by more than one route.

Many foreign substances absorbed by a lactating mother are excreted into her milk. Substances such as ethanol, DDT, chloroform, bromides, and many antibiotics appear in milk. The process involved appears to be passive diffusion in most cases, although some substances (e.g., tetracyclines) may be present in higher concentrations in the milk than in the plasma.

Urinary Excretion

The first step in urine formation is glomerular filtration. Fluid and dissolved solutes are forced from the glomerular capillaries into Bowman's capsule due to the hydrostatic pressure of the blood. This process is filtration (bulk flow), not diffusion, therefore both hydrophilic and lipophilic substances enter the glomerular filtrate with equal ease. Very large molecules such as the plasma proteins are unable to pass through the pores; therefore molecules bound to plasma proteins are not filtered. (As mentioned earlier, however, as the concentration of unbound substance decreases, more molecules are released from plasma proteins. Therefore substances that bind with plasma proteins can still be eliminated.)

As the filtrate passes through the lumen of the proximal convoluted tubule, the loop of Henle, the distal convoluted tubule, and the collecting duct, molecules can move from the tubule lumen to the blood (i.e., be reabsorbed) by passive diffusion or by active transport. In addition, molecules from the capillary blood surrounding the tubules can move into the lumen (i.e., be secreted) by passive diffusion or active transport.

Passive diffusion of substances tends to occur in the direction of reabsorption rather than secretion because the solutes in the filtrate become more concentrated as water is reabsorbed and the concentration gradient favors movement from the tubule lumen to the blood. Since the molecules have to diffuse across the lipid membranes of the tubular epithelial cells, lipophilic substances are passively reabsorbed to a greater degree than hydrophilic substances. Therefore lipophilic compounds are not readily excreted in the urine, but hydrophilic substances are.

As mentioned previously, pH influences the ionization of weak organic acids and bases and therefore affects the solubility of these substances. Consequently, urinary pH can influence the rate of excretion of weak organic acids and bases. Weak organic bases (e.g., amphetamine) are only slightly ionized in alkaline urine. Therefore they are more lipophilic and are passively reabsorbed. When the urine is acid these substances are ionized to a greater extent (i.e., are more hydrophilic) and therefore excreted more rapidly. The converse is true for weak organic acids (e.g., barbiturates). When the urine is alkaline these substances are ionized and so are excreted rapidly. When the urine is acid they are less ionized and therefore reabsorbed by passive diffusion. Therefore, in the treatment of barbiturate intoxication, administration of sodium bicarbonate will make the urine alkaline and hasten the excretion of the barbiturate.

Many foreign substances, particularly those that are ionized, are actively secreted into the urine. For example, the following are among the drugs that are secreted into the urine: dihydromorphine, neostigmine, quinine, acetazolamide, furosemide, penicillin, phenylbutazone, and salicylate.

Biliary Excretion

Many substances are excreted in the bile. Liver cells actively transport some substances into the bile, for example, probenecid, penicillin, chlorothiazide, ouabain, digoxin, digitoxin, and quaternary ammonium compounds such as procaine amide ethobromide. Small molecules (molecular weight less than 300) are minimally excreted into the bile. Substances conjugated with glucuronic acid are excreted into the bile to a great extent. Thus, a lipophilic substance may undergo conjugation with glucuronic acid in the liver and subsequently be excreted into the bile. (Conjugation makes the substance hydrophilic and also increases the size of the molecule. Therefore passive reabsorption of the substance from the intestinal tract does not occur to any appreciable extent. If a lipophilic substance is excreted in the bile without undergoing conjugation, however, it may be largely reabsorbed from the intestine by passive diffusion.)

After biliary excretion a foreign substance or its metabolite may be altered in the gastrointestinal tract. In some instances the product is toxic. Some of the substance or its product may be reabsorbed and the rest is eliminated in the feces.

MECHANISMS OF ACTION OF TOXINS

Toxic effects are produced when molecules of the foreign substance interact with specific sites (receptors) in target tissues. This interaction is referred to as the *toxodynamic phase* (or in the case of drugs, the *pharmacodynamic phase*) of action. The effects that are produced are not necessarily restricted to the target tissue. Many types of chemical interactions are possible between xenobiotics and body components. Often the exact mechanism of action of a foreign substance is not known. Some of the more important mechanisms are discussed here.

Interference with Enzyme Action

The metabolic processes of the body are unable to proceed without the activity of enzyme catalysts. Many toxic agents exert their effects by combining with enzymes and inactivating them. A foreign substance may react very specifically with one particular enzyme or it may interact with many enzymes. The resulting inhibition of enzyme action may be reversible or irreversible. Sometimes a blocked metabolic pathway can be bypassed. The toxic effects depend on which particular enzyme is inhibited and how vital that enzyme is for functioning of the body.

Irreversible (Noncompetitive) Enzyme Inhibition

Some toxic substances form strong covalent chemical bonds with enzymes. In some cases the toxin combines with the same site on the enzyme at which the substrate would combine (the active site) and thus prevents the enzyme from combining with its substrate. In other cases the poison combines with some portion of the enzyme other than the active site, but the combination alters the shape of the enzyme so that its catalytic activity is lost.

Some enzymes contain sulfhydryl (–SH) groups, which in many cases are essential for the activity of the enzyme. Ions of heavy metals such as silver, mercury, lead, and arsenic combine with sulfhydryl groups and thereby inactivate many enzymes. Some enzymes contain metal ions (e.g., iron, copper) that are essential for enzyme activity. Some poisons inactivate enzymes by combining with the metal. For example, cyanide and sulfide combine with ferric iron and inactivate the enzyme cytochrome oxidase (see below under Interference with Cellular Respiration). Fluoride and oxalate combine with magnesium and calcium ions and therefore inhibit enzymes that require these ions.

An example of a very specific interaction of a poison with a particular enzyme is the inactivation of acetylcholinesterase by organophosphate pesticides (e.g., paraoxon, the metabolite of parathion). The phosphate group forms a covalent bond with the enzyme at its active site and irreversibly blocks the activity of the enzyme. The normal substrate for acetylcholinesterase is acetylcholine, a chemical mediator for the transmission of nerve impulses across synapses and across the neuromuscular junction. Acetylcholinesterase catalyzes the hydrolysis of acetylcholine and thereby terminates synaptic transmission. When acetylcholinesterase activity is inhibited acetylcholine persists at the synapses and neuromuscular junctions, causing continuous prolonged stimulation. Cholinergic nerve fibers (i.e., those that release acetylcholine at synapses and neuroeffector junctions) include both parasympathetic and sympathetic preganglionic fibers, all parasympathetic postganglionic fibers, a few sympathetic postganglionic fibers (e.g., those to sweat glands), and motor fibers to skeletal muscles. Therefore, following poisoning with substances that inhibit acetylcholinesterase prolonged stimulation of the ciliary muscles in the eyes causes miosis and blurring of vision. Vomiting, diarrhea, and abdominal cramps result from persistent stimulation of gastrointestinal smooth muscle. In addition, excessive salivation and lacrimation occur from protracted parasympathetic stimulation. Parasympathetic stimulation also causes increased tracheobronchial secretions and bronchoconstriction so that moist rales are heard and affected people experience dyspnea. Diaphoresis occurs from prolonged stimulation of sweat glands by cholinergic sympathetic fibers. Initially the continuous stimulation of motor endplates causes fine muscle tremors, but ultimately gross convulsions occur. Lack of coordination of respiratory-muscle activity impairs ventilation, causing hypoxia and carbon dioxide retention. Exhaustion, coma, and finally death ensue.

Reversible (Competitive) Enzyme Inhibition

When a foreign substance is structurally similar to the substrate normally acted upon by an enzyme, the xenobiotic can compete with the normal substrate for occupation of the active site. As a result of the combination of the enzyme with the foreign substance, the normal reaction is blocked. The binding of the foreign substance is reversible and inhibition of the enzyme can be partially overcome by increasing the concentration of the normal substrate. A substance that interferes with the use of an essential substrate because of its structural similarity is called an *antimetabolite*. In some cases an antimetabolite blocks an enzyme but is not acted upon by the enzyme. In other cases an antimetabolite may be substituted for the normal metabolite in a biochemical reaction, resulting in an abnormal, nonfunctional product. A number of antimetabolites that interfere with nucleic acid synthesis are used in the treatment of cancer.

Interference with Cellular Respiration

Many poisons exert their effects by interfering with cellular respiration, thus depriving the cells of energy in the form of ATP. (See Chapter 10 for a discussion of cellular respiration and the consequences of its impairment.) These poisons are usually highly toxic.

Arsenic salts and oxides interfere with energy metabolism. As stated previously, arsenic inactivates many enzymes by combining with their sulfhydryl groups. The enzyme complex that catalyzes the conversion of pyruvic acid to acetyl CoA is inhibited by arsenic and therefore energy production from carbohydrate oxidation is impaired. This block can be bypassed in tissues that can utilize fatty acids as a source of acetyl CoA. Nervous tissue does not have the capacity of other tissues to utilize fatty acids, however, so that subacute and chronic arsenic poisoning produce symptoms of sensory and motor dysfunction and degeneration of peripheral nerves.

Cyanide is much more toxic than arsenic (i.e., smaller doses are lethal) because the block caused by cyanide cannot be bypassed. As mentioned earlier, cyanide combines with ferric iron and inhibits cytochrome oxidase. As a result, the transfer of electrons from the respiratory chain to oxygen is blocked and oxidative phosphorylation (i.e., the aerobic production of ATP) stops. The iron in hemoglobin is in the ferrous state and so cyanide does not bind with it. If hemoglobin iron is oxidized to the ferric state (methemoglobin), however, it will form a complex with cyanide.

Some poisons uncouple phosphorylation; that is, they do not stop electron transfer along the respiratory chain but interfere with the use of the energy released by this process. Instead of being used to form ATP, the energy is dissipated as heat. Therefore such poisons produce fever, as well as depriving the cell of ATP. As a result, the rate of utilization of food molecules and oxygen increases. Dinitrophenol and a weed killer, dinitroorthocresol, are examples of poisons that uncouple phosphorylation. In the past dinitrophenol was sometimes used to treat obesity, but this practice has been stopped because dinitrophenol is too toxic.

Interference with Oxygen Transport

Poisons that convert hemoglobin to methemoglobin decrease the oxygen-carrying capacity of the blood and can produce hypoxia because methemoglobin cannot combine with oxygen (see Chapter 10). The erythrocytes can reduce methemoglobin back to hemoglobin, but this ability is limited. Therefore when excessive amounts of methemoglobin are formed the erythrocytes cannot keep up, and hypoxia results. Aromatic amines, azo compounds, nitro compounds, nitrites, and a number of drugs such as sulfonamides, acetanilide, antipyrine, para-aminosalicylic acid, nitrofurantoin, quinine, and primaquine can cause the formation of methemoglobin.

Infants are less able than adults to reconvert methemoglobin to hemoglobin due to immaturity of the necessary enzyme system in the erythrocytes. Also, fetal hemoglobin is more susceptible than adult hemoglobin to conversion to methemoglobin. Therefore, chemicals that produce methemoglobin are more toxic to infants than adults.

A second way that poisons can interfere with oxygen transport is by binding to hemoglobin at the same place where oxygen is normally bound. The classic example is carbon monoxide poisoning. Combination of hemoglobin with carbon monoxide produces carboxyhemoglobin. Hemoglobin has a greater affinity for carbon monoxide than it does for oxygen, therefore exposure to relatively low concentrations of carbon monoxide can result in a considerable decrease in the oxygen-carrying capacity of the hemoglobin. In addition, when both carbon monoxide and oxygen are bound to hemoglobin, the oxygen is not as readily released to the tissues.

The signs and symptoms of carbon monoxide poisoning are due to hypoxia. Up to 10% of the hemoglobin can be combined with carbon monoxide without the occurrence of symptoms. Mild to moderate degrees of intoxication cause headache, dizziness, visual disturbances, and possibly syncope. The pulse and respiratory rate are increased. With severe poisoning (i.e., when the hemoglobin is more than 50% saturated with carbon monoxide) the person goes into coma and may have convulsive seizures. Concentrations of carbon monoxide that are high enough to produce coma do not cause cyanosis, but rather produce a typical cherry-red complexion due to the color of carboxyhemoglobin. With increasing levels of carbon monoxide in the blood (i.e., increasing degrees of hypoxia), cardiac function and respiration are depressed. Death occurs when the hemoglobin is 60% to 80% saturated with carbon monoxide.

Interference with Neurotransmission

Poisons can interfere with neurotransmission in several ways, by blocking any one of several steps involved in the transmission of impulses across synapses and neuroeffector junctions.

Synaptic Transmission
Synaptic transmission normally occurs in the following manner (Fig. 25-7). A chemical transmitter agent is synthesized in the terminal knob of an axon and stored in vesicles within the knob.

When a nerve impulse reaches the end of an axon the chemical transmitter is released into the synaptic cleft. The transmitter diffuses across the gap and binds with specific receptor sites on the membrane of the postsynaptic neuron. As a result of this binding the permeability of the membrane is altered, depolarization occurs, and an impulse may be generated in the postsynaptic neuron. In the case of a neuroeffector junction, the binding of the transmitter to receptor sites on the effector cell brings about whatever action is appropriate to the effector (i.e., secretion by a gland or contraction of a muscle). Some chemical transmitter substances in the central nervous system cause inhibition rather than excitation when they bind to receptor sites. In the peripheral nervous system acetylcholine is the transmitter substance except at sympathetic neuroeffector junctions, where norepinephrine is released. Several other chemicals, in addition to acetylcholine and norepi-

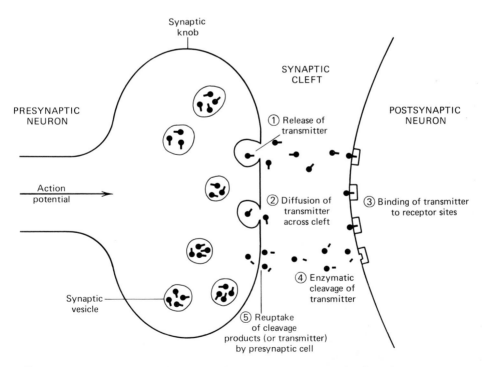

Figure 25-7. *Transmission of nerve impulses across synapses is mediated by chemical transmitters. See text for explanation.*

nephrine, act as transmitter substances in the central nervous system.

Stimulation of the postsynaptic neuron or effector cell will continue for a long time if the chemical transmitter is not removed or inactivated. Inactivation of acetylcholine is brought about by hydrolysis catalyzed by the enzyme acetylcholinesterase, as previously mentioned. The acetate and choline that are formed are taken up by the presynaptic neuron and resynthesized to acetylcholine. Norepinephrine and some central nervous system transmitter substances (e.g., dopamine) are actively removed from the synaptic cleft and taken up again by the presynaptic terminal knob. Following reuptake the neurotransmitter is stored for future use or degraded by the enzyme monoamine oxidase.

Interference with Synaptic Transmission

Poisons can interfere with nervous system function by inhibiting the formation of transmitter substances, inhibiting transmitter release, inhibiting the breakdown of transmitter substances, or by binding with receptor sites. Binding with receptor sites blocks the action of the transmitter substance. In some cases the foreign substance may act as a false transmitter and may cause stimulation when it binds to postsynaptic receptor sites.

A substance called methionine sulfoxime, for example, inhibits enzymes that are involved in the synthesis of gamma-aminobutyric acid (GABA). GABA is an inhibitory transmitter in the brain; interference with its synthesis can result in convulsive seizures.

Tetanus toxin appears to exert its action by interfering with the release of glycine, an inhibitory transmitter substance in the spinal cord. Consequently inhibitory inputs to the motor neurons are eliminated and the influence of excitatory inputs prevails unchecked. The results are hypertonic muscular paralysis, convulsions, and often death.

Botulinum toxin (the agent responsible for one type of food poisoning) prevents the release of acetylcholine at the neuromuscular junctions. The cranial nerves are affected first, causing diplopia (double vision) from lack of stimulation of the external ocular muscles, difficulty swallowing, flaccidity of the jaw muscles, and difficulty talking. Subsequently flaccid paralysis occurs in the muscles of the trunk and limbs. Death results from paralysis of the respiratory muscles. Both tetanus toxin and botulinum toxin are produced by bacteria (see Chapter 28) and both are extremely potent. Less than 0.0001 mg of botulinum toxin can kill an adult.

As an example of inhibition of transmitter breakdown, the inactivation of acetylcholinesterase by organophosphate pesticides has already been described.

Curare exerts its action by binding with receptor sites on the motor endplates and blocking stimulation of the muscles by acetylcholine. The result is paralysis.

Numerous drugs, for example adrenergic agents, adrenergic blocking agents, cholinergic agents, cholinergic blocking agents, and many antidepressants, exert their actions by influencing synaptic neurotransmission in some way.

Alteration of Cell Membranes

Many substances that are very lipophilic appear to exert their actions by interacting with the lipids of cell membranes. Very lipophilic substances tend to accumulate in cell membranes, as well as body fat depots, because they are not soluble in the extracellular fluid or the aqueous environment inside cells. Lipophilic compounds may simply dissolve in cell membranes or they may react chemically with membrane lipids. As a result, membrane functions are impaired and permeability is altered.

Accumulation in Cell Membranes

General anesthetics (e.g., ether, cyclopropane, and halothane) are very lipophilic and possibly exert their effects by accumulating in the cell membranes. As mentioned previously, the brain has a high lipid content. It also has a good blood supply. Therefore these substances are preferentially taken up by the brain. Accumulation of lipophilic substances in the cell membranes may interfere with movement of oxygen and/or glucose into the cells and therefore depress cellular activity by interfering with energy metabolism. As mentioned in Chapter 9 the central nervous system is especially sensitive to a lack of oxygen or glucose. In addition, ion transport may be altered.

Higher brain centers and those parts that control consciousness are depressed by lower concentrations of anesthetic agents than are required to depress the vital centers in the brainstem. Not only substances used as anesthetics, but other lipophilic substances such as volatile petroleum products and hydrocarbons in gasoline, can depress the central nervous system by this mechanism of action.

Interaction with Membrane Components

Spatial relationships are important in cell functioning. The enzymes involved in a series of steps in a metabolic pathway may be located adjacent to one another on a membranous structure within the cell. Alteration of the membrane may disrupt the normal spatial relationships and therefore impair various metabolic processes.

For example, carbon tetrachloride is believed to exert its toxic effects by reacting with membrane lipids and altering their structure. In particular, carbon tetrachloride interacts with organelle membranes within the cell, such as the endoplasmic reticulum. This reaction results in disintegration of the membranous structures and loss of activity of enzymes located on their surfaces. The microsomal enzymes that are involved in oxidation reactions appear to play a role in carbon tetrachloride toxicity. Carbon tetrachloride is particularly toxic to the liver, which is rich in these enzymes. As a result of carbon tetrachloride poisoning fat accumulates in the liver and varying degrees of necrosis occur. Fat accumulates because of breakdown of the mechanisms necessary for

formation of very-low-density lipoproteins in the liver cells and transport of the lipoproteins from the liver cells into the plasma.

Alteration of DNA

Some xenobiotics react with DNA (deoxyribonucleic acid) or are incorporated into the DNA molecule during replication. As a result of this structural alteration, cell division may be impaired. In other cases, cell division occurs normally but the genetic information carried by the DNA is altered. That is, the xenobiotic has a *mutagenic effect* (see Chapter 3). This effect is often not immediately noticeable, but may only be seen in the offspring after several generations. Another possible effect of interaction of foreign substances with DNA is the development of cancer at a later time. In other words, a foreign chemical can have a *carcinogenic effect* (see Chapter 20).

Alkylating agents, such as nitrogen mustards, are examples of chemicals that react with DNA. Alkylating agents are very reactive chemically and preferentially interact with amino groups and hydroxyl groups, which are present in the DNA molecule. Alkylating agents can form chemical bonds with the bases in DNA, thereby interfering with the transcription of RNA from the DNA template and inhibiting protein synthesis. Consequently many cell functions are impaired and tissue growth is arrested. With some alkylating agents, one molecule can react with two bases in the DNA at the same time. If the two bases are on opposite strands, cross-linking of the two DNA strands occurs and prevents normal DNA replication. As a result, cell division is inhibited.

Alkylating agents are particularly harmful to tissues containing rapidly dividing cell populations, such as hematopoietic tissue, gastrointestinal epithelium, and neoplastic tissue. They are sometimes used as anticancer drugs for this reason. As a result of damage to the gastrointestinal epithelium, nausea, vomiting, and diarrhea can occur. Depression of hematopoietic tissue results in leukopenia, which lowers a person's resistance to infection; thrombocytopenia, which produces a bleeding tendency; and anemia.

Hypersensitivity Reactions

Some xenobiotics can lead to the development of hypersensitivity, or allergy, in exposed people. Hypersensitivity is discussed in Chapter 30.

Some substances are deposited in the skin and produce extreme sensitivity to sunlight (photosensitization). Photosensitization is discussed in Chapter 23.

SUGGESTED ADDITIONAL READING

Chilcote RR et al: Sudden death in an infant from methemoglobinemia after administration of "sweet spirits of nitre." *Pediatrics* **59:** 280–282, 1977.

Chisolm JJ: Lead poisoning. *Sci Am* **224**(2): 15–23, 1971.

Kerr ML: Salicylate poisoning in children. *J Emerg Nurs* **5**(3): 20–24, 1979.

Mennear JH: The poisoning emergency. *Am J Nurs* **77**(5): 842–844, 1977.

Savage RL: Drugs and breast milk. *J Hum Nutr* **31:** 459–464, 1977.

Turk MS: House plant poisoning in children. *J Emerg Nurs* **5**(3):8–13, 1979.

26

Endogenous Toxins

Normal constituents of the body can be toxic if they are produced at a faster rate than they can be metabolized or excreted. When liver disease is present, the ability of the body to metabolize and/or excrete potentially toxic substances is decreased. With renal disease, toxic substances may accumulate in the body as a result of impaired excretion. In some cases potentially toxic substances (e.g., bilirubin) may be produced at an abnormally fast rate and may accumulate in the body despite normal hepatic and renal function.

OVERPRODUCTION OF NORMAL METABOLITES

Several situations can lead to overproduction of a normal body constituent, with its subsequent accumulation in the tissues. A major metabolic pathway may be blocked as a result of a genetic defect, so that a precursor substance is metabolized by a minor secondary route to a greater extent than normal. Consequently the secondary product is overproduced and may be toxic. (See Chapter 6 under Inborn Errors Due to Blocked Metabolic Pathways.) In uncontrolled diabetes mellitus, faulty glucose metabolism leads to excessive catabolism of fat, which results in overproduction of ketone bodies (see Chapter 18). Several factors can cause accumulation of bilirubin in the body; overproduction is one cause.

Hyperbilirubinemia

The normal metabolism of bilirubin is shown in Figure 26-1. Bilirubin is a metabolic product of heme breakdown. Most of the heme is derived from hemoglobin following destruction of red blood cells, but about 15% to 20% is derived from other hemoproteins, such as myoglobin, cytochromes, and some enzymes. Heme is degraded to biliverdin, a green pigment, with the release of carbon monoxide and iron. The biliverdin is subsequently converted to bilirubin, a yellow pigment. These reactions can be carried out in reticuloendothelial cells in the liver, spleen, kidneys, and other tissues. This *unconjugated bilirubin* that is formed is moderately lipophilic, is only slightly water soluble, and cannot be excreted by the kidneys. (Unconjugated bilirubin is also called *indirect bilirubin* because in a laboratory test for bilirubin it will only react after it has been dissolved by the addition of alcohol.) Because of its lipophilic nature it can cross membranes relatively easily.

After being released into the plasma, most of the unconjugated bilirubin binds strongly with albumin because of its poor water solubility. A small fraction remains unbound. The unbound pigment is rapidly taken into liver cells by facilitated diffusion. Inside the hepatocytes bilirubin is conjugated with glucuronic acid to form bilirubin glucuronide, or *conjugated bilirubin* (also called *direct bilirubin* because it reacts immediately with Ehrlich's reagent in the van den Bergh test). The conjugation reaction is catalyzed by the enzyme glucuronyl transferase.

Conjugated bilirubin is water soluble. A small amount of it escapes into the plasma and though it can be excreted by the kidneys, conjugated bilirubin is normally not detectable in the urine. Most of the conjugated bilirubin is secreted into the bile by what appears to be an active process. Only minute amounts of unconjugated bilirubin are present in bile.

After excretion into the intestinal tract, bilirubin glucuronide is acted on by bacterial enzymes. Some is hydrolyzed back to unconjugated bilirubin and subsequently is converted to a series of compounds called *urobilinogens*. Some of the urobilinogens are eliminated in the feces, but some are absorbed from the intestinal tract, carried to the liver, and excreted into the bile. Urobilinogens are water soluble; therefore small amounts are also excreted by the kidneys.

Jaundice

The normal concentration of bilirubin in the plasma is 0 to 1.5 mg/100 ml; of that amount 0 to 0.3 mg/100 ml is direct bilirubin. *Hyperbilirubinemia* is an abnormally high concentration of bilirubin in the blood. It may be a result of an increased amount of unconjugated bilirubin, conjugated bilirubin, or both. *Jaundice*, or *icterus*, is a yellow discoloration of the skin, sclerae, and mucous membranes due to the deposition of excess bilirubin in the tissues. Jaundice usually becomes visible when the serum bilirubin level is greater than 2.5 to 3 mg/100 ml. In dark-skinned people it may only be noticeable in the sclerae.

Hyperbilirubinemia and jaundice can result from excessive production of bilirubin, decreased uptake of bilirubin by the liver cells, impaired conjugation of bilirubin, or impaired excretion of conjugated bilirubin. The most common cause of increased bilirubin production is excessive breakdown of red blood cells; the result is *hemolytic jaundice*. In this condition the plasma level of unconjugated bilirubin is increased. The rate of uptake, conjugation, and excretion of bilirubin by the liver increases but cannot keep up with the load. As a result of increased excretion, the amount of urobilinogen being formed in the intestinal tract and absorbed is increased. Therefore urinary excre-

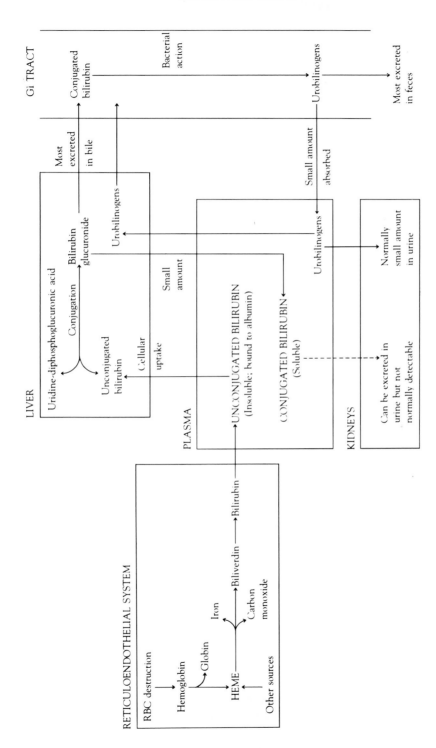

Figure 26-1. *Summary of bilirubin metabolism.*

tion of urobilinogen is increased. Unconjugated bilirubin is *not* excreted in the urine.

Impaired uptake of bilirubin by hepatic cells is rare. It may occur in a genetic disorder called Gilbert's syndrome. In addition, hepatic uptake may be inhibited by some drugs. The plasma level of unconjugated bilirubin is increased; urinary urobilinogen is not increased.

Impaired conjugation of bilirubin may be caused by some drugs and sometimes occurs in Gilbert's syndrome. It also occurs in an inherited disorder called Crigler-Najjor syndrome, in which there is a partial or complete lack of the enzyme glucuronyl transferase. When the enzyme is completely lacking, unconjugated bilirubin reaches high levels in the blood and frequently causes kernicterus in affected infants (see below under Bilirubin Toxicity). Since no bilirubin is conjugated it cannot be excreted. Therefore, the bile is colorless, the stools pale, and no urobilinogen is excreted in the urine. When the enzyme deficiency is partial the hyperbilirubinemia is less severe and kernicterus does not usually occur. The bile is pigmented and some urobilinogen appears in the urine. Administration of phenobarbital can induce increased glucuronyl transferase when the defect is only partial but has no effect when the enzyme is completely lacking.

Glucuronyl transferase activity can be inhibited by a steroid, pregnene-3α, 20β-diol, which some women excrete in their milk during the first few days postpartum. Therefore, some breast-fed infants may exhibit hyperbilirubinemia as a result of this factor.

Excretion of conjugated bilirubin may be impaired because of liver cell damage or blockage of bile canaliculi within the liver (*intrahepatic cholestasis*) or because of obstruction of the bile ducts outside the liver (*extrahepatic cholestasis*). Intrahepatic cholestasis may be the result of a genetic disorder, of drugs that interfere with the secretion of substances across the hepatic cell membrane, or of liver diseases such as viral hepatitis and cirrhosis. Several conditions can cause extrahepatic chole-

stasis; cholelithiasis is the most common cause (see Chapter 21). The result is *obstructive jaundice*.

When biliary excretion is impaired the plasma level of conjugated bilirubin rises. Since conjugated bilirubin is water soluble it is excreted in the urine, giving the urine a dark color. On the other hand, the stools are pale due to a lack of bile pigments and the amount of urobilinogen in the urine decreases. Although the hyperbilirubinemia of cholestasis is initially due to conjugated bilirubin, the retained bile impairs liver cell function and eventually the plasma level of unconjugated bilirubin also rises.

Icterus Neonatorum

In the neonatal period, bilirubin metabolism is in transition from the fetal period (in which excretion of lipid-soluble unconjugated bilirubin takes place through the placenta) to the adult period (in which excretion of water-soluble conjugated bilirubin takes place through the liver). Because of immaturity of the liver, uptake and conjugation of bilirubin by hepatic cells occurs at a much slower rate in newborns than in adults. In addition, the load of bilirubin to be excreted may be high because fetal red blood cells have a shorter life span than adult red blood cells and because unconjugated bilirubin is reabsorbed from the intestinal tract. (Conjugated bilirubin cannot be reabsorbed from the intestinal tract, but unconjugated bilirubin can be. Meconium contains a large amount of unconjugated bilirubin. In addition, a larger portion of the conjugated bilirubin that is excreted in the bile and subsequently hydrolyzed back to unconjugated bilirubin is not converted to urobilinogens because newborns lack the intestinal bacteria that are necessary for this conversion.) Consequently, the plasma level of unconjugated bilirubin is usually elevated in the newborn.

Fifty to sixty percent of term infants and about 80% of preterm infants become jaundiced during the first week of life because of the factors just described. This jaundice is called *physiological jaundice*, or *icterus neonatorum*. Physiological jaundice does not usually appear in the first 24 hours after birth because it takes time for the bilirubin to accumulate. For term infants, the highest plasma bilirubin level occurs between the second and fifth days after birth, with a peak level of 5 to 6 mg/100 ml. The level declines after the fifth day, but may remain slightly elevated until about the end of the second week after birth. For preterm infants, the peak level may be as high as 8 to 12 mg/100 ml and it occurs between the fourth and seventh days.

A variety of conditions can cause severe hyperbilirubinemia in newborns (i.e., a plasma bilirubin level greater than 12 mg/100 ml). The most common cause is hemolytic disease of the newborn, usually from Rh or ABO incompatibility (see Chapter 30). The jaundice in this case is called *icterus gravis neonatorum* and may appear within 24 hours of birth. Kernicterus can occur if adequate therapy is not instituted soon enough.

Bilirubin Toxicity

Although both conjugated and unconjugated bilirubin can cause jaundice, conjugated bilirubin is nontoxic because it is water soluble, does not enter the brain, and can be excreted in the urine. Unconjugated bilirubin is toxic, however, particularly to nervous tissue. Bilirubin is rarely toxic to adults but is a serious neurotoxin for infants for two reasons. First, bilirubin enters the brain more easily in infants than in adults, presumably due to immaturity of the blood-brain barrier in newborns. Secondly, the infant brain is not fully developed and therefore is more susceptible to damage by bilirubin.

Plasma bilirubin levels greater than 18 to 20 mg/100 ml in infants are associated with a high incidence of kernicterus. *Kernicterus* is a neurological disorder caused by deposition of unconjugated bilirubin in the brain. The basal ganglia, cerebellum, hippocampus, and eighth cranial nerve nuclei are particularly affected. The exact mechanism of bilirubin toxicity is not known, but it appears to interfere with oxygen utilization by the brain cells. Although kernicterus rarely occurs at plasma bilirubin concentrations less than 18 to 20 mg/100 ml, a variety of factors can increase the risk of kernicterus so that it may occur at lower bilirubin levels. For example, prematurity, hypoxia, and acidosis increase the susceptibility to brain damage due to hyperbilirubinemia. Drugs or other substances that compete with bilirubin for binding with albumin can increase the risk of kernicterus. In addition, male infants appear to be more susceptible than females.

Early signs of kernicterus may be subtle and commonly include lethargy, poor sucking ability, and loss of the Moro reflex. As the condition progresses respiratory distress, twitching of the face or limbs, and opisthotonos (a spasm in which the head and heels are bent backward and the body arched forward) may occur, accompanied by bulging of the fontanels and a shrill high-pitched cry. With further progression, convulsive seizures occur and the infant may die. Those that survive severe degrees of kernicterus are usually seriously brain damaged, although the full extent of the damage may not be apparent until the child is about 3 years old. By that time the child often exhibits choreoathetosis (involuntary irregular movements and repetitive slow gross movements), mental retardation, dysarthria (poor speech articulation from disturbances of muscular control resulting from nervous system damage), hearing loss, and strabismus (squint). Convulsive seizures are common. Mild degrees of kernicterus may cause mild to moderate neuromuscular incoordination, partial deafness, and behavioral problems which may only become apparent when the child starts school.

IMPAIRED METABOLISM

Normal body constituents can accumulate if their metabolism is impaired. A substance may accumulate in the tissues if an enzyme necessary for its metabolism is defective because of a genetic disorder (e.g., galactose in galactosemia). In diabetes mellitus, glucose accumulates in the extracellular fluid (ECF) because it cannot be metabolized normally. Consequently the ECF becomes hyperosmotic (i.e., the glucose exerts a toxic effect). The liver is an important organ for the metabolism of many substances. Therefore many potentially toxic substances can accumulate in the body when liver function is impaired.

Hepatic Encephalopathy

Hepatic encephalopathy is a syndrome that usually occurs secondarily to advanced liver disease and is characterized by mental changes and altered consciousness, muscle twitching, and a peculiar "flapping" tremor (asterixis).

Signs and Symptoms

Inability to concentrate, forgetfulness, and general malaise are usual in the early stages of hepatic encephalopathy. Inappropriate behavior and slurred speech may be observed. Muscle twitching, incoordination, and tremors occur. As the condition progresses speech becomes incoherent. Clouding of consciousness and confusion are apparent. Eventually the person lapses into stupor and finally into deep coma. The EEG is abnormal.

Etiological Factors

Hepatic encephalopathy is usually associated with chronic liver disease but occasionally results from acute hepatic failure. The acute hepatic failure is usually a result of viral hepatitis but occasionally results from an idiosyncratic drug reaction, infarction, or poisoning with carbon tetrachloride or phosphorus. Gastrointestinal bleeding, ingestion of large amounts of dietary protein, and administration of sedatives can all precipitate hepatic encephalopathy in people with chronic liver disease. Hepatic encephalopathy is also common following portacaval shunt.

The exact cause of hepatic encephalopathy is not known. Possibly the liver normally secretes some substance that is required by the brain; with liver disease this substance is lacking. Most researchers, however, believe that hepatic encephalopathy is caused by some toxin or toxins that would normally be cleared by the liver.

The exact nature of the toxin(s) is not known, but it appears to be a nitrogenous compound arising from the gastrointestinal tract. The fact that hepatic encephalopathy may be provoked by increased protein intake (protein contains nitrogen) and gastrointestinal bleeding (blood contains protein) supports this view. Gastrointestinal bacteria also seem to play a role in the development of hepatic encephalopathy. Many people show improvement following oral administration of antibiotics that reduce the number of bacteria in the intestine.

Some researchers believe that ammonia is involved in the pathogenesis of hepatic encephalopathy. The level of ammonia in the blood and cerebrospinal fluid is increased in people with liver disease, with or without coma. In addition to being formed within the body from deamination of amino acids, ammonia that is formed by intestinal bacteria is absorbed. Normally ammonia is metabolized to urea in the liver, but when the liver is diseased this function is impaired. In addition, when blood is shunted around the liver, large amounts of ammonia absorbed from the intestinal tract enter the general circulation without going through the liver. The exact mechanism of action of ammonia is not known; several mechanisms have been proposed but they have not been verified. Among the mechanisms suggested are interference with ATP production, which could occur at several steps in the pathway of glucose oxidation, and impairment of acetylcholine synthesis.

Other researchers have suggested that short-chain fatty acids may be the toxic agents. Another proposal is that an imbalance in the relative amounts of various amino acids may be responsible for hepatic encephalopathy.

Another theory is that various phenolic amines are taken up by the nervous system and act as false neurotransmitters. These amines can be produced in the intestine by the action of bacterial enzymes on dietary amino acids and subsequently absorbed into the portal circulation. Normally they would be cleared from the portal blood by the liver, but when liver function is impaired and blood is shunted around the liver large amounts of these substances enter the general circulation. The false neurotransmitters are taken up by the nervous system and replace the normal transmitter substances. Subsequently, when nerve impulses reach the presynaptic terminals, these false transmitters are released. They are not as effective as the normal transmitters and therefore the postsynaptic action is weak.

FAILURE TO EXCRETE NORMAL METABOLITES

Many by-products of metabolism are excreted in the urine. Therefore, when renal function is impaired, many normal metabolites accumulate in the body and can exert toxic effects. The kidneys are not merely organs that excrete urine, however. They perform vital functions in the regulation of the composition of the internal environment. Therefore, disruption of renal function leads to serious disturbances of homeostasis. The inability of the kidneys to maintain the normal volume and composition of the body fluids under conditions of normal intake is called *renal failure*.

Renal Failure

Acute renal failure develops suddenly. It is usually due to *acute tubular necrosis* (ATN), although it may also develop as a result of acute glomerulonephritis or acute pyelonephritis. ATN is most commonly caused by acute renal ischemia resulting from shock (see Chapter 14). It may also be caused by poisons (e.g., mercuric ion, carbon tetrachloride) that destroy tubular epithelial cells.

Chronic renal failure develops slowly and progressively as a result of many diseases that destroy the kidney parenchyma and lead to its replacement with scar tissue. Initially the renal disease may affect mainly the glomeruli (e.g., glomerulonephritis), the renal tubules (e.g., pyelonephritis), or the blood vessels (e.g., nephrosclerosis), but eventually the entire nephron is destroyed. The early stages are often asymptomatic, although hypertension may be present and urinalysis may reveal proteinuria, hematuria, or the presence of white blood cells. As the nephrons are destroyed, the *renal reserve is diminished.* The kidneys are able to excrete normal loads, but are unable to cope with large amounts of electrolytes or other substances that need to be excreted.

Further progression of the disease produces *renal insufficiency*. The remaining functional nephrons are overloaded and hypertrophy. Although their reabsorptive capacity is increased, only a small portion of the filtered solutes are reabsorbed, resulting in an osmotic diuresis. In addition, the glomerular blood flow and glomerular filtration rate for each functional nephron increases. The increased flow of fluid through the tubules impairs the urine concentrating mechanism (see Chapter 12). Therefore, signs of renal insufficiency are polyuria (excessive excretion of urine), nocturia (excessive urination at night), and inability to concentrate the urine.

When about 90% of the nephrons have been destroyed, *end-stage renal failure* and *uremia* develop. This stage is characterized by oliguria (diminished output of urine in relation to fluid intake), water retention, and inability to excrete normal metabolites. The serum creatinine and blood urea nitrogen (BUN) levels rise. Inability to concentrate or dilute the urine results in production of urine that is isoosmotic with plasma, as reflected by a urine specific gravity that is fixed near 1.010.

Uremia

Uremia literally means "urine in the blood"; it is a syndrome that reflects abnormal functioning of all organ systems as a result of altered composition of body fluids due to renal failure. Some of the manifestations of uremia are a result of fluid retention (see Chapter 12 under ECF Volume Excess) and electrolyte imbalances that occur as a result of inadequate renal function. Hyperkalemia, hyperphosphatemia, and hypocalcemia are particularly likely to occur (see Chapter 16). Failure to excrete hydrogen ions leads to metabolic acidosis (see Chapter 15). Many of the signs and symptoms of uremia, however, are attributable to toxic effects of retained nitrogenous by-products of protein and amino acid metabolism.

Oxidation of carbohydrates and fats yields carbon dioxide and water, which can be excreted through the lungs and skin. Many products of protein and amino acid metabolism, however, cannot be oxidized to carbon dioxide and water and must be excreted primarily through the kidneys. Therefore, with renal failure the plasma levels of many nitrogenous by-products of protein metabolism are elevated; the major substance is urea. An excess of urea or other nitrogenous substances in the blood is called *azotemia*. Other nitrogenous substances that are present in increased amounts are guanidino compounds, including guanidine, methylguanidine, creatine, creatinine, guanidinoacetic acid, guanidinosuccinic acid, and diphenylguanidine. All these substances have been considered as possible toxins in the uremic syndrome, although their mechanisms of action are not known. Metabolic by-products of the aromatic amino acids (phenylalanine, tyrosine, and tryptophan) often contain a benzene or indole ring and these substances are also possible toxins.

In acute renal failure the uremic syndrome develops abruptly, within a week. In chronic progressive renal disease the onset of signs and symptoms is usually slow and insidious. The manifestations of uremia become more severe as the degree of renal failure increases.

Nervous System Manifestations

Many of the clinical manifestations of uremia reflect central, peripheral, and autonomic nervous system dysfunction. These manifestations progressively include lethargy; nighttime insomnia and daytime drowsiness; inability to focus attention or concentrate; difficulty expressing ideas; poor memory; headaches; slurred speech; restlessness; irritability and emotional withdrawal; hypothermia and feelings of coldness; muscle twitching and cramps; peculiar sensations in the legs, including creeping, crawling, pricking, and itchy sensations that are relieved by movement ("restless legs" syndrome); a burning sensation in the feet; hiccoughs; asterixis; psychotic personality changes; bizarre behavior; anxiety; disorientation; confusion; hallucinations; numbness of extremities; ataxia; nystagmus; aphasia; deafness; vertigo; and finally coma and convulsive seizures.

Digestive System Manifestations

Anorexia, nausea, and vomiting occur early in uremia and are presumably due to autonomic nervous system disturbances. Consequently malnutrition, weight loss, and emaciation are common, particularly with chronic renal disease. In the late stages stomatitis, diarrhea, and gastrointestinal ulcerations may occur. The exact cause of these lesions of the alimentary canal is not known. One theory is that they are at least partly due to irritation from ammonia produced by the action of bacterial enzymes on urea. With renal failure, large amounts of urea are excreted in the saliva and into the gastrointestinal tract. Decomposition of salivary urea by oral bacteria produces an ammoniacal odor to the breath and causes an unpleasant taste, particularly at the posterior part of the tongue.

Cutaneous Manifestations

Pruritus is a common early symptom of uremia. It is probably caused by ammonia produced by bacterial action on urea excreted in the sweat. In advanced stages of uremia, urea excreted in the sweat crystallizes on the skin, producing urea frost. Petechial hemorrhages may be apparent due to altered platelet function (see below).

Circulatory System Manifestations

Hypertension is a common complication of renal disease and frequently accompanies uremia. Several factors, including altered sodium and water metabolism and activation of the renin-angiotensin-aldosterone system, are probably involved in the pathogenesis of this hypertension (see Chapter 13).

Pericarditis occurs fairly commonly in people with uremia and causes dyspnea and chest pain. The cause of uremic pericarditis is not known. The effusion accompanying pericarditis may produce acute cardiac tamponade and shock.

Myocardial dysfunction may also occur and can have a variety of causes. Electrocardiographic abnormalities, abnormal rhythms, and decreased myocardial contractility can be caused by electrolyte imbalances. Cardiac hypertrophy, left ventricular failure, and atrial fibrillation commonly occur secondarily to hypertension and do not necessarily result from uremia per se.

Progressive anemia accompanies chronic renal failure. This anemia is of a normochromic, normocytic type and is mainly due to decreased production of erythropoietin, which results in decreased red blood cell formation. (See Chapter 10 for a discussion of anemia and erythropoietin.) In addition, the survival time of the red blood cells is shortened in uremia. The altered chemical composition of the blood appears to cause hemolysis, but the exact nature of the hemolytic factor is not known.

Abnormal platelet function gives rise to a bleeding tendency in uremia (see also Chapter 7). The platelet abnormality includes decreased platelet aggregation and decreased release of platelet factor 3. It appears to be due to guanidinosuccinic acid and hydroxyphenylacetic acid, two compounds that are present in abnormally high concentrations in uremia. The mechanism of action of these toxins is not known. Other unknown compounds may also be involved. These substances can be removed from the blood by dialysis, with subsequent correction of the platelet defect. A few people with uremia may have thrombocytopenia or abnormalities of plasma clotting factors, but platelet dysfunction is now accepted as the major cause of the bleeding tendency.

Metabolic Disturbances

A variety of metabolic disturbances occur in uremia. Calcium and phosphate imbalances, hyperplasia of the parathyroid glands, and metabolic bone disease are commonly associated with chronic renal disease. This syndrome is called renal osteodystrophy and is believed to be related to impaired metabolism of vitamin D by the diseased kidneys (see Chapter 16).

Plasma levels of amino acids are altered in uremia. The levels of some amino acids are increased, while others are decreased. These changes are partly due to altered dietary intake and partly due to altered metabolism of amino acids. The altered metabolism is possibly due to enzyme inhibition by uremic toxins.

Glucose tolerance is impaired in uremia; cellular uptake of glucose in response to insulin is decreased. Plasma insulin levels are usually increased from impaired degradation of insulin by the kidneys.

Lipid metabolism is also abnormal in uremia. Hyperlipidemia occurs from an accumulation of very-low-density lipoproteins (VLDL) in the plasma. (See Chapter 17 for a discussion of lipid metabolism.) Possibly the liver produces increased amounts of VLDL in response to the elevated insulin level. In addition, the removal of VLDL from the plasma by adipose and other tissues may be decreased. The lipoprotein-lipase enzyme system, which mediates this process, may be inhibited by uremic toxins.

Immunological responses are depressed in uremia, possibly partly because of inhibition by some retained metabolic waste product and partly due to malnutrition (see Chapter 29). Therefore, people with uremia are prone to infection.

SUGGESTED ADDITIONAL READING

Gorrell JF: Hemolytic-uremic syndrome: an overview and a pediatric case report. MCN 3(4): 235–241, 1978.

Lander A: Periarteritis nodosa with associated renal failure: managing a multi-symptom condition. Nurs Mirror 147(17): 26–29, 1978.

UNIT SEVEN

BIOLOGICAL STRESSORS

27
Infectious Agents

Many microorganisms inhabit the human body. Usually these microorganisms are harmless and in some cases they may be beneficial. Occasionally microorganisms invade the tissues and cause disease. The living together or close association of two organisms is called *symbiosis*. Symbiosis in which both organisms are benefited by the association is called *mutualism*. In *commensalism* one organism benefits without causing harm or giving benefit to the other organism. In *parasitism* one organism (the parasite) derives benefit from the association at the expense of the other organism (the host).

The microorganisms that normally inhabit the skin and mucosa of many parts of the body in a mutualistic or commensal type of association are referred to as *normal flora,* or *resident flora.* Under some circumstances, when body defenses are lowered, resident flora may invade the tissues and multiply there, causing damage. In other words, the microorganisms may establish a parasitic relationship and cause infection. In addition, microorganisms that are not normally present in or on the body may invade the tissues and cause infection. The interactions between microorganisms and the human host are discussed in Chapter 28. This chapter describes the characteristics of organisms that parasitize human beings.

A wide variety of microorganisms can cause infection. Some are noncellular particles (viruses), some are unicellular prokaryotic organisms (bacteria), and some are eukaryotic organisms (fungi and protozoa). In addition to microbial parasites, many macroscopic multicellular animals such as helminths (worms) can parasitize human beings.

VIRUSES

The Nature of Viruses

Viruses are chemical particles composed of a core of nucleic acid (the *nucleoid*) surrounded by a protein coat (the *capsid*). The nucleic acid together with its protein coat is called the *nucleocapsid.* In addition, some viruses have an outermost lipoprotein membrane called an *envelope.*

Viruses differ from cells in several ways. Unlike cells, which contain both DNA and RNA, viral particles contain only one type of nucleic acid. It may be either DNA or RNA, but never both. Viruses lack the machinery necessary for energy production and biosynthesis. Consequently viruses are *obligate intracellular parasites,* which can only

replicate within a host cell. The virus provides the genetic material and utilizes the biosynthetic and energy-generating mechanisms of the host cell in order to replicate. At one stage during replication viruses lose their envelope and protective protein coat and exist as nucleic acid only. Unlike cells, which contain many enzymes, some viruses have no enzymes while other have only a few. Like chemicals, but unlike cells, viruses can be crystallized. A complete viral particle, found extracellularly and capable of surviving in crystalline form and infecting a living cell, is called a *virion.*

Viruses have a variety of shapes and sizes. Some are shaped like rods, bricks, bullets, or tadpoles; many appear spherical. A capsid is made up of many identical subunits called capsomeres. The geometric arrangement of the capsomeres is icosahedral, helical, or complex combinations of these two forms. Viruses that appear spherical are actually icosahedrons. An icosahedron is a geometric form with 12 apexes and 20 faces, each of which is an equilateral triangle. (A geodesic dome is an example of an icosahedron.) In a helical virus the capsomeres are arranged spirally to form a cylindrical capsid.

Viruses are much smaller than cells and only the largest of them can be seen with a light microscope. Most can be visualized only with an electron microscope. They range in size from about 20 nanometers (nm; 10^{-9} meter) in diameter to dimensions of 230 by 300 nm. In contrast, bacterial cells have dimensions ranging from about 0.3 micrometers (μm; 10^{-6} meter) in diameter to lengths of 10 μm (1 μm = 1,000 nm). A human red blood cell has a diameter of about 8 μm. The relative sizes of several microorganisms are shown in Figure 27-1.

Viruses infect not only human beings but also animals, plants, and even bacteria. The viruses that infect bacteria are called *bacteriophages,* or phages for short. Much of the knowledge of viruses has come from the study of bacteriophages. Most phages contain DNA as their nucleic acid; a few contain RNA. All plant viruses contain RNA. Some human and animal viruses contain DNA and

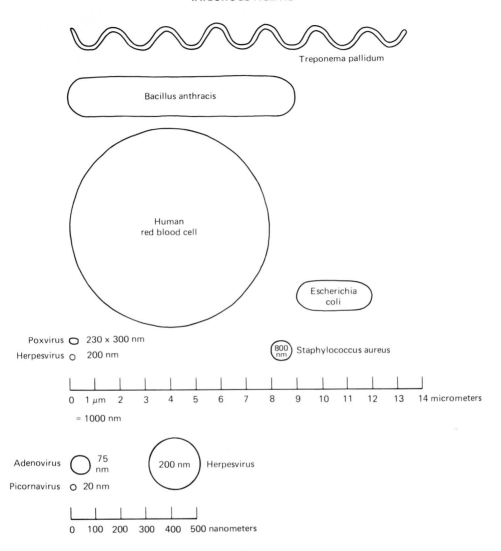

Figure 27-1. *The relative sizes of some representative microorganisms.*

others contain RNA. Only the viruses of clinical importance will be described here.

Classification of Viruses

Several classification schemes have been proposed for viruses and the classification frequently changes. Generally viruses are classified according to their size, shape, and type of nucleic acid and whether or not they have an envelope. Those without an envelope are said to be naked.

DNA Viruses
The following groups of viruses contain deoxyribonucleic acid (DNA).

Poxviruses. These viruses have a complex structure and appear brick-shaped. They are enveloped

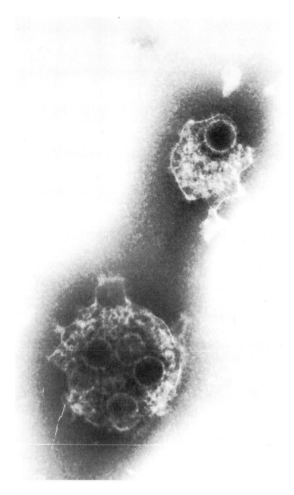

Figure 27-2. *Herpes simplex virus* ($\times$ 106,260). *(Courtesy of Dr. D. McLean and Ms. Kathy Wong, Division of Medical Microbiology, University of British Columbia, Vancouver, B.C., Canada.)*

and have dimensions of about 230 by 300 nm. Members of this group include the agents responsible for smallpox (variola), vaccinia, cowpox, and molluscum contagiosum. Pox viruses characteristically replicate in the skin, producing skin lesions.

Herpesviruses. Viruses of this group are icosahedral with diameters of about 200 nm. They are enveloped. Herpes simplex virus (Fig. 27-2),

varicella-zoster virus, cytomegalovirus, and Epstein-Barr virus (EB virus) are included in this group. Herpes simplex type 1 causes oral infections and is responsible for "cold sores." Herpes simplex type 2 causes genital lesions. Keratoconjunctivitis, encephalitis, meningitis, tracheobronchitis, and pneumonia can also be caused by herpes simplex. Varicella-zoster virus is responsible for chickenpox and herpes zoster. EB virus is associated with infectious mononucleosis and with Burkitt's lymphoma. Many herpesviruses persist in the host for a long time after the initial infection. (See the discussion of latent infections in Chapter 28.)

Adenoviruses. These viruses are naked icosahedrons with diameters of about 75 nm. About 32 types are known. They were first isolated from adenoids of children and cause a variety of respiratory infections.

Papovaviruses. These viruses are naked icosahedral particles about 50 nm in diameter. The name is derived from the first two letters of the three members of this group: *pa*pilloma, *po*lyoma, and *va*cuolating viruses. Papilloma viruses cause warts in human beings. Polyoma viruses are oncogenic (i.e., tumor producing) in mice, hamsters, and rats. The most important vacuolating virus is simian virus 40 (SV 40), which infects monkeys and is capable of causing tumors in baby hamsters.

RNA Viruses
The nucleoids of the following viruses are composed of ribonucleic acid (RNA).

Orthomyxoviruses. These viruses have dimensions ranging from 80 to 200 nm. The nucleocapsids have helical symmetry and are enclosed in envelopes of variable shape (i.e., the viral particles are *pleomorphic*). Spikes containing proteins called neuraminidase and hemagglutinin protrude from the envelope. Hemagglutinin attaches to receptors on the surfaces of red blood cells and causes agglutination (clumping of the cells). Influenza viruses are members of this group (Fig. 27-3).

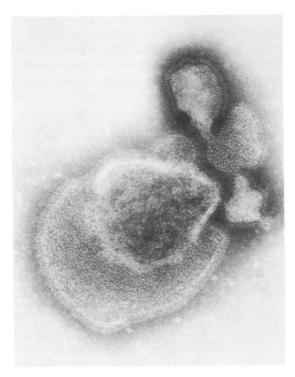

Figure 27-3. *Influenza virus (× 148,665). Note irregular shape and spikes on envelope. (Courtesy of Dr. D. McLean and Ms. Kathy Wong, Division of Medical Microbiology, University of British Columbia, Vancouver, B.C., Canada.)*

Paramyxoviruses. These viruses are similar to orthomyxoviruses but are slightly larger. Members of this group include parainfluenza viruses, which cause respiratory infections; mumps virus; measles (rubeola) virus; and respiratory syncytial viruses.

Rhabdoviruses. These viruses are bullet-shaped, with dimensions of about 70 by 175 nm. The nucleocapsid is helical and is enclosed in an envelope. Rabies virus is in this group.

Togaviruses. Viruses in this group are icosahedral with diameters of 50 to 70 nm. They are enveloped. Arboviruses (*arthropod borne*) types A and B are in this group. Type A arboviruses cause Eastern and Western encephalitis. Type B arboviruses cause yellow fever, dengue, and St. Louis encephalitis. Although rubella (German measles) virus is not arthropod borne (i.e., is not carried by an insect vector), it also has the characteristics of a togavirus.

Arenaviruses. These viruses are pleomorphic enveloped particles with diameters of 100 to 300 nm. The nucleocapsid is helical. The viruses of lymphocytic choriomeningitis and Lassa Fever are in this group.

Coronaviruses. These enveloped viruses have diameters of 80 to 120 nm. Bulbous surface projections give the particles the appearance of a corona. Members of this group cause upper respiratory infections.

Picornaviruses. These viruses are naked icosahedral particles 20 to 30 nm in diameter. This group is further subdived into rhinoviruses and enteroviruses. *Rhinoviruses* are the most frequent causative agents of the common cold. About 100 types are known. *Enteroviruses* include polioviruses, coxsackie viruses, and ECHO viruses (*enteric cytopathic human orphan* viruses). When the ECHO viruses were first isolated from children's feces they could not be linked with any disease (thus the designation orphan viruses). It is now known that ECHO viruses can cause aseptic meningitis, encephalitis, paralysis, and respiratory infections. Coxsackie viruses cause a variety of conditions, including aseptic meningitis, myocarditis, and respiratory illnesses. Polioviruses are responsible for poliomyelitis.

Double-stranded RNA viruses. Reoviruses and rotaviruses contain double-stranded RNA molecules rather than the usual single-stranded RNA. They are naked icosahedral particles 60 to 80 nm in diameter. Reoviruses are prevalent but the exact syndromes caused by these viruses are not known. They may be responsible for mild respiratory and gastrointestinal infections. Rotaviruses are fairly common causes of acute gastroenteritis in children (Fig. 27-4).

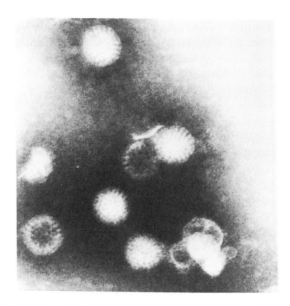

Figure 27-4. *Rotavirus particles from feces of a child with gastroenteritis (× 178,200). (Courtesy of Dr. D. McLean and Ms. Kathy Wong, Division of Medical Microbiology, University of British Columbia, Vancouver, B.C., Canada.)*

Replication of Viruses

As stated earlier, viruses can only replicate within host cells. Unlike a cell, which divides to give rise to two identical daughter cells, a single virion directs the synthesis of dozens of new virions within a host cell. The various components of the virus are made separately and then assembled to form new virions, something like mass production on a factory assembly line. Viral replication involves several phases.

Attachment and Entry
into the Host Cell

Attachment, or adsorption, of a virion to a host cell involves binding of specific sites on the virion to receptors on the surface of the host cell. The ability of a given virus to infect a particular cell depends partly on the presence of specific receptors. The virion is unable to attach to cell types that do not have such receptors.

Entry of the virion into the cell may be by a process similar to phagocytosis or pinocytosis. The engulfed virion is temporarily within a membrane-bound vesicle. Subsequently the viral nucleic acid or nucleocapsid is released into the cytoplasm as a result of the action of degradative enzymes. In the case of some enveloped viruses the envelope may fuse with the cell membrane, with release of the nucleocapsid into the cytoplasm.

Eclipse Phase

After the virus enters a host cell, there is a period called the *eclipse* during which no intact, infectious virus can be detected. The eclipse phase begins with the uncoating of the virus. Various enzymes act on the virus particle, stripping off the envelope (if one is present) and capsid. This process releases the viral nucleic acid and any enzyme that might be present in the virion. The viral nucleic acid then directs the synthesis of new viral components. The process is slightly different for RNA viruses than for DNA viruses.

Replication of DNA viruses. Following infection, replication and transcription of host-cell DNA is usually inhibited. (Some oncogenic viruses, however, may stimulate synthesis of host-cell DNA.) In addition, synthesis of host-cell proteins may be inhibited. Consequently host-cell functions are shut down and energy is directed to the synthesis of new viral particles.

The viral DNA acts as a template for the transcription of messenger RNA. (See the section on DNA and RNA in Chapter 3.) In some cases the enzyme necessary for the process is part of the virion. The first messenger RNA that is transcribed (early mRNA) codes for enzymes that are necessary for the replication of the viral DNA. Messenger RNA transcribed later (late mRNA) codes for structural proteins and enzymes for the virion. Synthesis of viral enzymes and structural proteins takes place on host-cell ribosomes. (See Chapter 3, the section on Translation, for a description of protein synthesis.) In most cases synthesis of viral DNA takes place in the nucleus of the host cell. Replication of poxvirus DNA, however, takes place in the cytoplasm. Replication of a DNA virus is shown schematically in Figure 27-5.

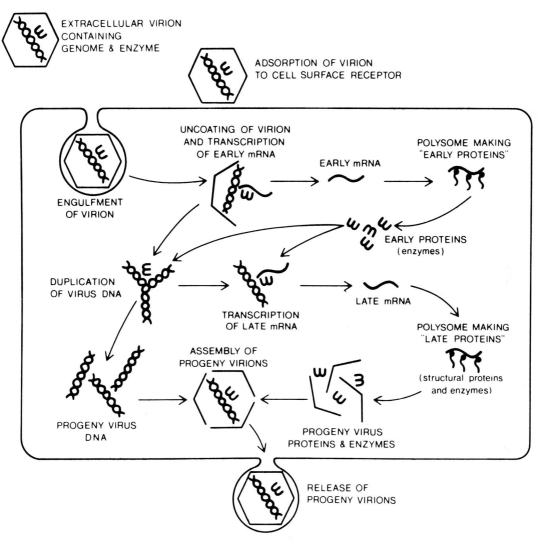

EXTRACELLULAR VIRION
CONTAINING
GENOME & ENZYME

ADSORPTION OF VIRION
TO CELL SURFACE RECEPTOR

UNCOATING OF VIRION
AND TRANSCRIPTION
OF EARLY mRNA

EARLY mRNA

POLYSOME MAKING
"EARLY PROTEINS"

ENGULFMENT
OF VIRION

EARLY PROTEINS
(enzymes)

DUPLICATION
OF VIRUS DNA

TRANSCRIPTION
OF LATE mRNA

LATE mRNA

POLYSOME MAKING
"LATE PROTEINS"

(structural proteins
and enzymes)

ASSEMBLY OF
PROGENY VIRIONS

PROGENY VIRUS
DNA

PROGENY VIRUS
PROTEINS & ENZYMES

RELEASE OF
PROGENY VIRIONS

Figure 27-5. *Steps in the replication of a DNA virus. (From Drew WL (ed):* Viral Infections: A Clinical Approach. *Philadelphia, F. A. Davis Co., 1976.)*

Replication of RNA viruses. As in the case of DNA viruses, infection with RNA viruses inhibits the synthesis of host-cell RNA and protein and the cell machinery is used instead to form new viral particles. In some cases (e.g., poliovirus) the infecting RNA molecule serves as messenger RNA for the synthesis of viral proteins. In other cases (e.g., influenza viruses) the RNA of the infecting particle acts as a template for the synthesis of a complementary strand of messenger RNA.

Host cells do not contain the enzyme necessary for replication of the viral RNA. Therefore the viral messenger RNA must code for this enzyme (RNA synthetase) or the enzyme must be present in the virion. For most RNA viruses, replication of the RNA involves the formation of a double-stranded RNA intermediate. First a new strand complementary to the infecting strand is synthesized. This complementary strand then acts as a template for the synthesis of new viral RNA molecules.

Some oncogenic RNA viruses replicate their RNA through the production of a DNA intermediate. These viruses contain an enzyme called reverse transcriptase, which catalyzes the synthesis of DNA using the viral RNA as a template. (Until the discovery of this enzyme in 1970 it was thought that transcription could only occur in the direction of DNA to RNA and not the reverse.) The DNA intermediate then appears to be integrated into the host-cell DNA as a *provirus*. The provirus DNA is replicated and passed on to daughter cells along with the chromosomes when the host cell divides. The provirus DNA provides the template for transcription of viral RNA and an infected cell must pass through mitosis before synthesis of new viral particles takes place.

Maturation and Release

The eclipse phase ends and the maturation phase begins when newly formed virus particles first appear. Assembly of new nucleocapsids begins when a pool of newly synthesized viral nucleic acid and proteins accumulate in the cell. With some viruses assembly is spontaneous; components "fit together" as in crystallization. With others, assembly of the viral particles is mediated by specific enzymes.

After the viral particles are formed they are released from the host cell. In some cases many virions are released at once, causing death and lysis of the host cell. In other cases, virions are extruded through the cell membrane of the host cell one at a time by a process of budding. This process occurs over a period of time and usually does not cause death of the host cell. In the process of budding, viral protein is incorporated into the cell membrane. Then as the nucleocapsid is extruded, part of this altered membrane goes with it, forming the envelope. Some DNA viruses are released when the host cell dies and disintegrates.

PROKARYOTIC MICROORGANISMS

Prokaryotic organisms include bacteria and blue-green algae. Since blue-green algae do not cause human disease they will not be considered here. Prokaryotic cells differ from eukaryotic cells in several respects. A *prokaryotic cell* does not have a true nucleus; that is, the nuclear material is not separated from the cytoplasm by a nuclear membrane. A *eukaryotic cell* has a true nucleus, with the nuclear material separated from the cytoplasm. Prokaryotic cells tend to be smaller than eukaryotic cells and do not contain cellular organelles such as mitochondria. The ribosomes (protein-synthesizing machinery) of prokaryotic cells are smaller than the cytoplasmic ribosomes of eukaryotic cells. Unlike the ribosomes of eukaryotic cells, prokaryotic ribosomes are not attached to an endoplasmic reticulum.

All higher organisms are composed of eukaryotic cells. The structural differences between prokaryotic and eukaryotic cells form the basis for the selective toxicity of some antibiotics that inhibit bacterial growth without harming human cells. For example, antibiotics such as chloramphenicol, tetracyclines, streptomycin, kanamycin, neomycin, and lincomycin interfere with various steps in protein synthesis in bacterial cells because they bind to specific sites on prokaryotic ribosomes. Since eukaryotic ribosomes are different, protein synthesis by cytoplasmic eukaryotic ribosomes is not affected. (Some organelles of eukaryotic cells, such as mitochondria, however, contain prokaryotic-type ribosomes. This fact may account for some of the side effects of certain antibiotics.)

The Nature of Bacterial Cells

Bacteria are very small unicellular organisms. (Although most bacteria exist as single cells, some form filaments in which many cells are held together in a common sheath. None of the filamentous bacteria is pathogenic for human beings.) Bacterial cells occur in three basic shapes: spherical, cylindrical or rod shaped, and helical or spiral (Fig. 27-6). Spherical bacteria are referred to as

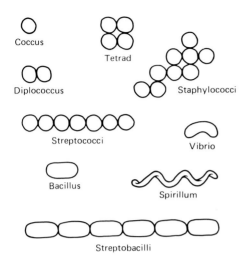

Figure 27-6. *Shapes and arrangements of bacterial cells.*

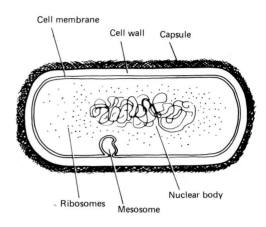

Figure 27-7. *Schematic representation of a generalized bacterial cell.*

cocci (singular: coccus) and cylindrical bacteria as *bacilli* (singular: bacillus). Some short, thick oval-shaped bacilli are referred to as *coccobacilli.* Helical cells may be curved like a comma, as in a *vibrio,* or form several curves as in *spirilla* (singular, spirillum) and *spirochetes.* The long axis of a spirillum remains rigid when the cell is in motion, but the long axis of a spirochete bends when the cell is in motion.

Some bacterial cells tend to stick together after they divide, resulting in characteristic arrangements of cells. Cocci that tend to remain associated in pairs are called *diplococci;* cells that occur in groups of four are called *tetrads.* Cells that divide along only one plane and remain associated after cell division form long chains, as in *streptococci* and *streptobacilli.* Cells that divide along several planes at random form clusters, as in *staphylococci.*

Structure

The structure of a bacterial cell is shown in Figure 27-7. In common with other cells, bacterial cells have a *cell membrane* that encloses the cytoplasm. In addition, most bacterial cells have a *cell wall* that surrounds the cell membrane. The mycoplasma or pleuropneumonialike organisms (PPLO)

are an exception; they lack a cell wall. Most bacteria have a rigid cell wall, which maintains the shape of the organism, but some (e.g., spirochetes) have a flexible cell wall. (All plant cells have a cell wall, but animal and human cells do not have a cell wall. Plant cell walls have a different structure than bacterial cell walls.) The cell wall prevents the cell from bursting when it is in a hypotonic solution. Since many bacteria grow in dilute solutions that are hypotonic relative to the cell cytoplasm, this function of the cell wall is important.

The cell walls of bacteria contain a complex mucopeptide that is found only in prokaryotes and nowhere else in nature. In addition, some bacteria (gram-negative organisms) have a lipopolysaccharide and a lipoprotein in their cell wall. Components of the cell wall are sometimes responsible for the symptoms of disease. (See the discussion of endotoxin in Chapter 28.) Some antibiotics (e.g., penicillin) exert their effect by interfering with the synthesis of the cell wall in growing cells. As a result the cell wall is weakened and the cells are easily lysed.

In addition to the cell wall, some bacteria have an outermost layer called a *capsule.* The capsule is a loose-fitting gelatinous structure composed of either polysaccharide or polypeptides. The capsule is associated with the pathogenicity of some bacteria (e.g., *Streptococcus pneumoniae*). Encapsulated cells resist phagocytosis by host cells (see Chapter 28).

The cell membrane of bacterial cells is a lipoprotein structure similar to the cell membranes of other types of cells. As in other organisms, the cell membrane regulates the passage of certain substances into and out of the cell. Some bacteria secrete enzymes into the surrounding medium. These enzymes break down large molecules (e.g., polysaccharides) that cannot penetrate the cell wall and cell membrane into their subunits, which are much smaller molecules that can be transported into the cell.

As stated earlier, prokaryotic cells lack mitochondria. Instead, many enzymes concerned with catabolism of food molecules and production of energy are associated with the inner surface of the cell membrane.

A *mesosome*, an irregular convoluted infolding of the cell membrane, is present in some bacteria. The mesosome possibly is involved in the formation of the cross wall and the partitioning of the parent cell DNA into the daughter cells during cell division.

As mentioned previously, the nuclear material of prokaryotic cells is not separated from the cytoplasm by a nuclear membrane. Most of the genetic material in a bacterial cell is contained in a single large circular molecule of DNA that is attached to the cell membrane. In contrast, eukaryotic cells contain a much larger amount of DNA, which is packaged into a number of chromosomes. Although the bacterial DNA is sometimes referred to as a chromosome, it does not have the complex structure of eukaryotic chromosomes. Therefore it is sometimes referred to as a *nuclear body*. In addition to the large molecule of DNA, some bacterial cells contain small fragments of DNA that are not integrated into the chromosome. Some of these extrachromosomal genetic elements are called episomes and others are referred to as plasmids. An *episome* can exist either as an extrachromosomal element or integrated into the chromosome. A *plasmid* occurs in the cytoplasm and is never integrated into the chromosome. An example of a plasmid that is found in some bacteria is *drug-resistance factor* (R factor). This factor can be transferred from one bacterium to another and contains genetic information that confers resistance to certain antibiotics.

Some bacteria have *flagella* (singular: flagellum) and are motile (i.e., are capable of spontaneous movement). Bacteria that lack flagella are immotile. Spirochetes have an *axial filament* that is attached to both ends of the cell and functions in locomotion.

Under certain conditions, some bacteria (particularly certain species of bacilli) undergo a process called sporogenesis or sporulation and form an *endospore*. In this process a vegetative (i.e., actively metabolizing) cell forms within it a round or oval body that is surrounded by a capsule. Gradually the rest of the cell disintegrates, leaving only the endospore. Endospores have no metabolic activity and are usually resistant to a variety of conditions that would kill vegetative cells, such as drying, freezing, and exposure to heat, chemicals, and radiation. When conditions are right, the endospore germinates and gives rise to a vegetative cell again. Bacterial endospores are *not* reproductive structures, since a single bacterium forms only one endospore and the endospore in turn gives rise to a single bacterium. Rather, an endospore is a dormant phase in the life cycle of a bacterial cell.

Growth Requirements

As a group, bacteria can grow under a wide variety of conditions. Individual species, however, have a narrower range of environmental conditions in which they can grow and multiply. Bacterial growth is influenced by nutritional factors and by physical factors such as temperature, pH, osmotic pressure, and oxygen.

Nutritional factors. The nutritional requirements of bacteria vary. In general, the materials necessary for the synthesis of cell components and for the production of energy must be available. All organisms require a source of carbon for the synthesis of cell components. Some organisms, which are said to be *heterotrophic*, use organic compounds (e.g., sugars) as a source of carbon for biosynthesis and as a source of energy. Organisms that use carbon dioxide as their major source of carbon for biosynthesis are said to be *autotrophic*. These organisms usually obtain energy either from the sun (through photosynthesis) or by metabolizing inorganic compounds such as hydrogen gas (H_2), ammonia (NH_3), reduced iron (Fe^{2+}), nitrite (NO_2^-), or hydrogen sulfide (H_2S).

In addition to carbon, other elements found in cell components, such as nitrogen, phosphorus, and sulfur, must be available. Nitrogen is necessary for incorporation into amino acids, purines, and pyrimidines. Some bacteria require these compounds preformed, but many bacteria can synthesize them if a simple nitrogen source such as ammonia or nitrate (NO_3^-) is available. Phosphorus is necessary for synthesis of nucleic acids, phospholipids, and ATP (adenosine triphosphate). Most bacteria can use phosphate. Sulfur is required for incorporation into sulfur-containing amino acids, coenzymes, and other cellular components. Many bacteria can use sulfate for this purpose. Some bacteria also require various vitamins.

Physical factors. The optimum temperature for most bacteria is between 15 and 50°C, but some (psychrophiles) grow well at lower temperatures, and others (thermophiles) grow best at higher temperatures. Most pathogenic bacteria are adapted to growing in the human body and grow best at temperatures between 35 and 40°C.

Most bacteria can tolerate pH ranges from 5 (acidic) to 8 (basic), but they grow best at a neutral pH (7). A few bacteria can tolerate a very acidic environment.

The osmotic pressure of a medium depends on the number of solute particles in the solution (see Chapter 11 under Movement of Fluids Between Compartments). Most bacteria can grow in media having a rather broad range of solute concentrations because the cell is able to keep the internal concentration of substances fairly constant by means of active transport. As mentioned earlier, the cell wall prevents the cell from rupturing when

it is in a hypotonic medium. If bacterial cells are placed in solutions that are too hypertonic, however, water is drawn out of the cell by osmosis and growth is inhibited.

Bacteria vary in their oxygen requirement, reflecting differences in the metabolic pathways utilized to generate energy. Some bacteria must have oxygen for growth; these organisms are *obligate aerobes*. Oxygen is toxic for some bacteria; these organisms grow only in the absence of oxygen and are called *obligate anaerobes*. Some bacteria are *facultative anaerobes*; they can grow with or without oxygen, although usually they grow more quickly when oxygen is available. Some bacteria require a little oxygen, but grow best when the oxygen concentration is low (lower than in atmospheric air). These bacteria are said to be *microaerophilic*.

Energy Metabolism

As with human cells and the cells of all other organisms, the energy currency of bacterial cells is ATP (see Chapter 10 under Cellular Respiration). As with human cells, many bacterial cells metabolize glucose by the pathway known as glycolysis. Under anaerobic conditions, some bacteria convert pyruvic acid to lactic acid, as human cells do, but other bacteria metabolize pyruvic acid to different end products, depending on the particular enzyme(s) present in the bacterial cell. For example, some bacteria convert pyruvic acid to acetaldehyde, butyric acid, formic acid, ethanol, butanol, isopropanol, or other substances. When the final electron (i.e., hydrogen) acceptor is an organic molecule, as in these cases, the whole glycolytic process is called fermentation. When the sequence of reactions in which an inorganic substance is the final electron (hydrogen) acceptor is used, the process is called respiration.

Many bacteria have the enzymes necessary for the operation of the TCA cycle (Krebs cycle) and respiratory chain for the production of ATP. The final electron acceptor in the respiratory chain is usually oxygen, but some organisms (facultative anaerobes) can use other inorganic compounds, such as nitrate, sulfate, or carbon dioxide, as the final electron acceptor if oxygen is not available.

Obligate anaerobes lack the cytochromes of the respiratory chain and many of the enzymes of the TCA cycle. If they are exposed to oxygen, the oxygen combines with hydrogen to form hydrogen peroxide (H_2O_2), which is toxic to all cells. Most aerobic organisms have an enzyme called catalase which splits hydrogen peroxide into water plus oxygen, but obligate anaerobes lack this enzyme.

As mentioned earlier, autotrophic bacteria can oxidize inorganic compounds to generate energy. These bacteria are not important clinically, but some (e.g., methane bacteria) are important in waste disposal and others are involved in the nitrogen cycle, which is important in food production. The methane bacteria, for example, derive energy from the oxidation of hydrogen gas, as follows:

$$4H_2 + CO_2 \rightarrow CH_4 \text{ (methane)} + 2H_2O$$

Methane bacteria are anaerobic, but some bacteria that oxidize inorganic compounds are aerobic (e.g., sulfur bacteria).

Reproduction

Bacteria reproduce by an asexual process called *binary fission,* in which one cell divides to produce two progeny cells. Before a cell divides, it increases in size and duplicates its cellular components, such as DNA. In the first stage of division the cell membrane invaginates into the center of the cell, producing a transverse septum. As this process occurs, one DNA molecule is pushed (or pulled) into one side of the dividing cell, and its replica is pushed into the other side. The cell wall then grows in toward the center between the folds of the membrane, producing a cross wall that is thicker than the rest of the cell wall. The cross wall divides the cell into two. Cell separation is then achieved by cleavage of this thickened cross wall, with each half forming part of the wall of each progeny cell.

Classification of Bacteria

A thorough discussion of bacterial classification is beyond the scope of this book. The classification of bacteria is complicated and is undergoing change. Generally the older, more cumbersome classification schemes are being replaced with simpler schemes in which bacteria are placed in descriptive groups according to staining properties, shape, oxygen requirement, and so on. Only the groups of clinical importance will be briefly outlined here. It should be realized, however, that many other groups of bacteria also exist.

An important staining procedure, which divides bacteria into two major groups, is the *Gram stain.* In this procedure a basic purple dye (usually gentian violet or crystal violet) is applied to cells that have been heat fixed on a slide. All bacterial cells able to take up the dye stain purple. Then a dilute iodine solution is added; this solution decreases the solubility of the purple stain within the cell. Next an organic solvent, such as ethanol, is added. This solvent removes the purple dye from some species of bacteria but not from others. Finally, a red stain is applied. The bacteria that are decolorized by the organic solvent are *gram-negative;* they appear red due to the red stain. The bacteria that retain the purple dye after treatment with the organic solvent are *gram-positive;* they appear purple. The reason that some bacteria retain the purple dye and others do not is related to differences in the chemical structure of the cell wall. Certain other properties of the cell are also correlated with these differences.

Each distinct kind of bacterium is recognized as a species and is named according to the binomial system of nomenclature, in which each species is given a two-word name. The first word, called the genus (plural: genera), is capitalized; the second word, called the species, is not. Both words are type-set in italics. Sometimes the genus is abbreviated. For example, *Escherichia coli* becomes *E. coli.*

Gram-Positive Cocci

Members of the genera *Staphylococcus* and *Streptococcus* are clinically important gram-positive cocci. They are nonmotile, non-spore-forming organisms.

Staphylococci. These bacteria typically occur in grapelike clusters and most are facultative anaerobes. There are two species of staphylococci. *Staphylococcus epidermis* is a nonpathogenic organism often found on the skin as part of the resident flora. *Staphylococcus aureus* is found on the skin of some people and is pathogenic. Several strains of *S. aureus* exist; some are more virulent than others. Virulent stains produce an enzyme called coagulase that clots plasma.

Staphylococci are specifically associated with infections of the skin, such as boils, carbuncles, and impetigo; and with osteomyelitis, staphylococcus enteritis, and one type of food poisoning (see Chapter 28). They may also cause systemic diseases such as endocarditis, meningitis, pneumonia, cystitis, and pyelonephritis.

Streptococci. These cocci occur in varying sizes arranged in long or short chains. Most are facultative anaerobes but a few are strict anaerobes. Some species have a capsule. Not all species are pathogenic.

Streptococci are classified into three groups according to their behavior when they are cultured on blood agar. *Alpha-hemolytic* species or viridans secrete a hemolysin that produces a narrow greenish zone of hemolysis around each colony. *Beta-hemolytic* species secrete a hemolysin that produces a wide clear zone of hemolysis around each colony. *Gamma* species do not hemolyze red blood cells. In addition, streptococci are classified into Lancefield groups designated by letters A through O based on antigenic properties of the cell-wall carbohydrate.

Group A beta-hemolytic streptococci have the species name *Streptococcus pyogenes*. This species is responsible for most streptococcal diseases. Streptococcal diseases can be classed as suppurative, or primary infections, and nonsuppurative diseases that are regarded as complications following primary infections. Suppurative infections include acute pharyngitis, puerperal fever, and skin infec-

tions such as impetigo, cellulitis, and erysipelas. Nonsuppurative complications are scarlet fever, rheumatic fever, acute glomerulonephritis, and erythema nodosum.

Group B beta-hemolytic streptococci have the species name *S. agalactiae*. This species is rarely pathogenic. It is found in the vagina of some women during pregnancy and can cause infections in the newborn.

Several species of alpha-hemolytic streptococci are found in the mouth and play a role in dental caries.

Group D streptococci include alpha-hemolytic and nonhemolytic species that are found mainly in the intestinal tract. *S. faecalis* is a gamma streptococcus that is sometimes responsible for urinary infections and for abdominal infections following bowel surgery.

Streptococcus pneumoniae (pneumococcus) usually occurs in pairs, although it can occur singly and in chains. It is alpha hemolytic. This organism is found in the respiratory tract of many people. Pathogenic strains have a capsule and commonly cause lobar pneumonia. They can also cause meningitis, otitis media, bronchitis, and peritonitis.

Gram-Negative Cocci

The clinically important gram-negative cocci are *Neisseria gonorrhoeae* (the gonococcus) and *Neisseria meningitides* (the meningococcus). These organisms are nonmotile, non-spore-forming diplococci. They are very delicate organisms that do not survive very long outside of the human host. *N. gonorrhoeae* causes the veneral disease gonorrhea. *N. meningitides* causes meningitis and septicemia in susceptible people.

Gram-Negative Enteric Bacilli

The group of bacteria referred to as enteric bacilli are gram-negative non-spore-forming rods that are facultative anaerobes. Some of them are pathogenic. Others are resident flora of the intestinal tract which are not normally pathogenic but can become pathogenic under certain circumstances. *Escherichia coli*, *Klebsiella pneumoniae*, and

Enterobacter aerogenes are sometimes referred to as *coliforms*. The presence of these organisms in water or food is used an indicator of fecal contamination.

E. coli is a normal resident of the intestinal tract and is not usually pathogenic. It can cause serious infections, however, if it is introduced into the urinary tract. Certain strains can produce diarrhea, particularly in infants.

Enteric bacilli of the genus *Salmonella* are pathogenic. *S. typhi* and *S. paratyphi* cause the systemic diseases typhoid fever and paratyphoid fever. Some species of *Salmonella*, most notably *S. typhimurium*, cause gastroenteritis (salmonellosis).

Species of *Shigella* are enteric bacilli that cause bacillary dysentery. *Shigella dysenteriae* is the most virulent species and is capable of causing septicemia as well as intestinal infection.

Most *Pseudomonas* species are found in water, soil, and sewage but one, *P. aeruginosa*, is sometimes found in the human intestinal tract. *P. aeruginosa* is an opportunistic pathogen that is responsible for many hospital-acquired infections, particularly in people with burns (see Chapter 24) and those recovering following kidney transplants.

Klebsiella pneumoniae (Friedländer's bacillus) is carried in the throat or intestinal tract of about 10% of the population. This organism is sometimes responsible for hospital-acquired infections, such as septicemia in children and secondary bacterial pneumonia or upper respiratory infections in people with respiratory diseases.

Species of *Proteus* also inhabit the intestine. These organisms produce an enzyme called urease that splits urea to form ammonia. *Proteus vulgaris* is sometimes responsible for secondary intestinal and urinary tract infections.

Gram-Negative Anaerobic Bacilli

Members of the genus *Bacteroides* are nonmotile, non-spore-forming gram-negative bacilli that are obligate anaerobes. They are the most numerous group of microorganisms resident in the human intestinal tract. Some species are also found in the oral cavity. *Bacteroides* species are sometimes responsible for wound infection.

Members of the genus *Fusobacterium* are gram-negative rods that are pointed at one or both ends. They are also obligate anaerobes. They are commonly found in the oral cavity and by themselves do not appear to cause infection. They appear in increased numbers in association with an oral spirochete, however, in periodontal disease such as Vincent's angina.

Non-spore-forming Gram-Positive Bacilli

Two important genera in this group are *Lactobacillus* and *Corynebacterium*. Lactobacilli are nonmotile, non-spore-forming gram-positive rods that are microaerophilic or anaerobic. They tend to prefer acid conditions. Lactobacilli are resident flora of the mouth, intestinal tract, and vagina. They are associated with dental caries.

The most important member of the genus *Corynebacterium* is *C. diphtheriae*, the organism responsible for diphtheria. *C. diphtheriae* is an aerobic, nonmotile, gram-positive pleomorphic bacillus. Individual cells may be straight or curved, may be clubbed at one or both ends, or may be swollen in the middle.

Spore-forming Gram-Positive Bacilli

Bacillus and *Clostridium* are two major genera of this group. *Bacilli* are found in soil, water, and vegetation. *Bacillus anthracis* is the only pathogenic species. It causes anthrax, a disease primarily of sheep, horses, and cattle that can be transmitted to human beings. *B. anthracis* is one of the largest pathogenic bacteria known. It is a nonmotile facultative anaerobe that forms endospores. Some strains have a capsule.

Clostridium species inhabit water, soil, and vegetation. A few inhabit the intestinal tracts of people and animals. Except for one species (*C. histolyticum*), clostridia are obligate anaerobes. Their spores, however, can tolerate oxygen and are very resistant to heat. Pathogenic clostridia are *C. tetani*, which causes tetanus; *C. botulinum*, which is responsible for botulism, one type of food poisoning; and *C. perfringens*, which causes gas gangrene.

Gram-Negative Aerobic Coccobaccilli

Members of this group are nonmotile, non-spore-forming organisms that are capable of forming capsules. The group includes members of the genera *Hemophilus*, *Bordetella*, *Brucella*, and *Francisella*.

Several species of *Hemophilus* are resident flora of the upper respiratory tract. The major pathogenic species is *H. influenzae*. Encapsulated strains of this species are primary pathogens that cause meningitis in young children and can also cause pneumonia, bronchitis, otitis media, and epiglottitis. Nonencapsulated strains of *H. influenzae* commonly cause secondary infections of the upper respiratory tract following invasion by viruses.

Bordetella species are also common inhabitants of the upper respiratory tract. *Bordetella pertussis* causes whooping cough.

Brucella species are primarily pathogenic to animals and infect people secondarily. The major species are *B. abortus*, which infects cattle; *B. suis*, which infects swine; and *B. melitensis*, which infects sheep and goats. Human beings can be infected by all three species; the disease they cause is called brucellosis. Human disease caused by *B. melitensis* is also referred to as undulant fever.

Francisella tularensis is the most important species of the genus *Francisella*. It causes the disease tularemia, which affects rodents (particularly rabbits) but can also be transmitted to people.

Mycobacteria
Mycobacteria are nonmotile, non-spore-forming aerobic bacilli. They are difficult to stain but when they do take up basic dyes they resist decolorization with acid alcohol (i.e., they retain the dye). Therefore they are referred to as *acid-fast*. (Most bacteria do not retain the dye.) The important species in this group are *Mycobacterium tuberculosis*, which causes tuberculosis in people; *Mycobacterium bovis*, which causes tuberculosis in cattle; and *Mycobacterium leprae*, which causes leprosy.

Spiral and Curved Bacteria
Members of this group include the vibrios and spirella. The most important pathogenic organism is *Vibrio cholerae*, a small aerobic, motile, gram-negative curved rod that causes cholera.

Spirillum minus is a motile, gram-negative, tightly coiled organism that is found mainly in wild rats. It can be transmitted to human beings by the bite of a rat and is one cause of rat-bite fever.

Spirochetes
Unlike the vibrios and spirella, which have rigid cell walls, spirochetes have a flexible cell wall. Also, they have a different mode of locomotion, as mentioned previously. The important genera in this group are *Treponema* and *Borrelia*.

Treponema species are 6 to 14 μm long and have regularly spaced coils 1 μm apart. The most important is *Treponema pallidum*, the causative agent of the venereal disease syphilis. This organism is very sensitive to drying and cannot survive very long outside the human body. *T. pertenue* causes a nonvenereal disease called yaws.

Pathogenic *Borrelia* species are 10 to 30 μm long and have irregularly spaced coils. *B. recurrentis*, which is transmitted from one person to another by body lice, and *B. duttonii*, which is transmitted to people by ticks, cause relapsing fever.

Mycoplasmas
Mycoplasmas are unusual in that they lack a cell wall. They are the smallest cells capable of an independent existence. *Mycoplasma pneumoniae*, which causes primary atypical pneumonia, is the only species that is pathogenic for human beings.

Rickettsiae
Rickettsiae are small pleomorphic coccobacilli that can only reproduce within a host cell. The cell membranes of rickettsiae are "leaky" and allow the loss of nutrients from the cell. This fact may be the basis of their inability to multiply outside a susceptible host cell.

Rickettsiae infect arthropods such as ticks, mites, fleas, and lice. They are transmitted to humans through the bites of these animals. *R. prowazekii* causes epidemic typhus fever, *R. mooseri* causes endemic typhus fever, and *R. tsutsugamushi* causes scrub typhus. *R. rickettsiae* is responsible for Rocky Mountain spotted fever, and *Coxiella burnetii* is the etiological agent of Q fever.

Chlamydiae

Chlamydiae are spherical organisms that are slightly smaller than rickettsiae. These organisms do not have an energy-generating mechanism. Therefore they are obligate intracellular parasites, depending on the host cell for ATP. Agents in this group are responsible for trachoma, lymphogranuloma venereum, and psittacosis (ornithosis).

EUKARYOTIC MICROORGANISMS

Eukaryotic microorganisms include protozoa, fungi, and algae. Algae are not pathogenic and will not be considered here. As mentioned earlier, in eukaryotic cells the nucleus is separated from the cytoplasm by a nuclear membrane and organelles such as mitochondria and an endoplasmic reticulum are present in the cytoplasm.

Fungi

Fungi are simple plants that lack chlorophyll and are not capable of photosynthesis. Most are *saprophytes*; that is, they exist on dead or decaying organic matter. Some are parasitic on living plants or animals but only a few species are pathogenic for human beings. Most of the fungi that infect people live mainly in the soil and are not obligate parasites. Fungi range in size from microscopic unicellular organisms to macroscopic multicellular organisms. Fungal cells and filaments are surrounded by rigid cell walls.

Unicellular fungi of the class Ascomycetes or Deuteromycetes are called *yeasts*. Fungi that exist as multicellular filamentous organisms are called *molds*. Some fungi are capable of existing either as unicellular or multicellular organisms, depending on environmental conditions, and are called *dimorphic fungi*.

The single-celled reproductive form of a mold is called a *spore*. When a spore reaches a suitable environment it germinates and forms a process called a *germ tube*. The tube continues to elongate and forms a multinucleate filament called a *hypha*. In some fungi the nuclei of the filament are separated into individual cells by cross walls called *septa* (singular: septum). The filament branches and forms many hyphae that become entwined; the resulting mass of hyphae is called a *mycelium* (Fig. 27-8). The part of the plant that extends down into the medium is the vegetative mycelium. The part that projects above the surface is the aerial mycelium. The reproductive structures are usually found in the aerial mycelium. Fungi form both asexual and sexual spores. Specialized structures that bear sexual spores are called fruiting bodies.

Yeasts often reproduce by an asexual process called budding, although they are capable of forming sexual spores under certain conditions. The budding cell is sometimes called a blastospore. In the process of budding the nucleus moves toward the edge of the cell and divides. The cytoplasm protrudes at this point, forming a bud. One daughter nucleus moves into the bud while the other remains in the parent cell. The bud enlarges and becomes constricted at its base. Finally it separates from the parent cell to become an independent small yeast cell.

Fungi prefer a moist environment for growth. Most are aerobic, but some yeasts are facultative anaerobes. Most fungi grow best at temperatures ranging from 20° to 35°C. Fungi can grow at a

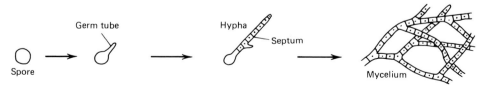

Figure 27-8. *Growth of a mold.*

wide range of pH, but they grow best in an acid medium. The molds have a pH optimum of 5.0 to 6.0, whereas yeasts grow best at a pH of 4.5 to 5.0.

There are four classes of fungi: Phycomycetes, Basidiomycetes, Ascomycetes, and Deuteromycetes (Fungi Imperfecti). Most of the clinically important fungi are in the class Deuteromycetes.

Phycomycetes

This class includes aquatic and terrestrial organisms. Some of the water molds are unicellular and do not produce a mycelium. Those that do develop mycelia lack septa. Usually they reproduce asexually, but some can reproduce both sexually and asexually.

The common black bread mold, *Rhizopus nigricans*, is a familiar example of the terrestrial members of this class. This mold reproduces asexually by means of single-celled spores called sporangiospores, which form within sacs called sporangia (singular: sporangium) at the tips of hyphae. *Rhizopus* species can also reproduce by a sexual process when two mycelia of opposite sex come together. Each forms a special side branch and cells in contact fuse to form a zygospore.

Basidiomycetes

This class includes the rusts and smuts that infect grains, as well as mushrooms and puffballs. They produce sexual spores on a specialized structure called a basidium.

Ascomycetes

This class is the largest and includes most of the yeasts as well as morels, cup fungi, powdery mildews and some molds. Yeasts of the genus *Saccharomyces* are used in bread making, brewing, and wine making. *Neurospora* is a mold that is used in genetics research.

Ascomycetes reproduce sexually by the formation of spores called ascospores. The ascospores develop in a saclike structure called an ascus, usually with four or eight spores per ascus. Yeasts can form ascospores under certain conditions, but usually reproduce asexually by budding, as described previously.

Deuteromycetes (Fungi Imperfecti)

Fungi of this class have no demonstrated sexual, or perfect, stage in their life cycle. Asexual spores are formed by any of a variety of processes. The spores are usually called conidia and are borne on specialized hyphae. Occasionally sexual spore formation is observed in some members of this group and they are reclassified, usually as Ascomycetes. Molds of the genera *Penicillium* and *Aspergillus* are important fungi that usually reproduce asexually and are classed as Deuteromycetes, but occasionally sexual forms are found and they are classed as Ascomycetes.

Penicillium chrysogenum and *Penicillium notatum* produce the antibiotic penicillin. Some species of *Penicillium* are used in the manufacture of certain cheeses (e.g., Roquefort and Camembert). Other *Penicillium* species cause clothing mildew and spoilage of fruits. Some *Aspergillus* species cause granulomatous respiratory disease. (See Chapter 8 for a discussion of granuloma formation.)

Cryptococcus species are yeastlike organisms. *Cryptococcus neoformans* is a pathogen that particularly affects the lungs, brain, and meninges. Members of the genus *Candida* are dimorphic fungi. *Candida* species, particularly *C. albicans*, are often found as resident flora of the mouth, intestinal tract, and vagina. They are opportunistic pathogens that sometimes cause serious infection. *Candida* infection (referred to as candidiasis or moniliasis) mainly affects debilitated people or those receiving broad-spectrum antibiotics. The antibiotics decrease the number of bacterial flora, which usually inhibit the growth of *Candida*. *Candida* can infect the skin, nails, and mucous membranes and can also cause serious systemic disease. Oral candidiasis (thrush) and vaginal candidiasis are common.

Fungi of the genera *Microsporum*, *Trichophyton*, and *Epidermophyton* cause superficial infections, called *tineas* (ringworm) of the skin, hair, and nails.

Inhalation of the spores of several fungi can lead to systemic disease. *Histoplasma capsulatum* can multiply within various reticuloendothelial cells and produces histoplasmosis. Lesions resembling those of tuberculosis occur in the lungs. In addition the liver, spleen, and lymph nodes may be involved. *Coccidioides immitus* causes coccidioidomycosis, a disease that starts as an upper respiratory infection but may become disseminated throughout the body. Blastomycosis is a pulmonary disease caused by *Blastomyces dermatitides*.

Protozoa

Protozoa (singular: protozoon) are heterotrophic unicellular organisms that do not have a cell wall. Most are microscopic, but some are quite large and can be seen without the aid of a microscope. Protozoa require large amounts of moisture. Many saprophytic species are found in marine, freshwater, and terrestrial habitats. Some species are parasites. Some protozoa ingest particulate matter (e.g., bacteria) by phagocytosis. Others (Mastigophora and Sporozoa) usually assimilate organic substances through their cell membranes.

The active feeding, vegetative form of a protozoon is called a *trophozoite*. Some protozoa also exist as *cysts*, protective forms that are formed when conditions for growth are unfavorable. When a cyst is formed the organism becomes dehydrated and surrounded by a thick membrane. Cysts are resistant to many conditions that would kill trophozoites and are often responsible for the spread of protozoan infections. When growth conditions are suitable, the cyst imbibes water and the organism becomes a trophozoite again.

Protozoa are divided into four groups: Sarcodina, Ciliophora, Mastigophora, and Sporozoa.

Sarcodina

Members of this group are ameboid organisms that move by means of pseudopodia (false feet). Some marine forms have hard exoskeletons or shells. Amebae, which belong to this group, reproduce asexually by binary fission following mitotic division of the nucleus. Mitotic nuclear divisions also occur during encystment, producing several nuclei within one cyst. When excystment occurs, each nucleus may give rise to a new trophozoite. Some Sarcodina species reproduce sexually.

Several amebae inhabit the human intestinal tract. One of them, *Entamoeba histolytica*, is pathogenic and causes amebic dysentery.

Ciliophora (Ciliates)

These organisms have hairlike structures called cilia for locomotion. They have a permanent ovoid shape of fixed dimensions and are structurally quite complex. Ciliophora have two nuclei, a large macronucleus that directs the cell's activities and a small micronucleus that is responsible for cell reproduction. These organisms usually reproduce asexually but can also reproduce sexually by conjugation.

Most members of this group are free-living. A few species inhabit the intestinal tracts of animals and one, *Balantidium coli*, occasionally infects humans. It can cause a chronic, recurrent type of dysentery.

Mastigophora (Flagellates)

Organisms in this group are ovoid or elongated cells that have one or more flagella as means of locomotion. Some have an undulating membrane, a protoplasmic membrane running like a fin along the organism. Its margin is formed by a flagellum that may continue free beyond the undulating membrane.

Several species of Mastigophora inhabit the human intestinal tract. One of them, *Giardia lamblia*, dwells in the upper intestinal tract and is often harmless, but can cause persistent diarrhea, inflammatory changes in the mucosa of the small intestine, and malabsorption.

Trichomonas vaginalis is a flagellate that infects the vagina in females and the genitourinary tract in males. In males the infection is usually asymptomatic.

Members of the genera *Trypanosoma* and *Leishmania* are referred to as hemoflagellates. They are transmitted by insects and infect the blood and tissues of humans. These organisms have complex life cycles that involve alternate existence in human (or animal) and insect hosts. *Trypanosoma gambiense* and *Trypanosoma rhodesiense* cause African sleeping sickness (trypanosomiasis).

Leishmania donovani causes kala-azar (visceral leishmaniasis).

Sporozoa

Members of this group have no external means of locomotion but some immature forms have an ameboid type of motion by means of pseudopodia. All organisms in this group are parasitic. Sporozoa have complex life cycles involving both sexual and asexual developmental stages.

The clinically important Sporozoa are members of the genus *Plasmodium*, which cause malaria. The most common type is tertian malaria, caused by *Plasmodium vivax*. The least common type is quartan malaria, caused by *Plasmodium malariae*. Falciparum malaria (formerly called estivoautumnal malaria), which is caused by *Plasmodium falciparum*, is the most serious type.

Plasmodium species have a complex life cycle involving an asexual phase called *schizogony*, which occurs in the human (intermediate) host, and a sexual phase called sporogony, which takes place in female *Anopheles* mosquitoes (the definitive host). The organism is injected into the bloodstream when a person is bitten by an infected mosquito. Within the human host the parasite first has one or more cycles of development in the cells of the liver. Then it invades the red blood cells, where it undergoes further stages of development. When a female *Anopheles* mosquito bites an infected person and takes a blood meal, the parasite enters the mosquito and undergoes further development.

SUGGESTED ADDITIONAL READING

Costerton JW, Geesey GG, Cheng K-J: How bacteria stick. *Sci Am* **238**(1): 86–95, 1978.

Clowes RC: The molecule of infectious drug resistance. *Sci Am* **228**(4): 18–27, 1973.

Holland JJ: Slow, inapparent and recurrent viruses. *Sci Am* **230**(2): 33–40, 1974.

Marples MJ: Life on the human skin. *Sci Am* **220**(1): 108–115, 1969.

Watanabe T: Infectious drug resistance. *Sci Am* **217**(6): 19–27, 1967.

28

Host-Microbe Interactions

The mere presence of microorganisms in or on the body does not signify disease. As mentioned in Chapter 27, many microorganisms inhabit the body surfaces and the lumen of the intestinal tract as resident flora. The resident flora normally have a benign commensal or mutualistic type of relationship with the human host. Some are saprophytes (i.e., obtain nutrition from nonliving organic material). For example, some live on dead cells in the outer layers of the skin and others live on food in the lumen of the intestinal tract.

Microorganisms cause *infections* when they invade the tissues and multiply there, stimulating a host response. The infection may or may not be accompanied by overt symptoms of disease. A *local* infection is one that is restricted to a particular anatomical site. A *generalized*, or *systemic*, infection is one in which microorganisms and/or their products are spread throughout the body. A *focal* infection is a localized site of infection from which microorganisms and/or their products are spread to other parts of the body. An initial infection caused by one kind of microorganism is a *primary* infection. A *secondary* infection is an infection by a second microorganism following a primary infection by another kind of microorganism (e.g., streptococcal pneumonia following influenza infection). A *mixed* infection is one caused by more than one kind of microorganism. *Sepsis* is the presence of pathogenic (i.e., disease-producing) microorganisms or their toxins in the blood or tissues.

Some pathogenic microorganisms only exist as parasites in a human or animal host (e.g., *Neisseria gonorrhoeae*, *Plasmodium vivax*). Other microorganisms, however, often exist as free-living organisms (e.g., *Pseudomonas aeruginosa*) or exist in a commensal or mutualistic type of relationship with the human host (e.g., *Escherichia coli*), but are capable of causing infection if host defenses are lowered. Such microorganisms are referred to as *opportunistic* pathogens. Hospital-acquired infections are commonly caused by opportunistic pathogens.

THE ENCOUNTER BETWEEN HOST AND MICROBE

Sources of Infectious Agents

Infections caused by microorganisms that are considered part of the normal resident flora are said to be *endogenous*. Endogenous infection occurs when the normal balance between the microorganism and the human host is upset due to impaired host defenses or when the microorganism is introduced into a part of the body where it does not normally occur (e.g., displacement of *E. coli* from the intestinal tract into the urinary tract). Infections caused by microorganisms that are not part of the normal resident flora are said to be *exogenous*. Exogenous infectious agents can be transmitted to the host from a variety of sources.

Reservoirs of Infection
A local environment that supports the survival and growth of pathogenic microorganisms and that

serves as a source of the microorganisms for transmission to susceptible hosts is called a *reservoir of infection*. A human or animal host that harbors the microorganism constitutes a *living reservoir*. People who harbor a pathogenic microorganism without symptoms of disease are called *carriers*. Some carriers have had the particular infectious disease but continue to harbor the microorganism for a long time after recovery. Other carriers, however, may never have had overt clinical disease.

Soil, water, and food serve as *inanimate reservoirs* of infection. Most of the microorganisms that inhabit the soil are not pathogenic for human beings, but soil is a natural reservoir for some pathogenic fungi and for the anaerobic spore-forming bacterium *Clostridium botulinum*. Some microorganisms whose primary source is the intestinal tract of human beings and/or animals are capable of surviving in the soil; the soil is a secondary reservoir for these organisms (e.g., *Clostridium tetani*). Most of the microorganisms normally found in water are not pathogenic for human beings, but water polluted with sewage serves as a reservoir for bacteria such as *Salmonella* and *Shigella* species and *Vibrio cholerae*, viral agents of poliomyelitis and infectious hepatitis, and the protozoan *Entamoeba histolytica*.

Food can be a primary reservoir when it is derived from infected animals or their products (e.g., eggs, milk). For example, *Salmonella* infections are common in poultry and not only the meat but also the eggs of infected birds can be directly infectious. Food can become contaminated in a variety of ways during handling. When the contaminants have the opportunity to multiply in the food before it is eaten, food serves as a secondary reservoir.

Transmission of Infection
When the causative agent of a disease may be passed directly or indirectly from one person to another, the disease is said to be communicable. When a disease is easily spread directly from one person to another it is said to be *contagious*. Not all infectious diseases are communicable. For exam-

ple, diseases due to endogenous infection are not communicable.

Direct contact.   Transmission by *direct contact* involves close association of an infected person (or animal) with a susceptible host. Some pathogenic microorganisms cannot survive outside the human host and can only be transferred by direct contact (e.g., the agents of syphilis and gonorrhea and some viruses). Infected people can transfer pathogenic microorganisms directly to other people by touching, kissing, and sexual intercourse. Diseases transmitted by sexual intercourse are called *veneral diseases. Droplet spread* of infection may also be quite direct when a susceptible person is in close proximity to an infected person. Droplets of saliva and mucus containing microorganisms become dispersed in the air during coughing, sneezing, singing, and speaking. These droplets may then be inhaled by another person who is close by.

Direct transfer of infection from parent to offspring can occur by several means and is referred to as *vertical spread.* (Transfer of infection from one person to another who is not an offspring is referred to as *horizontal* spread.) Vertical spread can occur through the egg, sperm, placenta, or milk, or by contact. Viruses are the agents most commonly transmitted vertically. A number of viruses can cross the placenta, most notably rubella virus. *Treponema pallidum*, the spirochete responsible for syphilis, and the protozoan *Toxoplasma gondii* can also penetrate the placental barrier. An infant can also become infected during birth as a result of contact with microorganisms in the birth canal. For example, if the mother has gonorrhea the bacterial agent (*Neisseria gonorrhoeae*) may infect the conjunctiva of the newborn.

Pathogenic microorganisms can also be spread from infected animals to human beings by direct contact. For example, rabies virus is transmitted directly to a human host by the bite of an infected animal.

Indirect contact.   Transmission by *indirect contact* occurs when a susceptible person comes in contact with infectious material derived from an infected host. It can only occur when the microorganism is capable of surviving outside the human host. Inanimate articles such as eating utensils, clothing, or bedding that are contaminated with pathogenic microorganisms are called *fomites.* Contaminated water and food, including milk, can also convey infection. In addition, infection can be spread by contaminated airborne particles. Particles of dried secretions from the nose and throat (*droplet nuclei*) remain suspended in the air for a long time. Organisms that are resistant to drying (e.g., staphylococci and the tubercle bacillus) can survive in these droplets and subsequently be inhaled by other people. Organisms from the skin and excreta can be found in dust particles. Dust particles settle fairly quickly but can be resuspended in the air (e.g., by shaking blankets) and may be inhaled or settle on wounds.

Vectors are another means of transmission of infectious disease by indirect contact. A *vector* is a carrier (especially an animal) that transfers an infectious agent from one host to another. Vectors are usually arthropods of the class *Insecta* (e.g., mosquitoes, flies) or *Arachnida* (e.g., mites, ticks). An arthropod in whose body the microorganism multiplies or develops before becoming infectious to a human host is said to be a *biological vector.* For example, the malaria parasite is only capable of infecting human beings after it completes part of its life cycle within the female *Anopheles* mosquito (see Chapter 27 under Protozoa). Therefore the mosquito is a biological vector. An arthropod that passively transfers microorganisms from one host to another but is not essential to the life cycle of the parasite is called a *mechanical vector.* For example, a fly in contact with fecal material picks up microorganisms and carries them on its body surface. Subsequently the fly may land on food or on a human being and deposit some of the microorganisms.

Entry of Microorganisms into the Body

To gain entry into the body, microorganisms must penetrate the skin covering the external surface or

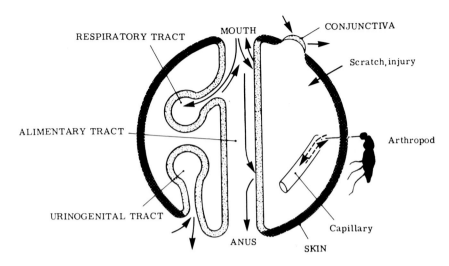

Figure 28-1. *Body surfaces as sites of microbial entry and shedding. (From Mims CA:* The Pathogenesis of Infectious Disease. *New York, Academic Press, 1977.)*

the mucous membranes lining the respiratory, gastrointestinal, and urogenital tracts or the conjunctiva (Fig. 28-1). These barriers constitute the body's *first line of defense* against microbial invasion. When these barriers are intact the microorganism must establish itself at the body surface before it can gain entry.

The normal resident flora of the skin, oral cavity, intestinal tract, and vagina also offers some protection against invasion by exogenous microorganisms. Many microorganisms are deposited on body surfaces but are unable to compete with the resident flora and establish themselves. In addition, the resident flora stimulate the development of the antimicrobial defense mechanisms of the host. The needs of the resident flora for growth and multiplication are met in relation to the resistance of the human host to invasion and damage. As mentioned previously, resident flora can cause infection when this balance is upset. The resident flora are normally in a state of delicate balance with each other, as well as with the host. Growth of one member is held in check by growth of other members. When growth of some of the normal flora is inhibited by administration of antibiotics, overgrowth of one member of the resident

flora may occur because it is no longer held in check by the others. This situation is referred to as *superinfection.* The fungus *Candida albicans* is particularly likely to cause superinfection because it is not affected by antibiotics that kill the bacterial flora.

Cutaneous Entry

The intact skin forms a relatively tough, impermeable barrier to microorganisms. In many regions the dry, scalelike keratinized layer of the epidermis is too dry for some microorganisms. Also microorganisms are carried away with the squames as the superficial layers of the skin are shed. Growth of many microorganisms is inhibited by the fatty acids present in sebaceous secretions and by the acidity of the sweat. The pH of sweating skin is usually about 5.5, except in the axillae, groin areas, and interdigital skin of the feet. Some microorganisms may enter by way of hair follicles, but microscopic or macroscopic breaks in the continuity of the skin are the major sites of entry. Abrasions, lacerations, or burns are obvious breaches of the integrity of the skin. Artificially produced wounds due to needles (whether those of a tattoist or a nurse or a physician) can also provide sites of entry. If the needle, syringe, or solution is contaminated, microorganisms can be injected directly into deeper tissues.

Bites of animals (or humans) introduce microorganisms from the saliva into the wound. Large bites are uncommon, but small bites by arthropods occur frequently. In some cases the mouthparts of the arthropod are contaminated and the infectious agent is transmitted mechanically, but biological vectors have microorganisms in their saliva. Some insects (e.g., mosquitoes) may inject saliva directly into capillary blood.

Respiratory Entry

A variety of particles and microorganisms suspended in the air are inhaled with each breath. The respiratory tract has several cleansing mechanisms to remove these particles and microorganisms.

The nasal hairs filter out the largest particles. Slightly smaller particles are deposited on the nasal turbinates, which act as "baffle plates." Particles deposited here are trapped in mucus, swept to the back of the throat by ciliary action, and swallowed. Small particles (less than about 10 μm in diameter) are not deposited on the turbinates, but are carried further into the respiratory tract. Those less than 5 μm in diameter may reach the alveoli. In addition to the filtering system of the nose, protection against invading microorganisms is provided by lysozyme in the mucus (see below) and the acidity of the nasal secretions.

Most of the surface of the lower respiratory tract is covered by a membrane consisting of ciliated cells together with mucus-secreting goblet cells and subepithelial mucus-secreting glands. Particulate material deposited on this surface is trapped in the mucus and carried from the lungs to the pharynx by ciliary action. This mechanism is referred to as the *mucociliary escalator*. The alveoli do not have a mucociliary blanket but are lined with phagocytic macrophages that ingest foreign particles and microorganisms.

In order to gain entry by way of the respiratory tract, microorganisms must avoid being carried to the back of the throat by the mucociliary escalator

and subsequently swallowed. They must also avoid being phagocytosed and killed by alveolar macrophages. Some viruses, particularly influenza viruses and rhinoviruses, are able to attach to receptors on epithelial cells and avoid being swept away. *Mycoplasma pneumoniae* and *Bordetella pertussis* (the bacterium responsible for whooping cough) are also able to attach to the respiratory epithelium.

Bacteria that lack a mechanism for attaching to epithelial cells will only become established when the mucociliary cleansing mechanism is impaired. Mucociliary damage often occurs as a result of viral infection. Various bacteria, especially streptococci, are then able to establish a secondary infection. People with chronic bronchitis have altered mucociliary function (see Chapter 10 under Chronic Obstructive Pulmonary Disease) and frequently have lung infections. Cigarette smoking and atmospheric pollutants may impair mucociliary function. Ciliary activity is also impaired by dry air. Some respiratory pathogens, such as *Bordetella pertussis*, *Hemophilus influenzae*, and *Mycoplasma pneumoniae*, depress ciliary activity directly and thus avoid being removed from the respiratory passages.

Mechanisms by which microorganisms avoid phagocytosis or survive following phagocytosis are discussed later. The alveolar macrophages are damaged or destroyed following ingestion of inhaled silica or asbestos particles. Consequently people with silicosis or asbestosis are very susceptible to pulmonary infection, particularly by the agent of tuberculosis. (Silicosis and asbestosis are discussed in Chapter 21 under Foreign Bodies in the Respiratory Tract.)

Oropharyngeal Entry

As with the skin and intestinal tract, resident flora of the mouth and pharynx inhibit the growth of other transient microorganisms. The cleansing action of saliva forms the major defense against oropharyngeal infection. Saliva not only has a mechanical flushing action, but contains secretory antibodies (see Chapter 29) and an enzyme called *lysozyme*. Lysozyme breaks down the mucopeptide of bacterial cell walls and is particularly effective against gram-positive organisms.

In order to establish oropharyngeal infection, microorganisms have to avoid being washed away and swallowed, either by attaching to epithelial surfaces or finding their way into crevices. Virulent strains of *Streptococcus pyogenes* attach specifically to pharyngeal cells. Presumably other microorganisms that cause upper respiratory infections do likewise. During swallowing, material from the mouth, nose, and lungs that is brought to the pharynx is firmly wiped against the pharyngeal walls by the backward thrust of the tongue. This action may contribute to the development of infection. Oral infection may occur when the flow of saliva is decreased (e.g., in people who are dehydrated).

Intestinal Entry

Not only ingested food and fluids but also materials originating in the mouth, nasopharynx, and lungs are swallowed and enter the gastrointestinal tract. In order to survive in the gastrointestinal tract, microorganisms must be able to resist the actions of acid, enzymes, and bile. Most bacteria are unable to resist the acid conditions in the stomach, although the tubercle bacillus can. Bacteria such as *Salmonella* species and *Vibrio cholerae* are more likely to survive and establish infection when they are sheltered inside food particles or when secretion of acid by the stomach is impaired. Enteroviruses are resistant to acid and to bile salts.

Multiplication of microorganisms in the intestinal tract is counterbalanced by their passage to the exterior in the feces. When the rate of flow of intestinal contents is increased, as in diarrhea, the microorganisms have less time to multiply and the number of microorganisms in the feces decreases.

The flow of intestinal contents carries microorganisms right through the intestinal tract unless they have some means of attaching to the epithelial lining. Many pathogenic microorganisms appear to attach to specific receptors on intestinal epithelial cells. The normal mixing of the contents of the intestinal tract provides many opportunities for microorganisms to come into contact with epithelial cells and become attached. Mucus protects the epithelial cells and perhaps acts as a mechanical barrier that prevents the attachment of some microorganisms. In addition, it contains secretory antibodies.

The intestinal tract has a large population of resident flora. Many of the resident microorganisms are closely associated with the epithelial cells. As in other parts of the body, the normal flora help to prevent the establishment of other microorganisms. The normal resident flora possibly inhibit growth of other microorganisms by competing for nutrients or attachment sites or by the production of toxic substances.

After attachment to the epithelial cells, some pathogenic bacteria (e.g., *Salmonella typhimurium*) appear to be taken into intestinal cells by a process that resembles phagocytosis. In addition, microbial toxins can be absorbed.

Urogenital Entry

Urine is normally sterile. The flushing of the urinary tract by the flow of urine normally makes it difficult for microorganisms to gain entry and become established.

In males, microorganisms normally do not ascend more than one-third the length of the urethra without being washed out. They rarely reach the bladder unless they are introduced by means of an instrument such as catheter. The gonococcus is able to attach very firmly to urethral epithelial cells and avoid being washed out. It is also resistant to spermine and zinc, substances present in prostatic secretions that inhibit many other bacteria.

In females, microorganisms easily ascend the short urethra and urinary tract infections are common. Microorganisms may be introduced into the female bladder as a result of urethral deformations occurring during sexual intercourse.

Urine is a good medium for the growth of many bacteria and urinary tract infection is particularly likely when residual urine remains in the bladder after urination or if free flow of urine is obstructed. (Urinary tract obstruction is discussed in Chapter 21.) Damage to the epithelial lining of the urinary tract (e.g., from mechanical trauma by renal calculi) can provide a focus for the establishment of infection.

In prepubertal girls the vagina is lined with columnar epithelium and the vaginal secretion is alkaline. Under the influence of sex hormones at puberty, however, the epithelium changes to a more resistant stratified squamous type and contains glycogen. A lactobacillus (Döderlein's bacillus) colonizes the vagina and metabolizes the glycogen to lactic acid, creating an acidic environment that inhibits the growth of other microorganisms. Therefore, vaginal infections are uncommon unless conditions in the vagina are altered. Gonococci can invade columnar epithelium and transitional epithelium, but not stratified squamous epithelium. Therefore gonorrheal lesions usually occur in the cervix and urethra, but not the vagina. Vaginal infections due to *Neisseria gonorrhoeae* can occur in prepubertal girls, however. *Treponema pallidum*, the agent of syphilis, apparently gains entrance through minute abrasions in the epithelium and the primary lesion of syphilis usually occurs on the cervix. Before puberty and after menopause when the vaginal epithelium lacks glycogen and the secretion is alkaline, vaginal infection due to staphylococci and streptococci may occur.

Conjunctival Entry

The continuous flow of tears over the conjunctiva and the wiping action of the eyelids every few seconds mechanically washes inanimate foreign particles and microorganisms into the nasal cavity by way of the tear ducts. In addition, the tears contain lysozyme. Microorganisms have little opportunity to initiate infection unless they are able to attach to the conjunctival surface or unless the conjunctiva is abraded. Inanimate foreign particles can cause abrasions and provide opportunities for microorganisms to gain entry. The chlamydia responsible for inclusion conjunctivitis and trachoma probably attach to receptors on the cell surface.

Microorganisms are usually mechanically deposited on the conjunctiva (e.g., by fingers or towels). Airborne microorganisms are rarely deposited in the eyes. Swimming pools provide a good source and mode of transmission for infectious agents. As the water flows over the eyes, it not only deposits microorganisms on the conjunctiva but also causes slight mechanical and chemical damage that facilitates infection.

Host-Microbe Interactions in the Tissues

Once pathogenic microorganisms have entered the body, they may establish local infection at the site of entry or they may become disseminated throughout the body and establish themselves at sites remote from the site of entry. Whether or not invading microorganisms establish infection at the site of entry or at a distant site depends on the growth requirements of the organism, the local tissue environment, the strength of host defenses, and the ability of the microorganism to overcome host defenses. Many bacteria that usually cause local infections and many opportunistic pathogens that do not usually invade can cause systemic infection when host resistance is lowered. Host defenses include general, nonspecific responses and specific inducible immunological responses. The immunological responses are described in Chapter 29.

Intracellular versus Extracellular Parasites

Most pathogenic bacteria are *extracellular parasites;* that is, they multiply in the tissue spaces. Viruses, chlamydia, rickettsia, and some protozoa (e.g., the agents that cause malaria) are *obligate intracellular parasites;* that is, they can only reproduce within host cells. Some microorganisms (e.g., *Salmonella typhi, Mycobacterium tuberculosis,* and some species of *Brucella*) are *facultative intracellular parasites;* that is, they can reproduce either inside or outside of a host cell.

Obligate intracellular parasites must enter the blood or lymph in order to spread systemically. They must gain access to subepithelial lymphatic or blood vessels as free microorganisms or be taken up by leukocytes that will carry them to other parts of the body. The microorganism must reach a susceptible cell before it can replicate. If susceptible cells are only located at the body surface, systemic spread will be hindered. The microorganism may enter the blood but will not establish infection at sites other than the surface.

Extracellular parasites do not have to find susceptible cells and theoretically can multiply in any tissue to which they gain access. Such microorganisms are constantly exposed to the body's defense mechanisms, however. In contrast, intracellular parasites are exposed to general body defenses only while they are in transit from one host cell to another, although they must resist the defense mechanisms of the host cells. Infected cells, however, may be attacked by the immune system if their surfaces are altered (see Chapter 29).

Entry into cells. Many intracellular parasites enter host cells by being taken up by phagocytosis. As described in Chapter 27, many viruses appear to enter host cells by phagocytosis. Certain enveloped viruses, however, fuse with the cell membrane of the host cell and the nucleocapsid is set free in the cytoplasm. Some bacteria (e.g., *Shigella* and pathogenic *Salmonella* species) adsorb to the surface of the host cell, induce a local breakdown in the host-cell membrane, and enter the cytoplasm directly. The host-cell membrane is immediately reformed. Some protozoa enter host cells by active penetration, using their own lysosomal enzymes to penetrate host-cell membranes.

Growth in Epithelial Tissues

Many bacterial infections are usually confined to epithelial surfaces at the site of entry because the bacteria are normally not able to overcome host defenses and to spread systemically. With infections of the throat or respiratory tract caused by *Bordetella pertussis*, *Corynebacterium diphteriae*, or streptococci, the bacteria spread in the epithelium but do not invade deeper tissues, although diptheria toxin is disseminated systemically (see below). Streptococci may invade subepithelial tissues to a limited extent but rarely spread systemically. Similarly, staphylococcal skin infections remain localized unless host defenses are impaired. *Shigella* and most *Salmonella* species (except *S. typhi* and *S. paratyphi*) do not normally penetrate the intestinal epithelium. Gonococcal infections of the urethra or conjunctiva remain localized, with limited subepithelial spread.

Many viruses, particularly those that cause respiratory infections (e.g., rhinoviruses, influenza viruses, and parainfluenza viruses) and intestinal infections, multiply in the epithelial surface at the site of entry, produce a spreading infection in the epithelium, and are shed directly to the exterior. Epithelial cells are destroyed, stimulating an inflammatory response, but little or no invasion of subepithelial tissues occurs. The layer of liquid on the surface of the epithelium facilitates the spread of the viruses and the infection progresses rapidly. The infection is terminated partly because most available cells have been infected and partly because nonimmunological host-resistance factors prevent further invasion by the virus. An important resistance factor is a substance called *interferon* that is secreted by cells infected by viruses and protects other cells from infection. (Interferon is discussed in Chapter 29.)

Infection by rhinoviruses is limited to the upper respiratory tract partly because these viruses replicate best at 33 °C (the temperature of nasal mucosa) and do not replicate as well at the temperature of the body core (37 °C). Influenza and parainfluenza viruses can infect the lungs as well as the upper respiratory tract but infections are limited to epithelial surfaces because these viruses appear to be unable to replicate in other tissues. Systemic effects and damage to other organs that sometimes occur appear to be due to a circulating toxic substance.

Some fungi, referred to as *dermatophytes*, grow only in dead keratinized layers of epithelium. These fungi are unable to grow in living tissues and do not become disseminated systemically. Dermatophytes are responsible for ringworm of the skin, hair, and nails. *Candida albicans* is also usually restricted to epithelial tissues, but it can invade deeper tissues and become disseminated systemically if host defenses are impaired.

Subepithelial Invasion

Microorganisms that are transmitted by biting arthropod vectors and those that enter wounds are directly deposited in the subepithelial tissues. Other microorganisms must penetrate the epithelial cell layer and basement membrane to reach the subepithelial tissues (Fig. 28-2). The basement membrane acts as a filter and can delay subepithelial invasion to some extent.

The gel-like nature of the connective tissue matrix in the subepithelial tissues also physically hinders the direct spread of infection into adjacent tissues. Some bacteria, however, secrete enzymes that can digest various tissue components. Many of these enzymes probably have functions related to bacterial nutrition, but at the same time, they may facilitate local spread of the microorganisms. For example, streptococci produce hyaluronidase, which breaks down hyaluronic acid, and streptokinase, which activates fibrinolysin. Some bacteria produce collagenase, which digests collagen.

Microorganisms that reach the subepithelial tissues are exposed to three important internal *second-line defenses*: antimicrobial substances in the tissue fluids, phagocytic cells, and the lymphatic system leading to the lymph nodes. These defenses are brought into play by the inflammatory response. (The inflammatory response is described in detail in Chapter 8.)

The tissue fluids normally contain small amounts of plasma proteins, including the smaller immunoglobulins (IgG) and components of the complement system (see Chapter 29). The in-

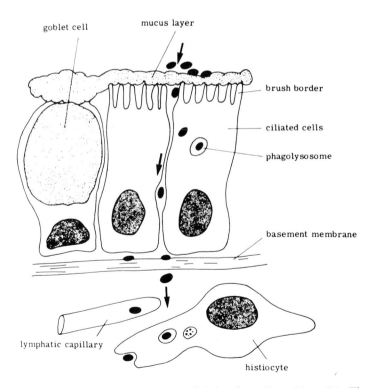

Figure 28-2. *Microbial invasion across an epithelial surface. (From Mims CA: The Pathogenesis of Infectious Disease. New York, Academic Press, 1977.)*

crease in vascular permeability during inflammation allows larger amounts of these substances to enter the tissue fluids.

Phagocytosis. The phagocytic cells are the most important host defenses. Two types of specialized phagocytic cells are present in the body: the polymorphonuclear leukocytes and the macrophages. Other types of cells are also capable of phagocytosis, but these cells are particularly active and are specialized for intracellular killing and digestion of ingested microorganisms.

Polymorphonuclear leukocytes are produced in the bone marrow and circulate in the blood. During inflammation they are attracted to the inflammatory site by chemotaxis and actively leave the blood vessels to enter the tissue spaces. Neutrophils are the most abundant, but small numbers of eosinophils and basophils are also present. Eosinophils are not as effective as neutrophils in the phagocytosis and killing of microorganisms. They are especially active in the phagocytosis of immune complexes, however, and increase in number (eosinophilia) in allergic diseases and in some helminthic and protozoal infections. Basophils are not involved in phagocytosis.

Macrophages are derived from circulating monocytes, which are formed in the bone marrow. Macrophages are widely distributed in the body and comprise what is called the *reticuloendothelial system* (RES). Fixed macrophages line blood sinusoids in the liver (Kupffer cells), spleen, bone marrow, and adrenal glands and lymph sinuses in the lymph nodes. Other fixed macrophages line the alveoli in the lungs (dust cells) and the pleural and peritoneal cavities. Microglia of the central nervous system are also fixed macrophages. Wandering cells of the RES include monocytes of the blood and histiocytes in loose connective tissue. These cells are chemotactically attracted to sites of inflammation and move through the tissues by ameboid motion.

A microorganism must become attached to the surface of a phagocytic cell before it can be ingested. Divalent cations such as calcium (Ca^{2+})

and magnesium (Mg^{2+}) are involved in this process. Some antibodies and complement components, referred to as *opsonins*, coat the surfaces of microorganisms and facilitate their attachment to and ingestion by phagocytic cells. Motile microorganisms often need to be immobilized by opsonins before they can be caught by phagocytic cells. The cell membrane of the phagocyte surrounds the microorganism and the microorganism is brought into the phagocytic cell within a membrane-bounded vacuole called a phagosome. Lysosomes then fuse with the phagosome and release a variety of potent enzymes that kill and digest the microorganism (Fig. 28-3). Macrophages contain different lysosomal enzymes than neutrophils. Therefore their ability to kill ingested microorganisms differs.

Microorganisms have developed a variety of strategies to overcome the phagocytic defense mechanism. Some bacteria kill the phagocytic cells. Pathogenic streptococci produce hemolysins (streptolysins) that not only lyse red blood cells but also kill neutrophils and macrophages. Streptolysin causes the lysosomal enzymes of the phagocytic cell to be released into the cytoplasm, causing destruction of the cell. Streptolysins may also inhibit the chemotaxis of neutrophils, so that fewer phagocytic cells arrive at the site of infection. Pathogenic staphylococci also produce hemolysins that can kill phagocytes. In addition, some staphylococci release a substance called leukocidin that kills phagocytic cells but does not cause hemolysis.

Some pathogenic microorganisms are able to resist phagocytosis because of their surface properties. Phagocytosis can occur after the microbial surface is coated with specific antibodies, but antibodies take time to develop and the host does not have them available at the first encounter with the microorganism. The capsules of a number of bacteria (e.g., *Streptococcus pneumoniae, Klebsiella pneumoniae,* and *Hemophilus influenzae*) render them resistant to phagocytosis. Some streptococci have surface proteins (M proteins) that are associated with resistance to phagocytosis, but it is not

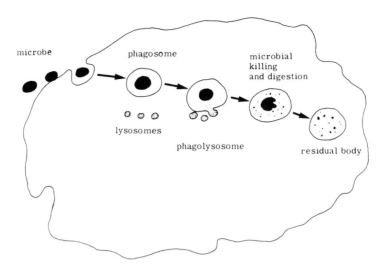

Figure 28-3. *Schematic representation of phagocytosis and intracellular digestion of microorganisms. See also Figure 8-2.* (From Mims CA: The Pathogenesis of Infectious Disease. New York, Academic Press, 1977.)

known how these proteins act. (The same M proteins are necessary for attachment of the bacterial cells to epithelial cells at the site of infection.)

Some pathogenic microorganisms are taken up by phagocytes but resist being killed or digested and may even multiply within the phagocytes. For example, the protozoan *Toxoplasma gondii* is ingested by macrophages but often the lysosomes fail to fuse with the phagosome. It is not known how the microorganism inhibits the fusion of the lysosomes. The toxoplasma multiply within the macrophage and eventually kill it. Some bacteria (e.g., *Mycobacterium tuberculosis*) are resistant to killing by the lysosomal enzymes, perhaps because of substances on the surfaces of the bacteria.

Many viruses are destroyed by neutrophils and macrophages but are able to multiply in susceptible host cells. Certain viruses (e.g., reovirus), however, can resist destruction in the phagolysosomes of phagocytic cells. The lysosomal enzymes uncoat the virus, but the viral nucleic acid escapes into the cytoplasm and initiates replication of the virus.

Macrophages have a longer life span than neutrophils. Therefore, macrophages are more important as host cells for intracellular parasites. Also, as mentioned previously, the lysosomal enzymes of the two cell types differ, so that some microorganisms that resist killing in macrophages may not resist killing in neutrophils.

Since white blood cells are the body's major defense against infection, it is not surprising that increased numbers are released into the blood and the white blood cell count usually rises during infection (*leukocytosis*). Leukocytes serve not only phagocytic functions but also immunological functions (see Chapter 29), and not every kind of white blood cell is increased in number with every kind of infection.

With most infections the main response is an increase in phagocytic cells and the neutrophil count rises (*neutrophilia*). Neutrophilia does not usually occur in tuberculosis or fungal and chlamydial infections. With *Salmonella* infections, brucellosis, pertussis, and some rickettsial, viral, and protozoal infections the neutrophil count falls (*neutropenia*) for reasons that are unclear. Neutropenia also occurs in very severe infections when the neutrophil stores and productive capacity of the bone marrow are inadequate to keep up with cell utilization. In this event neutropenia is an ominous prognostic sign.

The monocyte count may be increased (*monocytosis*) during recovery from acute bacterial infections, in some chronic infectious diseases, and when there is neutropenia. Monocytosis is common in tuberculosis, brucellosis, syphilis, and some rickettsial and protozoal infections.

Lymphocytes are involved in both the humoral and cell-mediated immune responses. As participants in cell-mediated immune responses they are important in the defense against intracellular parasites. The lymphocyte count is increased (*lymphocytosis*) in many viral and rickettsial infections and in tuberculosis, syphilis, brucellosis, and pertussis.

Lymphatics and lymph nodes. Lymphatic vessels form a complex network beneath the surface epithelium. The skin and intestinal wall have a particularly extensive superficial plexus of lymphatics. Microorganisms that reach the subepithelial tissues enter the lymphatics almost immediately and are carried to the local lymph nodes within minutes. Within the lymph node the microorganisms are exposed to the macrophages lining the sinuses of the node. Usually there is a second node before the lymph enters the venous system, so that microorganisms that escape phagocytosis in the first node may be trapped in the second node. The lymph nodes are also involved in the immune response (see Chapter 29).

Inflammatory products of microbial growth are also carried to the lymph nodes from the site of infection. Consequently an inflammatory response occurs in the nodes, causing some swelling and tenderness. The inflammatory response also brings neutrophils to the nodes to assist the macrophages with phagocytosis. Some of the swelling of the lymph nodes is due to recruitment of lymphoid cells from the blood to the nodes and division of cells within the nodes as part of the immune response.

The efficiency with which the lymph nodes remove microorganisms from the lymph and prevent them from reaching the blood in influenced by the rate of lymph flow and the concentration of microorganisms in the lymph. When large numbers of microorganisms are carried to the nodes, the phagocytic cells may not be able to handle them all. Certain viruses and the leprosy bacillus multiply in the endothelium of lymphatic vessels, so that their numbers are increased by the time they reach the lymph node. The efficiency of the nodes is also decreased when the rate of lymph flow is high, as during muscular exercise or inflammation of tissues (unless the lymphatics are blocked by fibrin; see Chapter 8). The rate of lymph flow from the intestines is increased after a large fatty meal.

As mentioned earlier, some microorganisms are able to resist phagocytosis or, if they are taken up by phagocytic cells, are not killed. Microorganisms that are able to multiply in the lymph nodes are discharged in the efferent lymph and enter the bloodstream. In some cases the microorganisms (particularly viruses) are able to multiply in the macrophages or lymphocytes without seriously damaging them and subsequently are disseminated by these cells in the course of their normal migratory movements. Multiplication of the infectious agent in the lymph node occurs with bubonic plague, brucellosis, and typhus, as well as many viral infections. Tubercle bacilli are usually arrested in the local lymph node after entering lymphatics at the site of primary infection. Occasionally, however, they spread to regional lymph nodes and then enter the blood by way of the thoracic duct, producing disseminated (miliary) tuberculosis.

Systemic Spread

Hematogenous spread. Microorganisms may gain access to the blood by way of the lymph, as just described, or may enter the blood directly. Direct entry into the blood occurs when the microorganisms are introduced by biting arthropod vectors, when blood vessels are damaged as a result of injury, or occasionally when the microorganisms damage the blood vessel wall. Microorganisms can be rapidly transported to any part of the body once they enter the blood.

Microorganisms may be carried free in the plasma or may be carried in association with blood cells. Poliovirus, yellow-fever virus, bacteria such as *Streptococcus pneumoniae* and *Bacillus anthracis,* all types of rickettsiae, and the protozoan agents of trypanosomiasis are carried free in the plasma and are exposed to antimicrobial factors in the blood. Some viruses (e.g., cytomegalovirus and herpes simplex, EB, measles, and smallpox viruses) are carried in or on white blood cells, particularly lymphocytes and monocytes. Intracellular bacteria such as tubercle bacilli and *Brucella* species and the protozoan *Leishmania donovani* infect monocytes and are carried in them. If the host cells are not damaged, the microorganisms within them are protected from phagocytic cells and antimicrobial factors in the plasma. Some microorganisms are carried in or on erythrocytes. These microorganisms are protected from phagocytosis as long as the host cell remains normal. The malaria parasite, in particular, lives in red blood cells. When progeny parasites are released, however, they exist free in the plasma for a short time until they are able to enter other red blood cells. Viruses do not usually infect red blood cells, but some (e.g., arboviruses) attach to the surface of red blood cells. Rickettsiae are frequently carried on erythrocytes as well as free in the plasma.

Microorganisms traveling in the blood tend to be arrested in capillaries and sinusoids where blood flow is slow. Subsequently they have the opportunity to establish infection in adjacent tissues. Circulating microorganisms often localize in organs such as the liver and spleen because they are phagocytosed by the fixed macrophages lining the sinusoids in these organs. Infected leukocytes that show surface changes or signs of damage are also arrested in these organs.

The spread of microorganisms through the body is outlined in Figure 28-4. To some extent, the site of entry influences the fate of microorganisms in the blood. Those entering blood vessels in the systemic circulation first encounter capillary beds in the lungs. They may localize in the lungs or be carried further. Microorganisms entering blood

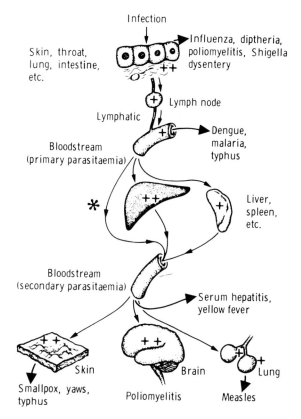

Figure 28-4. *The spread of infection through the body. Large arrows indicate sites of possible shedding to the exterior; + indicates sites of possible multiplication; * indicates multiplication in the bloodstream or vascular endothelium rather than in viscera (e.g., malaria, typhus). (From Mims CA: The Pathogenesis of Infectious Disease. New York, Academic Press, 1977.)*

vessels in the lungs are carried to capillary beds in the systemic circulation.

Microorganisms entering subepithelial blood vessels in the intestine are carried to the liver, where they are exposed to the Kupffer cells lining the sinusoids. Normally most bacterial products and bacteria that enter the portal circulation are removed by the Kupffer cells. If extracellular parasites are able to resist phagocytosis or to kill the phagocytes, they can lodge in the sinusoids and grow. Intracellular parasites that can resist being killed by the phagocytic cells after being taken up may cross through the macrophages and enter the hepatic cells, may grow in the macrophages, or both.

Blood flow also influences where microorganisms will localize. Microorganisms have more opportunity to settle in organs that receive a high portion of the cardiac output (e.g., the kidneys) than in organs that receive less blood flow.

In order to invade tissues without sinusoids, circulating microorganisms must first adhere to the blood vessel endothelium and then grow through the vessel wall, leak through the vessel wall, or be passively carried through it. Invasion is most likely to occur across capillaries or venules, where the vessel wall is thinnest and blood flow is slowest.

Circulating microorganisms often localize in the liver, spleen, and bone marrow because of phagocytosis by reticuloendothelial cells in the sinusoids of these organs, but little is known about the factors governing localization of microorganisms in particular capillary beds. In areas of inflammation, circulating microorganisms settle readily on the "sticky" capillary endothelium. Microorganisms must circulate in the blood for a relatively long time and in a fairly high concentration before localization in normal capillaries occurs. Therefore, the more quickly microorganisms are inactivated by antibodies in the plasma or removed by phagocytic cells, the less chance they have to localize in capillary beds.

In many systemic infectious diseases, microorganisms localize in the skin, causing characteristic rashes (*exanthems*). Inflammation in the dermis as a result of infection in the dermal vascular bed or its immediate vicinity produces macules and papules. A *macule* is a discolored spot that is not elevated above the surface. A *papule* is a small, circumscribed, solid elevation of the skin. An eruption consisting of both macules and papules is referred to as a *maculopapular rash*. In some viral infections (e.g., measles), the virus alone does little damage to the blood vessels and skin, but the interaction of sensitized lymphocytes or antibodies with viral antigens generates an inflammatory response that produces the rash. Thus, the maculopapular rash of measles only occurs when there is an adequate immune response.

Rickettsiae localize and grow in the endothelium of small blood vessels. As a result, swelling, thrombosis, small infarcts, and hemorrhages occur, producing a characteristic rash.

Some microorganisms produce toxins that localize in dermal blood vessels, causing damage and inflammation and producing a rash. For example, strains of *Streptococcus pyogenes* carrying a particular bacteriophage produce a toxin that enters the blood, localizes in dermal blood vessels, and produces the rash of scarlet fever.

When microorganisms leave the dermal blood vessels and spread to superficial layers of the skin, vesicles and pustules are formed. A *vesicle* is a small blister; it is a small circumscribed elevation of the epidermis that contains serous inflammatory exudate. When the exudate is pus, the lesion is a *pustule*. For example, with varicella and herpes simplex, the viruses replicate in the endothelium of dermal blood vessels, are shed into the dermis, and infect the epidermis. Focal necrosis and inflammation occur, producing vesicles filled with virus particles. The vesicles are secondarily infiltrated with leukocytes and become pustules, which later burst, dry, scab, and heal.

Some microorganisms, particularly viruses, that enter the circulation of a pregnant woman may cross the placental barrier and infect the fetus. The result may be abortion, stillbirth, or malformations of the fetus. Microorganisms do not appear to be passively transferred across the placenta. First they localize in the maternal vessels of the placenta, then they either grow across the junction (e.g., rubella and cytomegalovirus) or multiply, produce toxins, locally disrupt the integrity of the junction, and enter the fetal blood (e.g., *Treponema pallidum*).

In systemic viral infections, small numbers of virus particles cross the epithelial surface and reach the blood at an early stage to be spread through the body. The presence of viruses in the blood at this early stage of infection is called *pri-*

mary viremia. It is a common event and is not usually associated with any signs or symptoms. After reaching target tissues, the viruses replicate in susceptible host cells. Large numbers of progeny virus may then be released into the blood, causing a *secondary viremia* that spreads the infection to other tissues. For example, in measles small numbers of virions enter the bloodstream by way of the lymphatics after minimal multiplication near the site of entry in the respiratory tract. As a result of this primary viremia organs such as the liver and spleen are infected and more extensive virus multiplication occurs. A secondary viremia then carries the virus particles to the epithelial surfaces of the body, where further multiplication of the virus causes an exanthem and enanthem (an eruption on a mucous membrane). A similar sequence of events occurs in the rickettsial disease typhus.

The presence of bacteria in the blood is called *bacteremia.* Some bacteria that regularly cause generalized infections (e.g., *Salmonella typhi* and *Bacillus anthracis*) enter the blood in fairly large numbers and then establish focal infections in various organs. In contrast to the many viruses that regularly enter the blood, few bacterial species regularly do so, but bacteria that do not usually cause a systemic infection can enter the blood in small numbers and cause transient bacteremias. Usually the circulating bacteria are removed and inactivated by phagocytic cells, and the bacteremia is not serious. Bacteremia can be serious, however, when circulating bacteria settle in vulnerable tissues or when host resistance is impaired. For example, circulating bacteria may localize on abnormal heart valves to cause subacute bacterial endocarditis or on traumatized growing ends of bones to cause osteomyelitis. When host resistance is impaired, microorganisms may persist and multiply in the blood, producing systemic disease. This condition is called *septicemia* and it can lead to shock (see Chapter 14). Bacteria and fungi growing extracellularly tend to release toxins and cause serious disease when they invade the blood, but viruses are usually being carried passively in the blood and do not elaborate toxins. Therefore viremia is usually silent.

Other routes of spread. Microorganisms entering the peritoneal cavity or pleural cavities can rapidly spread from one visceral organ to another in the serous fluid. An injury or focus of infection in an abdominal organ can lead to entry of microorganisms into the peritoneal cavity. Microorganisms can enter the pleural cavity as a result of chest wounds or from foci of infection in the lungs. Inflammation of the pleural surface (pleurisy) often occurs during pneumonia and later the pleura may become infected.

Microorganisms in the blood may enter the cerebrospinal fluid (CSF) by crossing the blood-CSF junction in the meninges or choroid plexus. Once microorganisms enter the CSF they are passively carried with the flow of fluid from the ventricles to the subarachnoid space and throughout the central nervous system. Subsequently they may invade the brain and/or spinal cord.

Some viruses and toxins spread from peripheral parts of the body to the central nervous system by way of the peripheral nerves. For example, herpesviruses and rabies virus travel along nerves, but the exact pathway in the nerve is not known. Possible routes include movement through the tissue spaces between nerve fibers, sequential infection of Schwann cells, or carriage in the cytoplasm of the axon.

Effects of Infection on the Host

Fever commonly accompanies infection. The mechanism by which fever is produced is discussed in Chapter 24. Whether fever is harmful or beneficial is controversial (see below). Many of the signs and symptoms of infectious diseases are a result of the host response or of loss of function in an infected organ.

The effects of infection on the host are greatly influenced by the tissue involved. Damage to the heart from infection may cause serious functional changes, whereas damage to a skeletal muscle may have minimal consequences. Infection in the central nervous system is particularly serious; cell damage here may result in coma or paralysis. Cerebral edema as a result of inflammation in the confined space of the skull causes increased intracranial pressure, which can damage brain cells and disrupt brain function. In the lungs, edema caused by inflammation can seriously impair respiratory function. The liver and kidneys have large functional reserves and may be able to withstand considerable damage before function is seriously impaired.

Mechanisms of Tissue Damage

Invading microorganisms may cause direct damage to host cells, but often tissue damage in infected organs is produced indirectly.

Direct mechanisms. Intracellular parasites are particularly likely to cause direct damage to host cells. Most viruses, rickettsiae, and chlamydiae, for example, damage the host cells in which they replicate. As described in Chapter 27, viruses inhibit the synthesis of host-cell DNA, RNA, and protein, disrupting cell function. Some viruses cause lysis of host cells when progeny virions are released. Other intracellular parasites compete with host cells for nutrients or break down cell components.

In malaria the development of the parasites in the erythrocytes tends to become synchronized, so that release of progeny parasites (merozoites) causes almost simultaneous rupture of many red blood cells. This event is marked by severe chills and fever, which usually lasts for several hours and may be accompanied by headache, nausea, and vomiting. These episodes recur at regular intervals that are characteristic for the particular *Plasmodium* species and reflect the length of time required for the parasite to develop. Lysis of the red blood cells result in anemia. Red blood cell fragments, hemoglobin, and malarial metabolites are taken up by the RES and produce enlargement of the liver and spleen. (See the discussion of hemolytic anemia in Chapter 10.)

Bacteria that grow extracellularly often cause tissue damage by the liberation of toxins. Toxins that are secreted into the surrounding medium during the growth of microorganisms are called *exotoxins.* Toxins that are associated with the cell wall and are released when the bacteria die are called *endotoxins.*

Endotoxins are part of the outer layer of the cell wall of gram-negative bacteria. Since large numbers of gram-negative bacteria normally reside in the intestines, endotoxins are continuously being absorbed. These endotoxins enter the portal blood and are normally degraded by Kupffer cells in the liver. Small amounts of endotoxins may enter the blood after trauma or after genitourinary instrumentation without causing signs and symptoms, but large amounts of endotoxins entering the blood cause shock. (See Chapter 14, the section on Septic Shock.) Endotoxins are also pyrogenic (i.e., cause fever).

Exotoxins are mainly produced by gram-positive bacteria. They are proteins and some of them are known to be specific enzymes. Clostridia are anaerobic, gram-positive spore-forming bacilli that produce potent exotoxins. Several *Clostridium* species are associated with gas gangrene. Since these organisms are strict anaerobes they only grow in necrotic or devitalized tissues. Infection occurs following contamination of wounds by soil or intestinal contents containing spores. The bacteria produce several toxins that cause tissue necrosis. The most important is alpha toxin, which is an enzyme (phospholipase) that breaks down cell membranes, including those of red blood cells. Therefore massive hemolysis may occur in infected people.

Tetanus (lockjaw) results from the contamination of wounds by spores of *Clostridium tetani* (also found in soil and feces), with subsequent infection. This organism liberates a neurotoxin that causes hypertonic muscular paralysis. (See Chapter 25 under Interference with Neurotransmission.)

Clostridium botulinum also produces a potent neurotoxin, as described in Chapter 25. This organism does not cause infection but is responsible for one type of food poisoning. Spores germinate in improperly canned food, and as the microorganism multiplies it produces the toxin. After the contaminated food is eaten the toxin is absorbed from the intestinal tract.

A second type of food poisoning (the most common) is caused by an exotoxin produced by certain strains of *Staphylococcus aureus*. The bacteria grow in many foods (e.g., custard, deviled eggs, salad dressings, and cream), particularly when the food is stored for several hours with inadequate refrigeration. The toxin, called enterotoxin, is elaborated by the multiplying bacteria and is ingested with the food. The toxin is absorbed from the intestine and acts on the vomiting center in the brain, causing nausea and vomiting. It also causes abdominal cramps and diarrhea.

Intestinal infection caused by *Salmonella* species (salmonellosis) is also frequently referred to as food poisoning. In this case the disease is not caused by a toxin, but results from the ingestion of large numbers of bacteria in food or water. Some of the bacteria survive and multiply in the intestinal tract, causing damage to epithelial cells and producing inflammation. The results are vomiting, diarrhea, colicky abdominal pain, and fever.

The disease cholera is also caused by a toxin; the causative agent, *Vibrio cholerae*, does not invade tissues. The organism grows in the lumen of the intestine and attaches to the intestinal epithelium. It produces a toxin that acts on the epithelial cells, altering their function. As a result, large amounts of water and electrolytes pass through the intact epithelial cells into the small intestine. The consequences are profuse watery diarrhea, acidosis (because of loss of bicarbonate and potassium; see Chapter 15 under Metabolic Acidosis), hypovolemia, and shock.

The serious consequences of diphtheria are also a result of production of a toxin by the infecting bacteria. The toxin is disseminated in the blood and enters cells, where it acts by interfering with protein synthesis. All cells are susceptible to the toxin, but its effects on the heart (myocarditis), kidneys (tubular necrosis), and nervous system (myelin degeneration) are particularly serious. At the site of local infection in the upper respiratory tract, the toxin causes death of epithelial cells, producing an inflammatory reaction and formation of a tough membrane composed of fibrin and necrotic epithelium. The membrane, together with edema, commonly causes obstruction, with resultant asphyxia.

Indirect mechanisms. In some cases damage may be a result of mechanical effects, such as obstruction or pressure. For example, cerebral edema as a result of the inflammatory response causes increased intracranial pressure, as already mentioned. Obstruction of blood vessels can lead to tissue ischemia and infarction. For example, in falciparum malaria the surfaces of the parasitized red blood cells are altered and the red blood cells tend to plug small vessels in many organs, including the brain.

Often tissue damage is caused indirectly as a result of the immune response. Intracellular parasites often cause alterations on the surfaces of infected cells. For example, cells infected with viruses have viral antigens on their surfaces. Antibodies combine with these antigens, complement is activated, and destruction of the cell occurs. Infected cells can also be destroyed by sensitized lymphocytes as the result of a cell-mediated immune response (see Chapter 29).

Another mechanism by which the immune response leads to tissue damage is through the formation of immune complexes. The combination of antigens with antibodies is an important part of the host defense against infection. When the amount of circulating antibody is equal to or greater than the amount of antigen, large antigen-antibody complexes are formed and are quickly removed by retriculoendothelial cells. When the amount of antigen exceeds the amount of antibody, however, the antigen molecules are not completely coated with antibody and are not removed by reticuloendothelial cells. They continue to circulate in the blood and may localize in small blood vessels in various parts of the body. When they are deposited on the walls of small blood vessels an inflammatory reaction may occur. In the kidneys they filter through the glomerular capillaries. The smaller complexes pass through the basement membrane and enter the urine, but larger complexes may accumulate on the basement membrane and may lead to impaired glomerular function. When antigen-antibody reactions occur in the extravascular tissues an inflammatory reaction occurs.

Nutritional and Metabolic Effects

A variety of nutritional and metabolic effects accompany generalized acute infectious disease. Many of these effects are mediated by hormones or other substances released from body cells and are influenced by dietary intake and availability of nutrients from body stores. In addition host nutrients are used by the invading microorganisms for their growth and multiplication. The duration of the infection and the involvement of particular organs (e.g., liver or intestine) also influences the nutritional and metabolic effects.

During infection the plasma levels of iron and zinc decrease, mainly because of accumulation in the liver as storage forms. This response appears to be mediated by a substance released from active phagocytic cells. It occurs soon after exposure to pathogenic microorganisms, before the onset of symptoms (i.e., during the incubation period), and lasts for the duration of infection. With persistent infection iron remains trapped in storage forms and its incorporation into hemoglobin is somehow blocked, resulting in anemia.

The plasma level of amino acids also declines early in infection, possibly because of increased uptake by the liver. The liver produces increased amounts of "acute-phase" proteins, such as haptoglobin, alpha-antitrypsin, fibrinogen, complement, and ceruloplasmin. This response is possibly mediated by a hormonelike substance released from the phagocytic cells. The plasma level of acute phase proteins rises about the time of onset of fever. Ceruloplasmin is a glycoprotein that transports most of the copper in the plasma and the plasma copper concentration rises during infection.

Metabolism of amino acids and protein is altered throughout the course of infection. In addition to the increased production of certain proteins by the liver, increased production of leukocytes requires increased protein synthesis for new cellular components. Protein synthesis is also increased to produce lysosomal enzymes in phagocytic cells and to produce antibodies. At the same time, increased catabolism of skeletal muscle proteins occurs to provide alanine for gluconeogenesis and to provide amino acids for synthesis of essential proteins (see Chapter 17 under Starvation). Negative nitrogen balance begins shortly after the onset of fever, largely as a result of decreased intake from anorexia, while urinary losses continue at a normal or increased rate. During infection the body does not seem to be able to conserve nitrogen as well as it does during starvation. The negative nitrogen balance is accompanied by negative balances of other intracellular elements such as potassium, magnesium, and phosphate. The body swings into positive balances of these substances during convalescence.

Increased metabolism during fever results in increased caloric expenditure. Consequently glycogenolysis and gluconeogenesis increase. At the same time, glucose tolerance is decreased. With very severe infections, however, hypoglycemia may occur.

The altered metabolism of protein and carbohydrate during infection is probably mediated by complex interactions of several hormones. Early in infection the levels of catecholamines, glucocorticoids, and growth hormone are increased as a result of the stress response (see Chapter 2 under Physiological Responses to Stress). Fasting levels of glucagon and insulin are also increased. (See Chapter 18 for a discussion of how these hormones influence metabolism.)

Fluid and electrolyte disturbances frequently accompany infectious diseases. If the person has diarrhea, losses of water, sodium, chloride, bicarbonate, and potassium can lead to ECF volume deficit (see Chapter 12) and metabolic acidosis (see Chapter 15). Profuse diaphoresis may contribute to water and electrolyte losses in some cases. If vomiting occurs, hydrogen ions, chloride, and potassium are lost and metabolic alkalosis may occur (see Chapter 15). Ventilation increases at the onset of fever because the metabolic rate increases, producing an increased demand for oxygen. Consequently a transient respiratory alkalosis may occur from hyperventilation.

In the absence of diarrhea and/or vomiting, most severe generalized infections are accompanied by sodium and water retention resulting from increased secretion of mineralocorticoid hormones as part of the stress response. During early convalescence a period of diuresis occurs as the accumulated excess of fluid is lost. With infections of the central nervous system, inappropriate secretion of antidiuretic hormone may cause severe water retention, leading to water excess and dilutional hyponatremia (see Chapter 12).

OUTCOME OF THE HOST-MICROBE INTERACTION

Depending on the nature of the invading microorganism and on the strength of the host defenses, the result of the battle between the host and microbe may be complete elimination of the microorganism and recovery of the host or overwhelming infection and death of the host. In some cases the host may not be able to eliminate the microorganism from the body, but the microorganism is held in check with minimal pathological effects. In such cases the person may be considered to have recovered from the acute infection.

Factors Influencing the Outcome

The outcome of the host-microbe interaction will depend on the virulence of the microorganism and on the strength of the host resistance, both of which are influenced by several factors.

Microbial Factors

The ability of a microorganism to cause disease is referred to as its *pathogenicity*. The term *virulence* refers to the degree of pathogenicity of a microorganism. Virulence can be measured experimentally by determining the number of a particular microorganism required to cause an infection in 50% of the test animals (the infectious dose; ID_{50}) or by determining the number that can cause death of 50% of the test animals (the lethal dose; LD_{50}).

Serial passage of a microorganism through a host that it does not normally infect or repeated subculturing of the organism on artificial laboratory media often results in decreased virulence of the microorganism. A decrease in virulence produced in this manner is referred to as *attenuation*. The basis of attenuation is adaptation. Through genetic changes the microorganism adapts to conditions in the unnatural host and becomes more virulent for that host but, in the process, becomes less well adapted for growth in the original host.

Virulence is determined by the invasiveness and toxigenicity of a microorganism. *Invasiveness* refers to the ability of a microorganism to enter host tissues and when in the tissues to survive, to multiply, and to spread. The nutritional and physical factors required for microbial growth are described in Chapter 27. These factors are genetically determined. If the host tissues do not satisfy the requirements for growth of a particular microorganism, that microorganism will be unable to grow and to multiply. For example, if clostridial spores enter a tissue that has a good blood supply and is well oxygenated, they will be unable to germinate.

The ability of a microorganism to survive in the tissues and to spread will depend on its ability to resist host defenses. Several means by which microorganisms evade host defenses have already been described. For example, bacteria that have a capsule are resistant to phagocytosis. As mentioned earlier, the ability of some bacteria to secrete enzymes that break down tissue components also contributes to the ability to spread.

Toxigenicity refers to the ability of a microorganism to elaborate toxins that are harmful to the host. Toxins have been discussed in a previous section. In many cases the ability of a particular strain of bacteria to produce a toxin results from infection of the bacteria by a bacteriophage. Diphtheria toxin is an example.

Host Factors

The *genetic constitution* of the host influences susceptibility to infection. Genetic variation produces differences in the biochemical environment in the tissues of different people. Therefore some people may be more susceptible to particular pathogenic microorganisms and other people less susceptible, depending on how well the environment in the tissues suits the microorganisms.

Sickle cell trait, an inherited condition (see Chapter 6), confers resistance to falciparum malaria. The resistance possibly results from the fact that the use of oxygen by the developing parasites causes infected red blood cells to sickle, and such cells are quickly removed from the circulation by the reticuloendothelial system.

Immune responses are also under genetic control. Therefore inherited differences in immune responsiveness can also influence the outcome of a host-microbe encounter. In some cases inherited immunodeficiencies make a person more susceptible to infectious disease (see Chapter 29). On the other hand, the presence of certain immune response genes may be responsible for the manifestations of disease in some cases. For example, juvenile-onset diabetes is possibly due to a defective immune response to particular viruses, conferred by certain immune response genes (see Chapter 18).

Age is another host factor that influences susceptibility to infection. Generally the very young and the very old are more susceptible than people of other age groups, partly because immune responses are weaker in infants and the elderly. In some cases age-related differences in resistance are due to physical or physiological differences. For example, the airways of infants are narrow and are more easily blocked by edema and secretions, so that respiratory infections tend to be more serious in infants than in adults. In addition, infants are more prone to develop serious fluid and electrolyte disturbances caused by infections characterized by vomiting, diarrhea, and fever than adults are. Although fluid represents a high proportion of the body weight in infants, the total fluid volume is very small. For example, the total blood volume of an infant is about 0.6 liter as compared with about 4.8 liters in an adult. Therefore fluid losses from diarrhea in an infant can rapidly deplete the extracellular fluid.

Some virus infections tend to be more severe in adults than in children (e.g., varicella, mumps, poliomyelitis, and EB virus infections). The reason for the increased severity of these infections in adults is not known. It is possible, however, that some of the manifestations of these diseases result indirectly from an immune response, and adults generally have a stronger immune response than children.

The *nutritional status* of the host can also influence susceptibility to infection. Impaired integrity of skin and mucosal barriers as a result of vitamin A, B, and C deficiencies allows microorganisms easier access to body tissues. Protein deficiency impairs the immune response, particularly the cell-mediated immune response. Consequently malnourished people are very susceptible to tuberculosis and viral diseases in which cell-mediated immune responses play an important part in host defenses.

Hormonal factors can influence susceptibility to infection. Corticosteroid hormones are particularly involved in the inflammatory-reparative response (see Chapter 8 under Factors Influencing Healing). People with Cushing's syndrome have increased susceptibility to infection resulting from the antiinflammatory effect of excessive glucocorticoids. The consequences of infection are also very severe in people with Addison's disease because they are unable to produce adequate amounts of corticosteroids in response to the stress of infection and the adrenal glands may be exhausted, precipitating Addisonian crisis (see Chapter 19).

Susceptibility to infection is increased during pregnancy, partly because of hormonal changes, although the exact role of each hormone in this altered susceptibility is not clear. Also, the cell-mediated immune response is weaker during pregnancy.

Whether *fever* plays a role in the defense against invading microorganisms is controversial. High temperatures may be damaging to the microorganisms, but they are also damaging to host cells. The agents of syphilis and gonorrhea are killed by febrile temperatures, but in the natural course of these infections high fevers rarely occur. Before antibiotics were available, fever therapy was used in the treatment of syphilis and gonorrhea. (The fever was induced by infecting the people with one of the agents of malaria.)

If the fever is not too high, the elevated temperature increases leukocyte mobility, enhances phagocytosis and killing of ingested microorganisms, and increases the production of interferon. Therefore fever may be beneficial as a result of these mechanisms.

It has recently been suggested that fever coupled with the decrease in the plasma iron concentration is a coordinated host-defense mechanism. Iron is not only required for human metabolism but is also required for microbial metabolism, and many species of bacteria grow poorly when the concentration of iron in the medium is low. A low iron concentration appears to have a greater inhibitory effect on bacteria at febrile temperatures than at normal body temperature. Therefore, the combined effects of decreased availability of iron and increased body temperature may be a host defense against infection. If this is the case, excessive iron supplements may decrease host resistance.

Recovery

For recovery from infection to occur, multiplication of the microorganisms must first be brought under control. Antimicrobial forces must remove the infectious agents at a faster rate than they can multiply so that the number of microorganisms decreases. In addition, the antimicrobial factors must stop the spread of microorganisms through the body. Immune responses, complement, phagocytosis, and interferon are host factors that are important in recovery from infection. The relative importance of each factor varies for each type of infection. Once the microorganisms are completely destroyed, resolution of the inflammation occurs, if there has been no tissue damage. If tissues have been damaged, integrity is restored by regeneration or repair, as described in Chapter 8.

Persistent Infections

Persistent infections occur when host defenses are unable to overcome the invading microorganism and eliminate it from the body. In some cases the persistence of the microorganism is associated with signs and symptoms of disease and the disease process becomes *chronic* (e.g., tuberculosis, leprosy, syphilis, trachoma). At times the microorganism may be held in check by host defenses, but at other times the infectious agent may gain the upper hand. Often granuloma formation occurs (see Chapter 8).

In some cases, people may continue to harbor pathogenic microorganisms and to shed them to the exterior even though they have recovered from the acute infectious disease and are asymptomatic. These people are *carriers* and can transmit the infectious agent to other susceptible hosts. For example, *Salmonella typhi* sometimes colonizes scarred avascular areas of the gallbladder, where the bacteria are not very susceptible to antimicrobial forces that are carried in the blood of the host. Consequently, after a person recovers from typhoid fever bacteria may persist in the gallbladder for a long time. From this site bacteria are intermittently shed into the bile and are then discharged in the feces.

Latent Infections

In some cases of infection caused by intracellular parasites the infected person apparently recovers and has no signs and symptoms of disease, but the microorganisms remains dormant in the body for long periods of time and can later be reactivated. In these cases the infection is said to be *latent*. During the dormant period the microorganism is not detectable in the body fluids and is not shed to the exterior, so that the person is not infectious.

When the infection becomes reactivated, however, shedding to the exterior does occur and the microorganism can be transmitted to another susceptible host.

Herpesviruses commonly cause latent infections. For example, primary infection with herpes simplex virus type one usually occurs in early childhood and produces gingivostomatitis. In many cases the infection is subclinical (i.e., without clinical manifestations). Subsequently the virus persists in a nonreplicating, noninfectious form in the trigeminal ganglion supplying the mouth and related areas. At intervals later in life the virus becomes reactivated and replicates, producing a vesicular eruption around the lips or nostrils in the area supplied by the nerve. Several factors can induce the virus to replicate, including colds, fever, exposure to sunlight, menstruation, and emotional stress, and the vesicular lesion is usually referred to as a "cold sore" or a "fever blister."

Another example of a latent infection caused by a herpesvirus is varicella-zoster. Primary infection with the varicella-zoster virus, usually occurring in childhood, causes chickenpox. At this time the virus enters sensory nerves in the skin and ascends to the dorsal root ganglia. Here it enters the nuclei of affected neurons and becomes latent after recovery from chickenpox and elimination of virus from the rest of the body. Virus in the dorsal root ganglia is kept in check by cell-mediated immunity, but when host defenses are weakened, either due to advancing age or underlying illness, reactivation of the varicella-zoster infection occurs. The virus multiplies and invades adjacent nerve cells, causing inflammation and necrosis of the affected ganglion. This event is accompanied by neuralgia and paresthesias of the corresponding segmental dermatome. The virus migrates down the peripheral nerve to the skin and produces a rash like that of chickenpox but restricted to the distribution of the particular nerve.

Brill's disease is an example of latent rickettsial infection. Rickettsia sometimes remain dormant in lymph nodes or the reticuloendothelial system for 10 or more years following clinical recovery from typhus. Reactivation causes a mild illness, less severe than the original typhus. The causes of reactivation of the latent infection are not known.

Malaria is a protozoal example of latency. After clinical recovery the malaria parasite (particularly *Plasmodium vivax*) may persist in the liver without causing signs and symptoms and without infecting erythrocytes. The parasite in the liver may reinfect red blood cells and cause a fresh clinical attack of malaria many years later.

A type of latent infection also sometimes occurs with tuberculosis. Early in life infection by tubercle bacilli in a lung or a lymph node may be controlled, producing a healed primary focus of infection that is asymptomatic. Later in life when the cell-mediated immune response is weakened for any reason, the primary focus may become reactivated and cause clinical disease.

SUGGESTED ADDITIONAL READING

Bielan B: What that rash really means. *RN* 42(2): 58–63, 1979.

Castle M, Watkins J: Fever: understanding a sinister sign. *Nurs 79* 9(2): 26–33, 1979.

Goad DM: Superficial neonatal infection. *Nurs Times* 75(23): 965–966, 1979.

Kaplan MM, Webster RG: The epidemiology of influenza. *Sci Am* 237(6): 88–106, 1977.

Melnick JL, Dreesman GR, Hollinger FB: Viral hepatitis. *Sci Am* 237(1): 44–52, 1977.

Panrucker R: Botulism: a team effort to save the poison salmon victims. *Nurs Mirror* 147(24): 32–35, 1978.

29

Mechanisms of Inducible Host Resistance

Resistance to infection involves not only the nonspecific host defenses discussed in Chapter 28 but also specific immune responses induced by and directed against the invading microorganism. *Immunity* is a state of relative resistance to a particular disease. *Natural,* or *innate,* immunity refers to the specific resistance a person has to microorganisms not previously encountered. Innate immunity is governed by inherited physiological and biochemical properties of the host. Species immunity is a form of innate immunity that refers to the resistance of one species to a microorganism that can cause disease in another species. For example, human beings are resistant to the virus that causes foot-and-mouth disease in cattle. Within a species, innate immunity is responsible for racial and individual differences in susceptibility to a particular infectious agent. For example, Negroes and North American Indians have greater susceptibility to tuberculosis, and Polynesians have greater susceptibility to measles than Caucasians do, but Caucasians are more susceptible to influenza and diphtheria than Negroes are.

Acquired, or *adaptive,* immunity is a state of enhanced resistance to a microorganism or its antigens, developed as a result of previous exposure. Acquired immunity depends on the development of antibodies and reactive lymphoid cells that interact specifically with that microorganism and its antigens. Immunity is *acquired naturally* as a result of recovery from an infection or as a result of maternal transfer of antibodies across the placenta to the fetus and in the colostrum to the breastfed neonate. Immunity is *artificially acquired* as a result of vaccination or inoculation and by administration of immune serum or cells. When immunity is acquired as a result of a response of the body to the presence of an immunogen, it is said to be *active*. When immunity is acquired as a result of transfer of antibodies or specifically modified reactive immune cells to a person, without the active participation of the body, it is said to be *passive*. The types of resistance to infection are summarized in Table 29-1.

Although the importance of the immune response was first recognized in relation to protection against infectious diseases, it later became apparent that several other clinical phenomena are related to immune responses. Allergy, some transfusion reactions and maternal-fetal interactions, graft rejection, and autoimmunity are due to immune responses. These conditions are discussed in Chapter 30. In addition, immune responses may be involved in protection against cancer through recognition and destruction of abnormal cells by the immune system (see Chapter 20).

Table 29-1. Types of Resistance to Infection

NONSPECIFIC RESISTANCE
Skin and mucosal barriers
Phagocytosis
Interferon

SPECIFIC RESISTANCE
Natural (Innate) Immunity
   Species
   Races
   Individual
Acquired (Adaptive) Immunity
   Naturally acquired
      passive (maternal transfer)
      active (postinfection)
   Artificially acquired
      passive (serum therapy; cell transfer)
      active (vaccination)

THE IMMUNE RESPONSE

The immune response involves the ability of the immune system to recognize a substance as foreign to the body (i.e., *not-self*) and to initiate mechanisms to destroy and to eliminate the substance. The exact mechanism by which the immune system distinguishes between self and not-self is not understood. It appears that exposure of the immune system to circulating and tissue substances during fetal development results in a state of immunologic tolerance to these substances. In other words, the body recognizes these substances as *self* and does not normally initiate an immune response against them.

Any substance that is capable of eliciting an immune response (either humoral or cell-mediated) is called an *immunogen*. An *antigen* is any substance that induces the formation of antibodies that react specifically with it. The terms immunogen and antigen are often used interchangeably, but they are not always synonymous. Antigens are very large molecules, usually proteins or polypeptides; but polysaccharides, glycoproteins, or nucleic acids may also act as antigens in some cases. Lipids by themselves are not antigenic, but lipoproteins and lipopolysaccharides can be. The immune response is actually directed against small discrete portions of an antigen, called *antigenic determinant sites*, not against the whole molecule. An *antibody* is a protein (immunoglobulin) molecule that reacts specifically with the antigen that induced its synthesis or with a closely related antigen. Some small molecules, called *haptens*, are not capable of eliciting antibody formation by themselves, but when combined with a larger molecule, called a *carrier*, they impart antigenic specificity on the complex and do elicit antibody production. The antibodies formed may subsequently react with the hapten alone or with the hapten-carrier complex.

Immunological responses are classified as humoral or cell-mediated. *Humoral immunity* is mediated by antibodies that circulate in the blood and are present in the body fluids. Antibodies act at a distance from the lymphoid cells that produce them. *Cell-mediated immunity* (CMI) depends on the local action of specifically sensitized lymphocytes that circulate through the body. The components of the immune system not only interact with foreign substances but also interact with each other, with the phagocytic cells, and with complement in destroying invaders.

The Nature of the Immune System

The cells of the immune system include thymus-dependent cells (T cells), thymus-independent cells (B cells), and macrophages. These cells are variously categorized as being part of the hematopoietic system, the reticuloendothelial system, or the lymphoid system. They originate in hematopoietic tissue. T cells and B cells migrate to lymphoid tissue for further development and expression of their immune function. Macrophages are part of the reticuloendothelial system, as described in Chapter 28.

Lymphoid Organs

The lymphoid system consists of *primary,* or *central,* lymphoid organs and *secondary,* or *peripheral,* lymphoid organs. Central lymphoid organs are the thymus and bone marrow. Peripheral lymphoid organs are the lymph nodes, spleen, tonsils, and intestinal lymphoid tissue (Peyer's patches and appendix).

The thymus is a flat, bilobed organ located behind the sternum in the upper portion of the mediastinum. It is well developed at birth and remains very active during the first few years of life. It gradually atrophies after puberty. During fetal development hematopoietic stem cells migrate to the thymic rudiment, where they proliferate and differentiate into thymic lymphocytes or thymocytes (T lymphocytes, T cells).

Birds have a central lymphoid organ called the *bursa of Fabricius,* which is not present in mammals. Hematopoietic stem cells that migrate to the bursa of Fabricius develop into bursal or B lymphocytes (B cells). The bursal equivalent (i.e., the source of B lymphocytes) in human beings is not known with certainty. It was once thought that lymphoid tissue associated with the intestinal tract served as the human bursal equivalent, but more recently it has been suggested that the bone marrow is the source organ for B lymphocytes.

Lymphocytes derived from the bursal equivalent and thymus are distributed through the blood and lymph to peripheral lymphoid organs.

A lymph node is a small bean-shaped organ enclosed by a fibrous capsule. Extensions of connective tissue from the capsule (trabeculae) go deep into the node, dividing it into compartments. A network of reticular fibers supports large numbers of lymphocytes, which form the parenchyma of the node. In the cortex (outer part) of the node, lymphoid tissue is concentrated into discrete masses called lymph follicles or lobules. At the centers of the follicles are *germinal centers* consisting of actively dividing lymphocytes. Germinal centers are not present at birth but develop during the first year of postnatal life. In the medulla (inner part) of the lymph node the lymphocytes form strands of tissue called medullary cords. Several afferent lymph vessels enter through the capsule at intervals. They bring lymph into the marginal sinus just under the capsule. From the marginal sinus lymph flows through smaller channels (radial sinuses) that lie between the medullary cords and converge on the hilus. As the lymph flows through the node, foreign particles in it are removed by macrophages lining the sinuses. Lymph leaves the node through one or more efferent lymphatics at the hilus. Nerves and blood vessels enter the node at the hilus.

Lymph nodes are widely distributed throughout the body, with groups of them occurring at strategic locations such as the axilla, the groin, and adjacent to the large veins in the neck and abdominal and pelvic cavities. In addition, a few are located in the popliteal fossa (knee) and near the antecubital fossa (elbow).

The spleen is structurally similar to a lymph node except it is much larger and its sinusoids are filled with blood rather than lymph. Nodules of lymphoid tissue resembling a lymph node cortex constitute the white pulp of the spleen. Some of the nodules of white pulp contain germinal centers. The remainder of the spleen, which corresponds to the medulla of a lymph node, is called the red pulp. It consists of a system of venous sinuses between which are cords of tissue containing many macrophages and red blood cells.

Clusters of diffuse lymphoid tissue are present in the lamina propria of the intestinal wall. Distinct follicles with germinal centers are often apparent in these clusters.

Tonsils are aggregates of lymphoid tissue found under the epithelium of the pharynx and oral cavity.

Cells of the Immune System

The development of the cells of the immune system is outlined in Figure 29-1. Lymphocytes are responsible for the specificity of the immune response, whereas macrophages generally have a nonspecific accessory role. As already mentioned, lymphocytes are divided into two major categories: B cells and T cells. Probably several subpopulations exist within these two categories. Lymphocytes that have the ability to recognize immunogens as foreign and to react specifically with them are said to be *immunologically competent*.

During early embryonic development hematopoietic stem cells come from the yolk sac and the liver, but later they are supplied by the bone marrow. Those that migrate to the thymus differentiate into small lymphocytes with certain properties that characterize them as *T cells*. It is believed that the development of T cells is influenced by a thymic humoral factor called thymosin. Immunologically competent T cells then migrate to peripheral lymphoid organs. The T cells preferentially locate in the interfollicular and deep cortical areas of the lymph nodes and around arterioles in the spleen. Most of the lymphocytes in the blood are T cells; few T cells are found in the bone marrow. T cells have a relatively long life span (months) compared with B cells.

T cells constantly recirculate through the blood and lymph. The leave the blood mainly through venules in lymphoid tissue, spend a variable

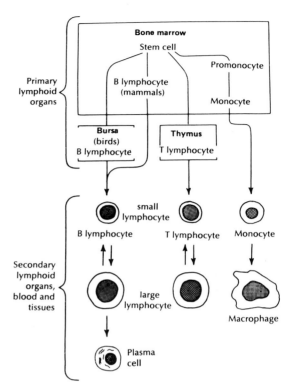

Figure 29-1. *Developmental pathways of mononuclear cells involved in immune responses. (From Freedman SO, Gold P (eds): Clinical Immunology, ed 2. Hagerstown, Md, Harper & Row, Publishers, 1976.)*

amount of time in the lymphoid tissue, then leave by way of efferent lymphatics to reenter the blood. A small portion of the cells leave capillaries in various parts of the body (especially the small intestine), move through the tissues, enter afferent lymphatic vessels, and are carried to local lymph nodes. T cells are involved with cell-mediated immunity, and their continual movement through the tissues and lymph nodes ensures that antigens or microorganism entering the body sooner or later encounter specifically reactive lymphocytes. This monitoring of tissues by lymphocytes is referred to as *immune surveillance*.

Stem cells in the bone marrow or some other bursal equivalent differentiate into small lymphocytes with certain properties that characterize them as *B cells*. From their source organ B lympho-cytes migrate to the peripheral lymphoid organs. They are found predominantly in the follicles and medullary cords of lymph nodes and in the spleen. Only a small portion of the circulating lymphocytes are B cells. A large number of B cells are found in the bone marrow, but very few are present in the thymus. When B cells are stimulated by antigen they develop further to form antibody-secreting cells called plasma cells (see later under Humoral Immunity).

Macrophages differentiate from monocytes and have a life span of several weeks or months. Mac-rophages appear to have several accessory roles in the immune response, although all the details of their actions and functions have not yet been es-tablished. They appear to be involved in "pro-cessing" antigens and possibly release factors that modulate the B cell response. Macrophages also act as effector cells in some types of cell-mediated immune responses. In addition, they produce some of the complement components.

Immunoglobulins

Proteins that function as antibodies are called *im-munoglobulins* (abbreviated Ig). Most of them are found in the gamma globulin fraction of the plasma proteins, but some are α_2- or β-globulins.

The basic structure, or monomeric unit, of an immunoglobulin molecule consists of four polypeptide chains. Two of the chains, which are identical, have a high molecular weight and are referred to as the heavy, or H, chains. The other two chains, which are also identical to each other, are of lower molecular weight and are referred to as light, or L, chains. In addition, a small amount of carbohydrate is present in the molecule. Each H chain has an L chain linked to it, and the two H chains are linked by disulfide bonds. This monomeric unit is depicted as having a Y shape (Fig. 29-2). Five major classes of immunoglobulins are known: IgG, IgM, IgA, IgD, and IgE. The various classes are distinquished by differences in the H chains; the light chains are common to all classes. Within each class are several subclasses.

Immunoglobulin G. Most of the circulating anti-bodies belong to the IgG class. IgG antibodies occur mainly in the blood, but small amounts are found in lymph, cerebrospinal fluid, synovial fluid, and peritoneal fluid. They are the only class of antibodies that cross the placenta.

IgG molecules are the smallest immunoglobu-lins and consist of one Y-shaped monomeric unit. Experimental hydrolysis of the IgG molecule yields two portions designated *Fab* (fragment, antigen-binding) and one portion designated *Fc* (fragment, crystallizable). The Fab portions represent the arms of the Y and contain the antigen-binding sites; since there are two of them, the IgG mole-cule is said to be divalent. The amino-acid se-quences of the polypeptide chains are variable at one end of the Fab portion, and this variation is responsible for the antigenic specificity of particu-lar IgG molecules. The amino-acid sequences of the remainder of the polypeptide chains are the same in all IgG molecules.

The Fc portion of the molecule represents the stem of the Y. It is involved in activation of com-plement (see below). It also contains a site that binds to receptors on the surfaces of neutrophils and macrophages. This binding site mediates the attachment of an antibody-coated microorganism to the phagocytic cell and thus facilitates phagocytosis. In addition, free antibodies can combine with phagocytic cells and confer immu-nological specificity on them. The Fc portion also contains a specific site that enables the IgG mole-cule to be transported across the placenta.

Immunoglobulin M. IgM antibodies are the largest immunoglobulin molecules and are found mainly in the blood. The human fetus is capable of producing IgM antibodies after the fifth to sixth month of development. These antibodies cannot cross the placenta; therefore, the presence of in-creased levels of IgM antibodies in the cord blood is suggestive of intrauterine infection or exposure to other antigens.

An IgM molecule consists of five monomeric units arranged radially and linked by disulfide bonds (Fig. 29-3). In addition, an extra polypep-

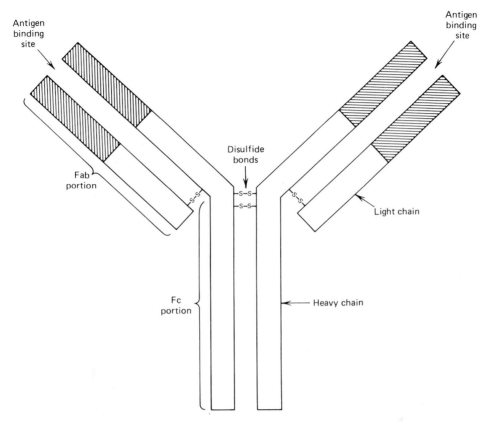

Figure 29-2. *Schematic representation of the basic structure of an immunoglobulin G molecule. Hatched areas denote portions of the polypeptide chains that have variable amino acid sequences.*

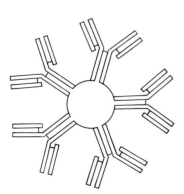

Figure 29-3. *Schematic representation of an immunoglobulin M molecule.*

tide chain, called the J chain, is present in the molecule. The functions of IgM antibodies are similar to those of IgG antibodies, but they are more efficient at activating complement and have a greater capacity for binding antibodies. Theoretically an IgM antibody has 10 antigen-binding sites, but experimentally it has been shown that an IgM antibody usually combines with only five antigens.

Immunoglobulin A. IgA antibodies exist in more than one form. In the blood they exist mainly as one monomeric unit, but polymeric units are also found. They are present in exocrine secretions such as colostrum, milk, tears, saliva, and mucus of the respiratory and intestinal tracts. The IgA molecules found in exocrine secretions differ slightly from the IgA molecules in the blood and are referred to as *secretory IgA*. Secretory IgA is made up of two monomeric units (i.e., it is a dimer) and contains one J chain. This dimer is synthesized by plasma cells, but as it is excreted, it acquires another polypeptide chain called secretory component (SC chain) that is produced by the epithelial cells of the mucosal surface.

Although most of the antibodies in exocrine secretions belong to the IgA class, small amounts of IgG and IgM antibodies are also present in these secretions. Secretory IgA is particularly important in protecting the host against infection of mucosal surfaces, apparently by preventing the attachment of microorganisms to the epithelial surfaces. Some bacteria, such as *Neisseria gonorrhoeae*, *N. meningitidis*, and some streptococci, produce enzymes called IgA proteases that break down IgA molecules and possibly serve to overcome this host defense mechanism.

Immunoglobulin E.   Normally only trace amounts of IgE are found in the blood. IgE is produced mainly by cells in the respiratory and intestinal mucosa. The Fc portion of IgE has a site that enables it to bind to mast cells and basophils. IgE is involved in allergic reactions (see Chapter 30).

Immunoglobulin D.   These molecules represent only a small fraction of the total immunoglobulins in the body. IgD has no known antibody activity, but it is present on the surface of B cells, particularly during the fetal and neonatal periods. It has been suggested that IgD may play a role during the development and maturation of the immune system.

Humoral Immune Response

Many antigens are associated with microorganisms and their products. Substances present on the surfaces of microorganisms, such as the components of the cell walls of bacteria or fungi, capsular components of bacteria, flagella of bacteria or protozoa, and envelope proteins or capsid proteins of viruses, can act as antigens. Soluble products secreted by microorganisms, such as enzymes and toxins, can also act as antigens. In addition, intracellular microbial substances can act as antigens after the microbial cell has been broken down. Therefore, a single microorganism can induce the synthesis of several different specific antibodies.

Microorganisms or their products that gain access to the tissues usually enter the lymph and are carried to the lymph nodes, where they encounter macrophages and lymphocytes and stimulate a humoral immune response. Alternatively, microorganisms may be ingested by macrophages in the tissues and transported to the lymph nodes within the macrophages. Microorganisms that enter the blood encounter macrophages and lymphocytes in the spleen, and the spleen is very important in the defense against blood-borne bacteria. (See the discussion of hyposplenism in the section on Secondary Immunodeficiency.)

Production of Antibodies

Most antigens require processing by the macrophages before B cells are stimulated, but some antigens may stimulate B cells directly. The exact mechanisms by which B cells are activated and specific antibodies are produced is not understood. It appears that within a macrophage the antigen is broken down, but the antigenic determinant site is preserved. The antigenic determinant site (possibly complexed with RNA) is then transferred to a B cell, and the B cell is activated.

In many cases T cells are involved in the activation of B cells, but the exact nature of this "helper" effect of T cells is not known. Some antigens, especially complex ones, require the mediation of T cells to stimulate antibody production and are referred to as T cell-dependent antigens. Simpler antigens can stimulate B lymphocytes without the mediation of T cells and are referred to as T cell-independent antigens.

B lymphocytes have immunoglobulin molecules on their surfaces, and these molecules act as receptors for antigens (or antigenic determinant sites). It is believed that many subpopulations of B cells exist, each with different surface receptors that bind specific antigens. It is further believed that these Ig receptors are spontaneously generated and that there are always a few cells that will react with almost any antigen that enters the body for the first time. The few lymphocytes that are capable of forming the required antibody are thus selectively activated.

The activated B cells, which are small lymphocytes, differentiate into larger blast cells (i.e., undergo blast transformation). Some of the blast cells then undergo mitotic divisions to produce a clone of cells that is committed to producing specific antibodies. These cells differentiate to become first large lymphocytes (immunoblasts and immature plasma cells) and then smaller mature plasma cells (see Fig. 29-1). The mature plasma cells synthesize large quantities of specific antibody that can react with the antigen that activated the precursor B cell. Plasma cells are rarely found in the peripheral blood. They remain in the lymphoid tissue and secrete antibodies into the lymph (or into an exocrine secretion, as in the case of secretory IgA). From the lymph the antibodies enter the blood and circulate throughout the body. Plasma cells probably die after a few days or a few weeks.

Some of the large lymphocytes may not differentiate into plasma cells, but instead they revert back to small lymphocytes that function as "memory" cells. These cells have long lives. On subsequent reexposure to the antigen they can respond quickly to bring about more antibody synthesis.

Usually an infection is initiated by a small number of microorganisms, and the amount of antigen present at the time of exposure is insufficient to provoke a detectable immune response. As the microorganism establishes itself and multiplies, however, the amount of antigen increases and stimulates an immune response. On first exposure to a particular antigen (the *primary immune response*) there is a latent period while lymphocytes differentiate and proliferate before antibody production begins. Initially the amount of antibody is too small to be detected, but over a period of days the number of antibody-producing cells increases, and the level of antibody in the blood rises. Free antibody becomes detectable about a week after the onset of infection. The first antibodies to be produced are of the IgM class. With continued antigenic exposure, mainly IgG antibodies are produced, and they are produced in larger quantities than IgM. The IgG response may be followed by the production of IgA.

Since an IgM molecule has a greater antigen-combining capacity than an IgG molecule and is a more powerful activator of complement, the production of IgM before IgG may favor earlier recovery from infection. The IgM level declines as some of the molecules are consumed in antigen-antibody reactions and some are catabolized. IgM antibodies are catabolized fairly quickly. Therefore, if a person's blood contains IgM antibodies to a particular microbial antigen, it indicates either recent infection or a persistent infection.

On subsequent reexposure to a particular microbial antigen there is an enhanced immune response (the *secondary immune response*). Within one to three days, larger amounts of antibodies, mainly of the IgG class, are produced. This *anamnestic* (without forgetting) or booster response is presumably mediated by the long-lived memory cells. As a result of this response, the microorganism is usually eliminated from the body quickly, without the development of disease symptoms.

IgG antibodies have a longer half-life than any other immunoglobulin (about 25 days); therefore, the level of IgG antibody in the blood falls slowly. Often IgG antibodies to a particular microbial antigen remain in the blood for many years, suggesting that antibody-forming cells are continually active. In some cases the microorganisms are not eliminated from the body after the original infection and continue to stimulate the immune system. (See the discussion of presistent infections in Chapter 28.) In other cases repeated reexposure to the microorganism boosts the immune response and maintains an elevated antibody level. In some cases antibodies remain in the blood for long periods of time when there is no evidence of persistent infection or reexposure. The mechanism for maintaining the antibody level in these cases is not understood.

Antimicrobial Effects of Antibodies

The antimicrobial effects of antibodies are mediated in a variety of ways. By binding with surface antigens on microbial cells, antibodies make the microorganisms more easily phagocytosed (i.e., the antibodies act as *opsonins*). Both neutrophils and macrophages have specific surface receptors for the Fc part of IgG and IgM antibodies. Therefore microbial cells that are coated with antibodies are effectively attached to the surfaces of phagocytic cells. Opsonization is particularly important in the defense against encapsulated bacteria and streptococci that have surface proteins that enable them to resist phagocytosis (see Chapter 28 under Subepithelial Invasion).

Free antibodies that combine with Fc receptors on macrophages are referred to as *cytophilic antibodies*. This combination enables macrophages to carry out immunologically specific phagocytosis by attaching to surface antigens on microbial cells.

Another way that antibodies exert an antimicrobial effect is by preventing the attachment of microbial cells to susceptible host cells or epithelial surfaces. As mentioned in Chapter 28, microorganisms attempting to establish themselves in the respiratory tract, intestinal tract, or urinary tract must attach to the epithelial surface to avoid being swept or washed away. Antibodies that coat the surfaces of microorganisms prevent this attachment. Secretory IgA is especially important in this regard. As mentioned in Chapter 27, viruses must attach to surface receptors on host cells before they can enter host cells and start replicating. Antibodies that coat the viral surface prevent this attachment and protect host cells from infection. Circulating antibodies that perform this function are particularly important in controlling systemic virus diseases that are associated with viremia (e.g., poliomyelitis). (See Chapter 28 under Systemic Spread.) The virus-antibody complexes are taken up and digested by phagocytic cells. Antibodies that counteract virus infectivity are called *virus neutralizing antibodies*.

Antibodies that combine with and neutralize microbial toxins are vital in the recovery from diseases that are caused by toxins (e.g., diphtheria, tetanus). These antibodies are called *antitoxins.*

Antibodies also exert an antimicrobial effect by activating complement (see below). Activation of complement induces inflammation, bringing more phagocytic cells and antibodies to the site of infection. Activation of complement by antibodies attached to the surfaces of microorganisms brings about lysis of the microbial cells (*immune cytolysis*). Host cells that have viral antigens on their surfaces can also be lysed by this mechanism, often before the virus has finished replicating.

Antibodies that combine with the surfaces of microorganisms may cause them to clump together (i.e., to *agglutinate*). Agglutination of smaller microorganisms makes them more readily phagocytosed. Antibodies that combine with soluble antigens may cause the antigens to precipitate, again facilitating phagocytosis. Motile microorganisms may be immobilized by the attachment of antibodies to their surfaces, perhaps making phagocytosis easier.

Cell-Mediated Immune Response

During an infection, both humoral and cell-mediated immune (CMI) responses are usually activated, but for a given pathogenic agent one type of reaction may be a more important defense mechanism than the other. Cell-mediated immunity appears to be particularly important in recovery from infection caused by intracellular parasites (e.g., viruses, tubercle bacilli).

The ability to generate a CMI response apparently occurs later in development than the ability to produce antibodies, but at or shortly after birth a human infant has functional B and T cells and an operative phagocytic system. Both antibody production and the CMI response tend to decrease during old age, probably because of a decline in the total number of immune reactive cells.

Cell-mediated immunity involves T lymphocytes. It is assumed that T cells have surface receptors that confer the ability to recognize antigens as foreign and to react specifically with them, but the nature of the T cell receptors is uncertain.

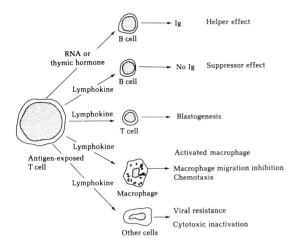

Figure 29-4. *Various lymphokines secreted by antigen-exposed T lymphocytes often function on other host cells rather than on the antigen. (From Barrett JT: Basic Immunology and Its Medical Application. St. Louis, C.V. Mosby Co., 1976.)*

Following appropriate antigenic stimulation, small T lymphocytes undergo blast transformation and cell division to produce a clone of cells with the same specific reactivity. Initially large or medium-sized lymphocytes are formed, but after further cell division small lymphocytes are formed again. Some of these cells may have long lives and serve as memory cells.

Activated T cells have several functions, many of which appear to be mediated by chemicals called *lymphokines* that are secreted by the T cells (Fig. 29-4). As mentioned previously, some T lymphocytes are involved as *helper cells* in the activation of B lymphocytes. The helper activity may be mediated by a hormonelike substance or an RNA from T cells. In addition, some *suppressor T cells* have an inhibitory effect on antibody production by B cells. Thus T lymphocytes exert a regulatory effect on B-cell function.

Sensitized T lymphocytes produce a lymphokine called *mitogenic*, or *blastogenic*, *factor* that induces blast transformation (blastogenesis) and division of other T cells. Thus the number of specifically sensitized lymphocytes is increased.

Lymphokines exert several effects on macrophages. One causes chemotactic attraction of macrophages to the site where the T cell has encountered the antigen. *Migration inhibition factor* (MIF) prevents movement of macrophages away from the site. *Macrophage aggregation factor* (MAF) causes agglutination of macrophages in vitro. MIF, MAF, and the chemotactic factor appear to be a single substance, which has the overall effect of attracting and retaining macrophages at sites of infection. Another lymphokine activates macrophages, causing them to increase their phagocytic activity. In addition the macrophages develop increased numbers of lysosomes and greater amounts of lysosomal enzymes, giving them greater digestive power. The activated macrophages express this increased reactivity not only against the microbial antigen that stimulated the T lymphocyte but also against other microorganisms. In other words, the activation of macrophages results from an immunologically specific encounter between a T lymphocyte and a microbial antigen, but it is expressed nonspecially against a wider range of microorganisms.

Another lymphokine produced by sensitized lymphocytes is *interferon*. Interferon is also produced by other cells. It inhibits replication of viruses (see below). T cells also produce a lymphokine called lymphotoxin, which has a cytocidal effect on nonspecific target cells.

In addition to secreting lymphokines, specifically sensitized T cells can cause destruction of target cells. This *cytotoxic effect* of T cells depends on direct contact of the sensitized lymphocyte with antigens on the surface of the target cell, but the exact mechanism by which the cell is killed is not known. The debris is disposed of by macrophages.

These functions of T cells may not all be carried out by the same cells. It appears that different subpopulations of T cells exist, which mediate different functions.

Interferon

Interferon is produced not only by antigen-stimulated T cells but also by many other cells in response to infection by viruses and other intracellular parasites, such as rickettsiae and some bacteria and protozoa. It was once thought to be a single protein, but it now appears that several proteins and glycoproteins have interferon activity. Interferon has been studied mainly in relation to viral infections. It is synthesized by host cells in response to double-stranded RNA, which is formed during viral replication (or experimentally in response to a variety of synthetic polynucleotides). Interferon is secreted into the surrounding medium and acts on other cells, inducing them to produce a second protein. The second protein does not prevent the entry of viruses into cells but prevents viral replication. This protection lasts for up to 24 hours and is nonspecific; that is, it is effective against any virus, not just the one that induced the synthesis of interferon. However, interferon is species specific, which means that interferon produced by one animal is not effective at protecting the cells of another animal, and animal interferon does not prevent viral infection of human cells.

The interferon response to viral infection occurs quickly, within hours. Interferon production reaches a peak within two to three days, before immunoglobulins are detectable. Therefore it is believed that interferon is an important factor in recovery from viral infections.

Complement

Complement is a system of eleven proteins normally present in the plasma. It is not specifically induced as immune responses are, but it works together with antibodies. Complement not only has an antimicrobial effect but also triggers inflammation.

The proteins of the complement system are numbered C1 through C9; C1 consists of three protein components, C1q, C1r, and C1s. When the complement system is triggered, the proteins are activated sequentially in a cascade fashion comparable to the clotting process. Activated components are indicated by a line over the number.

In the classical pathway, complement activation occurs when antibodies of the IgM or IgG classes bind with their specific antigens. As a result of antigen-antibody binding the immunolglobulin molecule is slightly altered, and a site on the Fc portion is able to bind and activate the C1 components. $\overline{C1}$ is an enzyme that activates C4. $\overline{C4}$ acquires an adhesiveness that allows it to bind to the antigen; it does not attach to the antibody or to C1. C2 binds to C4 and is also activated by $\overline{C1}$. The $\overline{C4,2}$ complex, which is called C3 convertase, then activates C3 by splitting it into a small fragment (C3a) that is released and a large fragment (C3b) that binds to $\overline{C4,2}$. The $\overline{C4,2,3}$ complex then acts on the other components, activating them in turn. In the process, a fragment called C5a is split from C5. When the antigen is on the surface of a microorganism or other cell, the complex of activated complement components damages the cell membrane, causing leakage of cell contents and cell death.

In addition to the cytolytic effect of activated complement, various complement components and fragments exert other effects. Some chemotactically attract neutrophils to the site and mobilize neutrophils from bone marrow. Some cause increased vascular permeability. Thus activated complement mediates inflammation. C3a and C3b cause the release of histamine from mast cells and are referred to as *anaphylatoxins.*

The C3b fragment is able to bind to a wide variety of substances, including immune complexes, particulate polysaccharides and lipopolysaccharides, basement membranes, and cell membranes. After it has bound to these substances, C3b can bind to specific receptors on neutrophils monocytes, erythrocytes, some B lymphocytes, and platelets. This phenomenon is called *immune adherence.* As a result of this property C3b can act as an opsonin. Many phagocytic cells have receptors for C3b as well as for the Fc portion of IgG. Therefore an antigen bound with both IgG and C3b is more likely to attach to phagocytic cells and be phagocytosed.

Complement can also be activated by an alternate (properdin) pathway, in which C1, C4, and C2 are bypassed. The properdin pathway can be triggered by particulate polysaccharides, lipopolysaccharides such as endotoxin, and aggregated IgA. These substances are believed to activate an undefined substance called initiating factor, which in turn activates properdin, a glycoprotein normally found in the plasma. Activated properdin then activates C3. The rest of the complement sequence, C5 through C9, is then activated.

Normally the complement system is held in check by several controls. Some of the components form unstable links and dissociate easily. In addition, an inhibitor of C̄1 and inactivators of C3b, C6, and anaphylatoxins are present in the plasma. Also, activated complement components are broken down rapidly, so they do not diffuse throughout the body and cause systemic effects.

The binding of complement to an antigen-antibody complex is referred to as *complement fixation,* and it is the basis of serological tests for the detection of specific antigens or antibodies (Fig. 29-5). Most often the test is used for the detection of antibodies in a person's serum. The binding of complement to the antigen-antibody complex is not a visible reaction; therefore, an indicator system is required. The test system consists of a specific antigen and serum believed to contain an antibody reactive with that antigen (or a specific antibody and serum believed to contain an antigen reactive with that antibody). The indicator system consists of sheep red blood cells as the antigen and an antiserum containing antibodies against sheep red blood cells. When complement is present the antiserum causes hemolysis of the sheep red blood cells, a visible reaction.

In performing the complement fixation test, the test serum is heated to inactivate any complement in it. The test antigen and test serum are them mixed, a measured amount of complement is added, and the mixture is incubated. Then the indicator system (i.e., sheep red blood cells and antiserum) is added. If the test serum contains antibodies that are specific for the test antigen (a positive test), complement is fixed in the test system and is not available for the indicator system. Therefore the sheep red blood cells are not lysed. If the test serum does not contain antibodies that are specific for the test antigen (a negative test), complement is not fixed in the test system. Therefore it is available for the indicator system, and lysis of the sheep red blood cells occurs.

The complement fixation test is used as an aid in the diagnosis of a number of viral diseases and systemic fungal diseases. It is also the basis of the Wasserman test for syphilis.

IMMUNODEFICIENCY

A deficiency of the host's immune mechanisms leads to increased susceptibility to infection. When the defect in the immune system is due to a genetic or developmental disorder, it is referred to as *primary immunodeficiency.* When it occurs as a secondary manifestation of an underlying disease process, it is referred to as *secondary immunodeficiency.* Immunodeficiency may involve a defect in the B-cell response, the T-cell response, or both. Increased susceptibility to infection may also result from defects in the phagocytic cells or in the complement system.

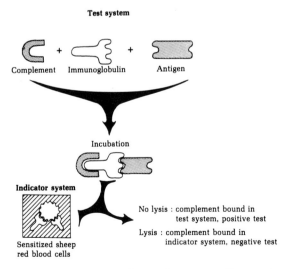

Test system

Complement + Immunoglobulin + Antigen

Incubation

Indicator system

Sensitized sheep red blood cells

No lysis : complement bound in test system, positive test

Lysis : complement bound in indicator system, negative test

Figure 29-5. *The complement fixation test. See text for explanation. (From Barrett JT:* Basic Immunology and Its Medical Application. *St. Louis, C.V. Mosby Co., 1976.)*

Deficiencies of humoral immunity are usually reflected by an abnormally low level of gamma globulins in the blood (*hypogammaglobulinemia*). The term *agammaglobulinemia* literally means an absence of gamma globulins in the blood, but it is usually used to denote conditions in which only a very small amount of gamma globulins are present (i.e., the gamma globulin level is extremely low). Some people use the terms agammaglobulinemia and hypogammaglobulinemia interchangeably. These terms are usually used when the levels of all classes of immunoglobulins are low. When the level of one or more classes of immunoglobulins is selectively decreased and the other classes of immunoglobulins are present in normal or increased amounts, the condition is called *dysgammaglobulinemia.* Dysgammaglobulinemia is relatively common but is not necessarily associated with increased susceptibility to infections.

Transient Hypogammaglobulinemia of Infancy

Although the newborn infant is capable of antibody synthesis, significant amounts of immunoglobulins are not formed until the infant has been challenged with antigens. As mentioned previously, IgG can cross the placenta and the neonate usually has a serum IgG level about the same as that of the mother. IgA and IgM are not able to cross the placenta, however, so the total amount of gamma globulin in a newborn infant is about two-thirds the normal adult level.

After birth the level of IgG in the infant's blood falls for about three months because the maternal IgG is catabolized and the infant does not begin significant synthesis of IgG until 2 to 3 months of age. Therefore between 3 and 6 months of age a temporary *physiologic hypogammaglobulinemia* occurs. The infant displays its greatest sensitivity to infectious disease at this time but is not unusually susceptible to infection. After this time the IgG level steadily increases and reaches about 75% of the adult level by 3 years of age. IgM is synthesized earlier in infancy than IgG and the IgM concentration increases rapidly after birth, reaching 50%

of the adult level within the first six months. The IgA, IgD, and IgE levels rise more slowly.

When an infant is slow to begin systhesis of IgG so that the physiologic hypogammaglobulinemia persists until 18 months of age or later, the condition is called *transient hypogammaglobulinemia.* The reason for the delayed synthesis of IgG is not known. Adequate levels of IgG are usually achieved by 3 to 4 years of age, but in the interim the serum gamma globulin level falls to very low levels, and the child may be susceptible to recurrent pyogenic infections.

Primary Immunodeficiency

Deficiency of Humoral Immunity

When B lymphocytes are lacking or are unable to synthesize immunoglobulins, humoral immunity is impaired. When all classes of immunoglobulins are involved affected people suffer repeated infections due to pyogenic bacteria such as *Streptococcus*, *Staphylococcus*, *Hemophilus*, and *Pseudomonas* species. They usually have normal resistance to viral and fungal diseases, since immunity to viruses and fungi is primarily mediated by T cells.

An example of primary humoral immunodeficiency is *infantile X-linked (Bruton type) agammaglobulinemia*, which as the name suggests, is an X-linked recessive inherited disorder. (See Chapter 4 for a discussion of X-linked inheritance.) This condition appears to result from a block in the development of B cells from precursor stem cells. B cells are usually absent from the peripheral blood, but the number of T lymphocytes is normal or increased. Since B lymphocytes normally comprise only a small fraction of circulating lymphocytes, the blood lymphocyte count is usually within the normal range. The levels of all classes of immunoglobulins in the blood are extremely low or may be absent. Plasma cells are absent from the lymph nodes, spleen, bone marrow, and gastrointestinal tract, and the lymph nodes are small.

The condition usually becomes apparent after six months of age, since before that time the affected infant is protected by maternal antibodies. Affected infants then develop repeated infections such as otitis media, sinusitis, furunculosis, pneumonia, and meningitis.

Deficiency of Cell-Mediated Immunity

Deficiency of cell-mediated immunity results from a lack of T cells or impaired T-cell function. Affected children are very susceptible to infections caused by viruses and fungi (e.g., *Candida albicans*). Childhood diseases such as chickenpox may be fatal. Respiratory infections due to bacteria and the protozoan *Pneumocystis carinii* are common. A high incidence of malignant neoplasia also occurs. (Cell-mediated immunity is believed to be part of the normal defense against cancer. See Chapter 20 under Effects of the Host on the Tumor.)

Two examples of deficient cell-mediated immunity are Nezelof's syndrome and DiGeorge's syndrome. *Nezelof's syndrome* is a genetic condition with an autosomal recessive mode of inheritance. It appears to be due to a block in the production of T cells from precursor stem cells. Connective tissue of the thymus gland is present, but normal lymphoid development of the gland fails to occur. Similarly, development of T-cell regions of peripheral lymphoid tissue is deficient. B-cell regions of lymphoid tissue do develop, and serum immunoglobulin levels are reasonably normal. IgE levels may be elevated, presumably due to absence of a T-cell suppressor action with regard to IgE antibody formation.

DiGeorge's syndrome is not an inherited condition but results from failure of embryonic development of the third and fourth branchial pouches. The third and fourth branchial pouches normally give rise to the parathyroid and thymus glands, but in DiGeorge's syndrome these glands are hypoplastic or absent. Tetralogy of Fallot and abnormalities of the aortic arch, mandibles, and ears may also occur. Peripheral lymphoid tissue is deficient in T cells, but B cells are present. A decreased number of T lymphocytes and an increased number of B lymphocytes are present in the peripheral blood. The level of immunoglobulins in the blood is normal.

Infants with DiGeorge's syndrome manifest neonatal hypocalcemia, which causes tetany (see Chapter 16). Children who survive the episodes of neonatal tetany develop repeated infections due to *Candida albicans*, *Pneumocystis carinii*, and various bacteria. When the thymus and parathyroid glands are completely absent, death usually occurs in infancy. In some cases a small thymus gland and hypoplastic parathyroid glands may be found in ectopic locations in the neck; the clinical course of this incomplete form of the syndrome is more benign.

Combined Immunodeficiency

Severe combined immunodeficiency disease (SCID) is the term appled to a heterogeneous group of disorders characterized by a profound deficiency of both the B-cell and T-cell systems. Both humoral and cell-mediated immunity are impaired. In some cases the disorder is inherited as an X-linked recessive trait (sex-linked agammaglobulinemia), and in some cases it has an autosomal recessive mode of inheritance (Swiss-type agammaglobulinemia).

The thymus is small and poorly developed and peripheral lymphoid tissue lacks follicles and germinal centers. In many cases the defect appears to be failure of a stem cell to develop into B cells and T cells, and the lymphocyte count is low (lymphopenia). In some cases the lymphocyte count is normal, but humoral and cell-mediated immune responses are deficient, suggesting a functional abnormality of the B and T cells rather that a stem-cell defect. Usually agammaglobulinemia occurs, but in some cases dysgammaglobulinemia may be present.

Affected infants develop a variety of infections due to viral, fungal, protozoal, and bacterial agents, beginning at about 3 months of age. Most have diarrhea. They fail to thrive and usually do not survive past two years of age.

Wiskott-Aldrich syndrome is an X-linked recessive disorder characterized by thrombocytopenia, eczema (atopic dermatitis), and multiple infections. The humoral immune response to polysaccharide antigens is impaired, but affected people respond normally to protein antigens. It has been suggested that this defect may be due to a failure of the macrophages to process polysaccharide antigens. Dysgammaglobulinema occurs. Typically the serum IgM level is decreased. The IgG level may be normal and the IgA and IgD levels slightly increased. The IgE level is usually elevated, reflecting the chronic atopic dermatitis. (See Chapter 30 for a discussion of atopic dermatitis.) Cell-mediated immunity is also impaired. The nature of the defect in the T-cell system is not known, but the peripheral lymphoid tissue has a deficiency of T cells. The thrombocytopenia is due to excessive destruction of platelets as a result of an intrinsic defect in the platelets.

Secondary Immunodeficiency

Primary immunodeficiency is relatively uncommon, but secondary immunodeficiency occurs quite frequently. Secondary immunodeficiency accompanies a variety of infections, malignant conditions, conditions characterized by protein deficiency, and hyposplenism. In addition, exposure to ionizing radiation can cause immunodeficiency (see Chapter 23). Also, various drugs suppress the immune system.

In a number of infectious diseases the host shows a depressed immune response to antigens unrelated to those of the infecting microorganism. Intracellular parasites that replicate in macrophages or lymphocytes are particularly likely to cause immunosuppression. Either humoral or cell-mediated immune responses may be impaired. Secondary immunodeficiency has been observed in viral diseases such as measles, rubella, mumps, varicella, yellow fever, infectious hepatitis, and infectious mononucleosis; in bacterial infections such as leprosy, syphilis, tuberculosis, and brucellosis; and in fungal infections such as histoplasmosis, blastomycosis, and coccidioidomycosis. Transient or persistant immunological abnormalities occur with the congenital rubella syndrome, possibly as a result of aberrant development of the immune system due to viral infection of the lymphoid tissues.

Cancer is frequently accompanied by immunodeficiency, particularly when the neoplasm involves lymphocytes or plasma cells (immunoproliferative diseases). People with immunoproliferative disorders may have defects of humoral or cell-mediated immunity or both, but people with other types of cancer tend to have defects in the cell-mediated immune response. The mechanism responsible for this immunodeficiency is unclear. As a result of the impairment of cell-mediated immunity, reactivation of latent infections may occur and herpes zoster is common in people with cancer. (Latent infections are discussed in Chapter 28.) In addition to the immunodeficiency caused by the cancer, drugs and radiation used in cancer therapy cause immunosuppression.

Children with protein-energy malnutrition (see Chapter 17) usually have deficient cell-mediated immunity. The thymus gland is small and atrophic, and the lymph nodes may be depleted of T cells. In some cases humoral immunity is also impaired, and the plasma levels of several complement components may be low. Herpesvirus infections and sepsis due to gram-negative bacteria frequently occur in these children.

Protein-losing gastroenteropathy is a syndrome characterized by the loss of proteins through the intestinal tract in association with a variety of intestinal diseases. Affected people often have severe hypogammaglobulinemia but respond normally to antigenic challenge. Some people may lose lymphocytes as well as proteins. Consequently they have lymphopenia and deficient cell-mediated immunity.

The spleen is a critical line of defense against blood-borne bacteria to which the host has little or no preexisting antibody, and people with hyposplenism are vulnerable to fulminant septicemia. The spleen is the main site of clearance of blood-borne bacteria and the initial site of synthesis of specific antibodies. Well-opsonized bacteria can be cleared from the blood by the liver, but the spleen is more capable of removing poorly opsonized bacteria. When opsonizing antibodies are lacking, clearance of blood-borne bacteria is delayed and depends of splenic function. Young children who have had their spleen removed are particularly at risk to develop fatal septicemia, although postsplenectomy sepsis can also occur in adults. The causative agents are usually encapsulated bacteria such as pneumococci, meningococci, and *Hemophilus influenzae*. (Recall that encapsulated bacteria resist phagocytosis unless they are coated with opsonizing antibodies.) Functional hyposplenism can occur even when the spleen is of normal size or enlarged. Children with sickle cell anemia, for example, are susceptible to septicemia particularly when the spleen is enlarged, and not later when it is atrophic.

SUGGESTED ADDITIONAL READING

Burke DC: The status of interferon. *Sci Am* **236**(4): 42–50, 1977.

Capra JD, Edmundson AB: The antibody combining site. *Sci Am* **236**(1): 50–59, 1977.

Edelman GM: The structure and function of antibodies. *Sci Am* **223**(2): 34–42, 1970.

Jerne NK: The immune system. *Sci Am* **229**(1): 52–60, 1973.

Mayer MM: The complement system. *Sci Am* **229**(5): 54–66, 1973.

Notkin AL, Koproski H: How the immune response to a virus can cause disease. *Sci Am* **228**(1): 22–31, 1973.

Powell KR: Host defense mechanisms: the immune compromised host. *Pediatr Nurs* **4**(5): 13–16, 1978.

30

Altered Immune States

HYPERSENSITIVITY

Type I, Anaphylactic Reactions
Systemic Anaphylaxis
Local Anaphylaxis (Atopy)

Type II, Cytotoxic Reactions

Type III, Immune Complex Reactions
Poststreptococcal Glomerulonephritis
Thrombocytopenic Purpura
Serum Sickness

Type IV, Cell-Mediated Reactions
Allergy of Infection
Allergic Contact Dermatitis

ISOIMMUNE REACTIONS

Blood Incompatibilities
Hemolytic Disease of the Newborn
Transfusion Reactions

Histoincompatibility
Graft Rejection
Graft versus Host Reaction

AUTOIMMUNE REACTIONS

Sequestered Antigens

Bypass of T Cells
Autoimmune Thyroiditis

Loss of Suppressor Activity
Systemic Lupus Erythematosus

Immune responses are normally beneficial, providing the host with resistance to infection, as discussed in Chapter 29. In some cases, however, altered reactivity of the immune system causes harm. The word *allergy* was originally defined as an altered response to an antigen, whether it was underreactivity or overreactivity. Since most allergic reactions are overresponses (i.e., hypersensitivity) and hypersensitivity was the most widely studied form of allergy, the two terms gradually came to be used as synonyms. Now most people use the words

allergy and hypersensitivity interchangeably. *Hypersensitivity* is a state of altered reactivity in which the body reacts with an exaggerated response to a foreign agent (i.e., antigen). A substance capable of inducing allergy or specific hypersensitivity is called an *allergen*. Allergens are a special group of antigens that are harmless to most people but that may cause disease in predisposed people who are exposed to them.

Immune responses can also cause harm when the immune system fails to recognize self and directs immune responses against constituents of the body's own tissues. This condition is called *autoimmunity*, and the tissue constituents against which the immune response is directed are called *autoantigens*. Antibodies directed against the body's own tissue constituents are called *autoantibodies*.

Normal body constituents that exist in alternative forms in a species and that induce an immune response when one form is transferred to members of the species who lack it are called *isoantigens*, or *alloantigens* (e.g., blood group antigens). Antibodies produced by one individual that react with isoantigens of another individual of the same species are called *isoantibodies*, or *alloantibodies*. Isoantigens and isoantibodies assume importance with regard to blood transfusions and tissue grafts. They can also be responsible for disease when maternal isoantibodies attack fetal isoantigens.

HYPERSENSITIVITY

The initial exposure of a predisposed person to an allergen does not produce a reaction. After a sensitization period of about one week, however, reexposure to the allergen causes a hypersensitivity reaction. The sensitization period is necessary to allow for the synthesis of immunoglobulins and/or the development of sensitized T lymphocytes. The initial exposure to the allergen (or dose administered) is called the *sensitizing dose*. The subsequent exposure to the allergen (or dose administered) is called the *shocking*, or *challenging*, dose or exposure.

Hypersensitivity reactions are traditionally classified as immediate type or delayed type, depending on the speed and nature of the reaction in the skin when a sensitized person is skin-challenged with the antigen. *Immediate hypersensitivity* is mediated by immunoglobulins (i.e., it is a humoral response). The reaction appears suddenly and disappears within one to four hours. The response to the skin test is a wheal and erythema (wheal and flare). When an allergen to which a person is sensitized is introduced into the skin the site becomes reddened (erythematous) within minutes. As edema fluid collects in the area, the central portion becomes raised and blanched (i.e. a wheal forms), while the periphery remains erythematous.

Delayed hypersensitivity is mediated by T cells. (See Chapter 29 for a discussion of T cells.) When an allergen is introduced into the skin, the reaction develops slowly, becoming maximal 48 to 72 hours after administration of the allergen. The reaction site on the skin is characterized by erythema and induration (hardening and thickening of the skin). In immediate hypersensitivity there is infiltration of the area with neutrophils, but in delayed hypersensitivity monocytes predominate.

An alternative classification of hypersensitivities, devised by Gell and Coombs, divides hypersensitivity reactions into four types. Type I, anaphylactic reactions, are mediated by IgE antibodies. Type II, cytotoxic reactions, are mediated by IgG antibodies. Type III, immune complex reactions, are mediated by IgG and/or IgM antibodies. Type IV, cell-mediated reactions, depend on sensitized T lymphocytes and correspond to the traditional delayed-type hypersensitivity.

A particular allergen can sometimes produce more than one type of allergic reaction, depending on its nature, the route by which it enters the body, and the amount that enters.

Type I, Anaphylactic Reactions

Anaphylaxis literally means "without protection." Whereas immunity implies protection, or prophylaxis, anaphylactic reactions are harmful, not beneficial. Anaphylactic reactions appear to be mediated primarily by antibodies of the IgE class, which are also called *reagins*. The sensitizing dose of a soluble allergen induces the production of specific IgE antibodies by plasma cells. IgE-producing plasma cells are particularly abundant in the germinal centers in the tonsils and adenoids and in the mucosa and submucosa of the respiratory, gastrointestinal, and urinary tracts. The Fc portion of the IgE molecules binds to the surfaces of mast cells and basophils. Mast cells are granular cells that are found in most tissues. They are especially abundant in the lungs and uterus, around blood vessels, and in connective tissue. Basophils are one type of granulocytic white blood cell. They appear to be circulating equivalents of mast cells. The granules of mast cells and basophils contain several physiologically active chemicals. IgE antibodies are said to be *homocytotropic* because they have an affinity for one type of cell. When specific antigens (allergens) react with IgE antibodies on the surfaces of mast cells and basophils, the reaction triggers degranulation of the cells, with the release of chemical mediators into the extracellular fluid. The chemical mediators include histamine, slow reacting substance of anaphylaxis (SRS-A), and eosinophil chemotactic factor of anaphylaxis (ECF-A).

Histamine causes vasodilation, increased vascular permeability, contraction of nonvascular smooth muscle (especially in the gastrointestinal tract and bronchial tree), and increased gastric, nasal, and lacrimal secretions. It is rapidly broken down by enzymes that are present in the plasma, and therefore its systemic effects are short-lived. SRS-A does not exist preformed in the mast cells, but the immunologic reaction triggers its synthesis, and then it is released. Therefore it is released later than the other substances, after a lag period. SRS-A also increases vascular permeability and causes contraction of some types of nonvascular smooth muscle. ECF-A chemotactically attracts eosinophils to the site of the allergic reaction. Not only is the number of eosinophils increased in the tissues at the site of the reaction but increased numbers of eosinophils are also found in the blood in association with hypersensitivity disorders. The exact role of the eosinophils is not known. It has been observed, however, that eosinophils contain an enzyme that can inactivate SRS-A. Therefore eosinophils possibly function as part of a control mechanism to limit the intensity of the allergic reaction.

Type I allergic reactions include systemic anaphylaxis and atopy, or local anaphylaxis. Systemic anaphylaxis is an acute severe reaction that can cause death in 15 to 120 minutes. It occurs within seconds or minutes after exposure to an allergen to which a person is specifically hypersensitive. The term *atopy* refers to hypersensitivity states to which there is an inherited predisposition. It includes asthma, hay fever, atopic dermatitis, and acute urticaria. Urticaria can be caused by a variety of other factors in addition to allergy.

Systemic Anaphylaxis

Systemic anaphylaxis occurs when a challenging dose of an allergen is received in such a way as to favor a massive release of histamine and other chemical mediators at one instant. It usually follows injection of a soluble allergen. The major causes of systemic anaphylaxis are injections of therapeutic or diagnostic agents and insect stings. Many drugs can cause anaphylactic reactions. Most are low-molecular-weight substances that are not antigenic in themselves but act as haptens. Penicillin is probably the drug that most frequently causes systemic anaphylaxis.

Systemic anaphylaxis may affect the skin, the respiratory tract, the gastrointestinal tract, and the cardiovascular system; but all these systems are not necessarily involved in every case. The first manifestation is often pruritis (itching), which is most severe over the face, upper chest, axillae, and groin, followed by erythema (redness) and generalized urticaria. *Urticaria*, or hives, is a cutaneous eruption consisting of sharply circumscribed, elevated areas of edema of the skin. The wheals are of varying sizes and shapes (Fig. 30-1).

Laryngeal edema and bronchospasm cause tightness or pain in the chest, laryngeal stridor, wheezing, dyspnea, and cyanosis. Vomiting, diarrhea, and severe abdominal cramps may occur because of gastrointestinal smooth muscle spasm. Women may have laborlike pains due to contraction of uterine smooth muscle.

Hypotension and circulatory collapse (*anaphylactic shock*) may occur and in some cases

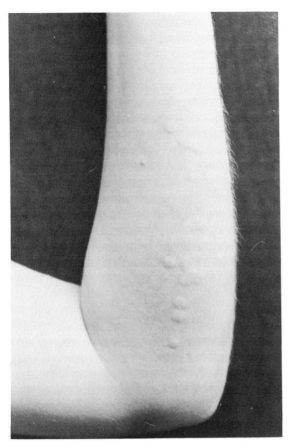

Figure 30-1. *Urticaria.*

are the only manifestations of systemic ana-phylaxis. The shock is primarily the result of a sharp reduction in plasma volume (i.e., hypovolemia) because the increased vascular permeability results in a loss of fluid from the intravascular compartment to the interstitial space.

The usual causes of death in systemic anaphylaxis are asphyxia due to laryngeal edema and intense bronchospasm or circulatory failure (i.e., shock). In nonfatal cases signs and symptoms may resolve within minutes of the initiation of treatment or may persist for up to 24 hours.

Local Anaphylaxis (Atopy)

In atopic allergies exposure to the allergen occurs through the respiratory tract, gastrointestinal tract, or skin. Common inhalant allergens are pollens of trees, grasses, and weeds, mold spores, animal danders and feathers, and house dust. The most common food allergens are fish, shellfish, grains, nuts, eggs, cow's milk, strawberries, oranges, tomatoes, and chocolate. Stings of bees, wasps, hornets, and yellow jackets cause a localized anaphylactic reaction in some cases.

Entry of allergens appears to be facilitated at times when mucosal permeability is increased due to infection or nonspecific irritation. The gastrointestinal tract appears to be an important early route of sensitization, possibly because immaturity of the infant gastrointestinal tract permits proteins to enter the circulation. The respiratory tract is a more important route later in life. Deficiency of IgA antibodies may also influence absorption of allergens across the mucosal surfaces. Binding of allergens by IgA antibodies on the mucosal surface might normally prevent absorption of the allergens and their subsequent binding to IgE antibodies.

Asthma. This condition is characterized by recurrent attacks of paroxysmal dyspnea with wheezing due to spasmodic contraction of the bronchi. (See also Chapter 10 under Chronic Obstructive Pulmonary Disease.) The etiology of asthma is complex and not completely understood. Excessive bronchial irritability mediated by the autonomic nervous system, and emotional factors, as well as allergic factors, contribute to asthma. A panic-fear reaction to the initial mild symptoms of asthma may establish a vicious cycle of increased asthma and increased panic. Vigorous exercise, especially running, for 10 to 15 minutes can induce an asthmatic attack by an unknown mechanism. It is postulated that vigorous exercise causes trauma to lung tissue, with the release of bronchoconstrictor substances.

Allergy-mediated asthmatic attacks usually follow inhalation of an allergen, but sometimes may occur after absorption of soluble allergens from the gastrointestinal tract. Although IgE antibodies appear to be the major mediators of the allergic reaction, IgG antibodies may also be involved in some people with asthma. An immediate response, a late response, or both may occur after inhalation of an allergen. IgG antibodies are believed to be important in the pathogenesis of the late response. The *immediate asthmatic response* has its onset within 10 to 20 minutes of allergen inhalation, reaches a peak between 20 and 30 minutes, and resolves between one and three hours after inhalation of the allergen. The *late asthmatic response* begins 4 to 6 hours after exposure to the allergen, reaches a peak between 8 and 12 hours, and subsides within 24 hours.

The initial manifestation of an asthma attack is a feeling of mild tightness across the chest, accompanied by a persistent nonproductive cough. At this stage the expiratory phase of breathing is prolonged and scattered expiratory wheezes are heard throughout the chest. As the attack progresses the cough changes to bronchospasm, and the person experiences subjective dyspnea and acute respiratory discomfort. As the bronchospasm becomes increasingly severe the rhonchi become more audible, and eventually wheezing occurs during inspiration as well as expiration. The accessory muscles of respiration may be used, and the chest may be hyperinflated. The cough becomes productive of thick sputum. Severe attacks lasting for more than 30 minutes may be accompanied by a constant dull aching pain over the lower rib cage or across the anterior chest wall, probably because of spasm of thoracic muscles. During a very severe attack, the airways may become so obstructed by mucous plugs and bronchospasm that very little air passes through them and very few rhonchi are produced. Restlessness, apprehension, fatigue, irritability, lightheadedness, and headache may occur, probably because of the effects of hypoxia on the cerebral cortex.

Allergic rhinitis. Nonseasonal, or perennial, allergic rhinitis occurs continuously or intermittently throughout the year. It is caused by an allergen that is always present in the environment (e.g., house dust). Seasonal allergic rhinitis, or hay fever, occurs at a particular time of the year, usually the spring or summer. Pollens are the allergens commonly involved.

Because of the efficient filtering and cleansing function of the nose, most pollens and other allergens are trapped in the nasal mucus, and only a small portion of inhaled particles reach the lower airways (see Chapter 28 under Respiratory Entry). Lysozyme in the nasal mucus breaks down the outer coatings of the pollen grains, releasing soluble protein antigens that trigger the allergic response. Histamine is the most important chemical mediator of the reaction. It acts on small blood vessels in the nose, causing dilatation and increased permeability, which produces edema of the nasal mucosa. In addition, a profuse watery nasal discharge is produced. Histamine released by mast cells in the submucosa leads to intense itching of the nasal passages, soft palate, and eustachian tubes. Reflex sneezing occurs as a result of stimulation of the olfactory nerve or of the fifth cranial (trigeminal) nerve by histamine. Some people may experience itching and burning of the eyes, accompanied by excessive lacrimation and swollen eyelids. Mild to moderate anterior headache may occur, due to edema of the nasal or paranasal mucous membranes. Profound lassitude and fatigue, transient feelings of irritability or depression, or generalized malaise may accompany acute seasonal allergic rhinitis. Despite the word "fever" in the term hay fever, fever does not occur with uncomplicated allergic rhinitis.

When allergic rhinitis is of long duration, the chronic edema of the nasal tissues leads to epithelial hypertrophy and increased activity of the mucous glands. Eventually polyp formation or permanent thickening of the membranes lining the sinus cavities may occur. Polyps may obstruct the openings of the paranasal sinuses, leading to secondary infection. Anosmia (absence of the sense of smell) occurs when polyps or edematous membranes prevent odors from reaching the olfactory nerve endings.

Atopic dermatitis. Atopic dermatitis is an eczematous skin eruption that occurs most commonly in infancy and childhood but may persist into adulthood and may even appear for the first time after 20 years of age. It is frequently associated with respiratory allergy, and most people with atopic dermatitis have a family history of asthma or hay fever. Although total serum IgE levels are increased in people with atopic dermatitis, the lesions are not the typical wheal and flare associated with IgE mediated reactions, and the immunological mechanism of atopic dermatitis is not known. Many nonimmunological factors, including emotional stress, influence the development of atopic dermatitis.

Intense pruritis precedes and accompanies the eruptions of atopic dermatitis. In infancy the lesions are vesicular, exudative, and crusted and occur most commonly on the scalp and cheeks, although scattered patches may occur over the trunk and extremities. In severe cases the entire body may be covered by a generalized eruption. In childhood the eruptions tend to occur mainly on the antecubital fossae, popliteal fossae, wrists, ankles, and flexures of the buttocks. The lesions are drier and lichenification occurs (i.e., thickening of the epidermis with exaggeration of its normal markings). In adolescents and adults the lesions tend to occur on flexural surfaces and are dry and lichenified (Fig. 30-2).

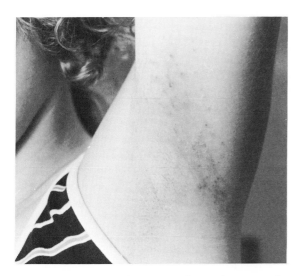

Figure 30-2. *Atopic dermatitis. Chronic lesions in the axilla of a 15-year-old girl.*

Food allergy. Food allergies may affect the gastrointestinal tract or may affect distant sites, such as the skin and bronchi. Acute urticaria may follow the ingestion of food to which a person is hypersensitive. Manifestations of gastrointestinal allergy include oral inflammation, perioral erythema, edema, and pruritis, nausea, intestinal cramps, gaseous distension, diarrhea, and perianal itching.

Type II, Cytotoxic Reactions

In cytotoxic reactions antibodies, usually of the IgG class, bind to the surfaces of cells. The Fab portion of the immunoglobulin binds to specific antigens on the cell surface. The antibody may act as an opsonin, causing the cell to be phagocytosed, or complement may be activated, causing lysis of the cell. The antigen may be an intrinsic component of the cell or may be an exogenous antigen or hapten that has attached to the cell surface. Type II reactions include blood transfusion reactions, hemolytic disease of the newborn (see below), autoimmune hemolytic anemias, some forms of thrombocytopenic purpura, and some forms of drug allergies. For example, penicillin binds to the surface of erythrocytes and acts as a hapten. The penicillin-erythrocyte complex acts as an immunogen that elicits the formation of IgG antibodies. As a result, the red blood cells may be hemolyzed. Penicillin-induced hemolytic anemia is rare and usually only occurs with administration of more than 10 million units of penicillin per day. With lower doses not enough penicillin attaches to the red blood cells to trigger erythrocyte destruction.

Type III, Immune Complex Reactions

Immune complex reactions involve IgG or IgM antibodies and often complement. Cells and tissues are injured indirectly, as "innocent bystanders." Insoluble antigen-antibody complexes and large soluble antigen-antibody complexes are rapidly removed from the circulation by reticuloendothelial cells. Intermediate-sized soluble immune complexes that are formed when antigen is present in moderate excess of antibody, however, may not be removed by the phagocytic cells. They continue to circulate in the blood and may coat blood cells or may localize in small blood vessels in various parts of the body. Subsequently complement may be activated, producing inflammation and destroying cells. Examples of immune complex disorders include poststreptococcal glomerulonephritis and some types of thrombocytopenic purpura. Some aspects of serum sickness are also due to immune complex reactions.

Poststreptococcal Glomerulonephritis

Acute glomerulonephritis is a frequent sequela of upper respiratory or skin infections caused by certain types of group A β-hemolytic streptococci. Antibodies are directed against a streptococcal antigen, and antigen-antibody complexes form in the blood. These circulating complexes filter through the glomerular capillaries but are trapped on the glomerular basement membrane. Complement is activated, resulting in inflammation and infiltration of the area with polymorphonuclear neutrophils. Swelling of the endothelium and basement membrane tends to obliterate the glomerular lumens. Increased permeability of the glomerular capillaries allows protein and red blood cells to enter the filtrate. Damage occurs diffusely throughout the kidneys and in most cases is reversible, although healing may take as long as two years in some cases.

Acute glomerulonephritis usually appears one to two weeks after the streptococcal infection. In addition to hematuria and proteinuria, hyaline, granular, and red cell casts may be present in the urine. Impaired glomerular function leads to fluid retention, as manifested by oliguria, edema (usually noticeable as periorbital and facial puffiness), and hypertension. The impaired glomerular function is also reflected by an increase in the blood urea nitrogen (BUN) and creatinine levels (azotemia). Other signs and symptoms include mild fever, headache, and malaise. The erythrocyte sedimentation rate is usually increased. The serum complement level is decreased during the acute phase, reflecting increased utilization of complement, but the level rises to normal with recovery. In most cases complete clinical recovery occurs within three to four weeks.

Thrombocytopenic Purpura

A variety of bacterial, viral, and rickettsial infections, as well as hypersensitivity to drugs or their breakdown products, can cause destruction of platelets, producing thrombocytopenia. (See Chapter 7 under Platelet Abnormalities for a discussion of the clinical consequences of thrombocytopenia.) The drugs (or their metabolites) act as haptens and are believed to combine with plasma proteins. Antibodies are formed against the hapten-protein complex or against the invading microorganisms. Antigen-antibody complexes then coat the platelets, complement is activated, and the platelets are destroyed as innocent bystanders. In some cases complement may not be activated but the platelets coated with immune complexes are sequestered in the spleen and are destroyed by reticuloendothelial cells.

Serum Sickness

The administration of a large amount of antigenic material that persists in the body for a long time can lead to the development of serum sickness. Since the substance remains in the blood for a long time, one dose serves as both the antibody-inducing stimulus and the reaction-provoking exposure. Some aspects of serum sickness appear to be due to an anaphylactic-type reaction, and others appear to be due to immune complexes.

Serum sickness was encountered quite frequently in the preantibiotic era when equine immune serum was used in the treatment of pneumonia and diphtheria. It still occasionally occurs after administration of tetanus antitoxin. The antigens are horse serum proteins. Although the reaction is called serum sickness because it was first described after the administration of horse serum, nonprotein drugs that are designed to have a prolonged action, such as some penicillin preparations, can also elicit a serum sickness type of reaction. Antilymphocyte serum used in the immunosuppression of graft recipients can also cause serum sickness.

After administration of the serum or other persistent antigen, antibody synthesis begins. When the level of antibodies is sufficient to interact with the remaining antigen in the proper proportions, the serum sickness reaction is manifested. The onset is usually 6 to 12 days after injection of the antigen (or hapten in the case of drugs). The first sign of serum sickness is often generalized swelling of the lymph nodes (lymphadenopathy), presumably due to increased antibody production. Other manifestations that soon follow are urticaria, fever, and arthralgias. The urticaria is mediated by IgE antibodies, but the joint pain (arthralgia) and stiffness appears to be the result of deposition of immune complexes in the joints. Usually the large and medium joints are involved. In more severe cases the joints are swollen, with effusion into the synovial spaces. Occasionally angioedema of the face and extremities occurs. (Angioedema is produced by essentially the same process as urticaria, but the swelling is more extensive and involves the subcutaneous tissues as well as the skin.) Peripheral neuritis, particularly involving the cervical portion of the brachial plexus, develops in a few people. Occasionally the shoulder girdle, arm, and hand are affected. The cause of the peripheral neuritis in serum sickness is not known. In experimental serum sickness produced in animals, glomerulonephritis occurs due to deposition of immune complexes on the glomerular basement membrane, but nephritis is not a prominent feature of human serum sickness. Serum sickness is a transient, self-limited disease, which may disappear in a few days or may persist for a few weeks.

Type IV, Cell-Mediated Reactions

Delayed-type hypersensitivity is mediated by sensitized T cells. Type IV hypersensitivity occurs with some microbial infections and also occurs after dermal contact with a wide variety of substances.

Allergy of Infection
When certain soluble products of microbial growth are injected intradermally into a person who has previously been exposed to the particular microbial agent, gradual reddening and thickening of the skin around the injection site occurs. The response is a typical delayed hypersensitivity reaction and reaches its peak after 48 to 72 hours. This reaction is the basis of the tuberculin skin test. Allergies of infection persist long after recovery from the infection. For this reason, a positive skin test is rarely diagnostic of existing disease (except in very young children) but merely indicates that the person has been previously exposed to the infectious agent. Delayed-type dermal hypersensitivity occurs with a variety of viral, bacterial, and fungal infections, including mumps, lymphogranuloma venereum, smallpox, tuberculosis, leprosy, brucellosis, diphtheria, salmonellosis, streptococcal infections, histoplasmosis, blastomycosis, and coccidioidomycosis. Cell-mediated hypersensitivity contributes to the tissue damage that occurs in these diseases.

Allergic Contact Dermatitis
Dermal contact with a wide variety of chemicals can cause allergic contact dermatitis. The contact allergens are usually low-molecular-weight compounds such as drugs, dyes, plastics, industrial chemicals, mercurial compounds, chromates, nickel, and some plant compounds (e.g., oleoresins of poison ivy, poison sumac, and poison oak). These low-molecular-weight compounds act as haptens. They penetrate the skin and combine with skin proteins to form complete antigens.

Specific lymphocytes encounter the antigen in the tissue and are stimulated. It is not known whether the T lymphocytes are stimulated directly or whether macrophages or some other type of cell process the antigen first and then stimulate specific lymphocytes. The stimulated lymphocytes travel to the regional lymph node, where they proliferate and differentiate into small lymphocytes with either memory or effector function. (See the discussion of T cells and cell-mediated immunity in Chapter 29.) The memory and effector cells then circulate in the body, and the person is hypersensitive to the specific hapten. This sensitization process takes five to seven days.

On subsequent exposure to the hapten an allergic reaction is elicited. Memory cells undergo an accelerated process of antigen recognition, proliferation, and differentiation into new populations of memory and effector cells, increasing the level of hypersensitivity. The exact mechanism by which the effector cells cause the skin reaction is not known. In the tuberculin-type delayed hypersensitivity it appears that antigenic stimulation causes sensitized effector cells to release lymphokines. Some lymphokines chemotactically attract monocytes and macrophages to the area and hold them there, while another causes direct damage to tissue cells (see Chapter 29). The mechanism in contact dermatitis appears to be different, however, and is not dependent on lymphokines to produce inflammation. It has been hypothesized that antigen stimulation causes sensitized effector cells to release substances that stimulate basophils and mast cells. These cells then release substances that induce inflammation. At the same time the sensitized T cells release lymphokines that attract and activate macrophages, which then clear the inflammation.

The acute reaction in allergic contact dermatitis is characterized by pruritis, erythema, vesicle formation, exudation of fluid, and localized edema of the skin. Nonspecific inflammatory changes accompanied by infiltration of mononuclear cells occur in the dermis. In the epidermis spongiosis occurs (separation of the cells of the spongy, or malpighian, layer by edema), followed by intraepidermal vesiculation. When the lesions become chronic (e.g., as a result of repeated contact due to occupational exposure), crusting, scaling, and lichenification occur, and the rash becomes more eczematous.

ISOIMMUNE REACTIONS

The cells of the body have a variety of genetically determined protein and glycoprotein substances on their surfaces. Since every person is genetically distinct, with the exception of monozygotic twins, the cells of different people have different surface components that can act as antigens when introduced from one person into another. This fact forms the basis of blood incompatibilities and of rejection of tissue grafts.

Blood Incompatibilities

Many isoantigens exist on the surfaces of red blood cells. These isoantigens can be grouped together into about 19 different blood group systems; the most important are the ABO and the Rh systems. People with type A blood have A antigens on their red blood cells; people with type B have B antigens; people with type AB have both A and B antigens on their blood cells; and people with type O have neither antigen (Fig. 30-3). Naturally occur-

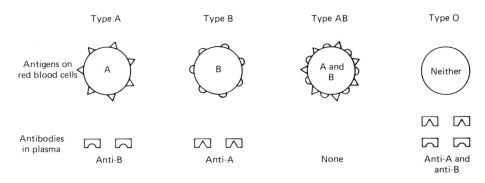

Figure 30-3. *ABO blood types.*

ring isoantibodies to these antigens exist in the plasma. People with type A blood have anti-B antibodies; people with type B blood have anti-A antibodies; and those with type O blood have both anti-A and anti-B antibodies. People with type AB blood have neither type of antibody. The naturally occurring antibodies are of the IgM class, but artificial immunization with the A and B antigens results in a strong IgM response that is followed by production of IgG antibodies.

The Rh blood group system is much more complex and consists of about 30 antigens. The Rh_0 (D) antigen is the most potent, and the term Rh positive usually refers to the presence of this antigen on the surfaces of the red blood cells. The Rh antigens are much less abundant on the erythrocyte surface than the A and B antigens are. Unlike the ABO system, isoantibodies to Rh antigens are not normally present in the blood. If Rh-negative people are transfused with Rh-positive blood, however, they will develop anti-Rh antibodies of the IgG class. Similarly, an Rh-negative mother can become sensitized and can develop anti-Rh antibodies when fetal Rh-positive erythrocytes enter the maternal circulation.

Hemolytic Disease of the Newborn

Hemolytic disease of the newborn (*erythroblastosis fetalis*) is caused by blood group incompatibility between the mother and fetus. About two-thirds of the cases are due to ABO incompatibility, whereas Rh incompatibility causes about one-third of the cases. Rh incompatibility causes more severe disease, however, so that it assumes greater clinical significance than ABO incompatibility. Other blood group incompatibilities are rare causes of hemolytic disease of the newborn.

Hemolytic disease of the newborn can occur when the mother is Rh negative and the father is Rh positive. The genes for the Rh antigens are dominant; therefore, if the father is homozygous, all the children will be Rh positive. If the father is heterozygous, the probability is that half of the children will be Rh positive (see Chapter 4 under Patterns of Inheritance). Hemolytic disease of the newborn occurs when an Rh-negative woman who is carrying an Rh-positive child has anti-Rh antibodies in her blood. The mother usually does not have these antibodies with the first pregnancy unless she has been previously transfused with Rh-positive blood. Small numbers of fetal erythrocytes may enter the maternal circulation during pregnancy, but larger numbers enter when the placenta separates at the time of delivery. Consequently the Rh-negative mother produces anti-Rh antibodies. In the next Rh-positive pregnancy, these antibodies cross the placenta and attack the fetal red blood cells. Maternal sensitization can also occur during ectopic pregnancy or abortion.

When maternal antibodies combine with fetal red blood cells, complement may be activated, causing intravascular hemolysis. Alternatively the erythrocytes coated with antibodies may be taken up by reticuloendothelial cells in the liver and spleen and be destroyed extravascularly. The clinical manifestations of hemolytic disease of the newborn depend on the amount of red blood cell destruction, which is generally proportional to the amount of antibody present in the maternal blood. Slight degrees of hemolysis may only be apparent as mild anemia. With a greater degree of red blood cell destruction, anemia is more severe, immature nucleated red blood cells appear in the peripheral blood, and the spleen may be enlarged due to intensive extramedullary hematopoiesis. (See also Chapter 10 under Anemia.) The excessive destruction of erythrocytes causes hyperbilirubinemia, which produces jaundice (*icterus gravis neonatorum*). If the hyperbilirubinemia is severe, kernicterus can occur (see Chapter 26 under Bilirubin Toxicity). Congestive heart failure may occur when hemolysis causes severe anemia. When congestive heart failure develops in utero massive edema may develop (*hydrops fetalis*), and the child may be stillborn. After birth such severe edema does not occur because pulmonary edema causes death before such massive edema can develop, but the fetus is not dependent on the lungs for oxygen.

Hemolytic disease of the newborn due to Rh incompatibility can be prevented by administering anti-Rh immune globulin to the mother immediately following delivery (or abortion) so that she will not form antibodies. It is assumed that the administered antibodies cause rapid removal of the fetal cells from the maternal circulation before they have the opportunity to evoke antibody synthesis. It is possible, however, that the antigenic sites on the fetal erythrocytes are blocked by the administered antibody or that the normal immune response is suppressed by feedback inhibition due to the administered antibodies. Administration of anti-Rh immune globulin is of no value if the mother has already formed antibodies.

Hemolytic disease of the newborn due to ABO incompatibility can occur when the mother has anti-A or anti-B isoantibodies of the IgG class and the child has type A or B blood. The usual anti-A and anti-B antibodies are of the IgM class, which cannot cross the placenta; but if the mother has been hyperimmunized, she may have antibodies of the IgG class, which can cross the placenta. IgG antibodies occur more frequently in people with type O blood than in people with type A or B, and the A antigen is stronger than the B antigen; therefore, hemolytic disease most frequently affects type A infants who have type O mothers.

In contrast to hemolytic disease due to Rh incompatibility, hemolytic disease due to ABO incompatibility may occur with the first pregnancy. Hemolysis is rarely severe, possibly because the A and B antigens are present in many tissues, not just on the erythrocytes. Therefore tissue antigens compete with erythrocyte antigens for maternal antibodies. Clinically the ABO incompatibility is usually manifested by mild anemia and jaundice. The jaundice usually develops in the first 24 hours of neonatal life. Hyperbilirubinemia is only occasionally severe enough to require exchange transfusion to prevent kernicterus.

Transfusion Reactions

People can exhibit many types of reactions to blood transfusions; not all reactions have immunological causes. Immunological reactions may be due to plasma proteins, erythrocytes, leukocytes, or platelets.

A large proportion of untoward responses to transfusions are *allergic reactions*, characterized by urticaria, angioedema, and bronchospasm. Signs and symptoms usually occur within 30 minutes of the onset of transfusion. Occasionally systemic anaphylaxis may occur. Allergic reactions may be due to reagins in the recipient that react with soluble antigens in the donor blood or, alternatively, from reagins in the donor blood reacting with allergens to which the recipient is exposed but ordinarily not sensitive. Also, plasma proteins of the donor may elicit an immune response in the recipient because of genetic differences in plasma proteins from different people. Some transfusion reactions have been caused by complement-fixing anti-IgA antibodies in the recipient that react with IgA in the donor blood.

Hemolysis due to blood group incompatibilities rarely occurs when blood is properly crossmatched. The hemolytic reaction is usually due to isoantibodies in the recipient reacting with donor red blood cells, because antibodies in the donor blood are diluted by the recipient's plasma and are distributed over a large number of the recipient's erythrocytes. ABO incompatibilities usually result in intravascular hemolysis. Symptoms occur shortly after the transfusion is started and consist of a sensation of pain or heat along the vein through which the blood is being infused, restlessness, and apprehension. Subsequently the face may be flushed and the person may have chills, fever, nausea, vomiting, and pain in the extremities or lumbar region. In severe cases constricting chest pain, air hunger, hypotension, and shock may occur. In some cases primary immunization to blood group antigens may take place, and acute hemolysis may occur after a delay of 7 to 10 days. In the rare cases of hemolysis occurring because of isoantibodies in the donor blood reacting with the recipient's erythrocytes, anemia, jaundice, and hemoglobinuria may develop a few hours after the start of the transfusion.

Rh incompatibilities usually cause sequestration and destruction of erythrocytes in the spleen rather than intravascular hemolysis. In some cases this event is asymptomatic. In other cases the only manifestations may be mild jaundice and failure to increase the red cell count after transfusion.

Naturally occurring isoantibodies against antigens on white blood cells are extremely rare but may develop in people who have had multiple transfusions. They may also occur in multiparous women as a result of isoimmunization from fetal leukocytes during pregnancy. With transfusion reactions due to *leukocyte incompatibility* the onset of symptoms is usually 30 to 90 minutes after the start of the transfusion. Flushing, palpitations, tachycardia, and a feeling of tightness in the chest are often the first symptoms. Subsequently chills and fever occur, presumably due to release of endogenous pyrogen from the destroyed transfused leukocytes (see Chapter 24 under Fever Resulting from Altered Set Point).

Transfusion reactions due to *platelet incompatibility* are manifested by petichiae and hemorrhages occurring five to seven days after the transfusion (*posttransfusion purpura*). This type of reaction usually occurs in multiparous women, and it is assumed that isoantibodies against platelets are formed as a result of immunization with fetal platelets during pregnancy. As determined by serological techniques, the antibodies are directed against donor platelets, but for reasons that are not understood both donor and recipient platelets are destroyed.

Histoincompatibility

A tissue or organ graft is said to be *histoincompatible* if the recipient recognizes the graft as foreign and rejects it. If the graft is not perceived as being foreign, it will survive in the recipient and is said to be *histocompatible*. Transplants between genetically dissimilar individuals of the same species are called *allografts*, or *allogeneic grafts*. (The term *homograft* may also be used.) Transplants between individuals of different species are called *xenografts*, or *xenogeneic grafts*. (They may also be called *heterografts*.) Allografts and xenografts are histoincompatible. Grafts taken from and returned to the same individual are called *autografts*, or *autogeneic grafts*. Transplants between identical twins or highly inbred animals that are genetically identical are called *syngrafts*, or *syngeneic grafts*. (The term *isograft* may also be used.) Autografts and syngrafts are histocompatible.

Graft rejection is based on immunological reactions, and the antigens that are responsible for graft rejection are referred to as histocompatibility, or transplantation, antigens. Some of the histocompatibility antigens are more potent than others. The most potent ones cause the most rapid graft rejection and are called major histocompatibility antigens, while the weaker ones are called minor histocompatibility antigens. The histocompatibility antigens are present in all cells, but their concentrations vary from one type of tissue to another. These antigens are presumably functional components of the cells, but their actual functions are not known. The major histocompatibility antigens in human beings are designated HLA (*h*uman *l*eukocyte *a*ntigens), because it is believed that leukocytes contain all or nearly all of the major antigens.

The formation of the major histocompatibility antigens is genetically controlled by the *major histocompatibility complex* (MHC), which consists of four loci on chromosome six. These loci are designated HLA-A (formerly called "La" and first locus), HLA-B (formerly "Four" and second locus), HLA-C (formerly AJ locus), and HLA-D. Each locus has multiple alleles; 19 are known at the A locus and 24 at the B locus. So far six alleles have been detected at the C locus, but probably more will be found. Very little is known about the D locus yet. Based on the number of alleles that are known at the four loci, over 200 million genotypes are possible. Therefore the probability of two unrelated people being histocompatible is very remote. To minimize the possibility of graft rejection, tests are made to select a donor whose major histocompatibility antigens are as similar as possible to those of the recipient, and the recipient is treated with immunosuppressive drugs.

Graft Rejection

Cell-mediated immune responses appear to be primarily responsible for graft rejection, but humoral immunity may also be important in some cases. *Hyperacute graft rejection* occurs if the blood of donor and recipient are ABO incompatible or if the recipient has become sensitized and formed antibodies to other blood group or tissue antigens as a result of previous transfusions, multiple pregnancies, or some other cause. Hyperacute graft rejection is avoided by appropriate crossmatching, but occasionally it occurs because the techniques used may not be sensitive enough to detect some antibodies. Hyperacute rejection of a transplanted organ usually becomes apparent immediately after the vascular connection is made. The organ becomes swollen and assumes a bluish purple color. Blood may fail to pass through the organ and may clot within the vessels. In hyperacute rejection of a skin graft revascularization fails to occur and the graft dries and sloughs.

In *first-set rejection* the transplanted organ or tissue is initially accepted. It becomes normally revascularized, its color appears normal, and it soon resumes its normal physiological function (e.g., excretion of urine by a kidney). The recipient becomes sensitized to tissue antigens in the graft, however, and develops specific immunity (mainly of the cell-mediated type) against the transplantation antigens. This process takes 5 to 10 days. Destruction of the graft then occurs. Cells in the donor tissue may be directly destroyed by T lymphocytes. In addition, immunological reactions in blood vessels may lead to vascular occlusion, with subsequent necrosis of the graft. Skin grafts become a dark purple color and then turn black as the tissue becomes necrotic. Rejection of a transplanted organ is characterized by failure of organ function (e.g., oliguria or anuria in the case of kidney rejection). Swelling of the organ may cause pain and tenderness. Fever and general malaise are other manifestations of graft rejection. The rejection process is completed between 11 and 20 days post transplantation. (The process may be delayed by immunosuppressive therapy, however.)

Second-set rejection occurs after a subsequent reexposure of the recipient to tissue of the same or an antigenically related donor. The events are similar to those in first-set rejection but occur at an accelerated rate because the recipient has been previously sensitized. Both immunoglobulins

against donor antigens and sensitized T cells contribute to the graft rejection.

Graft versus Host Reaction

When immunologically competent tissues are transplanted into an immunologically deficient recipient, lymphocytes in the donor tissue may react against the host. This situation is referred to as a *graft versus host* (GVH) reaction or GVH disease. It does not occur when skin or other tissue lacking mature lymphoid cells is transplanted, but it is a major problem with bone marrow transplants. The target organs that are mainly affected by GVH disease are the skin, gastrointestinal tract, liver, and lymphoid tissue. The exact mechanism by which destruction of these organs occurs is not known.

A GVH reaction may become evident one to six weeks after bone marrow transplantation. A generalized maculopapular rash is usually the first sign and in some cases is the only manifestation. In severe cases desquamation may occur. Degeneration of gastrointestinal mucosal glands and mucosal denudation may occur and causes anorexia, nausea, vomiting, diarrhea, abdominal pain, and malabsorption. Liver damage is manifested by hepatomegaly, hyperbilirubinemia, and elevated serum levels of liver enzymes. The spleen may be enlarged, while the thymus, lymph nodes, and intestinal lymphoid tissue atrophy.

AUTOIMMUNE REACTIONS

Autoimmunity is a condition characterized by a specific humoral or cell-mediated immune response against constituents of the body's own tissues. Autoimmune reactions to antigens present in only one particular organ or tissue are said to be *organ-specific* or *tissue-specific* (e.g., thyroiditis). Autoimmune diseases in which the autoimmune response is directed against antigens that are common to various organs and tissues are referred to as *generalized* or *non-organ-specific* autoimmune diseases (e.g., systemic lupus erythematosus). Although an autoimmune pathogenesis is suspected in many diseases, in very few cases is it established that the disease is initiated by an autoimmune mechanism.

Autoimmunity appears to be a state in which the natural immunological tolerance, or unresponsiveness, to self-constituents is inoperative. The mechanisms by which the immune system distinguishes between self and not-self and develops tolerance to self-antigens are not completely understood, and a review of all the theories is beyond the scope of this book. It has been suggested that two general mechanisms are responsible for immunological tolerance. One mechanism involves irreversible loss of competent lymphocytes that are reactive against self-antigens when they arise during fetal life. The other mechanism involves suppression of immunologically competent lymphocytes that are always present.

Like other physiological processes, immune responses appear to be homeostatically regulated. Several mechanisms limit antibody production. The presence of antibody to a particular antigen appears to inhibit production of more antibody by a negative feedback mechanism. The amount of antigen also influences the immune response. Large amounts of antigen, especially one that is poorly metabolized (e.g., pneumococcus polysaccharides), often cause immunological unresponsiveness rather than antibody production. In addition, interactions between lymphocytes appear to be important in regulating the immune response. Cooperation between T and B lymphocytes is often necessary to produce an immune response. As mentioned in Chapter 29, interaction with helper T cells is necessary before B cells respond to some antigens. Some T cells (suppressor cells) interact with B cells and other T cells in a negative manner to prevent an immune response.

A state of immunological unresponsiveness can be induced in both T cells and B cells. Low doses of antigen induce unresponsiveness in T cells while B cells remain competent, but high concentrations of antigens induce unresponsiveness in both types of cells. Without continued antigenic stimulation the cells return to competency, but T cells remain unresponsive longer than the B cells.

Thus, there are certain conditions under which T cells are tolerant, but B cells are competent with regard to a particular antigen. Since the B cells require help from the T cells, however, they normally do not initiate an immune response to the antigen.

Three mechanisms have been suggested for the pathogenesis of autoimmune disorders: stimulation of competent T cells and/or B cells by self-antigens that are normally sequestered from the immune system; a bypass of either T-cell specificity or the need for T cells in the presence of competent B cells; or a loss of suppressor activity which ordinarily limits the ability of lymphoid cells to respond to self-antigens. One or a combination of these mechanisms may be responsible for a particular autoimmune disorder.

Sequestered Antigens

In order to maintain a state of immunological unresponsiveness the immune system must be continually exposed to the antigen. Therefore, when antigens are not accessible to the blood and lymphatic system (i.e., when they are sequestered), tolerance may be lost. If these sequestered components are exposed to the immune system as a result of tissue damage, both T and B lymphocytes could react against the antigen. An example is the lens of the eye.

Bypass of T Cells

It is believed that in some cases tolerance to self-antigens is due to T-cell unresponsiveness, or tolerance, while B cells remain responsive, or competent. If the requirement for help from these tolerant T cells were to be bypassed in some way, the B cells might start forming autoantibodies.

One way that the tolerant T cells might be bypassed is by an alteration in the structure of the autoantigen (Fig. 30-4). T cells appear to respond to different antigenic determinant sites than the B cells. Therefore alteration of the autoantigen might present a new determinant site that would elicit a response from a different set of T lympho-

A.

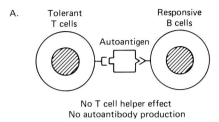

B.

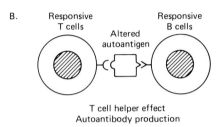

C.

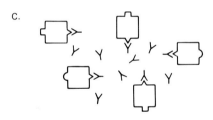

Figure 30-4. *Alteration in the structure of an autoantigen might expose antigenic determinant sites that are capable of stimulating reactive T cells, which would then cooperate with B cells. Thus the tolerant T cells would be bypassed and autoantibodies would be produced. See text for explanation.*

cytes than the tolerant ones. These responsive T cells would then cooperate with responsive B cells, resulting in the production of autoantibodies that could react with the normal autoantigen as well as with the altered autoantigen. The autoantigen may be altered as a result of interaction of normal body constituents with exogenous agents, such as radiation, thermal changes, chemicals, drugs, or microorganisms (especially viruses).

Tolerant T cells might also be bypassed because of infection with microorganisms that have anti-genic determinants that are similar to autoanti-gens. Responsive T cells then cooperate with re-sponsive B cells, resulting in the production of antibodies that not only react with the foreign an-tigen but also with the autoantigen. For example, rheumatic fever is believed to arise this way. Acute rheumatic fever follows infection with group A streptococci, usually of the β-hemolytic type. It appears that antibodies to a streptococcal antigen cross-react with an autoantigen in cardiac muscle.

Another way that tolerant T cells can be bypassed is by the administration of adjuvants. *Adjuvants* are substances that, when mixed with an antigen, enhance the immune response. Adjuv-ants may operate by prolonging the duration of antigen exposure by influencing its absorption or excretion; by stimulating macrophages or other cells that process the antigen; or by nonspecifically stimulating B cells or T cells or the cooperative activities between them. Adjuvants that act as nonspecific T-cell stimuli may stimulate T cells that can cooperate with responsive B cells, result-ing in the production of autoantibodies.

Autoimmune Thyroiditis

Autoimmune thyroiditis is also called Hashimoto's thyroiditis or chronic lymphocytic thyroiditis. In this condition an immune response involving both humoral and cell-mediated immunity is directed against self-components of the thyroid gland. Autoantibodies that react with thyroglobulin, a second antigen in the thyroid colloid, and an anti-gen in the cytoplasm of the follicular cells are pro-duced. The thyroid gland is infiltrated with lym-phocytes, macrophages, and plasma cells; and lymphoid follicles with germinal centers form within the gland. Concurrently destruction of epithelial cells and loss of colloid occurs. Late in the course of the disease severe hypothyroidism develops. (Hypothyroidism is discussed in Chapter 19.) Thyroglobulin is present in very small amounts in the circulation, and it is hypothesized that the normal tolerance to thyroglobulin is due to unresponsive T cells, while B cells remain com-petent. The cause of human autoimmune thy-roiditis is not known, but results of experiments with animals suggest it could arise as a result of tolerant T cells being bypassed.

Loss of Suppressor Activity

In cases where autoimmunity appears to arise as a result of an altered antigen or cross-reacting antigen, the autoimmune response is tissue or organ specific. In generalized autoimmune diseases in which many different autoantibodies are found, however, it is suspected that immunological regulation is disturbed. It has been suggested that a disturbance in the equilibrium between helper and suppressor T cells may lead to the development of autoimmunity. Decreased activity of suppressor T cells could lead to increased activity of helper T cells and of B cells, with subsequent autoantibody production. Evidence for this theory comes from experiments with mice. In addition, recent studies indicate that suppressor T cell function is depressed or absent in people with systemic lupus erythematosus.

The factors responsible for the loss of suppressor T-cell function are not well understood, but genetic factors appear to be involved. Viruses are also involved in autoimmune disease in mice. The role of viruses in human autoimmune disorders has not been established, but a viral etiology is suspected in some cases. Autoimmunity, in general, is more common in females than males, possibly because androgens have a protective effect. Experiments with mice suggest that the equilibrium between helper and suppressor T cells may be modulated by sex hormones, with androgens favoring suppression. Just how the sex hormones mediate this effect is not known. Experiments with mice also suggest that not only autoimmunity but also malignant proliferation of B cells may arise as a result of disturbed T-cell control of B-cell function.

Systemic Lupus Erythematosus

Systemic lupus erythematosus (SLE) is an autoimmune disease characterized by the production of many autoantibodies to a variety of tissue components, including nuclear and cytoplasmic constituents of cells, blood clotting factors, platelets, erythrocytes, and lymphocyte surface components. Antinuclear antibodies are particularly characteristic. The nuclear antigens include double-stranded (native) DNA, single-stranded (denatured) DNA, nucleoproteins (DNA-histone complex), and two extractable nuclear antigens (ENA). One of the extractable nuclear antigens is a ribonucleoprotein, and the other is an acidic protein that is devoid of DNA and RNA and is referred to as the Sm antigen. It is mainly the antibodies to double-stranded DNA that distinguish SLE from other conditions in which auto-antibodies are produced. Antibodies to double-stranded RNA are also found in some cases and give rise to speculation about a viral etiology for SLE. Double-stranded RNA does not normally occur in mammalian cells but it is found during the replication of RNA viruses and is the nucleic acid constituent of reoviruses and rotaviruses (see Chapter 27).

The presence of LE cells in the bone marrow and peripheral blood is a common finding in people with SLE. An LE cell is a phagocytic leukocyte, usually a neutrophil, that has engulfed nuclear material complexed with antinuclear antibodies. LE cells are not diagnostic of SLE since they may also be associated with rheumatoid arthritis, hepatitis, scleroderma, polyarteritis nodosa, and drug sensitivities and are not found in all people with SLE.

Systemic lupus erythematosus may occur at any age but usually appears in the second or third decade of life. It affects women much more often than men. Affected people appear to have a genetic predisposition to SLE. The primary event in the etiology of SLE is unknown, but one hypothesis is that SLE results from diminished suppressor T-cell activity. It is possible, however, that the diminished T-cell activity observed in SLE is a secondary event, perhaps related to a viral etiology.

SLE usually follows a course of exacerbations and remissions. Many organs and systems may be affected, but in any one person not all systems are necessarily involved. The system initially affected often tends to be the one predominantly involved throughout the course of the disease. Tissue damage in SLE appears to be caused mainly by deposition of immune complexes and activation of complement, particularly along basement membranes (e.g., in the kidneys and skin) and in the walls of blood vessels. Inflammation of affected blood vessels (vasculitis) may progress to necrosis and scarring. Disruption of the blood supply causes further tissue damage. In addition to clinical manifestations related to involvement of one or more organs or systems, fever, malaise, weakness, anorexia, and weight loss are common in SLE.

Skin lesions often occur in SLE. The most characteristic is an erythematous eruption on the bridge of the nose and cheeks in a "butterfly" pattern. The skin lesion was originally described as appearing like the bite of a wolf and gives the condition its name (*lupus* is the latin word for wolf). Skin lesions may also occur on other exposed areas, such as the hands, neck, and other parts of the face. Exposure to ultraviolet light causes exacerbation of the skin lesions, perhaps because ultraviolet radiation causes cell damage, which exposes nuclear material to antinuclear antibodies. In addition to skin lesions, shallow painful ulcerations of the oral and pharyngeal mucosa may occur. Loss of hair (alopecia) may occur in some cases, but the hair usually grows back.

Kidney involvement is common in SLE. It may take the form of focal or diffuse glomerulonephritis, nephrotic syndrome, or progressive renal failure.

Most people with SLE have muscle and joint pain and in some cases inflammatory arthritis may occur. The arthritis develops rapidly, mainly involves joints of the hands and feet, and may last only a few days. At times it is difficult to differentiate between SLE and rheumatoid arthritis, but the fixed joint deformities of rheumatoid arthritis do not occur in SLE.

Involvement of serous membranes in SLE may cause pleurisy or pericarditis. Pericarditis may be accompanied by pericardial effusion and cardiac tamponade. The endocardium and myocardium may also be involved.

Raynaud's phenomenon occurs in some people with SLE. Other cardiovascular abnormalities include recurrent thrombophlebitis, thrombotic occlusion of arteries and arterioles, and cardiac arrhythmias.

Hematological manifestations of SLE include neutropenia, autoimmune hemolytic anemia, and thrombocytopenic purpura. Results of serological tests for syphilis may be falsely positive. Serum complement levels are usually depressed during exacerbations of SLE, presumably because of consumption of complement in reactions with immune complexes.

SLE can also affect the central nervous system. Neurological manifestations include convulsive seizures, disturbances of mental function (e.g., depression, excitability, forgetfulness, or psychosis), and cranial nerve disorders.

SUGGESTED ADDITIONAL READING

Clarke CA: The prevention of "rhesus" babies. *Sci Am* **219**(5): 46–52, 1968.

Cullins LC: Preventing and treating transfusion reactions. *Am J Nurs* **79**(5): 935–937, 1979.

Gephardt D: Anaphylaxis from insect stings. *J Emerg Nurs* **4**(3): 19–23, 1978.

Hartley B: I've got a wolf by the ears. *Canad Nurse* **70**(1): 28–31, 1974.

Hartley B: Systemic lupus: a patient perspective. *Canad Nurse* **74**(2): 16–20, 1978.

Todd S, Mackarness R: Allergy to food and chemicals—1: the scope of the problem. *Nurs Times* **74**(11): 438–441, 1978.

Tovey LAD: Complications of blood transfusions. *Nurs Times* **74**(47): 1928–1930, 1978.

Wieczorek RR, Horner-Rosner B: The asthmatic child: preventing and controlling attacks. *Am J Nurs* **79**(2): 258–262, 1979.

Glossary

Acid A substance that can donate protons (i.e., hydrogen ions).

Acidemia A decrease in the pH of the arterial blood.

Acidosis An abnormal condition that tends to produce an increase in the hydrogen-ion concentration (or a decrease in pH) of the extracellular fluid.

Acinus A general term used in anatomical nomenclature to designate a small saclike dilatation, particularly one found in various glands.

Acute Having relatively severe manifestations and running a short course.

Adaptation The process of adjusting to environmental conditions.

Agglutination The clumping of cells in a fluid.

Alkalemia An increase in the pH of the arterial blood.

Alkalosis An abnormal condition that tends to produce a decrease in the hydrogen-ion concentration (or an increase in pH) of the extracellular fluid.

Allele Any one of two or more alternative forms of genes that occupy corresponding loci on homologous chromosomes.

Analgesia The absence of pain; usually denotes relief of pain without loss of consciousness.

Anaplasia A loss of differentiation of cells and of their orientation to one another and to their axial framework and blood vessels.

Anasarca Massive generalized edema.

Anemia A reduction below normal in the number of erythrocytes or in the concentration of hemoglobin in the blood.

Anencephaly Congenital absence of the cranial vault with cerebral hemispheres completely missing or reduced to small masses attached to the base of the skull.

Anhidrosis An abnormal deficiency of sweat.

Anion An ion with a negative charge.

Anorexia Lack or loss of appetite for food.

Anoxia Absence of oxygen in the tissues.

Antibody An immunoglobulin molecule that reacts specifically with a substance (antigen) that induced its synthesis or with a closely related antigen.

Antigen Any substance that induces the formation of antibodies with which it reacts specifically.

Anuria Absence of excretion of urine from the body.

Aphasia Defect or loss of power of expression by speech, writing, or signs or of comprehending spoken or written language due to injury or disease of brain centers.

Aplasia Lack of development of an organ or tis-

567

sue or of the cellular products from an organ or tissue.

Apnea　Absence of breathing.

Ascites　An accumulation of serous fluid in the peritoneal cavity.

Asterixis　An abnormal flapping tremor consisting of involuntary jerking movements, especially in the hands.

Asymptomatic　Showing or causing no symptoms.

Ataxia　Failure of muscular coordination.

Atelectasis　Collapse of part or all of the lung.

ATP　Adenosine triphosphate, the energy "currency" of cells.

Atrophy　A decrease in the size of a cell, tissue, or organ.

Azotemia　An excess of urea or other nitrogenous substances in the blood.

Bacteremia　The presence of viable bacteria in the circulating blood.

Bacteriophage　A virus that infects bacteria.

Base　Any substance that can accept protons.

Benign　The mild character of an illness or the nonmalignant character of a neoplasm.

Buffer　A substance that prevents rapid or great change in the pH of a solution.

Cachexia　Malnutrition and emaciation occurring in the course of a chronic disease.

Carcinogen　An environmental agent that can produce cancer.

Carcinoma　A malignant neoplasm arising from epithelial tissue.

Cation　An ion with a positive charge.

Centromere　A constricted portion of a chromosome at which the chromatids are joined and by which the chromosome is attached to the spindle during cell division.

Chromatid　Each of the two strands formed by longitudinal duplication of a chromosome that becomes visible during prophase of mitosis or meiosis; the two chromatids are joined by the still undivided centromere.

Chromosome　A structure in the cell nucleus that contains a linear thread of DNA (the genetic material), associated proteins, and RNA.

Chronic　Persisting over a long period of time; denoting a disease of slow progress and long continuance.

Clonic　Pertaining to or of the nature of clonus; marked by alternate contraction and relaxation of muscle.

Coenzyme　An organic substance that enhances or is necessary for the action of enzymes.

Commensalism　Symbiosis in which one organism benefits without causing harm or giving benefit to the other organism.

Congenital　Existing at birth; referring to conditions that are present at birth, regardless of their cause.

Contamination　Soiling with infectious matter.

Convalescence　The stage of recovery after a disease, a surgical operation, or an injury.

Convulsion　A violent involuntary contraction or series of contractions of skeletal muscles.

Cyanosis　A bluish discoloration of the skin and mucous membranes due to excessive concentration of reduced hemoglobin in the blood.

Desquamation　The shedding of epithelial elements, chiefly of the skin, in scales or small sheets.

Diarrhea　Abnormally frequent discharge of more or less fluid fecal material from the bowel.

Differentiation　Specialization; the acquiring or the possession of character or function different from that of the original type.

Diploid　Having two full sets of homologous chromosomes, as normally found in the somatic cells.

Disjunction　The moving apart of bivalent chromosomes at the first anaphase of meiosis.

Diuresis　An increase in the volume of urine formed.

DNA　Deoxyribonucleic acid, the carrier of genetic information.

Dominant　In genetics, a trait or allele that is capable of expression when carried by only one of a pair of homologous chromosomes.

Dysarthria Imperfect articulation of speech due to disturbances of muscle control that results from damage to the central or peripheral nervous system.

Dysplasia An alteration in the size, shape, and organization of differentiated cells.

Dyspnea A subjective feeling of shortness of breath and difficulty in breathing.

Ecchymoses Nonelevated rounded or irregular blue or purplish patches due to hemorrhage in the skin or mucous membranes; they are larger than petechiae.

Edema The accumulation of an abnormally large amount of fluid in the interstitial space.

Electrolyte Any acid, base, or salt that dissociates into ions when dissolved in water.

Embolus A mass of undissolved material traveling in the blood; it may be solid, liquid, or gaseous.

Endogenous Developing or originating within the organism.

Endotoxin A toxin associated with the cell wall of gram-negative bacteria that is liberated when the bacteria die.

Enzyme A protein that acts as a catalyst in biochemical reactions.

Epistaxis Nosebleed.

Erythema Redness of the skin.

Etiology Causation; specifically, the cause of disease.

Exacerbation An increase in the severity of a disease or in any of its signs or symptoms.

Exogenous Originating or produced outside the organism.

Exotoxin A toxin secreted into the surrounding medium during the growth of microorganisms.

Familial Occurring in or affecting more members of a family than would be expected by chance.

Fever Elevation of the body temperature above the normal range.

Fibrinolysin A plasma enzyme that breaks down blood clots.

Fibrosis The formation of fibrous tissue, usually as a reparative or reactive process.

Focus (plural: *foci*) The center or the starting point of a disease process.

Fomite A contaminated inanimate article.

Gene A unit of heredity; in most cases conceptualized as a particular sequence of nucleotides in DNA that codes for a single polypeptide chain.

Genome The total gene complement of a haploid set of chromosomes found in higher life forms, or the functionally similar but simpler linear arrangements found in bacteria and viruses.

Genotype The genetic constitution of an individual; may refer to the entire genetic constitution or to the alleles present at one or more specified loci.

Gluconeogenesis The formation of glucose from noncarbohydrate molecules.

Glucosuria The presence of glucose in the urine.

Glycogenesis The formation or synthesis of glycogen.

Glycogenolysis The hydrolysis of glycogen to glucose.

Glycolysis The energy-yielding conversion of glucose to pyruvic acid by the cells.

Glycoprotein Any of a class of conjugated proteins consisting of a protein with a carbohydrate group.

Glycosuria The excretion of an abnormally large amount of sugar in the urine.

Gynecomastia Excessive development of the male mammary glands.

Haploid Having a single set of chromosomes, as normally carried by a gamete, or having one complete set of nonhomologous chromosomes.

Hapten A substance of low molecular weight that by itself does not elicit the production of antibodies, but when combined with a larger carrier molecule imparts antigenic specificity on the complex and does elicit the production of antibodies.

Hemarthrosis   Extravasation of blood into a joint or its synovial cavity.

Hematocrit   The percentage of the volume of a blood sample that is occupied by erythrocytes.

Hematoma   A localized mass of extravasated blood, usually clotted, in an organ, space, or tissue.

Hematuria   Blood in the urine.

Hemiplegia   Paralysis of one side of the body.

Hemoconcentration   Decrease in the volume of plasma in relation to the number of red blood cells.

Hemolysis   The alteration, dissolution, or destruction of red blood cells in such a manner that hemoglobin is liberated into the medium in which the cells are suspended.

Hemostasis   The arrest of bleeding by physiological or surgical means.

Homeostasis   The maintenance of constant conditions in the internal environment.

Hypalgesia   Decreased sensitivity to pain.

Hyperalgesia   Excessive sensitivity to pain.

Hyperbilirubinemia   An abnormally high concentration of bilirubin in the blood.

Hypercalcemia   An abnormally high concentration of calcium in the blood.

Hypercapnia   An excess of carbon dioxide in the arterial blood.

Hypercholesterolemia   An abnormally high concentration of cholesterol in the blood.

Hyperchloremia   An abnormally high concentration of chloride ions in the blood.

Hyperemia   An excess of blood in a part.

Hyperglycemia   An abnormally high concentration of sugar, especially glucose, in the blood.

Hyperkalemia   An abnormally high concentration of potassium in the plasma.

Hyperlipidemia   An excess of lipids in the blood.

Hyperlipoproteinemia   An excess of lipoproteins in the blood.

Hypermagnesemia   An abnormally high concentration of magnesium in the plasma.

Hypernatremia   An abnormally high concentration of sodium in the blood.

Hyperoxia   An excess of oxygen in the system.

Hyperphosphatemia   An abnormally high concentration of phosphates in the blood.

Hyperplasia   An increase in the number of normal cells in a normal arrangement in a tissue or organ.

Hyperpnea   An increase in the rate and depth of breathing.

Hyperpyrexia   A highly elevated body temperature.

Hypertension   A persistently high arterial blood pressure.

Hyperthermia   An abnormally high body temperature.

Hypertriglyceridemia   An excess of triglycerides in the blood.

Hypertrophy   An increase in the size of an organ or part due to an increase in the size of its constituent cells.

Hyperventilation   Alveolar ventilation in excess of the body's need for carbon dioxide elimination.

Hypervolemia   An abnormal increase in the circulating blood volume.

Hypervolia   An increased volume or water content of a body fluid compartment.

Hypocalcemia   An abnormally low concentration of calcium in the blood.

Hypocapnia   An abnormally low concentration of carbon dioxide in the arterial blood.

Hypochloremia   An abnormally low concentration of chloride in the blood.

Hypoglycemia   An abnormally low concentration of sugar, especially glucose, in the blood.

Hypokalemia   An abnormally low concentration of potassium in the plasma.

Hypolipidemia An abnormally decreased amount of lipid in the blood.

Hypolipoproteinemia An abnormally decreased amount of lipoproteins in the blood.

Hypomagnesemia An abnormally low concentration of magnesium in the plasma.

Hyponatremia An abnormally low concentration of sodium in the blood.

Hypophosphatemia An abnormally low concentration of phosphates in the blood.

Hypoplasia Underdevelopment of tissue or an organ, usually due to a decrease in the number of cells.

Hypotension An abnormally low arterial blood pressure.

Hypovolemia An abnormally decreased volume of circulating blood.

Hypovolia A decreased volume or water content of a body fluid compartment.

Hypoxemia Deficient oxygenation of the arterial blood.

Hypoxia An abnormally low oxygen content in tissues or a decreased availability of oxygen to the cells.

Iatrogenic Any adverse condition in a patient resulting from treatment by a physician or surgeon.

Icterus Jaundice.

Idiopathic Of unknown causation.

Immunity A state of relative resistance to a particular disease.

Immunogen Any substance that is capable of eliciting a humoral or cell-mediated immune response.

Infarct An area of necrosis in a tissue due to ischemia.

Infarction The formation of an infarct.

Infection Invasion of the body tissues by microorganisms, with multiplication of the microorganisms in the tissues.

Insidious Coming on in a stealthy manner; of gradual and subtle development.

Involution A retrograde change, the reverse of evolution; applied especially to a lessening of the size of a tissue caused by a reduction in the number of its component cells, without degeneration.

Ion An atom or group of atoms that carries an electrical charge.

Ischemia Deficiency of blood in a part, due to functional constriction or actual obstruction of a blood vessel.

Jaundice A yellow discoloration of the skin, sclera, and mucous membranes due to the deposition of excess bilirubin in the tissues.

Kernicterus A neurological disorder caused by deposition of bilirubin in the brain.

Ketonemia An excess of ketone bodies in the blood.

Ketonuria Ketone bodies in the urine.

Ketosis A condition characterized by an abnormally elevated concentration of ketone bodies in the body tissues and fluids.

Latent Not manifest, but potentially discernible.

Leukocytosis An increase in the number of leukocytes in the blood.

Leukopenia A reduction in the number of leukocytes in the blood below normal.

Linkage Association of genes in inheritance due to the fact they are in the same chromosome.

Lipogenesis The formation of fat; the transformation of nonfat food materials into body fat.

Lipolysis The splitting up (hydrolysis) or chemical decomposition of fat.

Locus (plural: *loci*) In genetics, the specific site of a gene in a chromosome.

Macromolecule A very large molecule having a polymeric chain structure, as in proteins, polysaccharides, and nucleic acids.

Macule A small discolored patch or spot on the skin, neither elevated above nor depressed below the skin's surface.

Malaise A vague feeling of bodily discomfort.

Malignant Tending to become progressively worse and to result in death; in the case of a neoplasm, having the properties of anaplasia, invasion, and metastasis.

Melena   The passage of dark colored, tarry stools, due to the presence of blood altered by the intestinal juices.

Metaplasia   The replacement of one type of fully differentiated cells by another type of fully differentiated cells in a part of the body where the second cell type does not normally occur.

Monosomy   The absence of one chromosome from the complement of an otherwise diploid cell.

Mutagen   Any agent that causes the production of a mutation.

Mutant   An individual possessing one or more genes that have undergone mutation.

Mutation   A permanent transmissible change in the genetic material, usually in a single gene.

Mutualism   Symbiosis in which both organisms are benefited by the association.

Necrosis   The pathologic death of one or more cells, or a portion of tissue or organ, resulting from irreversible damage.

Neoplasm   A mass of cells forming a new and abnormal growth of tissue in which the growth is uncontrolled and progressive.

Neuroglycopenia   A diminished supply of glucose to the central nervous system, resulting in functional impairment.

Oliguria   Secretion of a diminished amount of urine.

Opsonin   An antibody or other substance that combines with microbial cells and renders them more susceptible to phagocytosis.

Orthopnea   Difficulty breathing while lying flat.

Osmosis   The net movement of water (solvent) from a more dilute solution to a more concentrated solution when the movement of solute is restricted by a membrane.

Osteoporosis   A condition in which bone mass is decreased but the composition (mineralization) of bone remains normal.

Oxidation   The loss of electrons from an atom or molecule.

Papilledema   Edema of the optic disc.

Papule   A small, circumscribed, solid elevation of the skin.

Paraplegia   Paralysis of both lower extremities and, generally, the lower trunk.

Parasitism   An association between two living organisms in which one organism (the parasite) benefits at the expense of the other (the host).

Parenchyma   The distinguishing or specific cells (the functional elements) of a gland or organ as distinct from the connective tissue framework, or stroma.

Paresthesia   An abnormal spontaneous sensation, such as of burning, pricking, tickling, or tingling.

Pathogenic   Causing disease.

Pathogenesis   The mode of origin or development of any disease or morbid process.

Peptide   A compound of two or more amino acids in which the carboxyl group of one is united with the amino group of the other, with the elimination of a molecule of water, thus forming a peptide bond.

Petechiae   Round, pinpoint, nonraised, purplish red spots, due to very small hemorrhages into intradermal or submucous tissues.

pH   Symbol for the negative logarithm of hydrogen-ion concentration, when the concentration is expressed in molarity.

Phenotype   The physical, biochemical, or physiological manifestation of a genetic trait that reflects gene interaction and gene-environment interaction.

Photosensitization   The development of heightened reactivity of a substance or a living cell or tissue to light, especially sunlight or ultraviolet light.

Pleomorphism   Occurring in more than one form or shape.

Polycythemia   An increase above the normal in the number of erythrocytes in the blood.

Polydipsia   Excessive thirst persisting for long periods of time.

Polyploid Having more than two full sets of homologous chromosomes.

Polyuria Excessive excretion of urine.

Prodrome An early or premonitory symptom of a disease.

Proteinuria The presence of an excess of plasma proteins in the urine.

Proteolysis Protein hydrolysis; the decomposition of protein.

Pruritis Itching.

Purpura Brownish red discolorations of the skin, slightly larger than petechiae, caused by hemorrhage into the tissues; also, a condition characterized by hemorrhages into the skin.

Pustule A small circumscribed elevation of the skin, containing pus.

Pyogen An agent that causes pus formation.

Pyrogen An agent that causes fever.

Quadriplegia Paralysis of all four limbs.

rad radiation absorbed dose; the amount of energy absorbed from ionizing radiation per unit mass of tissue.

Recessive In genetics, incapable of expression unless the responsible allele is carried by both members of a pair of homologous chromosomes.

Reduction A gain of electrons by an atom or molecule.

Remission A diminution or abatement of the symptoms of a disease; also the period during which such abatement occurs.

RNA Ribonucleic acid.

Sarcoma A malignant neoplasm arising from mesenchyme and its derivatives (i.e., connective tissue, blood vessels, and lymph vessels).

Sepsis The presence of pathogenic microorganisms or their toxins in the blood or tissues.

Septicemia Systemic disease caused by the persistence and multiplication of microorganisms in the circulating blood.

Sequela A morbid condition following as a consequence of a disease.

Sequester To detach or separate abnormally a small portion from the whole.

Serum The fluid portion of the blood obtained after removal of the fibrin clot and blood cells.

Shock A state of circulatory failure such that tissues are damaged due to inadequate blood flow.

Steatorrhea Excessive amounts of fat in the feces.

Stomatitis Inflammation of the oral mucosa.

Stress The nonspecific response of the body to any demand.

Stressor A stimulus or agent that produces stress.

Stroma The supporting tissue or matrix of an organ.

Substrate A substance on which an enzyme acts; that is, a reactant in a reaction catalyzed by an enzyme.

Suppuration The formation of pus.

Symbiosis The living together or close association of two organisms.

Syncope Fainting; a transient loss of consciousness due to cerebral ischemia.

Template A pattern or mold; in genetics, a strand of DNA which specifies the synthesis of a complementary strand of RNA.

Teratogen An agent that causes the production of physical defects in offspring in utero.

Tetany A disorder marked by intermittent tonic muscular contractions, accompanied by fibrillary tremors, paresthesias, and muscular pains, due to hypocalcemia or alkalosis.

Thrombocytopenia An abnormally low number of platelets in the circulating blood.

Thrombophlebitis Inflammation of a vein associated with thrombus formation.

Thrombosis The development or formation of a blood clot in the blood vessels or the heart during life.

Thrombus A clot in a blood vessel or one of the cavities of the heart formed during life from constituents of blood.

Tonic Characterized by continuous tension or contraction, especially muscular tension.

Transcription A process whereby the genetic information contained in DNA is used to order a complementary sequence of bases in an RNA chain.

Translation The process whereby the genetic information present in a messenger RNA molecule directs the order of the specific amino acids during protein synthesis.

Trisomy The presence of an additional (third) chromosome of one type in an otherwise diploid cell.

Uremia A syndrome resulting from altered composition of the body fluids due to renal failure.

Varix (plural: *varices*) An enlarged and tortuous vein, artery, or lymphatic vessel.

Varicose Of the nature of or pertaining to a varix; unnaturally and permanently distended.

Vector A carrier (especially an arthropod) that transfers an infectious agent from one host to another.

Vesicle A small blister; a small circumscribed elevation of the epidermis containing a serous liquid.

Wheal A smooth, slightly elevated area on the body surface, which is redder or paler than the surrounding skin.

Xanthoma A yellow papule, nodule, or plaque in the skin, due to deposits of lipids.

Xenobiotic A substance not normally found in the body; a foreign compound.

Xerophthalmia Dryness of the cornea and conjunctiva due to vitamin A deficiency.

Bibliography

GENERAL

Frohlich ED: (ed): *Pathophysiology: Altered Regulatory Mechanisms in Disease.* Philadelphia, JB Lippincott Co, 1972.

Guyton AC: *Textbook of Medical Physiology*, ed 5. Philadelphia, WB Saunders Co, 1976.

Landau BR: *Essential Human Anatomy and Physiology*, Glenview, Ill, Scott, Foresman and Co, 1976.

Langley LL, Telford IR, Christensen JB: *Dynamic Anatomy and Physiology*, ed 4. New York, McGraw-Hill Book Co, 1974.

Robbins SL, Angell M: *Basic Pathology*, ed 2. Philadelphia, WB Saunders Co, 1976.

Selkurt EE (ed): *Physiology*, ed 3. Boston, Little, Brown & Co., 1971.

Sodeman WA Jr, Sodeman WA: *Pathologic Physiology: Mechanisms of Disease*, ed 5. Philadelphia, WB Saunders Co, 1974.

Timiras PS: *Developmental Physiology and Aging.* New York, Macmillan Co, 1972.

Vander AJ, Sherman JH, Luciano DS: *Human Physiology*, ed 2. New York, McGraw-Hill Book Co., 1975.

SPECIFIC

Chapter 1

Atkinson DE: Biological feedback control at the molecular level. *Science* **150:** 851–854, 1965.

Baumgardt BR: Food intake, energy balance and homeostasis, in Sink JD (ed): *The Control of Metabolism.* University Park, Pa. Pennsylvania State University Press, 1974.

Boyden S: Cultural adaptation to biological maladjustment, in Boyden SV (ed): *The Impact of Civilisation on the Biology of Man.* Toronto, University of Toronto Press, 1970.

Dubos R: *Man Adapting.* New Haven, Conn, Yale University Press, 1965.

Engel GL: Homeostasis, behavioral adjustment and the concept of health and disease, in Grinker RR (ed): *Mid-century Psychiatry.* Springfield, Ill, Charles C Thomas Publisher, 1953.

Helson H: *Adaptation-Level Theory.* New York, Harper & Row, 1964.

Horrobin DF: *Principles of Biological Control.* Aylesbury, England, Medical and Technical Publishing Co, 1970.

Jones RW: *Principles of Biological Regulation: An Introduction to Feedback Systems.* New York, Academic Press, 1973.

Langley LL: *Homeostasis: Origins of the Concept.* Stroudsburg, Pa, Dowden, Hutchinson and Ross, 1973.

Lasker GW: Human biological adaptability. *Science* **166:** 1480–1486, 1969.

Lehninger AL: *Bioenergetics*, ed 2. Menlo Park, Calif, WA Benjamin, 1971.

Martin HW, Prange AJ Jr: Human adaptation: a

conceptual approach to understanding patients. *Canadian Nurse* **58**(3): 234–243, 1962.

Prosser CL: Principles and general concepts of adaptation, in Lee DHK, Minard D (eds): *Physiology, Environment and Man*. New York, Academic Press, 1970.

Roy C: Adaptation: a conceptual framework for nursing. *Nurs Outlook* **18**: 42–45, 1970.

Yamamoto WS, Brobeck JR (eds): *Physiological Controls and Regulations*. Philadelphia, WB Saunders Co, 1965.

Chapter 2

Aschoff J: Adaptive cycles, in Lee DHK, Minard D (eds): *Physiology, Environment and Man*. New York, Academic Press, 1970.

Cannon WB: *Bodily Changes in Pain, Hunger, Fear and Rage*, ed 2. Boston, Charles T Branford Co, 1929.

Dohrenwend BS, Dohrenwend BP (eds): *Stressful Life Events: Their Nature and Effects*. New York, John Wiley & Sons, 1974.

Dubos R: *Man Adapting*. New Haven, Conn, Yale University Press, 1965.

Engel GL: Homeostasis, behavioral adjustment and the concept of health and disease, in Grinker RR (ed): *Mid-century Psychiatry*. Springfield, Ill, Charles C Thomas Publisher, 1953.

McGrath JE: (ed): *Social and Psychological Factors in Stress*. New York, Holt, Rinehart & Winston, 1970.

Mims C: Stress in relation to the processes of civilisation, in Boyden SV (ed): *The Impact of Civilisation on the Biology of Man*. Toronto, University of Toronto Press, 1970.

Rabkin JG, Struening EL: Life events, stress and illness. *Science* **194**: 1013–1020, 1976.

Roddie IC, Wallace WFM: *The Physiology of Disease*. London, Lloyd-Luke, 1975.

Selye H: *Stress in Health and Disease*. Boston, Butterworths, 1976.

Selye H: *The Stress of Life*, rev ed. New York, McGraw-Hill Book Co, 1976.

Wolf S, Goodell H (eds): *Harold G. Wolff's Stress and Disease*, ed 2. Springfield, Ill, Charles C Thomas Publisher, 1968.

Chapter 3

Levitan M, Montagu A: *Textbook of Human Genetics*. New York, Oxford University Press, 1971.

Nora JJ, Fraser FC: *Medical Genetics: Principles and Practice*. Philadelphia, Lea & Febiger, 1974.

Strickberger MW: *Genetics*, ed 2. New York, Macmillan Co., 1976.

Watson JD: *Molecular Biology of the Gene*, ed 3. Menlo Park, Calif, WA Benjamin, 1976.

Chapter 4

Moody PA: *Genetics of Man*, ed 2. New York, WW Norton & Co, 1975.

Nora JJ, Fraser FC: *Medical Genetics: Principles and Practice*. Philadelphia, Lea & Febiger, 1974.

Stern C: *Principles of Human Genetics*, ed 3. San Francisco, WH Freeman and Co, 1973.

Strickberger MW: *Genetics*, ed 2. New York, Macmillan Co, 1976.

Chapter 5

Berry AC, Mutton DE, and Lewis DGM, Mosaicism and the trisomy 8 syndrome. *Clin Genet* **14**: 105–114, 1978.

Erickson JD: Down syndrome, paternal age, maternal age and birth order. *Ann Hum Genet* **41**: 289–298, 1978.

McKusick VA, Claiborne R (eds): *Medical Genetics*. New York, HP Publishing Co, 1973.

Moody PA: *Genetics of Man*, ed 2. New York, WW Norton & Co, 1975.

Nora JJ, Fraser FC: *Medical Genetics: Principles and Practice*. Philadelphia, Lea & Febiger, 1974.

Riccardi VM: *The Genetic Approach to Human Dis-*

ease. New York, Oxford University Press, 1977.

Chapter 6

Bacchus H: *Essentials of Metabolic Diseases and Endocrinology.* Baltimore, University Park Press, 1976.

Brady RO: Inherited metabolic diseases of the nervous system. *Science* **193:** 733, 1976.

Hsia DYY (ed): *Galactosemia.* Springfield, Ill, Charles C Thomas Publisher, 1969.

Kelley VC (ed): *Metabolic, Endocrine and Genetic Disorders of Children,* vol 2, 3. Hagerstown Md, Harper & Row, 1974.

Nyhan WL (ed): *Heritable Disorders of Amino Acid Metabolism: Patterns of Clinical Expression and Genetic Variation.* New York, John Wiley & Sons, 1974.

Chapter 7

Biggs R (ed): *Human Blood Coagulation, Haemostasis and Thrombosis,* ed 2. Oxford, England, Blackwell Scientific Publications, 1976.

Davie EW, Fujikawa K: Basic mechanisms in blood coagulation. *Ann Rev Biochem* **44:** 799–829, 1975.

Gazes PC: *Clinical Cardiology.* Chicago, Year Book Medical Publishers, 1975.

Holmberg L, Nilsson IM: Von Willebrand's disease. *Ann Rev Med* **26:** 33–44, 1975.

Russell RW (ed): *Cerebral Arterial Disease.* Edinburgh, Churchill Livingstone, 1976.

Tullis JL: *Clot.* Springfield, Ill, Charles C Thomas Publisher, 1976.

Chapter 8

Cappell DF, Anderson JR (eds): *Muir's Textbook of Pathology,* ed 9. London, Edward Arnold (Publishers), 1971.

Gartland JJ: *Fundamentals of Orthopaedics.* Philadelphia, WB Saunders Co, 1974.

Marin GA, Ostrow JD: Cirrhosis of the liver, in Brooks FP (ed): *Gastrointestinal Pathophysiology.* London, Oxford University Press, 1974.

Menaker L (ed). *Biologic Basis of Wound Healing.* Hagerstown, Md, Harper & Row, 1975.

Peacock EE Jr, Van Winkle W Jr: *Surgery and Biology of Wound Repair.* Philadelphia, WB Saunders Co, 1970.

Ross R: Wound healing. *Sci Am* **220**(6): 40–50, 1969.

Walter JB, Israel MS: *General Pathology,* ed 4. Edinburgh, Churchill Livingstone, 1974

Willis RA, Willis AT: *Principles of Pathology and Bacteriology,* ed 3. London, Butterworth and Co, 1972.

Chapter 9

Crue BL Jr (ed): *Pain: Research and Treatment.* New York, Academic Press, 1975.

Gastaut H, Broughton R: *Epileptic Seizures: Clinical and Electrographic Features, Diagnosis and Treatment.* Springfield, Ill, Charles C Thomas Publisher, 1972.

Melzack R, Wall PD: Pain mechanisms: a new theory. *Science* **150:** 971–978, 1965.

Niedermeyer E: *Compendium of the Epilepsies.* Springfield, Ill, Charles C Thomas Publisher, 1974.

Plum F, Posner JB: *The Diagnosis of Stupor and Coma,* ed 2. Philadelphia, FA Davis Co, 1972.

Weisenberg M (ed): *Pain: Clinical and Experimental Perspectives.* St. Louis, CV Mosby Co, 1975.

Chapter 10

Cherniack RM, Cherniack L, Naimark A: *Respiration in Health and Disease,* ed 2. Philadelphia, WB Saunders Co, 1972.

Flenley DC: Hypoxia in lung disease, in Stretton TB (ed): *Recent Advances in Respiratory Medicine,* vol 1. Edinburgh, Churchill Livingstone, 1976.

Howell JBL: Airways obstruction, in Stretton TB (ed): *Recent Advances in Respiratory Medicine*, vol 1. Edinburgh, Churchill Livingstone, 1976.

Lambertson CJ: Effects of excessive pressures of oxygen, nitrogen, carbon dioxide, and carbon monoxide: implications in aerospace, undersea, and industrial environments, in Mountcastle VB (ed): *Medical Physiology*, vol 2, ed 13. St. Louis, CV Mosby Co, 1974.

Lehninger AL: *Bioenergetics*, ed 2. Menlo Park, Calif, WA Benjamin, 1971.

Linman JW: *Hematology: Physiologic, Pathophysiologic, and Clinical Principles*. New York, Macmillan Co, 1975.

Silverman WA: The lesson of retrolental fibroplasia. *Sci Am* **236**(6): 100–107, 1977.

Thurlbeck WM: *Chronic Airflow Obstruction in Lung Disease*. Philadelphia, WB Saunders Co, 1976.

White RJ, Woodings DF: Impaired water handling in chronic obstructive airways disease. *Brit Med J* **2**: 561–563, 1971.

Chapter 11

Cheek DB: Extracellular volume: its structure and measurement and the influence of age and disease. *J Pediatr* **58**: 103–125, 1961.

Edelman IS, Liebman J: Anatomy of body water and electrolytes. *Am J Med* **27**: 256–274, 1959.

Feldschuh J, Enson Y: Prediction of the normal blood volume—relation of blood volume to body habitus. *Circulation* **56**: 605–612, 1977.

Friis-Hansen B: Body water compartments in children: Changes during growth and related changes in body composition. *Pediatrics* **28**: 169–181, 1961.

Koushanpour E: *Renal Physiology: Principles and Functions*. Philadelphia, WB Saunders Co, 1976.

Ljunggren H, Ikkos D, Luft R: Studies on body composition. *Acta Endocrin* **25**: 187–223, 1957.

Maxwell MH, Kleeman CR (eds): *Clinical Disorders of Fluid and Electrolyte Metabolism*, ed 2. New York, McGraw-Hill Book Co, 1972.

Murray JF: *The Normal Lung, The Basis for Diagnosis and Treatment of Pulmonary Disease*. Philadelphia, WB Saunders Co, 1976.

Parker HV, et al: Body water compartments throughout the lifespan, in Wolstenholme GEW, O'Connor M (eds): *Ciba Foundation Colloquia on Aging*, vol 4. London, J and A Churchill, 1958.

Pitts RF: *Physiology of the Kidney and Body Fluids*, ed 3. Chicago, Year Book Medical Publishers, 1974.

Rushmer RR: *Cardiovascular Dynamics*, ed 4. Philadelphia, WB Saunders Co, 1976.

Winters RW (ed): *The Body Fluids in Pediatrics*. Boston, Little, Brown & Co, 1973.

Chapter 12

Collins RD: *Illustrated Manual of Fluid and Electrolyte Disorders*. Philadelphia, JB Lippincott Co, 1976.

Goldberger E: *A Primer of Water, Electrolyte and Acid-Base Syndromes*, ed 5. Philadelphia, Lea & Febiger, 1975.

Koushanpour E: *Renal Physiology: Principles and Functions*. Philadelphia, WB Saunders Co, 1976.

Leaf A, Cotran RS: *Renal Pathophysiology*. New York, Oxford University Press, 1976.

Maxwell MH, Kleeman CR (eds): *Clinical Disorders of Fluid and Electrolyte Metabolism*, ed 2. New York, McGraw-Hill Book Co, 1972.

Pitts RF: *Physiology of the Kidney and Body Fluids*, ed 3. Chicago, Year Book Medical Publishers, 1974.

Rushmer RF: *Cardiovascular Dynamics*, ed 4. Philadelphia, WB Saunders Co, 1976.

Winters RW (ed): *The Body Fluids in Pediatrics*. Boston, Little, Brown & Co, 1973.

Chapter 13

Birkenhäger WH, Schalekamp MADH: *Control Mechanisms in Essential Hypertension.* Amsterdam, Elsevier Scientific Publishing Co., 1976.

Freis ED: *Introduction to the Nature and Management of Hypertension.* Bowie, Md, Robert J Brady Co, 1974.

Freis ED: Salt, volume and the prevention of hypertension. *Circulation* **53:** 589–595, 1976.

Gavros H, Oliver JA, Cannon PJ: Interrelations of renin, angiotensin II, and sodium in hypertension and renal failure. *Ann Rev Med* **27:** 485–521, 1976.

Haber E: The role of renin in normal and pathological cardiovascular homeostasis. *Circulation* **54:** 849–861, 1976.

Heineman HO, Lee JB: Prostaglandins and blood pressure control. *Am J Med* **61:** 681–695, 1976.

Levine RS, et al: Tracking correlations of blood pressure levels in infancy. *Pediatrics* **61:** 121–125, 1978.

Lindheimer MD, Katz AI, Zuspan FP (eds): *Hypertension in Pregnancy.* New York, John Wiley & Sons, 1976.

London GM, et al: Total effective compliance, cardiac output and fluid volumes in essential hypertension. *Circulation* **57:** 995–1000, 1978.

Master AM, Dublin LI, Marks HH: The normal blood pressure range and its clinical implications. *J Am Med Ass* **143:** 1464–1470, 1950.

National Heart, Lung, and Blood Institute: Report of the Task Force on blood pressure control in children. *Pediatrics* **59**(suppl): 797–820, 1977.

Pickering G: *Hypertension, its Causes, Consequences and Management,* ed 2. Edinburgh, Churchill Livingstone, 1974.

Scher AM: Carotid and aortic regulation of arterial blood pressure. *Circulation* **56:** 521–528, 1977.

Weidmann P, Maxwell MH: Hypertension, in Massry SG, Sellers AL (eds): *Clinical Aspects of Uremia and Dialysis.* Springfield Ill, Charles C Thomas Publisher, 1976.

Chapter 14

Bell GH, Emslie-Smith D, Paterson CR: *Textbook of Physiology and Biochemistry,* ed 9. Edinburgh, Churchill Livingstone, 1976.

da Luz PL, et al: Pulmonary edema related to changes in colloid osmotic and pulmonary artery wedge pressure in patients after acute myocardial infarction. *Circulation* **51:** 350–357, 1975.

Dunkman WB, et al: Clinical and hemodynamic results of intraortic balloon pumping and surgery for cardiogenic shock. *Circulation* **46:** 465–476, 1972.

Forrester JS, et al: Filling pressures in the right and left sides of the heart in acute myocardial infarction. *N Engl J Med* **285:** 190–192, 1971.

Gorlin R: Current concepts in cardiology: practical cardiac hemodynamics. *N Engl J Med* **296:** 203–205, 1977.

Hinshaw LB, Cox BG (eds): *The Fundamental Mechanisms of Shock.* New York, Plenum Press, 1972.

Ledingham IMcA (ed): *Shock: Clinical and Experimental Aspects.* New York, American Elsevier Publishing Co, 1976.

Murray JF: *The Normal Lung: The Basis for Diagnosis and Treatment of Pulmonary Disease.* Philadelphia, WB Saunders Co, 1976.

Schumer W, Nyhus LM (eds): *Treatment of Shock: Principles and Practice.* Philadelphia, Lea & Febiger, 1974.

Steenblock UHM, Wolff G: Effect of hemorrhagic shock on intrapulmonary right-to-left shunt ($\dot{Q}_S/\dot{Q}_T$) and dead space (V_D/V_T). *Respiration* **33:** 133–142, 1976.

Swan HJC, et al: Hemodynamic spectrum of myocardial infarction and cardiogenic shock. *Circulation* **45:** 1097–1109, 1972.

Chapter 15

Leaf A, Cotran RS: *Renal Pathophysiology*. New York, Oxford University Press, 1976.

Masoro EJ, Siegel PD: *Acid-Base Regulation: Its Physiology, Pathophysiology and the Interpretation of Blood-Gas Analysis*, ed 2. Philadelphia, WB Saunders Co, 1977.

Maxwell MH, Kleeman CR (eds): *Clinical Disorders of Fluid and Electrolyte Metabolism*, ed 2. New York, McGraw-Hill Book Co, 1972.

Rose BD: *Clinical Physiology of Acid-Base and Electrolyte Disorders*. New York, McGraw-Hill Book Co, 1977.

Schwartz AB, Lyons H (eds): *Acid-Base and Electrolyte Balance: Normal Regulation and Clinical Disorders*. New York, Grune & Stratton, 1977.

Winters RW (ed): *The Body Fluids in Pediatrics*. Boston, Little, Brown & Co, 1973.

Chapter 16

Anast C, et al: Evidence for parathyroid failure in magnesium deficiency. *Science* **177:** 606–608, 1972.

Goldberger E: *A Primer of Water, Electrolyte, and Acid-Base Syndromes*, ed 5. Philadelphia, Lea & Febiger, 1975.

Leaf A, Cotran RS: *Renal Pathophysiology*. New York, Oxford University Press, 1976.

Maxwell MH, Kleeman CR (eds): *Clinical Disorders of Fluid and Electrolyte Metabolism*, ed 2. New York, McGraw-Hill Book Co, 1972.

Metz SA, et al: Neuroendocrine modulation of calcitonin and parathyroid hormone in man. *J Clin Endocrinol Metab* **47:** 151–159, 1978.

Newman JH, Neff TA, Ziporin P: Acute respiratory failure associated with hypophosphatemia. *N Engl J Med* **296:** 1101–1103, 1977.

Nordin BEC (ed): *Calcium, Phosphate, and Magnesium Metabolism*. Edinburgh, Churchill Livingstone, 1976.

O'Connor LR, Wheeler WS, Bethune JE: Effects of hypophosphatemia on myocardial performance in man. *N Eng J Med* **297:** 901–903, 1977.

Rose BD: *Clinical Physiology of Acid-Base and Electrolyte Disorders*. New York, McGraw-Hill Book Co, 1977.

Schwartz AB, Lyons H (eds): *Acid-Base and Electrolyte Balance: Normal Regulation and Clinical Disorders*. New York, Grune & Stratton, 1977.

Tsang RC, et al: Possible pathogenic factors in neonatal hypocalcemia of prematurity. *J Pediatr* **82:** 423–429, 1973.

Vora NM, et al: Comparative effect of calcium and of the adrenergic system on calcitonin secretion in man. *J Clin Endocrinol Metab* **46:** 567–571, 1978.

Chapter 17

Alleyne GAO, et al: *Protein-energy malnutrition*. London, Edward Arnold (Publishers), 1977.

Brooks FP (ed): *Gastrointestinal Pathophysiology*. New York, Oxford University Press, 1974.

Greenberger NJ, Winship DH: *Gastrointestinal Disorders: A Pathophysiologic Approach*. Chicago, Year Book Medical Publishers, 1976.

Kline MV, Coleman LL, Wick EE (eds): *Obesity: Etiology, Treatment, and Management*. Springfield, Ill, Charles C Thomas Publisher, 1976.

Mann GV: The influence of obesity on health. *N Engl J Med* **291:** 178–185, 226–232, 1974.

Mitchell HS, et al: *Nutrition in Health and Disease*, ed 16. Philadelphia, JB Lippincott Co, 1976.

Olson RE: (ed): *Protein-Calorie Malnutrition*. New York, Academic Press, 1975.

Sanford JP, Dietschy JM (eds): *The Science and Practice of Clinical Medicine*, vol 1. New York, Grune & Stratton, 1976.

Young VR, Scrimshaw NS: The physiology of

starvation. *Sci Am* **225**(4): 14–21, October 1971.

Chapter 18

Andreani D, Lefèbvre P, Marks V (eds): *Hypoglycemia.* Stuttgart, Georg Thieme Publishers, 1976.

Bacchus H: *Essentials of Metabolic Diseases and Endocrinology.* Baltimore, University Park Press, 1976.

Bajaj JS (ed): *Insulin and Metabolism.* Amsterdam, Elsevier/North-Holland Biomedical Press, 1977.

Beaumont JL, et al: Classification of hyperlipidemias and hyperlipoproteinemias. *Bull WHO* **43**: 891–908, 1970.

Berdanier CD, (ed): *Carbohydrate Metabolism: Regulation and Physiological Role.* Washington, DC, Hemisphere Publishing Corp, 1976.

Creutzfeldt W, Köbberling J, Neel JV (eds): *The Genetics of Diabetes Mellitus.* New York, Springer-Verlag, 1976.

Dietschy JM, Gotto AM Jr, Ontko JA (eds): *Disturbances in Lipid and Lipoprotein Metabolism.* Bethesda, Md, American Physiological Society, 1978.

Jackson WPU, Vinik AI: *Diabetes Mellitus: Clinical and Metabolic.* Capetown, South Africa, Juta and Co, 1977.

Kelley VC (ed): *Metabolic, Endocrine, and Genetic Disorders of Children*, vol 2. Hagerstown, Md, Harper & Row, 1974.

Lewis B: *The Hyperlipidaemias: Clinical and Laboratory Practice.* Oxford, Blackwell Scientific Publications, 1976.

Macdonald I (ed): *Effect of Carbohydrates on Lipid Metabolism.* Basel, S Karger, 1973.

Permutt MA, et al: Alimentary hypoglycemia in the absence of gastrointestinal surgery. *N Engl J Med* **228**: 1206–1210, 1973.

Sussman KE, Metz RJS (eds): *Diabetes Mellitus*, ed 4. New York, American Diabetes Association, 1975.

Chapter 19

Bacchus H: *Essentials of Metabolic Diseases and Endocrinology.* Baltimore, University Park Press, 1976.

Kashgarian M, Burrow GN: *The Endocrine Glands.* Baltimore, Williams & Wilkins Company, 1974.

Kryston LJ, Shaw RA (eds): *Endocrinology and Diabetes.* New York, Grune & Stratton, 1975.

Labhart A: *Clinical Endocrinology: Theory and Practice.* New York, Springer-Verlag, 1974.

Montgomery DAD, Welbourn RB: *Medical and Surgical Endocrinology.* London, Edward Arnold (Publishers), 1975.

Sterling K: Thyroid hormone action at the cell level. *N Engl J Med* **300**: 117–122, 173–177, 1979.

Williams RH (ed): *Textbook of Endocrinology*, ed 5. Philadelphia, WB Saunders Co, 1974.

Chapter 20

Anderson WAD, Kissane JM: *Pathology*, ed 7, vol 1. St. Louis, CV Mosby Co, 1977.

Bradley WP, et al: Correlations among serum protein-bound carbohydrates, serum glycoproteins, lymphocyte reactivity, and tumor burden in cancer patients. *Cancer* **40**: 2264–2272, 1977.

Braun AC: *The Story of Cancer: On Its Nature, Causes and Control.* Reading, Mass, Addison-Wesley Publishing Co, 1977.

Calman KC, Paul J: *An Introduction to Cancer Medicine.* New York, John Wiley & Sons, 1978.

International Union Against Cancer: *Clinical Oncology.* New York, Springer-Verlag, 1978.

Kilton LJ, et al: Bacteremia due to gram-positive

cocci in patients with neoplastic disease. *Am J Med* **66:** 596–602, 1979.

Morrison SD: Origin of anorexia in neoplastic disease. *Am J Clin Nutr* **31:** 1104–1107, 1978.

Van Lancker JL: *Molecular and Cellular Mechanisms in Disease*, vol 2. New York, Springer-Verlag, 1976.

Chapter 21

Brooks FP (ed): *Gastrointestinal Pathophysiology.* New York, Oxford University Press, 1974.

Cherniack RM, Cherniack L, Naimark A: *Respiration in Health and Disease*, ed 2. Philadelphia, WB Saunders Co, 1972.

Lapides J: *Fundamentals of Urology.* Philadelphia, WB Saunders Co, 1976.

Willis RA, Willis AT: *Principles of Pathology and Bacteriology*, ed 3. London, Butterworth and Co, 1972.

Chapter 22

Attinger EO, Monroe RG, Segal MS: The mechanics of breathing in different body positions. I. In normal subjects. *J Clin Invest* **35:** 904–911, 1956.

Attinger EO, Herschfus JA, Segal MS: The mechanics of breathing in different body positions. II. In cardiopulmonary disease. *J Clin Invest* **35:** 912–920, 1956.

Bourne GH (ed): *The Biochemistry and Physiology of Bone*, ed 2, vol. 1, 3. New York, Academic Press, 1971.

Bourne GH (ed): *The Structure and Function of Muscle*, ed 2, vol 1. New York, Academic Press, 1972.

Browse NL: *The Physiology and Pathology of Bed Rest.* Springfield, Ill, Charles C Thomas Publisher, 1965.

Chavarri M, et al: Effect of bedrest on circadian rhythms of plasma renin, aldosterone, and cortisol. *Aviat Space Environ Med* **48:** 633–636, 1977.

Chobanian AV, et al: The metabolic and hemodynamic effects of prolonged bed rest in normal subjects. *Circulation* **49:** 551–559, 1974.

Clauss RH, et al: Effects of changing body position upon improved ventilation-perfusion relationships. *Circulation* **37** (suppl 2): 214–217, 1968.

Deitrick JE, Whedon GD, Schorr E: Effects of immobilization upon various metabolic and physiologic functions of normal men. *Am J Med* **4:** 3–36, 1948.

Downs FS: Bed rest and sensory disturbances. *Am J Nurs* **74:** 434–438, 1974.

Fletcher GF, Cantwell JD: *Exercise and Coronary Heart Disease.* Springfield, Ill, Charles C Thomas Publisher, 1974.

Gibbs NM: Venous thrombosis of the lower limbs with particular reference to bed-rest. *Brit J Surg* **45:** 209–236, 1957.

Gallus AS: Venous thromboembolism: incidence and clinical risk factors, in Madden JL, Hume M (eds): *Venous Thromboembolism: Prevention and Treatment.* New York, Appleton-Century-Crofts, 1976.

Kottke FJ: The effects of limitation of activity upon the human body. *J Am Med Ass* **196:** 825–830, 1966.

Lampman RM, et al: Comparative effects of physical training and diet in normalizing serum lipids in men with type IV hyperlipoproteinemia. *Circulation* **55:** 652–658, 1977.

Letac B, Cribier A, Desplanches JF: A study of left ventricular function in coronary patients before and after physical training. *Circulation* **56:** 375–378, 1977.

Lipman RL, et al: Impairment of peripheral glucose utilization in normal subjects by prolonged bedrest. *J Lab Clin Med* **76:** 221–230, 1970.

Lynch TN, et al: Metabolic effects of prolonged bed rest: their modification by simulated altitude, *Aerospace Med* **38:** 10–20, 1967.

McMillan DE, Donaldson CL: Changes in serum proteins, viscosity, and protein-bound carbohydrates during prolonged bedrest. *Aviat Space Environ Med* **46**: 132–135, 1975.

McNeer JF, et al: The role of the exercise test in the evaluation of patients for ischemic heart disease. *Circulation* **57**: 64–70, 1978.

Melada GA, et al: Hemodynamics, renal function, plasma renin, and aldosterone in man after 5 to 14 days of bedrest. *Aviat Space Environ Med* **46**: 1049–1055, 1975.

Milic-Emili J: Distribution of ventilation, in Glaister DH (ed): *The Effects of Gravity and Acceleration on the Lung.* Slough, England, Technivision Services, 1970.

Murray JF: *The Normal Lung: The Basis for Diagnosis and Treatment of Pulmonary Disease.* Philadelphia, WB Saunders Co, 1976.

Rushmer RF: *Cardiovascular Dynamics,* ed 4. Philadelphia, WB Saunders Co, 1976.

Ryback RS, Lewis OF, Lessard CS: Psychobiologic effects of prolonged bed rest (weightless) in young, healthy volunteers (study II). *Aerospace Med* **42**: 529–535, 1971.

Sevitt S, Gallagher N: Venous thrombosis and pulmonary embolism. *Brit J Surg* **48**: 475–489, 1961.

Sheffield LT, et al: The exercise test in perspective. *Circulation* **55**: 681–682, 1977.

Vernikos-Danellis J, et al: Changes in glucose, insulin, and growth hormone levels associated with bedrest. *Aviat Space Environ Med* **47**: 583–587, 1976.

Vernikos-Danellis J, et al: Thyroid and adrenal cortical rhythmicity during bed rest. *J Appl Physiol* **33**: 644–648, 1972.

Vogt FB, Johnson PC: Plasma volume and extracellular fluid volume change associated with 10 days bed recumbency. *Aerospace Med* **38**: 21–25, 1967.

Vogt FB, et al: Tilt table response and blood volume changes associated with fourteen days of recumbency. *Aerospace Med* **38**: 43–48, 1967.

Warlow CP, et al: Platelet adhesiveness and fibrinolysis after recent cerebro-vascular accidents and their relationship with subsequent deep venous thrombosis of the legs. *Thrombos Haemostas* **36**: 127–132, 1976.

West JB: Regional distribution of blood flow, in Glaister DH (ed): *The Effects of Gravity and Acceleration on the Lung.* Slough, England, Technivision Services, 1970.

Winget CM, et al: Circadian rhythm asynchrony in man during hypokinesis. *J Appl Physiol* **33**: 640–643, 1972.

Ziegler MB, Lake RC, Kopin IJ: The sympathetic-nervous-system defect in primary orthostatic hypotension. *N Engl J Med* **296**: 293–297, 1977.

Chapter 23

Chaplin CG: Lightning stroke and electric shock, in Eliot RS (ed): *The Acute Cardiac Emergency.* Mount Kisco, NY, Futura Publishing Co, 1972.

Daniels F Jr: Radiant energy. Part A: Solar radiation, in Slonim N (ed): *Environmental Physiology.* St Louis, CV Mosby Co, 1974.

Diamond I, Schmid R: Neonatal hyperbilirubinemia and kernicterus: experimental support for treatment by visible light. *Arch Neurol* **18**: 699–702, 1968.

Estes FL: Radiant energy. Part B: Ionizing and nonionizing radiation, in Slonim NB (ed): *Environmental Physiology.* St Louis, CV Mosby Co, 1974.

Herndon JH Jr, Freeman RF: Human disease associated with exposure to light. *Ann Rev Med* **27**: 77–87, 1976.

Lucey J, Ferreiro M, Hewitt J: Prevention of hyperbilirubinemia of prematurity by phototherapy. *Pediatrics* **41**: 1047–1053, 1968.

McRee DI: Potential microwave injuries in clinical medicine. *Ann Rev Med* **27**: 109–115, 1976.

Resnekov L: Direct current shock, in Chung EH

(ed): *Cardiac Emergency Care.* Philadelphia, Lea & Febiger, 1975.

Smith AW, Cooper JN: *Elements of Physics*, ed 8. New York, McGraw-Hill Book Co, 1972.

Solem L, Fischer RP, Strate RG: The natural history of electrical injury. *J Trauma* **17**: 487–491, 1977.

Tilley DE, Thumm W: *Physics for College Students with Applications to the Life Sciences.* Menlo Park, Calif, Cummings Publishing Co, 1974.

Travis EL: *Primer of Medical Radiobiology.* Chicago, Year Book Medical Publishers, 1975.

Van Lancker JL: *Molecular and Cellular Mechanisms in Disease*, vol 2. New York, Springer-Verlag, 1976.

Chapter 24

Costrini AM, et al: Cardiovascular and metabolic manifestations of heat stroke and severe heat exhaustion. *Am J Med* **66**: 296–302, 1979.

Dinarello CA, Wolff SM: Pathogenesis of fever in man. *N Engl J Med* **298**: 607–612, 1978.

Feller I, Jones CA: *Nursing the burned patient.* Ann Arbor, Mich, Institute for Burn Medicine, 1973.

Knochel JP: Environmental heat illness: an eclectic review. *Arch Intern Med* **133**: 841–863, 1974.

Maclean D, Emslie-Smith D: *Accidental Hypothermia.* Oxford, Blackwell Scientific Publications, 1977.

Muir IFK, Barclay TL: *Burns and Their Treatment*, ed 2. London, Lloyd-Luke (Medical Books), 1974.

Rudowski W et al: *Burn Therapy and Research.* Baltimore, The Johns Hopkins University Press, 1976.

Sevitt S: *Reactions to Injury and Burns and Their Clinical Importance.* Philadelphia, JB Lippincott Co, 1974.

Sevitt S: A review of the complications of burns, their origin and importance for illness and death. *J Trauma* **19**: 358–369, 1979.

Simon HB, Daniels GH: Hormonal hyperthermia: endocrinologic causes of fever. *Am J Med* **66**: 257–263, 1979.

Chapter 25

Ariëns EJ, Simonis AM, Offermeier J: *Introduction to General Toxicology.* New York, Academic Press, 1976.

Briggs M, Briggs M: *The Chemistry and Metabolism of Drugs and Toxins.* London, William Heinemann Medical Books, 1974.

LaDu BN, Mandel HG, Way EL: *Fundamentals of Drug Metabolism and Drug Disposition.* Baltimore, Williams & Wilkins Co, 1971.

Recknagel RO, et al: New data in support of the lipoperoxidation theory for carbon tetrachloride liver injury, in Eliakim M, Eshchar J, Zimmerman HJ (eds): *International Symposium on Hepatotoxicity.* New York, Academic Press, 1974.

Schanker LS: Flow of environmental agents in reaching their site of action, in Lee DHK, Minard D (eds): *Physiology, Environment, and Man.* New York, Academic Press, 1970.

Westerman E: Accumulation of environmental agents or their effects in the body, in Lee DHK, Minard D (eds): *Physiology, Environment, and Man.* New York, Academic Press, 1970.

Chapter 26

Fisher JE: Acute hepatic failure: hepatic coma and the hepatorenal syndrome, in Becker FF (ed): *The Liver: Normal and Abnormal Functions*, part B. New York, Marcel Dekker, 1975.

Goresky CA, Fisher MM (eds): *Jaundice.* New York, Plenum Press, 1975.

Marin GA, Ostrow JD: Acute and chronic hepatic encephalopathy, in Brooks FP (ed): *Gas-*

trointestinal Pathophysiology. New York, Oxford University Press, 1974.

Massry SG, Sellers AL (eds): *Clinical Aspects of Uremia and Dialysis.* Springfield, Ill, Charles C Thomas Publisher, 1976.

Pitts RF: *Physiology of the Kidney and Body Fluids,* ed 3. Chicago, Year Book Medical Publishers, 1974.

Chapter 27

Boyd RF, Hoerl BG: *Basic Medical Microbiology.* Boston, Little, Brown & Co, 1977.

Drew WL (ed): *Viral Infections: A Clinical Approach.* Philadelphia, FA Davis Co., 1976.

Luria SE, et al: *General Virology,* ed 3. New York, John Wiley & Sons, 1978.

McLean DM, Wong KSK, Bergman SKA: Virions associated with acute gastroenteritis in Vancouver, 1976. *Canad Med Assoc J* **117:** 1035–1036, 1977.

Nester EW, et al: *Microbiology: Molecules, Microbes, and Man.* New York, Holt, Rinehart & Winston, 1973.

Chapter 28

Beisel WR: Magnitude of the host nutritional responses to infection. *Am J Clin Nutr* **30:** 1236–1247, 1977.

Boyd RF, Hoerl BG: *Basic Medical Microbiology.* Boston, Little, Brown & Company, 1977.

Hoeprich PD (ed): *Infectious Diseases.* Hagerstown, Md, Harper & Row, 1972.

Kluger MJ, Rothenburg BA: Fever and reduced iron: their interaction as a host defense response to bacterial infection. *Science* **203:** 374–376, 1979.

Mims CA: *The Pathogenesis of Infectious Disease.* New York, Academic Press, 1977.

Wilson ME, Mizer HE: *Microbiology in Patient Care,* ed 2. New York, Macmillan Co, 1974.

Chapter 29

Barrett JT: *Basic Immunology and Its Medical Application.* St. Louis, CV Mosby Co, 1976.

Eichner ER: Splenic function: normal, too much and too little. *Am J Med* **66:** 311–319, 1979.

Freedman SO, Gold P (eds): *Clinical Immunology,* ed 2. Hagerstown, Md, Harper and Row, 1976.

Mims CA: *The Pathogenesis of Infectious Disease.* New York, Academic Press, 1977.

Plaut AG: Microbial IgA proteases. *N Engl J Med* **298:** 1459–1463, 1978.

Chapter 30

Barrett JT: *Basic Immunology and Its Medical Application.* St Louis, CV Mosby Co, 1976.

Cohen S, Ward PA, McCluskey RT (eds): *Mechanisms of Immunopathology.* New York, John Wiley & Sons, 1979.

Freedman SO, Gold P (eds): *Clinical Immunology.* Hagerstown, Md, Harper & Row, 1976.

Linman JW: *Hematology: Physiologic, Pathophysiologic, and Clinical Principles.* New York, Macmillan Co, 1975.

Morimoto C, Abe T, Homma M: Altered function of suppressor T lymphocytes in patients with active systemic lupus erythematosus—in vitro immune response to autoantigen. *Clin Immunol Immunopathol* **13:** 160–171, 1979.

Newman B, et al: Lack of suppressor cell activity in systemic lupus erythematosus. *Clin Immunol Immunopathol* **13:** 187–193, 1979.

Polak L: Recent trends in the immunology of contact sensitivity. *Contact Dermatitis* **4:** 249–263, 1978.

Talal N (ed): *Autoimmunity.* New York, Academic Press, 1977.

Index